E–Health and Telemedicine:

Concepts, Methodologies, Tools, and Applications

Information Resources Management Association
USA

Volume II

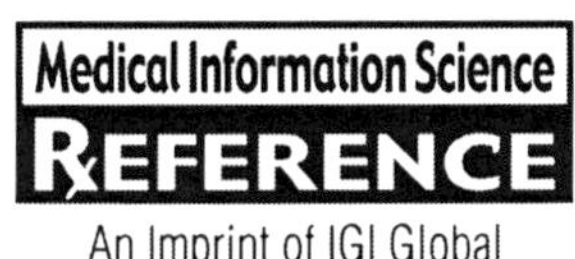

Managing Director: Lindsay Johnston
Managing Editor: Keith Greenberg
Director of Intellectual Propery & Contracts: Jan Travers
Acquisitions Editor: Kayla Wolfe
Production Editor: Christina Henning
Multi-Volume Book Production Specialist: Deanna Jo Zombro
Cover Design: Samantha Barnhart

Published in the United States of America by
      Medical Information Science Reference (an imprint of IGI Global)
      701 E. Chocolate Avenue
      Hershey PA, USA 17033
      Tel: 717-533-8845
      Fax: 717-533-8661
      E-mail: cust@igi-global.com
      Web site: http://www.igi-global.com

Library of Congress Cataloging-in-Publication Data

E-Health and telemedicine : concepts, methodologies, tools, and applications / Information Resources Management Association, editor.
      pages cm
  Includes bibliographical references and index.
  Summary: "This reference explores recent advances in mobile medicine and how this technology impacts modern medical care"-- Provided by publisher.
  ISBN 978-1-4666-8756-1 (hardcover) -- ISBN 978-1-4666-8757-8 (ebook) 1. Medical care--Technological innovation. 2. Medical informatics. 3. Telecommunication in medicine. I. Information Resources Management Association.
  R858.E223 2016
  610.285--dc23
                                    2015019904

British Cataloguing in Publication Data
A Cataloguing in Publication record for this book is available from the British Library.

For electronic access to this publication, please contact: eresources@igi-global.com.

List of Contributors

Table of Contents

Volume I

Section 1
Fundamental Concepts and Theories

This section serves as a foundation for this exhaustive reference tool by addressing underlying principles essential to the understanding of E-Health and Telemedicine. Chapters found within these pages provide an excellent framework in which to position E-Health and Telemedicine within the field of information science and technology. Insight regarding the critical incorporation of global measures into E-Health and Telemedicine is addressed, while crucial stumbling blocks of this field are explored. With 15 chapters comprising this foundational section, the reader can learn and chose from a compendium of expert research on the elemental theories underscoring the E-Health and Telemedicine discipline.

Section 2
Frameworks and Methodologies

This section provides in-depth coverage of conceptual architecture frameworks to provide the reader with a comprehensive understanding of the emerging developments within the field of E-Health and Telemedicine. Research fundamentals imperative to the understanding of developmental processes within E-Health and Telemedicine are offered. From broad examinations to specific discussions on methodology, the research found within this section spans the discipline while offering detailed, specific discussions. From basic designs to abstract development, these chapters serve to expand the reaches of development and design technologies within the E-Health and Telemedicine community. This section includes 11 contributions from researchers throughout the world on the topic of E-Health and Telemedicine.

Section 3
Tools and Technologies

This section presents an extensive coverage of various tools and technologies available in the field of E-Health and Telemedicine that practitioners and academicians alike can utilize to develop different techniques. These chapters enlighten readers about fundamental research on the many tools facilitating the burgeoning field of E-Health and Telemedicine. It is through these rigorously researched chapters that the reader is provided with countless examples of the up-and-coming tools and technologies emerging from the field of E-Health and Telemedicine. With 21 chapters, this section offers a broad treatment of some of the many tools and technologies within the E-Health and Telemedicine field.

Volume II

**Section 4
Cases and Applications**

This section discusses a variety of applications and opportunities available that can be considered by practitioners in developing viable and effective E-Health and Telemedicine programs and processes. This section includes 13 chapters that review topics from case studies to best practices and ongoing research. Further chapters discuss E-Health and Telemedicine in a variety of settings. Contributions included in this section provide excellent coverage of today's IT community and how research into E-Health and Telemedicine is impacting the social fabric of our present-day global village.

Section 5
Issues and Challenges

This section contains 17 chapters, giving a wide variety of perspectives on E-Health and Telemedicine and its implications. Within the chapters, the reader is presented with an in-depth analysis of the most current and relevant issues within this growing field of study. Crucial questions are addressed and alternatives offered along with theoretical approaches discussed.

Section 6
Emerging Trends

This section highlights research potential within the field of E-Health and Telemedicine while exploring uncharted areas of study for the advancement of the discipline. Introducing this section are chapters that set the stage for future research directions and topical suggestions for continued debate, centering on the new venues and forums for discussion. A pair of chapters on space-time makes up the middle of the section of the final 11 chapters, and the book concludes with a look ahead into the future of the E-Health and Telemedicine field. In all, this text will serve as a vital resource to practitioners and academics interested in the best practices and applications of the burgeoning field of E-Health and Telemedicine.

Preface

The constantly changing landscape of E-Health and Telemedicine makes it challenging for experts and practitioners to stay informed of the field's most up-to-date research. That is why Medical Information Science Reference is pleased to offer this three-volume reference collection that will empower students, researchers, and academicians with a strong understanding of critical issues within E-Health and Tele-medicine by providing both broad and detailed perspectives on cutting-edge theories and developments. This reference is designed to act as a single reference source on conceptual, methodological, technical, and managerial issues, as well as provide insight into emerging trends and future opportunities within the discipline.

E-Health and Telemedicine: Concepts, Methodologies, Tools and Applications is organized into six distinct sections that provide comprehensive coverage of important topics. The sections are:

1. Fundamental Concepts and Theories;
2. Frameworks and Methodologies;
3. Tools and Technologies;
4. Cases and Applications;
5. Issues and Challenges; and
6. Emerging Trends.

The following paragraphs provide a summary of what to expect from this invaluable reference tool.

Section 1, "Fundamental Concepts and Theories," serves as a foundation for this extensive reference tool by addressing crucial theories essential to the understanding of E-Health and Telemedicine. Introducing the book is *Project Initiation for Telemedicine Services* by Cynthia M. LeRouge, Bengisu Tulu, and Suzanne Wood; a great foundation laying the groundwork for the basic concepts and theories that will be discussed throughout the rest of the book. Another chapter of note in Section 1 is titled *Principles of Information Accountability: An eHealth Perspective* by Randike Gajanayake, Tony Sahama, and Renato Iannella. Section 1 concludes, and leads into the following portion of the book with a nice segue chapter, *Telemedicine Program for Management and Treatment of Stress Urinary Incontinence in Women: Design and Pilot Test* by Anna Abelló Pla, Anna Andreu Povar, Jordi Esquirol Caussa, Vanessa Bayo Tallón, Dolores Rexachs, and Emilio Luque.

Section 2, "Frameworks and Methodologies," presents in-depth coverage of the conceptual design and architecture of E-Health and Telemedicine. Opening the section is *Information Architecture for Pervasive Healthcare Information Provision with Technological Implementation* by Chekfoung Tan and Shixiong Liu. Through case studies, this section lays excellent groundwork for later sections that will get into present and future applications for E-Health and Telemedicine. The section concludes with an excellent work by Sabah Al-Fedaghi, titled *Design Principles in Health Information Technology: An Alternative to UML Use Case Methodology.*

Section 3, "Tools and Technologies," presents extensive coverage of the various tools and technologies used in the implementation of E-Health and Telemedicine. Section 3 begins where Section 2 left off, though this section describes more concrete tools at place in the modeling, planning, and applications of E-Health and Telemedicine. The first chapter, *Healthinfo Engineering: Technology Perspectives from Evidence-Based mHealth Study in WE-CARE Project* by Anpeng Huang and Linzhen Xie, lays a framework for the types of works that can be found in this section. Section 3 is full of excellent chapters like this one, including such titles as *A System for the Semi-Automatic Evaluation of Clinical Practice Guideline Indicators* by Alexandra Pomares Quimbaya, María Patricia Amórtegui, Rafael A. González, Oscar Muñoz, Wilson Ricardo Bohórquez, Olga Milena García, and Melany Montagut Ascanio; and *Ambulance Dispatching System with Integrated Information and Communication Technologies on Cloud Environment* by Jian-Wei Li, Chia-Chi Chang, Yi-Chun Chang, and Yung-Fa Huang. The section concludes with *Using a Smartphone as a Track and Fall Detector: An Intelligent Support System for People with Dementia* by Chia-Yin Ko, Fang-Yie Leu, and I-Tsen Lin. Where Section 3 described specific tools and technologies at the disposal of practitioners, Section 4 describes the use and applications of the tools and frameworks discussed in previous sections.

Section 4, "Cases and Applications," describes how the broad range of E-Health and Telemedicine efforts has been utilized and offers insight on and important lessons for their applications and impact. The first chapter in the section is titled *The Role and Use of Telemedicine by Physicians in Developing Countries: A Case Report from Saudi Arabia* written by Dana Alajmi, Mohamed Khalifa, Amr Jamal, Nasria Zakaria, Suleiman Alomran, Ashraf El-Metwally, Majed Al-Salamah, and Mowafa Househ. This section includes the widest range of topics because it describes case studies, research, methodologies, frameworks, architectures, theory, analysis, and guides for implementation. The breadth of topics covered in the chapter is also reflected in the diversity of its authors, from countries all over the globe, such as: *A Case for Enterprise Interoperability in Healthcare IT: Personal Health Record Systems* by Mustafa Yuksel, Asuman Dogac, Cebrail Taskin, and Anil Yalcinkaya. The section concludes with *Political Attitudes on the Dutch Electronic Patient Record* by Evert Mouw, a great transition chapter into the next section.

Section 5, "Issues and Challenges," presents coverage of academic and research perspectives on E-Health and Telemedicine tools and applications. The section begins with *Detection of Pre-Analytical Laboratory Testing Errors: Leads and Lessons for Patient Safety* by Wafa Al-Zahrani and Mohamud Sheikh. Chapters in this section will look into theoretical approaches and offer alternatives to crucial questions on the subject of E-Health and Telemedicine. For example, *Operative Role Management in Information Systems* written by Taina Kurki and Hanna-Miina Sihvonen. The section concludes with *Approaches to Evidence-Based Management and Decision-Making in Healthcare Organizations: Lessons for Developing Nations* by Nouf Al Saleem and Mohamud Sheikh.

Section 6, "Emerging Trends," highlights areas for future research within the field of E-Health and Telemedicine, opening with *Mobile Health Services: A New Paradigm for Health Care Systems* by Nabila Nisha, Mehree Iqbal, Afrin Rifat, and Sherina Idrish. This section contains chapters that look at what might happen in the coming years that can extend the already staggering amount of applications for E-Health and Telemedicine. The final chapter of the book looks at an emerging field within E-Health and Telemedicine, in the excellent contribution, *Coalitions: The Future of Healthcare in Public Private Partnerships* by Erinn N. Harris.

Although the primary organization of the contents in this multi-volume work is based on its six sections, offering a progression of coverage of the important concepts, methodologies, technologies, applications, social issues, and emerging trends, the reader can also identify specific contents by utilizing the extensive indexing system listed at the end of each volume. As a comprehensive collection of research on the latest findings related to using technology to providing various services, *E-Health and Telemedicine: Concepts, Methodologies, Tools and Applications*, provides researchers, administrators and all audiences with a complete understanding of the development of applications and concepts in E-Health and Telemedicine. Given the vast number of issues concerning usage, failure, success, policies, strategies, and applications of E-Health and Telemedicine in countries around the world, *E-Health and Telemedicine: Concepts, Methodologies, Tools and Applications* addresses the demand for a resource that encompasses the most pertinent research in technologies being employed to globally bolster the knowledge and applications of E-Health and Telemedicine.

Chapter 30
Services and Monitors for Dependability Assessment of Mobile Health Monitoring Systems

Alessandro Testa
Institute of High Performance Computing and Networking (ICAR), Italy

Antonio Coronato
Institute of High Performance Computing and Networking (ICAR), Italy

Marcello Cinque
Università di Napoli Federico II, Italy

Giuseppe De Pietro
Institute of High Performance Computing and Networking (ICAR), Italy

ABSTRACT

The problem of failure detection in mHealth monitoring systems is becoming more critical, and the use of wireless technologies and commodity hardware/software platforms pose new challenges to their correct functioning. Remote and continuous monitoring of patients' vital signs aims to improve the quality of life of patients. Such applications, however, are particularly critical from the point of view of dependability. Wireless channels can be affected by packet loss, and cheap and wireless-enabled medical devices can exhibit wrong readings, inducing the medical staff to make wrong decisions. In this chapter, the authors present the results of a Failure Modes and Effects Analysis (FMEA) conducted to identify the dependability threats of health monitoring systems and a set of services and monitors for the assurance of high degrees of dependability to mobile health monitoring systems. Moreover, the authors describe a case study realized to detect failures at runtime.

1. INTRODUCTION

Health monitoring systems have been shown to be effective in helping to manage chronic disease, post-acute care, and monitoring the safety of the older adult population. They can help older adults slow progression of chronic disease and ensure continued recovery after being discharged from an acute care setting. The implementation of such systems is gaining an increasing attention

DOI: 10.4018/978-1-4666-8756-1.ch030

in the academia and the industry, also due to the increasing healthcare costs and the aging of the world population (Hao et al., 2008).

To this purpose, cabled measurement equipment is already used to guarantee reliable and robust control of vital signs. However such systems complicate patient autonomy and mobility. Hence, wireless technologies and mobile devices are starting to be applied to build more comfortable and patient-friendly health monitoring systems (Paksuniemi et al., 2006).

Nevertheless, the use of wireless technologies and the adoption of commodity hardware/software platforms, such as smartphones, pose new challenges on the correct functioning of health monitoring systems. Wireless channels can be affected by packet loss, due to shadowing and absence of signal coverage. Smartphones can be subjected to unpredictable failures, which could affect the correct functioning of the system. Finally, cheap and wireless-enabled medical devices can exhibit wrong readings and temporary disconnections from the so-called Body Area Network (BAN (O'Donovan et al., 2009)). These issues may induce the medical staff to take wrong decisions, e.g., to administer wrong dosages of medicine, which can happen to be fatal for the patient.

For these reasons, the problem of failure detection and management in health monitoring systems is starting to be addressed in the literature, especially for mobile systems. However, several studies are based on simplistic failure assumptions or on basic fault-tolerance schemes (such as, sensor redundancy), which are not assured to cover all possible failure scenarios. For instance, sensor replication is ineffective against smartphone failures.

To overcome the limitations of current solutions, in this paper we propose the design of reliable mobile health monitoring system, based on the configurable and the automatic deployment of

system monitors, enriching the task of vital sign collection with the ability of detecting failures at runtime, hence enabling the realization of dependable health monitoring services. Differently from the previous attempts in the literature, we base our design on the results of a detailed Failure Mode and Effect Analysis of a typical mobile health monitoring system (Cinque et al., 2011) (Cinque et. al., 2012).

The FMEA allowed us to identify the failure modes of the main components composing such systems, by taking advantage of our past experience and detailed field studies on the dependability of mobile devices, wireless communication technologies, such as Bluetooth, and wireless sensor networks (WSNs). The characterization of the failure modes of the system components allowed us to identify the main responsibility of system monitors, along with their placement in a typical mobile health monitoring architecture. The driving idea behind our design is to keep monitors transparent to application developers, allowing them to implement dependable health monitoring applications only by using high-level collection and delivery services. Such services are in turn conceived to exploit the underlying system monitors to detect the failures and potentially react to them. In order to let the solution be adaptable to different application needs, monitors are conceived to be activated and configured automatically, based on a high-level and system-agnostic specification of the desired dependability level.

The rest of the paper is structured as follows: The related work is presented in Section 2; Section 3 describes the typical architecture of a mobile health monitoring system, while in Section 4 we discuss about the results on the realized FMEA. The proposed monitor-based dependable architecture is presented in Section 5. Section 6 presents a use example of a monitor. Finally, Section 7 reports our concluding remarks.

2. RELATED WORK

Currently, the research is progressively recognizing the need of novel solutions to build dependable health monitoring systems. These solutions mainly focus on two key issues: node failures and wireless network interference.

Regarding node failures, the power consumption of battery driven devices represent a remarkable issue, which is a limiting factor for long-term monitoring. Although the emerging of new technologies (Kansal et al., 2007) and new standards like the bluetooth low-energy profile, this issue cannot be considered definitively solved (Zhang et al., 2009). For this reason, the system must be able to detect low battery levels and to migrate onto spare devices.

In addition, both WSNs and BANs may suffer from intentional or unintentional node removal or unresponsive nodes. While in WSNs, this issue can be resolved with new path discovery or redundant paths, in BANs this may cause the loss of important vital signs being monitored by the failing sensor. A combination of node redundancy and multi-sensor data fusion was one of the solutions proposed to face these issues (Baskiyar, 2002)(Curiac et al., 2009). The introduction of redundant sensors measuring the same vital sign avoids the loss of any vital data if a node becomes compromised or faulty. In addition, they can serve to facilitate multiple paths when the routing becomes an issue.

Interference has the potential to cause significant delays and data loss and is a major concern with all wireless devices. Medical devices can interfere with each other in the BAN as well as being subject to environmental noise. This is due to the lack of harmonious regulations and standards, as demonstrated in (Hanna, 2009) (Spadotto, 2009). A solution would be to eliminate the wireless aspect of the intra-BAN network (Chen et al., 2011) (Hanson et al., 2009). BAN systems such as *MITHrill* (Chen et al., 2011), *SMART* (Chen et al., 2011), and *MobiHealth* (Van Halteren et al., 2004) all employ a wired connectivity between sensors and the aggregator. However, these solutions strongly limit the usability of the system, especially for elderly people, and makes it hard to interconnect all the sensors to commodity mobile devices, such as patients' smartphones, hence requiring ad-hoc aggregating devices which increase the overall cost of the system.

Some proposals in the literature have employed techniques to provide some form of fault tolerance to monitoring systems. *iROS* (Ponnekanti et al., 2003) uses an Event Heap for communication between various entities. The EventHeap is based on the tuple-spaces model proposed by Gelernter for *Linda* (Gelernter, 1985). Arnstein et al. propose a project (Arnstein et al., 2002) to enhance the robustness of ubiquitous systems by providing transaction-level persistence and support for disconnected operations. But the project does not address device or application failures.

Chetan et al. highlight the various challenges and issues that confront fault tolerant pervasive computing (Chetan et al., 2005); also, they propose some solutions to these problems but they do not address the specific issues of health monitoring systems.

Health monitoring systems within closed environments can be conceived as a special case of Ambient Intelligence (AmI) systems. Currently there is still a lack of a commonly accepted architectures to build dependable AmI systems. This issue was first considered in (Simoncini, 2003), where the author points out that the concepts of "architecture" and "system" need to be redefined in the context of AmI, in order to properly define dependability attributes, threats and means.

In (Bohn et al., 2005), authors define a dynamic AmI system able to adapt itself to the current situation. They claim that, in order to guarantee dependability requirements, the system architecture has to be manageable, controllable and it has to provide means for the prediction of the system correctness at runtime. In (Nehmer et al., 2006), authors proposed an integrated system approach for living assistance systems based on ambient intelligence technology. They claim that the construction of trustworthy, robust, and dependable living assistance systems is a challenging task which requires novel software engineering methods and tools, and novel approaches for dependable self-adapting software architectures, able to react to changes due to frequent failures and reconfiguration events, which become the norm, rather than the exception. In addition, self-adapting multi-modal human-computer interfaces must be devised, since even the wrong interaction with humans may represent an obstacle for the dependable operation of the system.

Georgalis et al. argue that the most important architectural property in an AmI architecture is the fault-tolerance (Georgalis et al., 2009). The fault tolerance, in the context of an AmI architecture, has to be able to isolate failures, to eliminate single points of failure, to restart failing services before that are used by the clients, and finally to provide mechanisms for notifying the fault level about the irreparable failure of a specific service.

Coronato and De Pietro (Coronato & De Pietro, 2010) pointed out that the design of Ambient Intelligence applications in critical systems requires rigorous software-engineering-oriented approaches. The authors proposed a set of formal tools and a specification process for AmI, which have been devised to lead the developer in designing activities and realizing software artefacts.

In (Duman et al., 2010) it is defined an Ambient Intelligent Environment (AIE) as a multitude of interconnected systems composed by embedded agent with computational and networking capabilities which form a ubiquitous, unobtrusive, and seamless infrastructure that surrounds the user. These intelligent agents are integrated into AIEs to form an intelligent "presence" to identify the users and be sensitive and attentive to their particular needs, based on a publish-subscribe communication infrastructure. The intelligent agents are dynamic and capable to keep a high level of dependability of a network structure preserving the resilience and the fault tolerance. They suggest,

as future work, to investigate the proposed AmI system in a truly distributed and real AIE with a richer set of sensors and actuators.

Some solutions focus on the dependable delivery of data. In (Chakraborly, 2007) authors propose a trust-based routing protocol able to ensure the delivery of event data from sensors to actuators in a Ambient Intelligence environment even in the presence of faults; the dependability is measured in terms of a trust value for the node. It is also performed a security analysis of the effects of malicious nodes.

Several new mHealth monitoring systems have been proposed in literature focusing on security and privacy issues but not on dependability issues within a WBAN (Lin et al., 2013)(Yan et al., 2010) (Triantafyllidis et al., 2012).

In (Lin et al., 2013) the authors present a new kind of mHealth monitoring system that is based on cloud computing; the paper is focused on security and privacy concepts since the authors design a cloud-assisted privacy preserving mHealth monitoring system to protect the privacy of the involved parties and their data. However dependability requirements such as coverage or connection resiliency are not considered.

Also in (Yan et al., 2010), it is implemented and evaluated a WBAN-based e-health monitoring system which is sensitive to security and privacy issues; it is proposed a mixed localization algorithm based on received sensor data and received signal strength indicator (RSSI) that is exploited to perform passive localization of monitored elderly people. However, the proposed system does not take in account failures like a packet loss or isolation of part of a WBAN.

Triantafyllidis et al. present the design and development of a pervasive health monitoring system integrates patient monitoring, through mobile wearable multisensing devices, and status logging for capturing various problems or symptoms met. The authors focus on security issues of a gateway device disregarding any failure that could occur in a WBAN that is the source of needed data.

There is some mHealth monitoring system based on reasoning techniques. Benlamri and Docksteader design the Mobile Ontology-based Reasoning and Feedback (MORF) health-monitoring system, which monitors a patient's health status using a mobile unit. Unlike previous cited papers, the system uses ontology based context model to process and determine a patient's health status; the system can process the incoming sensor data by means of ontologies and various reasoning methods. For this feature, this work is similar to our but also in this case no dependability assessment is performed.

Sneha and Varshney investigate an approach based on mobile ad hoc network to address the challenge of enhancing communication dependability in the context of health monitoring; they propose power management protocols to overcome issues of low battery power management of patient monitoring devices increasing communication dependability. They assert ensuring reliable end to end communication in a mHealth monitoring system is a critical requirement. However, their research is based on dependability issues that affect this kind of systems; also this work is far from our aim since only power consumption is considered as dependability parameter while we consider also coverage, connection resiliency and packet loss. Moreover they consider end-to-end dependability and not within a WBAN.

Therefore, several mHealth monitoring systems have been proposed in literature but dependability assessment remains an ongoing challenge.

Despite the presence of these reported solutions, several unexplored issues can limit the adoption of mobile health monitoring systems, such as cellular network connectivity, smart phone failures and many others. Each failure mode in turn needs proper countermeasures to be handled at runtime. Thus, not only a more comprehensive view of the failure modes of these systems is needed, but even a new architecture provided with monitors to observe the behavior of the system and to detect and mask the occurring failures.

3. MOBILE HEALTH MONITORING SYSTEMS

In the last years, several health monitoring systems have been proposed in the market. Among different implementations, we chose three of the most popular and presenting a sufficient variety of characteristics to conduct our experimentation: the *MedApps System*, the *Nicolet Ambulatory Monitor System* and a system used by the *Center for Technology and Aging*.

The *MedApps System* (Dicks, 2007) provides a healthcare connectivity platform that delivers scalable and flexible remote distribution using cellular, wireless and wired technologies with cloud-based computing. This system can work with multiple internal and external devices. Patient data is collected, analyzed and forwarded, via cell phone to servers, guaranteeing a more robust picture of the patients' health.

The *Nicolet Ambulatory Monitor System* (Carefusion, 2011) combines a flexible, high quality diagnostic unit, ideal for patients of all ages. It is a flexible, robust system specifically realized to provide the requirements of long-term monitoring. This system diagnoses patients' cerebral function (premature neonates to older adults) monitoring continuously ill patients at risk for brain damage and secondary injury.

Finally, authors in (Center for Technology and Aging, 2009) discuss two areas of opportunity for remote patient monitoring: i) Patient Safety and ii) Chronic Disease Management and Post-Acute Care Management. In alignment with the mission of the Center for Technology and Aging, they focus on technology-enabled innovations, such as wireless connectivity, mainly aimed at improving the health of older adults and promoting independent living in community-based, home, and long-term care settings.

Observing the underlying architectures of these systems, we can assert that a mobile health monitoring system is usually composed by a number of sensors (medical devices), a gateway device (a handheld device) and a medical station; typical communication means are Bluetooth (within the Body Area Network - Intra BAN communication), WiFi and cellular (external to the BAN - Extra BAN communication). Vital signs are sensed by sensors (i.e. oximeter, electrocardiogram - ECG, insulin pump, etc.) and transmitted to a mobile device over a bluetooth network. Afterwards, data are sent to a remote station deployed, for an example, in a hospital by means of either a WiFi or a cellular connection (the medical center location).

In this typical network, we can note that possible failures can occur in medical devices, in the bluetooth communication, in the mobile device, during the WiFi/cellular communication and finally in the local monitoring station of the caregiver.

Figure 1 depicts the components of a generic mobile health monitoring system.

4. THE FAILURE MODES AND EFFECTS ANALYSIS (FMEA)

4.1 FMEA Fundamentals

Failure Modes and Effects Analysis (FMEA) is a teambased, systematic and proactive approach for identifying the ways that a process or design can fail, why it might fail, and how it can be made safer (Latino et al., 2004). To properly evaluate a process or product for strengths, weaknesses, potential problem areas or failure modes, and to prevent problems before they occur, a FMEA can be conducted. The purpose of performing an FMEA, as described in US MIL STD 1629 (Department of Defense – USA, 1980), is to identify where and when possible system failures could occur and to prevent those problems before they happen. It represents a procedure for analysis of potential failure modes within a system for classification by the severity and likelihood of the failures.

Figure 1. A mobile health monitoring architecture

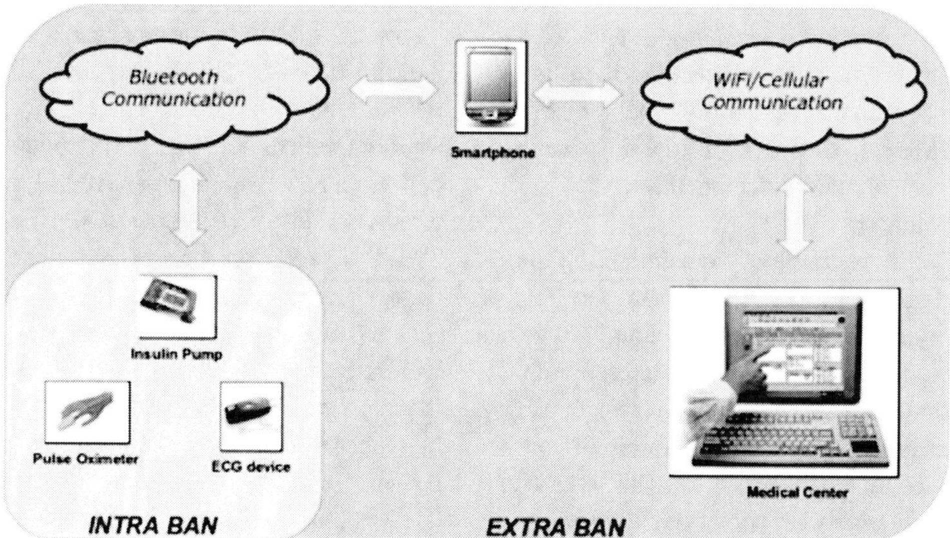

An FMEA provides a systematic method of resolving the questions: How can a process or product fail? What will be the effect on the rest of the system if such failure occurs? What action is necessary to prevent the failure? To realize a FMEA, the system is divided in components/ functions that are divided in subcomponents/ subfunctions; it considers a table in which the rows are composed by the subcomponents/sub- functions and the columns represent respectively the failure modes, the possible causes and the possible effects. If a particular failure could not be prevented, then the goal would be to prevent the issue from affecting health care organizations in the accreditation process. The FMEA team determines the effect of each failure by failure mode analysis and identifies single failure points that are critical.

It may also classify each failure according to the criticality of a failure effect (severity) and its probability of occurring (probability). There are some motivations why this analysis technique is very advantageous. FMEA provides a basis for identifying root failure causes and developing effective corrective actions; the FMEA identi- fies reliability and safety critical components; it facilitates investigation of design alternatives at all phases of design; it is used to provide other maintainability, safety, testability, and logistics analyses. FMEA is thus part of a larger system of quality control, where documentation is vital to implementation.

Since FMEA is effectively dependent on the members of the team which examines the failures, it is limited by their experience of previous failures. If a failure mode cannot be identified, then external help is needed from consultants who are aware of the many different types of product failure. In our case, we based the analysis both on our previous studies on different system components (such as WSNs, smart phones, and short range communica- tion technologies) and on FMEA results available on some subcomponents, such as medical devices (i.e. Pulse Oximeter, ECG Device, Insulin Pump).

4.2 FMEA Results

In this section we present the results of the FMEA we performed on mobile health monitoring sys- tems in (Cinque et al., 2011). The most frequent failure occurrences have been obtained from past experiences on real architectures and from the existing literature, trying to relate failure occur- rences with potential causes (faults).

Considering the general architecture, we omit the Medical Center location, since we assume it to be more reliable and under the direct control of the medical staff, who can immediately intervene in case of failures (e.g., they can connect to the system using a different machine). Hence, we want to focus on the components which have to be used by patients, who might not be technology experts and who need to rely on a monitoring system able to work even in case of accidental failures.

To perform the FMEA we identified four com- ponents/functions (Cinque et al., 2011): the node (i.e., the sensor used to monitor the patient), the Intra BAN communication, the Extra BAN com- munication, and the gateway (i.e., the smartphone of the patient).

Eight sub-components/subfunctions have been identified for the node component: the sensor board, the power supply unit, the CPU, and the OS (such as (Qnx., n.a.)(Threadx. n.a.) which are used in medical devices) are the general compo- nents of a node, and their analysis is based on our previous study on sensor networks (Cinque et al., 2007a). In addition, we considered the failures of some specific medical devices, such as the ECG sensor (divided in the ECG Device Adhesive, the ECG Device Electrolyte), the patient cable, and the Insulin Pump. The failures of such devices have been identified starting from existing studies, such as (James et al., 2004)(Sommerville, 2004). Clearly, other devices can be added to the analysis if used in a specific setting.

We report in Table 1 the FMEA results. Further we add for each failure mode the related severity and probability of occurrence that are

Table 1. Failure mode and effect analysis of a mobile health monitoring system

Component	Sub-Component	Potential Failure Mode	Potential Effects of Failure	Potential Causes of Failure	Sev.	Prob.
Node (the Medical Sensor)	Sensor Board	Stuck at Zero	The device is out-of-order it does not deliver any output to inputs	Sensing hardware	4	2
		Null Reading	The device delivers null output values	Sensing hardware	4	4
		Out of Scale Reading	The device delivers no meaningful values	Sensing hardware	3	4
	Power Supply	Stuck at Zero	The device is out-of-order; it does not deliver any output to inputs	Natural energy exhaustion	4	4
		Reset	The node resets itself to its initial conditions	Anomalous current request that cannot be supplied by batteries	3	1
	CPU	Stuck at Zero	The device is out-of-order; it does not deliver any output to inputs	Micro-controller	4	4
	OS	Software Hang	The device is powered on, but not able to deliver any output	Operating system's corrupted state	4	3
	ECG Device Adhesive	Incorrect reading	Wrong data values, irritation or rash of skin	Skin contact	2	3
	ECG Device Electrolyte	Incorrect reading	Wrong data values, irritation or rash of skin	Skin contact	2	3
	Patient Cable	Discontinuous readings	Noise, wrong data values	Defective wire	2	2
	Insulin Pump	Insulin overdose	Low blood sugar levels (hypoglycemia) which can be quite dangerous	Incorrect sugar level measured	3	4
		Insulin underdose	Patient at risk: sugar accumulates in the blood	Incorrect sugar level measured	1	3
		Power failure	Desidered dose was not given	Natural energy exhaustion	2	2
		No delivery failure	Desidered dose was not given	Corrupted rewinding mechanism	4	3
Intra BAN Communication	Transport and Routing	Packet Loss	The radio packet is not delivered	Packet corruption / Buffer overrun	3	2
		Isolation	The node is not longer connected to the sink node	Failure of all forwarding nodes	4	2
	Bluetooth Stack	Bluetooth stack failure	A Bluetooth module (e.g. L2CAP, BNEP, etc.) fails	Bluetooth stack's corrupted state	3	1
	Bluetooth Channel	Header corruption	Header delivered with errors	Packet corruption	2	1
		Header length mismatch	Header length deviates from the specified one	Packet corruption	2	1
		Payload corruption	Payload delivered with errors	Packet corruption	3	1

continued on following page

Table 1. Continued

Component	Sub-Component	Potential Failure Mode	Potential Effects of Failure	Potential Causes of Failure	Sev.	Prob.
Extra BAN Communication		Data Delivery Failures	The network is not able to deliver the required amount of measurements	The number of failed nodes is more than a given threshold	3	3
		Cellular/ WiFi network unavailable	Monitoring stopped	Area without cellular/WiFi signal	4	3
Gateway	**Device (The Smartphone)**	Freeze	The device's output becomes constant; the device does not respond to the users input.	Systems corrupted state	3	3
		Self-shutdown	The device shuts down itself; no service is delivered at the user interface.	Natural energy exhaustion or self-reboot due to corrupted state	4	2
		Unstable behavior	The device exhibits erratic behavior without any input inserted by the user	System/Application corrupted state	4	2
		Output failure	The device delivers an output sequence that deviates from the expected one	System/Application corrupted state	3	4
		Input failure	User inputs have no effect on device behavior	System/Application corrupted state; Natural energy exhaustion	1	1
	Bluetooth Application	Inquiry/Scan Failure	The scan procedure terminates abnormally	A Bluetooth module fails or device out of range	2	3
		Discovery Failure	The discover procedure terminates abnormally	A Bluetooth module fails or device out of range	2	3
		Connect Failure	The device is unable to establish a connection	A Bluetooth module fails or device out of range	4	3
		Packet Loss	Expected packets are not received	Packet corruption	3	1
		Data mismatch	Packets are delivered with errors in the payload	Memoryless channel with uncorrelated errors	3	1

represented by a value between 1 and 4. With lower value we identify a weak severity/probability instead with higher values a strong severity/probability (Stamatis, 2003). For example if a failure is classified with severity 4 and probability 4 it means that the failure is very dangerous and very probable. But if a failure is classified with severity 1 and probability 1 then there's almost nothing to worry.

Table 1 is structured by seven columns. Every row contains the description of a single failure mode. So, considering a possible failure mode that may occur in the health monitoring system, we identify from left to right the component (and the subcomponent if it exists) interested by failure mode, the failure mode, the possible effects of failure, the possible cause of failure and finally the severity and probability of occurrence, to highlight the more dangerous and frequent failures.

All of these analyzed failures cause abnormal vital sign readings, or even it can happen that a value is not received at the Medical Center location; in this case an inaccurate monitoring is provided, potentially resulting in a significant hazard to patients. Health monitoring systems must be aware of all the possible failures, in order to react to them or, at least, to detect them. For instance, in case of failure detection, a possible action can be to call to the patient's home or to call to an emergency contact to suddenly check the patient status and restore the normal operation of the system.

5. THE PROPOSED SERVICES

The problem of architecting mobile health monitoring systems with predictable and verifiable dependability properties still represents a critical open issue. The problem lies in the highly evolvable and dynamic nature of such systems, which, coupled with the unpredictability of hardware and software faults, exacerbates the definition of fault tolerance means, and compromises the application of fault forecasting techniques, due to the non-reproducibility of their behavior. In other terms, mobile health monitoring systems do not allow the application of techniques based on the a-priori knowledge of the system itself, even because, being these systems relatively young, there are no field failure data or experience reports available on their failure behavior, apart from the high-level FMEA reported in Section 4. Given the high dynamicity and heterogeneity of these systems (which behavior is strongly influenced by the mission they need to accomplish), we note that the knowledge on the system behavior needs to be acquired during the actual execution of the system, and to be adapted continuously to current system dynamics. This allows the tailor the intervention of fault tolerance means based on the current situation (what we call situation-aware fault tolerance).

In this section we present the proposed monitoring services conceived to build dependable mobile health monitoring systems, able to automatically detect failures and potentially react to them. The services are discussed with respect to a reference mobile health monitoring system, depicted in Figure 2. First we present the services offered to applications, and their role. Then, we introduce the concept of monitor and describe the monitor components introduced in the system.

The system is structured in four main parts: Intra-BAN, Gateway Services, Medical Center Services and External Applications.

5.1 Intra-BAN

The Intra-BAN is a particular network constituted by a set of biomedical sensors that communicate among each other and with the gateway. Being the majority of wireless medical devices available today equipped with the Bluetooth communication technology, we assume that devices are discovered with the Bluetooth Discovery service. Vital signs are then collected by means of the Bluetooth Connection service.

5.2 Gateway Services

The services offered on the Gateway side (mobile) are summarized in the following:

- **Bluetooth Connection:** This service provides the Bluetooth communication between a medical sensor of the Intra-BAN and the gateway device (i.e. a PDA, a notebook, etc...)
- **Bluetooth Discovery:** This service is used to discover the medical devices in the Intra-BAN.
- **Wifi Discovery:** This service is used to verify if there is an access point for the WiFi connection.

Figure 2. The proposed service schema

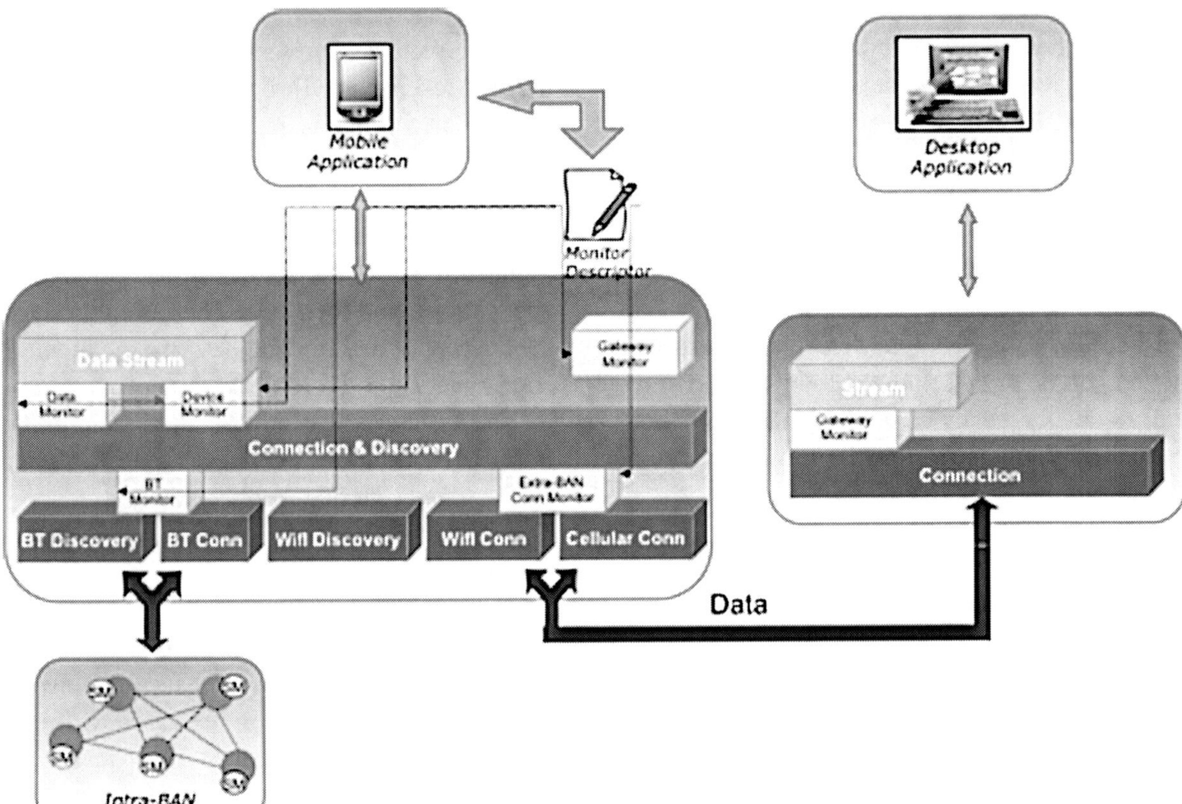

- **Wifi Connection:** This service provides the WiFi communication to transmit the data stream to the medical center.
- **Cellular Connection:** This service provides the cellular communication (GPRS, UMTS, etc...) to transmit the data stream to the medical center when a WiFi access point is not available.
- **Connection and Discovery:** This service is placed at an upper layer and it has the role to hide to applications the details on the communication technology (Bluetooth, WiFi and cellular). Further, it provides technology-agnostic discovery services, which are then specialized for Bluetooth and WiFi.
- **Data Stream:** It provides streaming services for vital sign data to the application.

5.3 Medical Center Services

The services offered for the Medical Center side (desktop) are:

- **Connection:** This service provides the needed communication interface to receive data from the Gateway and to send commands to manage the monitoring.
- **Stream:** It is the service that dialogues with the desktop application of Medical Center. It reports the data acquired by the medical devices.

5.4 External Applications

Finally, we have to consider external application for both side (mobile and desktop). These applica-

Table 2. Failures detected by the monitors

Monitor	Detected Failures
Sensor Monitor	stuck-at-zero; software hang; reset; power failure; isolation
Bluetooth Monitor	connect failure; bluetooth stack failure; header failures; payload corruption; inquiry/scan failure; discovery failure
Extra-BAN Monitor	cellular/wifi network unavailable
Data Monitor	packet loss; data delivery failure; data mismatch
Device Monitor	incorrect reading; discontinous reading; out of scale reading; null reading; insulin under/over dose; no delivery failure; device unavailable
Gateway Monitor (mobile-side)	self-shutdown; input failure; output failure; freeze; unstable behavior
Gateway Monitor (desktop-side)	gateway unavailable

tions generally include the GUI used by patients (on the mobile side) and by the medical staff (on the fixed side), and implement application specific data interpretation and reporting functions.

5.5 Monitors

Once introduced the general services of the mobile health monitoring system, we enrich the system with failure detection capabilities. To this aim, we introduce the concept of System Monitors.

A monitor is a service instantiated on-demand on the basis of the failures that have to be detected. By means of a Monitor Descriptor file (i.e. a XML file), the developer can set the failures that he wants to observe. This file is provided to the Mobile Application that, in turn, dynamically creates the requested monitors, which run in the background and are managed transparently from developers.

Monitors can act as lightweight model-checkers supporting formal runtime verification as shown in (Coronato et al., 2011).

Specifically, we introduce the following monitors to detect the failures reported in the FMEA study conducted in the previous section:

The Sensor Monitor is deployed on the medical device and it detects all of the failures that occur in a medical sensor node (ECG, Pulse Oximeter, Insulin Pump, etc...). This monitor can be considered as a failure logger for the medical device, since it can store the state of the node before of the failure, and report it to the gateway when the device is recovered. Since in the industry market there are medical sensors equipped of operating systems and programmability capabilities (i.e. TuffSat Oximeter (ThreadX, n.a.)), we can consider the possibility to add sensor monitors to the future releases of such sensors. On the other hand, the implementation of such monitor is already feasible in commodity WSN nodes, such as Berkley Motes (in (Salazar et al., 2010) authors identify a set of wireless sensors – IRIS, MICAz, TELOSb, SHIMMER and Imote2 - used for capturing and transmitting biomechanical and physiological signals, among other data related to healthcare, sports, motion capturing)

The Bluetooth Monitor detects the problems related to the Bluetooth connection such as, connection failures, Bluetooth channel failures and Bluetooth stack failures. It can also verify if there are problems during the discovery and inquiry phase of the medical devices equipped with the Bluetooth technology.

The Extra-BAN Monitor checks the availability of the WiFi and Cellular connections. It can be efficiently used to manage the handoff process between the two technologies. For instance, in the case of a patient leaving home, this monitor detects the WiFi connection failure and requires the establishment of a cellular connection. In contrast, when the patient comes back home, the Extra-BAN Monitor reveals the availability of the domestic network and switches from the cellular connection to a WiFi connection.

Figure 3. Failure detection by means of monitor

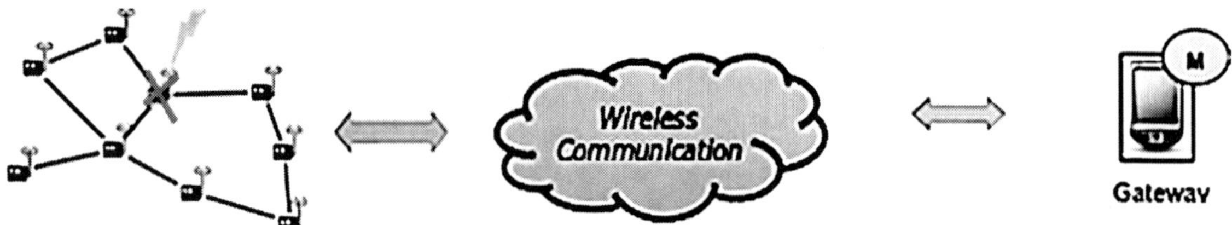

The Data Monitor checks if there are anomalies in the data stream acquired. For example, during the monitoring, some packet can be lost or a data delivery failure can occur.

The Device Monitor detects mainly if a medical device is unavailable. In this case, to better analyze the failure it is necessary to require extra information to the Sensor Monitor. Other failures that can be detected by this monitor are incorrect/discontinuous/out of scale/null reading failures and some failure related to a specific medical device (for instance, for insulin pump, it can control the injected dose, whereas out-of-scale readings can be detected for the ECG, depending on application specific threshold values specified in the Monitor Descriptor file).

The Gateway Monitor is present both in the Gateway and in the Medical Center. The aim of this monitor is to check if the gateway operates correctly. The Gateway Monitor in the Medical Center can only detect if the gateway becomes unavailable but it cannot know the cause. Instead the Gateway Monitor in the mobile side, can keep track of occurred failures, such as a freeze, self-shutdown, etc, following for instance the logging approach proposed in our earlier work (Cinque et al., 2007b).

from the real-world WSN. The monitor runs on a machine and listens for packets coming from all sensors through the sink node of the WSN. The detection of events (such as the stop of a node) is performed assuming that each sensor sends packets periodically, with a known rate, which is common to several WSN applications. Hence, for every node, the monitor sets a timeout, which is reset each time the monitor receives a packet from the given node. If the timeout expires for a node X, the monitor generates a Stop(X) event.

The use of time out may also detect temporary disconnections or delays. In this case, when packets from a node X are received again after a stop, the monitor generates a Start(X) event. Clearly, different failure detection approaches could be used as well, however this is not relevant for our experiment and out of the scope of the paper.

The monitor has been implemented as a java application running on a server (a Pentium 4 machine in our case) and connected via USB to a MIB520 Base station by Crossbow. As sensor nodes, we have adopted Iris Motes by Crossbow equipped with ZigBee RF Transceiver and TinyOS 2.0 operating system, running the BlinkToRadio application, just to perform a periodic sensing and sending of packets of all nodes to the sink.

6. USE OF A MONITOR

We have physically deployed a WSN topology in our lab to detect failures at runtime (Figure 3). We have designed and implemented a system monitor with the aim of detecting failure events

7. CONCLUSION AND FUTURE WORK

The advent of AmI systems applied to critical application scenarios, such as mobile health monitoring, requires facing new dependability threats that may arise during the functioning of the system and that may result fatal for the health of the patient. Moved by these considerations, in this paper we propose the design of an innovative mobile health monitoring system, based on the configurable adoption of system monitors, conceived to detect the failures occurring at runtime, and hence providing a means to react to them in due time, preventing catastrophic consequences. The responsibilities of the monitors in terms of the failures they have to detect, are defined starting from the results of a failure modes and effects analysis, which allowed us to focus on every single problem that may occur on these systems, and to define exactly where to deploy the monitors in order to deal with given failure modes. The approach can be used iteratively, to extend the system with further monitors or to readapt the existing ones, as soon as new failure modes are found. Future research activities will deal with the realization of a prototype system including the defined monitors, in order to assess on the field their capability at detecting the type of failures identified in the conducted failure mode analysis.

REFERENCES

Arnstein, L., Grimm, R., Hung, C., Kang, J. H., LaMarca, A., & Look, G. et al. (2002). Systems Support for Ubiquitous Computing: A Case Study of Two Implementations of Labscape. In *Proceedings of the First International Conference on Pervasive Computing (Pervasive '02)*. Springer-Verlag.

Baskiyar, S. (2002). A real-time fault tolerant intrabody network. In *Proceedings of Local Computer Networks,* (pp. 235-240). IEEE.

Benlamri, R., & Docksteader, L. (2010). Morf: A mobile health-monitoring platform. *IT Professional, 12*(3), 18–25. doi:10.1109/MITP.2010.3

Bohn, J., Coroama, V., Langheinrich, M., Mattern, F., & Rohs, M. (2005). Social, economic, and ethical implications of ambient intelligence and ubiquitous computing. In Ambient Intelligence. Springer.

Carefusion. (2011). *Carefusion nicolet.* Retrieved 2011 from http://www.carefusion.com/medical-products/neurology/neurodiagnostic-monitoring/eeg/nicolet-ambulatorymonitor.aspx

Center for Technology and Aging. (2009). *Technologies for remote patient monitoring in older adults.* Center for Technology and Aging.

Chakraborty, S., Poolsappasit, N., & Ray, I. (2007). Reliable Delivery of Event Data from Sensors to Actuators in Pervasive Computing Environments. In *Proceedings of 21st Annual IFIP WG 11.3 Working Conference on Data and Applications Security (DBSec'07)* (LNCS), (vol. 4602, pp. 77-92). Redondo Beach, CA: Springer.

Chen, M., Gonzalez, S., Vasilakos, A., Cao, H., & Leung, V. C. (2011). Body area networks: A survey. *Mob. Netw. Appl., 16,* 171–193. doi:10.1007/s11036-010-0260-8

Chetan, S., Ranganathan, A., & Campbell, R. (2005, Spring). Towards fault tolerance pervasive computing. *IEEE Technology and Society Magazine, 24*(1), 38–44. doi:10.1109/MTAS.2005.1407746

Cinque, M., Coronato, A., & Testa, A. (2011). A Failure Modes and Effects Analysis of Mobile Health Monitoring Systems. In *Proceedings of the 2011 International Conference on Systems, Computing Sciences and Software Engineering (SCSS), part of the International Joint Conferences on Computer, Information, and Systems Sciences, and Engineering (CISSE 11). Academic Press.*

Cinque, M., Coronato, A., & Testa, A. (2012). Dependable Services for Mobile Health Monitoring Systems. *International Journal of Ambient Computing and Intelligence*, 4(1), 1–15. doi:10.4018/jaci.2012010101

Cinque, M., Cotroneo, D., Di Martinio, C., & Russo, S. (2007a). Modeling and Assessing the Dependability of Wireless Sensor Networks. In *Proceedings of the 26th IEEE International Symposium on Reliable Distributed Systems (SRDS '07)*. IEEE Computer Society.

Cinque, M., Cotroneo, D., Kalbarczyk, Z., & Iyer, R. (2007b). How do mobile phones fail? A failure data analysis of symbian os smart phones. In *Proceedings of Dependable Systems and Networks*, (pp. 585–594). IEEE.

Coronato, A., & De Pietro, G. (2010). Formal design of ambient intelligence applications. *Computer*, 43(12), 60–68. doi:10.1109/MC.2010.335

Coronato, A., & De Pietro, G. (2011, July). Tools for the Rapid Prototyping of Provably Correct Ambient Intelligence Applications. *IEEE Transactions on Software Engineering*, 20.

Curiac, D., Volosencu, C., Pescaru, D., Jurca, L., & Doboli, A. (2009). A view upon redundancy in wireless sensor networks. In *Proceedings of the 8th WSEAS International Conference on Signal Processing, Robotics and Automation (ISPRA'09)*. WSEAS.

Department of Defense – USA (1980). *Us mil std 1629 1980: Procedure for performing a failure mode, effect and criticality analysis, method 102*. Author.

Dicks, K. E. (2007). *Telemedicine 2.0 has arrived. Future Healthcare Magazine*.

Duman, H., Hagras, H., & Callaghan, V. (2010). A multi-society-based intelligent association discovery and selection for ambient intelligence environment. ACM Trans. Autonom. Adapt. Syst., 5(2).

Gelernter, D. (1985, January). Generative communication in Linda. *ACM Transactions on Programming Languages and Systems*, 7(1), 80–112. doi:10.1145/2363.2433

Georgalis, Y., Grammenos, D., & Stephanidis, C. (2009). Middleware for Ambient Intelligence Environments: Reviewing Requirements and Communication Technologies. In *Proceedings of the 5th International on ConferenceUniversal Access in Human-Computer Interaction. Part II: Intelligent and Ubiquitous Interaction Environments (UAHCI '09)*. Springer-Verlag.

Hanna, S. (2009). Regulations and standards for wireless medical applications. In *Proc. of the 3rd Int. Symp. on Medical Information and Communication Technology*. Academic Press.

Hanson, M., Powell, H., Barth, A., Ringgenberg, K., Calhoun, B., Aylor, J., & Lach, J. (2009). Body area sensor networks: Challenges and opportunities. *Computer*, 42(1), 58–65. doi:10.1109/MC.2009.5

Hao, Y., & Foster, R. (2008). Wireless body sensor networks for health-monitoring applications. *Physiological Measurement*, 29(11), R27–R56. doi:10.1088/0967-3334/29/11/R01 PMID:18843167

James, C. B. H., Cook, R. & Konwinski, J. (2004). *Failure mode effects and criticality analysis (fmeca)*. Home ECG test kit.

Kansal, A., Hsu, J., Zahedi, S., & Srivastava, M. B. (2007). Power management in energy harvesting sensor networks. *ACM Transactions on Embedded Computing Systems*, 6.

Latino, R. J. & Flood, A. (2004). Optimizing fmea and rca efforts in healthcare. *Journal of Healthcare Risk Management*, *24*(3), 21–28. doi:.10.1002/jhrm.5600240305

Lin, H., Shao, J., Zhang, C., & Fang, Y. (2013). Cam: Cloud-assisted privacy preserving mobile health monitoring. *IEEE Transactions on* Information Forensics and Security, *8*(6), 985–997. doi:10.1109/TIFS.2013.2255593

Nehmer, J., Karshmer, A., Lamm, R., & Becker, M. (2006). Living assistance systems: an ambient intelligence approach. In *Proceedings of 28th International Conference on Software Engineering (ICSE'06)* (pp. 43-50). ICSE. doi:10.1145/1134285.1134293

O'Donovan, T., O'Donoghue, J., Sreenan, C., Sammon, D., O'Reilly, P., & O'Connor, K. A. (2009). A context aware wireless body area network (BAN). In *Proceedings of Pervasive Computing Technologies for Healthcare,* (pp. 1-8). Academic Press.

Paksuniemi, M., Sorvoja, H., Alasaarela, E., & Myllyla, R. (2006). Wireless sensor and data transmission needs and technologies for patient monitoring in the operating room and intensive care unit. In *Proceedings of Engineering in Medicine and Biology Society,* (pp. 5182-5185). IEEE.

Ponnekanti, S. R., Johanson, B., Kiciman, E., & Fox, A. (2003). Portability, extensibility and robustness in iROS. Pervasive Computing and Communications. 11-19.

Qnx. (n.d.). Retrieved from http://www.qnx.com/solutions/industries/medical/

Salazar, A. J., Silva, A. S., Borges, C. M., & Correia, M. V. (2010). An initial experience in wearable monitoring sport systems. In *Proceedings of Information Technology and Applications in Biomedicine (ITAB),* (pp. 1-4). IEEE.

Simoncini, L. (2003). Architectural Challenges for "Ambient Dependability". In *Proceedings of Object-Oriented Real-Time Dependable Systems.* IEEE.

Sneha, S., & Varshney, U. (2013). A framework for enabling patient monitoring via mobile ad hoc network. *Decis. Support Syst., 55*(1), 218–234. DOI: 10.1016/j.dss.2013.01.024

Sommerville, I. (2004). *Software Engineering* (7th ed.). Pearson Addison Wesley.

Spadotto, K. M. S. E., & Hawkins, J. (2009). ICT convergence, confluence and creativity: The application of emerging technologies for healthcare transformation. In *Proc. of the 3rd Int. Symp. on Medical Information and Communication Technology.* Academic Press.

Stamatis, D. H. (2003). Failure mode and effect analysis: FMEA from theory to execution (2nd ed.). ASQ Quality Press.

Threadx. (n.d.). Retrieved from http://www.qnx.com/solutions/industries/medical/

Triantafyllidis, A., Koutkias, V., Chouvarda, I., & Maglaveras, N. (2012). A pervasive health system integrating patient monitoring, status logging and social sharing. *IEEE Transactions on Information Technology in Biomedicine.* PMID:23193318

Van Halteren, A., Bults, R., Wac, K., Konstantas, D., Widya, I., Dokovski, N., et al. (2004). *Mobile Patient Monitoring: The Mobihealth System.* Academic Press.

Yan, H., Huo, H., Xu, Y., & Gidlund, M. (2010). Wireless sensor network based e-health system implementation and experimental results. *IEEE Transactions on* Consumer Electronics, *56*(4), 2288–2295. doi:10.1109/TCE.2010.5681102

Zhang, Y., & Xiao, H. (2009). Bluetooth-based sensor networks for remotely monitoring the physiological signals of a patient. *Trans. Info. Tech. Biomed., 13*.

KEY TERMS AND DEFINITIONS

Ambient Intelligence: The field to study and create embodiments for smart environments that not only react to human events through sensing, interpretation and service provision, but also learn and adapt their operation and services to the users over time.

Dependability: Dependability is a measure of a system's availability, reliability, and its maintainability.

Failure Analysis: The fault analysis is a top down, deductive analysis in which an undesired state of a system is analyzed combining a series of lower-level events.

Health Monitoring: In information technology and multimedia terms, health monitoring refers to the technique to check patient's vital sign by means of remote communications.

Monitor: A device used for observing, checking, or keeping a continuous record of something.

Resiliency: An ability to recover from or adjust easily to misfortune or change.

Wireless Sensor Networks: A network of RF transceivers, sensors, machine controllers, microcontrollers, and user interface devices with at least two nodes communicating by means of wireless transmissions.

Chapter 31
mHealth in Resource-Constrained Environments

Barbara Rita Barricelli
Università degli Studi di Milano, Italy

Yanet Devis
University of West London, UK

ABSTRACT

The use of mobile devices in telemedicine contributes to providing more effective and efficient remote healthcare in rural areas improving patients' life style and medical quality of service in this setting. The idea of creating mobile applications for this scenario led the authors to face important sociotechnical challenges in terms of innovation and design for resource-constrained environments. In this paper the authors present the outcomes of MANTRA (Mobile ANticoagulant TheRApy) Project developed for and evaluated in Venezuela. Through the evaluation of this project under those settings the authors developed an approach to mHealth in the remote management of chronic diseases by supporting the communication between doctors.

1. INTRODUCTION

Rural areas are very often resource-constrained environments where direct access to the Internet, through landlines or mobile phones may be challenging. In such settings, also the quality of health services is often affected by these limitations. In such conditions some chronic diseases are hard to be treated anticoagulant therapy management is one of those because it demands a regular monitoring of patients' conditions made by doctors or health professionals.

Anticoagulant therapy prevents the formation of thrombus. People at risk of developing thrombosis have to take anticoagulant treatment (warfarin) once a day in a dosage that needs to be adjusted on the basis of the International Normalised Ratio (INR) test results (Cohen et al., 2007). The INR test measures the prothrombin time (PT) – how long it takes for the blood to clot. The dose of warfarin is increased or decreased with the intention of keeping the INR value within an appropriate range. When the treatment starts the INR value is tested every 2-3 days but once its

DOI: 10.4018/978-1-4666-8756-1.ch031

level has stabilised it is tested between 7 and 20 days. Since the INR tests are usually performed in surgeries the patients have to make frequent visits to meet doctors to take the test and receive a prescription of warfarin.

In this paper we present MANTRA (Mobile ANticoagulant TheRApy), a project aimed at studying the feasibility and acceptability of the introduction of mobile technology in the management of anticoagulant therapy involving doctors in the design phases. The project was implemented as a proof of concept for a rural setting in Venezuela. We studied the existing literature and state of the art and performed a study on the end users profiles and the context/environment and designed, developed and evaluated two interactive high-fidelity prototypes for mobile devices (iPads) aimed at support the remote communication between doctors who operate in rural areas and doctors who practice in hospitals. This gave us the chance to derive a general approach to mHealth in the remote management of chronic diseases by supporting the communication among healthcare practitioners.

The paper is organized as follows. First, literature review and state of the art of telemedicine in anticoagulant therapy domain is presented and discussed. In Section 3 the MANTRA project is presented and its research context and methodology are illustrated. Section 4 presents the prototypes design and development and Section 5 illustrates the usability evaluations performed and their results. Finally, conclusion and future developments are presented.

2. LITERATURE REVIEW AND STATE OF THE ART

2.1. The Need for ICT Localization Integrating the Tradition and the New

The design and development of interactive systems for rural environments needs to consider the variety of cultures, e.g. different socio-political-econom-ical contexts, different languages and educational backgrounds. Thinyane et al. (2007) confirm the importance of localisation techniques in design and development and argue that it should be found "a way to make ICT solutions more sensitive to the local context, and therefore more effective" by capitalising on local knowledge and resources. Therefore, the positive impact of many existing ICTs has been attributed to their localisation for specific contexts and cultures. Given the subject handled by this study, the research focuses also on supporting the design and development of localised ICT solutions.

Choi et al. (2005) identified 52 cultural attributes in three different countries in a qualitative cross-national study of cultural influences on mobile data service design, which demonstrate that without any doubt the context and culture affect the way users interact with technology and systems. Research also shows that ICT solutions that simulate as closely as possible traditional local networks guaranteed a greater success in developing (Kolko et al., 2007).

All these findings and studies also suggest the need for a type of ICT localisation that integrates the traditional knowledge and tools from those cultures with new tools. However, when ICT projects are reviewed, or referred to developing countries, the benefits and implications for the targeted users tend to be the focus. One the other hand, others researches also emphasise the fact that the issues are more related with usability and efficiency of systems and processes.

An excellent piece of research by De Angeli et al. (2004) analysed the introduction of ATM machines in India to evaluate the socio-cultural impact. They concluded that "(...) as much as culture can influence technology, the reverse is also possible" (De Angeli A. et al., 2004). Based on these results and from a research perspective, it was necessary to consider the technology for the targeted rural community, "Wonken", before deciding how to design the prototypes.

In the literature, many have identified the need for a more culture oriented HCI research that emphasises cultural influences on design (Kampuri et al., 2006). However, the idea is not to develop radically new systems for each cultural group. Kapange (2006) suggested that ICT systems as they already exist in developed cultures can be adapted or localised for developing countries. Moreover, there may be some past implementations of ICT that could be highly relevant to new solutions currently being implemented. It is therefore crucial to learn from those which have already been in use (Mbarika, 2004). More importantly, one should also acknowledge that users influence technology as much as technology influences users, their culture and societies (Oostveen & van den Besselaar, 2004; Bijker, 1995), as shown by De Angeli et al. (2004). This reasoning led to conducting a heuristic evaluation of existing applications on the market, from the point of view of the end user target for those applications.

2.2. Targeting Technology for Rural Communities

mHealth is the more recent evolution of the well-known concept "telemedicine". Telemedicine is aimed at providing remote health care by the use of technology. In Bolivia and Ecuador, the telemedicine service covers approximately 25 rural communities, providing healthcare to 6,000 people and 24,000 people indirectly. This potential solution enables the strengthening of the capabilities of primary care local health professionals who are be able to access to medical specialist through teleconsultations providing diagnosis and treatment through the use of ICT (Tele Salud, 2013).

As to the procedures to be followed in developing systems for telemedicine applied to anticoagulant therapy, it has still not been adopted as common practice. In a pilot study by Gardiner et al. (2005), home telematics devices were tested with 19 anticoagulant patients over 5 months. The device was used to transmit the INR result to a

remote server. The prescription was then given by telephone to the patient, because the device was only able to receive from the server the date of the next test. Due to many severe technical and software problems and failures only 9 home telematics devices were tested. The study proved the feasibility of telemedicine for anticoagulant therapy but with many technical constraints. First of all this study promoted the use of home devices that are not mobile but need to be connected to landline and therefore cannot be used while travelling. Another problem is the lack of bidirectional communication via the home telematics device: the doctor needs to call the patients on the phone to communicate the next warfarin prescription and this procedure is obviously highly error prone.

In 2008, Salvador et al. (2008) proposed the use of telemedicine for first monitoring and then establishing self-management of anticoagulant therapy. The study involved 54 patients over more than two years and led to conclusions related to the feasibility of telemedicine in anticoagulant therapy and of the introduction of self-management approach, i.e. the use of decision systems to be used by the patients to self-prescribe warfarin. This research suffered from the same weakness as highlighted for the previous study (Gardiner et al., 2005) in that it provides devices that are supposed to be used at home and that are not usable while on a trip.

Another interesting and more current research developed in Denmark in 2011 (Christensen et al), tested a telemedicine system to be used on Personal Computers connected to the Internet. They involved 123 patients and proved, like the other research works presented above, the validity of the adoption of telemedicine for anticoagulant therapy. Like the other projects, this also presents problems that MANTRA project was aimed at overcoming. First of all, the difficulty for patients using a computer-based system and specifically a very complicated interface may lead to errors in communicating the INR test results. Secondly, the lack of bidirectional communication: the doctors have to send emails or call the patient on the phone to communicate the next prescription of warfarin.

One of the most important contributions that MANTRA proposes in this field is the adoption of mobile technology to support quick and successful remote communication between doctors by using simple and effective user interfaces designed involving the end users themselves.

2.3. Identifying Pertinent Cultural Traits for the Actors and Context

In summary, the issue is not only to understand context and culture separately. It should also involve the identification and interpretation of those pertinent cultural traits of the actors and the context itself. The understanding and interpretation of the relationship between context, culture and technology is thus well documented. The socio-technology approach is at the basis of the MANTRA Project, in that the technical solutions we designed and tested consider not only the requirements in terms of data management, data exchange and remote communication, but also the end users' and domain experts' profiles, needs, skills and expectations in order to support information and knowledge exchange and the construction of virtual communities aimed at collaborating for patients' own good (Hansen, 2006). Technical and social have been considered as interconnected entities and the coevolution phenomenon (Latour, 1993; Callon 1986; Law & Hassard 1999) has been taken into account when the prototypes have been designed and developed.

It is argued that technology acceptance and adoption depend to a great extent on how end users perceive the technology (Lin & Silva, 2005). It is only logical, therefore, that an understanding of users' cognitive frames helps increasing acceptance and adoption of the technology. Abdelnour-Nocera et al. (2007) also investigated how the usefulness of an Information System (IS) can be deeply influenced by socio-cultural factors. They found that users and designers may have differ-

ent perceptions of usefulness and consequently different expectations of a system. Then for a successful ICT design in a context for which the technologies were not initially developed, designers need to assess how the interpretive frames and practices of users in their local context can shape the usefulness of existing or proposed systems.

Ehn (1990) said once: "One of the oldest and widely accepted principles in the design of computer-based tools for users is the principle 'know the user'."

In the same manner, the "contextual inquiry", is an approach that consists of finding out about the end users' context and culture with their participation. It uses a mixture of ethnography and other field research approaches to provide designers with "(...) grounded and detailed knowledge of user work as a basis for their design." (Duncan & Beabes, 1995). The advantage with this approach is that users sometimes reveal important issues and concerns that researchers may find worth exploring and sometimes might not been elicited. Also, the focus should encompass the whole design project (global team interests) (Kleimann, 1996), rather than just focusing on a particular stage.

Contextual inquiries as an approach are applied in many forms using a variety of mixed methods. In addition to the most common methods used (survey questionnaires, interviews, focus groups), there are also other User Centre Design (UCD)-oriented methodologies in use in this approach that generate more details about the users' mental models, cognitive frame, initial and general perception of technologies envisaged. However, for the purpose of this project, the dissertation uses a more traditional approach, using un-structured interviews and questionnaires.

2.4. Features of Health Care Technologies and Their Implications

The MANTRA Project aimed at introducing the use of mobile devices and mobile telecommunication to enable the communication between doctors remotely collaborating. This effort is framed in what is called mHealth, i.e. mobile health. This is a term used for the practice of medicine and health, supported by mobile devices. According to Cipresso et al. (2012), the term is most commonly used in reference to using mobile communication devices, such as mobile phones, tablet computers and PDAs, for health services and information. In the last few years, a great number of consulting firms have investigated the development of mHealth around the world such is the case of Vital Wave Consulting (2009), who in 2009 published that the mHealth field emerged as a sub-segment of eHealth, which is the use of ICT for health services and information.

Currently the mHealth field has emerged as a means of providing greater access to larger segments of a population in developing countries, as well as improving the capacity of health systems in such countries to provide quality healthcare (Vital Wave Consulting, 2009). That supports the idea to found in Venezuela (a developing country), people willing to adapt to new technologies.

For Germanakos et al. (2005), mHealth applications include the use of mobile devices in collecting clinical health data, delivery of healthcare information to practitioners, researchers, and patients, real-time monitoring of patient vital signs, and direct provision of care (via mobile telemedicine). In the context of this project, the clinical health data collected and the delivery of information between doctors will be vital.

According to the analyst firm PricewaterhouseCoopers (2013), more "emerging-market doctors" offer mHealth services than colleagues in developed countries, due to the rarity of existing healthcare: there is a greater demand for change and there are a fewer entrenched interests to impede the adoption of new approaches. Nowadays, doctors are embracing some aspects of mHealth. This is supported by a 2012 survey of European doctors conducted by Manhattan Research (2012), an organization that found that 62% of medical

personnel have an iPad and spent over one-quarter of their professional time using them. In a similar way, a 2011 US survey showed that 30% of doctors had an iPad, and 28% expected to buy one to use it in their medical practice. And this is just for developed countries.

Mobile technologies have proved effective in outbreak-tracking in remote areas, like in Brazil's and Venezuela's Amazonas State, where the data gathering program provided nearly real time information on outbreaks of malaria and dengue fever which previously took months to collate (PricewaterhouseCoopers, 2012).

It is well know that doctors around the world tend to concentrate in urban areas, which has severely impact on developing countries where there are so few doctors overall, and is especially relevant in South African and South American countries, where a great amount of the population lives in the countryside. In such rural areas, most of the time the medical care (if any) is provided by last year medical students or interns (McKinsey & Company, 2007). The population of Venezuelan's rural areas lives exactly in this situation. In conclusion, there are many reasons why mHealth is so popular these days and why it should be studied, namely that it is seen as a solution for complex situations, as described above.

3. MANTRA PROJECT

The MANTRA Project lasted 12 months (January-December 2013) and was aimed at studying how to support the remote communication in Venezuela between doctors who operate in rural areas and hospital doctors who work in main cities. Due to the limited time available, the MANTRA Project has been designed as a proof of concept focused on investigating the opportunity of introducing the use of mobile technology in the practice of anti-coagulant therapy in resource-constrained areas.

3.1. Research Context

In the last couples of years, following the steps of developed countries, Venezuela has invested a lot of resources on enhancing telemedicine. However, despite best efforts, there are still gaps in the development process of telemedicine in rural areas, due to resource constraint. According to Dr. Tomás Sanabria, director of the Venezuelan health care foundation Fundación Maniapure ICT is making a huge difference to medical care in isolated villages. These uses of telemedicine mean that patients can be treated locally, and when needed, they can also be referred for further evaluation and care. Due to the arrangement with which has to adapt to new technologies, Venezuela seems a logical choice within which to carry out this research. However, there are still many flaws in the development of this technology (network connection, remote patient treatments, delay in replies, security data) and because of the delay time in the actual communication, telecommunication cannot be used properly for treating patients with anticoagulant therapy.

In Venezuela the rural areas are typically low-density populated and the social life of the community takes place in its centre where the medical surgery is located. People living in these areas refer to the doctors in the surgery for most of their medical needs but for specific treatments or services they have to move to the closest hospital. Usually, these areas are very isolated and the hospitals often very distant and this makes difficult for the patients to reach them.

For example, to reach Caracas city from the rural area of Woken takes 2-3 hours by car plus a 2-hour flight or a 15 hour journey by car. Patients on anticoagulant therapy who live in these rural areas need to personally go to the surgery in the village to take an INR test. In the surgery, a bioanalyst intern takes the blood sample and observes the clotting times without the use of digital devices (i.e. INR testing device) but only by using chemical reagents. Once the PT is known,

the intern calculates manually the correspondent INR value using a mathematical equation. The result has to be evaluated by rural doctors but this may take time because they usually have to serve several villages and may have to visit patients who cannot reach the surgery given their health condition. Once the rural doctor reviews the INR value, s/he needs to contact a hospital doctor to ask for a prescription of warfarin for the patients.

In Wonken rural doctors have access to a telemedicine environment on a computer connected to the Internet via a satellite connection. Each time they communicate with the hospital doctors, they have to send the patient clinical history, the latest prothrombin time and INR result and all the information needed to identify the patient. This information is sent to Caracas hospital and it usually takes about 24 to 48 hours to receive a reply. During the rainy season (from May to November) the satellite Internet connection is disrupted and so is the availability of the telemedicine service. Additionally, even telephone connection is very hard to use because only two landlines are available in the village. In this scenario, it is very challenging for the doctors to manage and keep track of INR values and prescriptions for their patients. It is not an objective of MANTRA Project in this setting to provide rural patients with mobile devices and INR testers because of the issues related to poor power infrastructure, geographical dispersion and very low IT literacy. On the contrary, MANTRA Project aims at addressing these communication problems and facilitating the remote asynchronous collaboration between doctors in order to offer a better medical service and indirectly make patients' life easier and safer.

In this scenario, the patient living in the village reaches the surgery where a rural doctor takes the INR test on her blood using an INR self-testing device. Once the result is returned, the rural doctor uses a dedicated mobile application on an iPad to send it to the hospital doctor. In case the Internet connection is not available at that moment, the result can be stored on the device and sent later. The hospital doctor receives the INR result on the iPad; s/he reviews it by browsing the patient's clinical history and sends this back to the rural doctor with the new warfarin prescription. The rural doctor receives the prescription on the application and gives it to the patient. One of the main changes proposed by the MANTRA Project is the idea of introducing in the rural medical practice the use of INR self-testing devices. INR self-testing devices are widely available but not currently integrated into the systems for managing anticoagulant therapy adopted by the hospitals/clinics and therefore are still quite expensive. INR self-testing devices allow easy checking of the INR value with a finger stick test. Using a lancet, a drop of blood is placed on a test strip that is then inserted into the device. The device uses three main methods to detect the INR value: 1) Monitoring of change in impedance of the sample when clotting occurs; 2) Mechanical endpoint clotting mechanism, monitored optically; 3) Mechanical clot detection.

With such devices the result is available within minutes. INR devices can be used in two ways: Self-testing: the result has to be communicated to a doctor who is in charge of deciding the prescription of warfarin and the date of the next INR check. Self-monitoring: the patients, after a proper and adequate training, self-check their INR value and adjust their own warfarin dosage.

However, in a resource-constrained setting like the one studied by the MANTRA Project, the INR self-testing devices could be used as a very useful tool for doctors working in the rural areas, to avoid mistakes in manual calculation of warfarin dosage. Several studies (e.g., Schneeweiss et al., 2012; Bussey et al., 1997; Cromheecke et al., 2000; Dorfman et al., 2005; Gardiner et al., 2005; Tripodi, 2004) report that the INR self-testing devices are reliable instruments and suitable alternative to conventional laboratory testing and that the INR results are typically very well reproducible and well interrelated.

3.2. Methodology

The general methodology of design research followed in the project is the one described in Vaishnavi, (2008) and depicted in Figure 1.

Its application in the MANTRA Project is described in what follows focusing on all the phases – Awareness of problem, Suggestion, Development, Evaluation and Conclusion.

3.2.1. Awareness of problem

This phase is aimed at studying the research context, the literature review and state of the art to understand open problems, challenges and opportunities. The study of the requirements is performed also by interviewing and in general involving representatives of the end users and/or domain experts.

In the MANTRA Project, our team focused on studying the research context. Specifically, we reviewed the literature on telemedicine in rural areas and on anticoagulant therapy management

We then analyzed the state of the art of existing mobile applications for self-monitoring of INR tests (designed for patients living in urban context and not supporting the communication with doctors) and we performed some informal interviews with British and Venezuelan healthcare professionals to understand better how the anticoagulant therapy management is organised in the two scenarios (UK and Venezuela).

From what found in this phase, we derived the profiles of two main user groups (presented in this paper in Section 4.1) that we used to perform a heuristic evaluation on the existing mobile applications for patients and also as reference for the design activity performed in the next phases.

We applied heuristic evaluation method (Nielsen & Molich, 1990) to test the usability of the first prototype. Two usability experts have been involved in the evaluations. For the evaluations we applied the 10 Nielsen's heuristics: Visibility of system status, match between system and real

Figure 1. A methodology of design research. Adapted from Vaishnavi and Kuechler (2004) and published in Barricelli (2011).

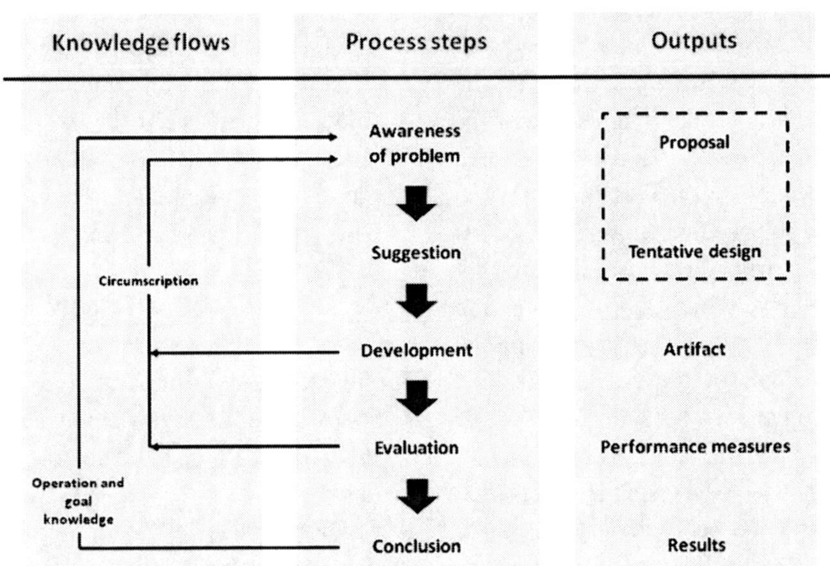

world, user control and freedom, consistency and standards, error prevention, recognition rather than recall, flexibility and efficiency of use, aesthetic and minimalist design, help users recognize, diagnose, and recover from errors, help and documentation. The results of the heuristic evaluations have been published and discussed in (Barricelli et al., 2013; Devis, 2013). From the heuristic evaluation and the study of the requirements and the context we were able to go on with the project and start the following phase.

3.2.2. Suggestion

Once informed by the preliminary research and study done in the Awareness of problem phase, at this stage the research team is expected to draft some possible intervention proposals and to explore their feasibility. According to this, we created some paper prototypes of the two applications we wanted to prototype (one for the rural doctors and one for the doctors working in the hospitals). We also recorded some videos of use of the paper prototypes and used them to discuss with healthcare professionals in order to validate the scenario and user requirements and to understand how to proceed with the Development phase.

3.2.3. Development

At this stage, the outcomes of the previous two phases are used to develop one of the solutions proposed. To this aim, in the MANTRA Project, we implemented two high-fidelity prototypes. Such kind of prototypes are quite close to the final product, with many details that aim at reproducing the actual aspect of a final version of the product and that also offer some most-fully working functions.

The prototypes were built according to the requirements that emerged in the initial phase of the project and were designed and realized keeping in mind the two Personas. Their final aspect reflected the one of the paper prototypes in terms of functions and interfaces organisations but their look and feel was perfectly consistent with iOS guidelines (for iPad). The details of the development are presented and discussed in Section 4.

3.2.4. Evaluation and Conclusion

These two last phases are devoted to gather, analyse and discuss the results of evaluations of the outcomes of the Development phase, but more in general of the overall project flow.

The evaluation of the two high-fidelity prototypes of the MANTRA Project, we were able to involve four doctors in Venezuela (two rural doctors and two hospital doctors). The user tests were performed on remote setting and not onsite. The details of the evaluation method used, the participants and the analysis and discussion of results are given in Section 5.

4. PROTOTYPES DESIGN AND DEVELOPMENT

Our research background is framed in a socio-technical design domain, which means evaluating technical and interface design decisions in terms of the social context of use and associated practices and values. We started with the design of scenarios, use cases, Personas and proceeded with storyboards and paper prototypes and successively high-fidelity prototypes design and development.

4.1. Personas

One of the most used tools in Interaction Design to provide an understanding of the potential audience that a product could have is Persona. Promoted by Alan Cooper (1999) and successively widely promoted by both researchers and practitioners, Personas are used to inspire the designers and developers through the entire production process, from initial specifications to deployment. A Persona is a description of a fictional user for each user group identified during the initial requirements analysis.

Through literature review and state of the art analysis and informal semi-structured interviews with doctors and other healthcare practitioners living in Venezuela, we identified two Personas that represent the potential final users, one for a doctor who works in rural areas (Gaby) and the other for a doctor who works in hospital (Caroline). The description of these 2 Personas can be seen below.

Gaby is 26 years old and works as General Doctor in Maniapure village. Gaby knows very well how to use a tablet and her smartphone, because she uses them regularly to browse the Internet, to read eBooks and uses apps related with her profession. Gaby has several patients that have been diagnosed with Proximal Atrial Fibrillation, and because of the resource-constrained work environment she works in, she has to contact the hospital really often to ensure that the treatment prescribed for her patients is correct. So she has to send emails to the hospital doctor or call her/him, but getting a reply can take quite a long time. Gaby wishes that an easier way will exit to contact the doctor and to not wait so long for an answer, which will benefit the patient's health care.

The second Persona is Caroline who is 45 years old. She has been a Cardiologist for the last 18 years, working in Caracas hospital during this time. Caroline is extremely intelligent; she likes to read about medicine and often attends conferences. Because of her job she has patients in the hospital, but she also has to send her prescriptions to doctors working in rural areas. Unfortunately, she does not have enough time to go through her emails so frequently therefore she does not reply promptly. Caroline is used to use her computer to send emails and search in Internet but does not know how to do these tasks with her smartphone. She does not have a tablet but she is more than willing to learn how to use one. She would like there was an easier way to send prescriptions, and to do it from anywhere.

4.2. Paper Prototypes

Paperboard prototypes (McConnell, 1998) are an approach useful for developing early understanding of the user interface requirements. In this approach the developers or the end users can start by developing pictures of the screens, dialogs, toolbars and other elements they would like the user interface to have.

Sefelin et al. (2003) and Virzi et al. (1996) studies showed that paper- and computer-based (low-fidelity and high-fidelity) prototypes lead to almost the same quantity and quality of critical user statements but subjects prefer computer prototypes. Since the comfort of the participants is one of the major factors of a successful usability test, one may argue that these two results mean that a design team should always prefer a computer-based prototype. However, paperboard prototypes also eliminate some of the most common risks associated with prototyping: on the developer side, they eliminate the need of unnecessarily overextending the prototype and of spending too much time fiddling with the prototype tool. On the user side the paperboard prototypes eliminate the risk of the users thinking that the prototype is the finished product.

Nevertheless, one weakness of the paperboard prototype is the risk that some developers and users simply can't picture the software on the paper

mockups, and since the essence of the prototypes is to help users visualize the final product this is a heavy disadvantage. However, since we developed this project in a remote setting because we could not personally visit Venezuela to perform the evaluations, paper prototypes happened to be the right tool to be used.

We developed two vertical paper prototypes, one for the rural doctor and one for the hospital doctor. Figure 2 shows the screen that presents the clinical records about a specific patient (on the left) and the screen for recording the INR value for that patient (on the right) for the rural doctor.

In Figure 3 other two screens of the paper prototype for the hospital doctor are presented: On the left side, the page that allows the doctor to register a prescription for a specific patient; on the right side, the chart that shows the INR test results registered over time.

We recorded videos of the interaction with the paper prototypes and we showed them to healthcare practitioners, both in the UK and in Venezuela to evaluate them. The feedbacks we collected were used to improve the design of the

Figure 2. The screens of the paper prototype for the rural doctor that enable to browse patients' clinical records (on the left side) and to register the INR value for them (on the right side)

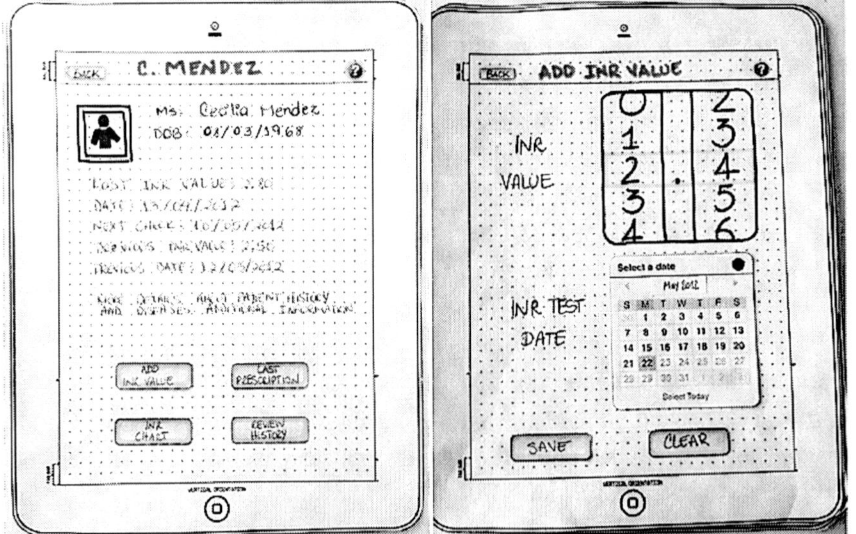

Figure 3. The two screens of the paper prototype for the hospital doctors devoted to prescription registration and INR chart visualization

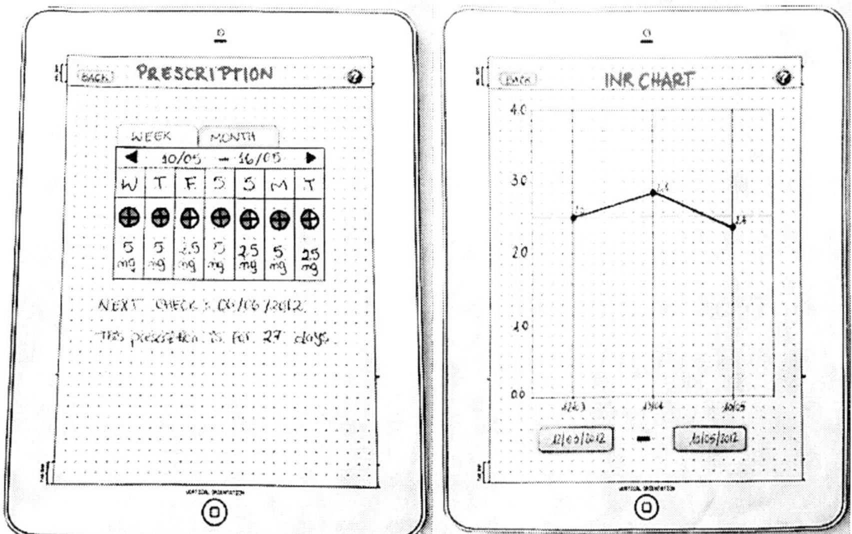

prototypes that have been then translated into interactive high-fidelity prototypes as described in the next section.

4.3. High-Fidelity Prototypes

Capitalizing on the outcomes of the design and informal evaluation of the paper prototypes, we developed two high-fidelity prototypes, one for rural doctors and one for hospital doctors.

We developed the prototypes of the apps for iPad with iOS 5.0+ operating system using Objective-C language in XCode IDE v4.6 and including the CorePlot plotting framework.

With their dedicated app (Figure 4) the rural doctors are able to record the INR test results for their patients, send them to the hospital doctors (immediately or when the Internet connection is available), receive the prescriptions, browse patients' INR values history and access a list of food with relative vitamin K content to be used for suggesting a correct diet to the patients. Hospital doctors can use their dedicated app to receive the INR test results from rural doctors, patients' INR

values history, and create and send the prescriptions to the rural doctors (Figure 5).

Given the differences between the ways anticoagulant therapy is managed in UK and Venezuela, we had to study the specific Venezuelan cultural settings and its influences in the development of the prototypes. For instance, we had to consider language localization issues that went beyond the mere language translation of the interface text. Among all the issues we want to cite two in particular: 1) We had to localize the colours used for the application and had to avoid the overuse the colour red because it is associated with the government's political party, even if it is common to see it for error feedbacks; 2) in Venezuela warfarin is distributed in tablets that have to be cut into parts to obtain different dosages of the medicine. Therefore, the prescription has to be visually represented like a full pill or a half pill depending on the milligrams prescribed (See Figure 5, Left). This constituted a big difference from the UK where warfarin is sold in tablets with different colours depending on the dosages. Another aspect, not directly related with cultural

Figure 4. Two screens of the high-fidelity prototype for the rural doctor

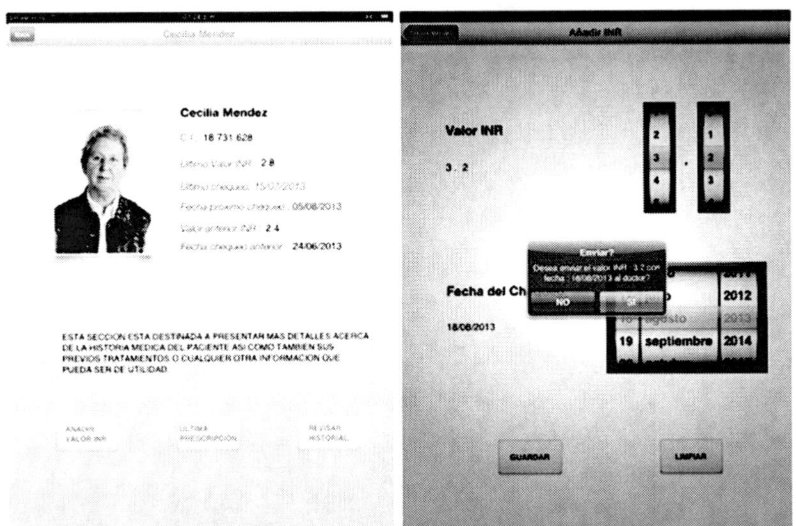

Figure 5. Two screens of the high-fidelity prototype for the hospital doctor

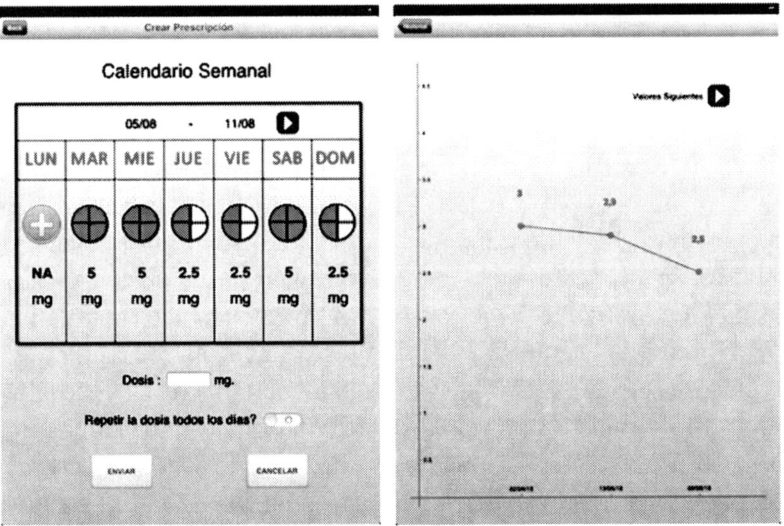

roots, that we had to consider was the development of features that allow doctors to access previous tests results visually represented in different ways, both as lists or charts. Because of the wide age range of the doctors and their variable ability in using touch devices, we took these aspects into account in designing the interfaces to make them accessible and usable.

5. USABILITY EVALUATION

Given the current critical situation in Venezuela and the fact that the rural areas are quite difficult to reach, we carried out the evaluation of the project remotely and asynchronously. We involved 4 doctors in the evaluation: two rural doctors currently working in the rural areas of Wonken and

Maniapure and two doctors working in a Caracas hospital. For the evaluations the doctors used their own iPads on which the prototypes have been previously installed by them following precise instructions.

We used a hybrid evaluation approach: A task-based cognitive walkthrough with the involvement of end users (the doctors) and no observers present during the interaction. We provided the participants with forms to answer post-task questions after the execution of each of the tasks.

A demographic pre-test questionnaire and a post-test CSUQ questionnaire (Lewis, 1993) were submitted to the participants. The pre-test was designed to collect information about the doctor, her/his expertise and knowledge of the domain and her/his expertise in using mobile technology. The CSUQ post-test questionnaire included items with 5-point Likert scale from "Strongly agree" (for 0) to "Strongly disagree" (for 1). We analysed the answers using the 4 factors defined by Lewis (1993): "Overall Evaluation" (Overall), "System Usefulness" (SysUse), "Information Quality" (InfoQual), and "Interface Quality" (IntQual). Overall is measured on items 1-10, SysUse on items 1-4, InfoQual on items 5-7 and IntQual on items 8-9.

The tasks in the walkthrough were different for the two prototypes. The details of the evaluation's results are presented in what follows.

5.1. Results: Rural Doctors

Two rural doctors between 25 and 35 years old, with 2 years of experience in rural areas and with an advanced level of competency in using touch devices were involved.

The rural evaluation consisted of 5 mandatory tasks/activities and 1 optional:

1. Go to the patient details.
2. Review the medical record of 3 previous INR values from one patient.
3. Save and send to the hospital doctor in Caracas the new INR value of one patient.
4. Check if you receive any notification, if yes then review the prescription.
5. Send all patients' INR values to Caracas.
6. Search food in the vitamin k list (optional)

Each activity had a maximum of two sub-tasks that helped to achieve the goal of the main activity. For each sub-task we asked between three and four questions. The estimated time of the assessment was 60 minutes.

After the questionnaire were collected the analysis of the results showed that the task with the highest number of usability principle broken was Review Prescription. Both doctors agreed that more information about the prescription should be displayed in this view; this information from patients in anticoagulant therapy will speed up the work. A similar issue was found when the rural doctors access to the patient's details, where they agreed that the information was well organized and simple to read, but they will include more personal facts from the patient, i.e. age or any specific note about the diagnosis of the patients to facilitate the process. Another issue was that one of the users couldn't recognize the meaning of the yellow icon in the Vitamin K Food List which whether is not represent a huge problem, it is something to think about. Moreover, one of the participants was concerned about the fact that once he sent the INR value he could not edit that value and send it again, however this user recognized that the app gave her enough warning beforehand to send any value to the doctor.

The results we collected through the post-test CSUQ questionnaire are presented in Table 1.

The results for the CSUQ questionnaire were quite good. Overall had 0.175, SysUse 0.125, InfoQual 0.21 and IntQual 0.18. The highest result was InfoQual because the users expressed the need to see more of the patient's data in the Patient Detail and Last Prescription screens.

Table 1. Level of satisfaction per item evaluated – Rural scenario

Questions	Score average
Overall, I am satisfied with how easy it is to use this system	0.125
I can effectively complete the tasks using this application	0.125
I feel comfortable using this application	0.25
It was easy to learn to use this application	0
Whenever I make a mistake using the application, I recover easily and quickly	0
The application gives error messages that clearly tell me how to fix problems	0.375
The organization of information on the application screens is clear	0.25
The interface of this application is pleasant	0
This application has all the functions and capabilities I expect it to have	0.375
Overall, I am satisfied with this application	0.25

5.2. Results: Hospital Doctors

The two hospital doctors involved were between 35-45 years old with 10-15 years of experience in the medical practice and their competency of touch devices use was self-reported as medium. For the hospital evaluation there are 3 mandatory tasks and 1 optional:

1. Go to the patient details.
2. Review the medical record of 3 previous INR values from one patient.
3. Check the last prescription registered and create and send the new prescription
4. Search food in the vitamin k list (optional)

Each activity has no more than two sub-tasks. Like before for each sub-task we asked between three and four questions, and 40 minutes was the time estimated to do the hospital evaluation.

From the results analyzed we concluded that both participants found issues creating the prescription, it took one to press the button 3 times to understand the right way to put a dosage in the prescription, and for the other user, she never saw the "repeat all week" switch so she manually complete the prescription for each day of the week. On the other hand, both users agreed that the application should give a warning before to delete a patient, to avoid possible mistakes. This finding didn't happen but the users commented that they need a double confirmation before to delete something.

For this part of the evaluation, neither of the users got any problem to complete the tasks and the usability issues found have a low severity, which generated a sense of security and satisfaction in the participants of this evaluation. All the participants found the organization of the elements in the screens satisfactory and also the clarity with which the information in the application is presented.

As to the CSUQ questionnaire, the average score is presented in Table 2.

In this case, we had Overall 0.26, SysUse 0.28, InfoQual 0.21 and IntQual 0.37. This time the satisfaction level was not high as the one of the rural doctors but this was not a surprise since the users pointed out several problems in the creation of a prescription. However, the users found the organization and clarity of the information presentation very clear and this explains the InfoQual low average score.

6. CONCLUSION

The results of the evaluations (both the walk-throughs and the final questionnaires) showed that all the participants positively evaluated the INR test-related features (recording, sending and reviewing INR values, and browsing history charts and lists). On the other hand, it emerged that important usability problems affected the prescription features (creation and review): all the doctors stated that the visualization of more information about the clinical history of the patients would help their practice, like other previous or current

Table 2. Level of satisfaction per item evaluated – Hospital scenario

Questions	% of satisfaction (scale from 0 to 1)
Overall, I am satisfied with how easy it is to use this system	0.125
I can effectively complete the tasks using this application	0.5
I feel comfortable using this application	0.5
It was easy to learn to use this application	0
Whenever I make a mistake using the application, I recover easily and quickly	0
The application gives error messages that clearly tell me how to fix problems	0.625
The organization of information on the application screens is clear	0
The interface of this application is pleasant	0.25
This application has all the functions and capabilities I expect it to have	0.5
Overall, I am satisfied with this application	0.125

diseases, other medicines that the patient is taking, and the date the anticoagulant therapy started.

As pointed out earlier in this paper, the objective of this research was to investigate the acceptability and feasibility of the introduction of mobile technology in the management of anticoagulant therapy. The feasibility of the MANTRA approach is proved by the design and development of the two prototypes, while the acceptability is positively proved by the evaluation's results. We collected many quotes from the participants who showed to like the aim of the research. Particularly the use of colours ("I like the use of colours"), the interface and the interaction style ("I also like the format."; "I like the fact that it is ease of use, and the use of images.") have been appreciated, together with the main goal of the applications ("Is easy to use, is a good idea").

The contribution of this research work, with respect to the literature review presented in Section 2, is the design and development of a mHealth solution for remote communication between healthcare practitioners in countries where rural areas are difficult to be reached and distances make quite impossible for them to move from place to place in reasonable time. We applied a research approach that merges social and technical requirements to address the end users' needs, to fit their cultural traits and to meet their expectations. Our proposed intervention is aimed at supporting the current practice of anticoagulant therapy making it more easily managed and integrating new mobile technologies without affecting the way of life of the patients. We tried to address the problems widely documented in literature for previous mHealth projects and we obtained positive results from the evaluation of our work.

The outcomes of the project, in terms of research context analysis, design and creation of the paper and interactive prototypes and evaluation method, could be used as general tools for other mHealth applications aimed at helping the remote management of chronic diseases especially where there is the need of supporting the communication between doctors who work in distant places.

The introduction of the MANTRA applications for the management of anticoagulant therapy in resource-constrained environments and the improvement in the communication between rural doctor and hospital doctor may lead to great advances in patients' health care and quality of life. What today is a complex medical treatment for rural areas that are currently affected by serious limitations in terms of infrastructures and funding may evolve into a more bearable and less costly one in terms of resources and time.

At this stage the MANTRA Project contributed with a proof of concept, given the fact that it has shown positive findings so far, and the users are willing to add to their practices, therefore further research is expected to take place. We will focus on the development of the final mobile applications by improving the high-fidelity prototypes using the results we obtained by the usability evaluations. These applications will be evaluated involving a larger group of doctors and expanded to other rural locations. We plan to perform the same evaluations described before directly in situ having the chance to observe the doctors in their daily medical practice.

ACKNOWLEDGMENT

The work of Barbara Rita Barricelli was supported by the Visiting Fellowship at University of West London funded by The Leverhulme Trust (UK). The authors wish to thank all the healthcare professionals who took part in this research and contributed with their expertise, wisdom and precious time.

REFERENCES

Abdelnour-Nocera, J. (2007). *The social construct of usefulness: An intercultural study of producers and users of a business information system.* Berlin, Germany: VDM Verlag.

Barricelli, B. R. (2011). *An architecture for end-user development supporting global communities.* PhD thesis. Università degli Studi di Milano, Italy.

Barricelli, B. R., Devis, Y., Abdelnour-Nocera, J., Wilson, J., & Moore, J. (2013). MANTRA: Mobile anticoagulant therapy management. In Proc. PervasiveHealth 2013 (pp. 278-281), IEEE.

Bijker, W. E. (1995a). *Of bicycles, bakelites, and bulbs: Toward a theory of sociotechnical change.* Cambridge, MA: MIT Press.

Bussey, H. I., Chiquette, E., Bianco, T. M., Lowder-Bender, K., Kraynak, M. A., & Linn, W. D. et al. (1997). A statistical and clinical evaluation of fingerstick and routine laboratory prothrombin time measurements. *Pharmacotherapy, 17*(5), 861–866. PMID:9324174

Callon, M. (1986). *Mapping the dynamics of science and technology: Sociology of science in the real world.* New York, NY: Sheridan House.

Christensen, H., Lauterlein, J. J., Sørensen, P. D., Petersen, E. R. B., Madsen, J. S., & Brandslund, I. (2011). Home management of oral anticoagulation via telemedicine versus conventional hospital based treatment. *Telemedicine and eHealth, 17*(3), 169-176.

Cipresso, P., Serino, S., Villani, D., Repetto, C., Selitti, L., & Albani, G. et al. (2012). Is your phone so smart to affect your states? An exploratory study based on psychophysiological measures. *Neurocomputing, 84,* 23–30. doi:10.1016/j.neucom.2011.12.027

Cohen, A. T., Agnelli, G., Anderson, F. A., Arcelus, J. I., Bergqvist, D., & Brecht, J. G. et al. (2007). Venous thromboembolism (VTE) in Europe - The number of VTE events and associated morbidity and mortality. *Thrombosis and Haemostasis, 98,* 756–764. PMID:17938798

Cooper, A. (1999). *The inmates are running the asylum.* Indianapolis, IN: SAMS Publishing.

Cromheecke, M. E., Levi, M., Colly, L. P., de Mol, B. J.-M., Prins, M. H., & Hutten, B. A. et al. (2000). Oral anticoagulation self-management and management by a specialist anticoagulation clinic: A randomised cross-over comparison. *Lancet, 356*(9224), 97–102. doi:10.1016/S0140-6736(00)02470-3 PMID:10963245

De Angeli, A., Athavankar, U., Joshi, A., Coventry, L., & Johson, G. I. (2004). Introducing ATMs in India: A contextual inquiry. *Interacting with Computers, 16*(1), 29–44. doi:10.1016/j.intcom.2003.11.003

Devis, Y. (2013). *Mobile health interface design and development for a rural environment (MANTRA Project).* M.Sc. Thesis. University of West London, UK.

Dorfman, D. M., Goonan, E. M., Boutilier, M. K., Jarolim, P., Tanasijevica, M., & Goldhaber, S. Z. (2005). Point-of-care (POC) versus central laboratory instrumentation for monitoring oral anticoagulation. *Vascular Medicine, 10*(1), 23–27. doi:10.1191/1358863x05vm587oa PMID:15920996

Duncan, A. S., & Beabes, M. A. (1995). *Contextual inquiry: Grounding your design in user's work. Conference companion on Human factors in computing systems.* Denver, CO: ACM Press. doi:10.1145/223355.223721

Ehn, P. (1990). *Work-oriented design of computer artifacts.* L. Erlbaum Associates Inc.

Gardiner, C., Williams, K., Mackie, I. J., Machin, S. J., & Cohen, H. (2005). Patient self-testing is a reliable and acceptable alternative to laboratory INR monitoring. *British Journal of Haematology, 128*(2), 242–247. doi:10.1111/j.1365-2141.2004.05300.x PMID:15638860

Germanakos, P., Mourlas, C., & Samaras, G. (2005). A mobile agent approach for ubiquitous and personalized eHealth information systems. In *Proc. Workshop on 'Personalization for e-Health' of the 10th International Conference on User Modeling* (pp. 67–70), Edinburgh, UK.

Hansen, T. R. (2006). Strings of experiments: Looking at the design process as a set of sociotechnical experiments. In *Proc. PDC '06 (pp. 1-10).* ACM. doi:10.1145/1147261.1147263

Kampuri, M., Bednarik, R., & Tukiainen, M. (2006). The expanding focus of HCI: Case culture. In *Proc. NordiCHI 2006: Changing Roles.* Oslo, Norway: ACM Press. doi:10.1145/1182475.1182523

Kapange, B. (2006). *ICTs in agricultural development: The case of Tanzania.* IST-Africa.

Kleimann, S. (1996). Response to "using contextual inquiry". *SIGDOC Asterisk J. Comput. Doc., 20*(1), 22–24. doi:10.1145/227614.228150

Kolko, E. B., Rose, J. E., & Johson, E. (2007). Communication as information-seeking: The case for mobile social software for developing regions. In *Proc. International World Wide Conference 2007: Technology for Developing Regions.* Alberta, Canada: ACM Press. doi:10.1145/1242572.1242689

Latour, B. (1993). *We have never been modern.* Cambridge, MA: Harvard University Press.

Law, J., & Hassard, J. (1999). *Actor network theory and after.* Oxford, UK: Blackwell.

Lewis, J. (1993). *IBM computer usability satisfaction questionnaires: Psychometric evaluation and instructions for use.* Retrieved March 14, 2014, from http://drjim.0catch.com/usabqtr.pdf

Lin, A., & Silva, L. (2005). The social and political construction of technological frames. *European Journal of Information Systems, 14*(1), 49–59. doi:10.1057/palgrave.ejis.3000521

Manhattan Research. (2012). *Taking the pulse U.S.* Retrieved March 14, 2014, from http://manhattanresearch.com/Products-and-Services/Physician/Taking-the-Pulse-U-S

Mbarika, V. W. A. (2004). On site: Is telemedicine the panacea for Sub-Saharan Africa's medical nightmare? *Communications of the ACM, 47*(7), 21–24. doi:10.1145/1005817.1005838

McConnell, S. (1998). *Software project survival guide.* Microsoft Press.

McKinsey & Company. (2007). *The 'bird of gold': The rise of India's consumer market.* McKinsey Global Institute.

Nielsen, J., & Molich, R. (1990). Heuristic evaluation of user interfaces. In *Proc. CHI 1990* (pp. 249-256). New York, NY: ACM Press.

Oostveen, A. (2004) From small scale to large scale user participation. In *Proc. Participatory Design Conference* (pp. 173–182). Toronto, Canada: ACM Press. doi:10.1145/1011870.1011891

Salvador, C. H., Ruiz Sanchez, A., de Mingo, M. A. G., & Rodriguez, M. (2008). Evaluation of a telemedicine based service for the FollowUp and monitoring of patients treated with oral anticoagulant therapy. *Trans. Info. Tech. Biomed.*, *12*(6), 696–706. doi:10.1109/TITB.2008.910750 PMID:19000948

Schneeweiss, S., Gagne, J. J., Patrick, A. R., Choudhry, N. K., & Avorn, J. (2012). Comparative efficacy and safety of new oral anticoagulants in patients with atrial fibrillation. *Circulation: Cardiovascular Quality and Outcomes*, *5*(4), 480–486. doi:10.1161/CIRCOUTCOMES.112.965988 PMID:22787066

Sefelin, R., Tscheligi, M., & Giller, V. (2003). Paper prototyping - what is it good for?: a comparison of paper- and computer-based low-fidelity prototyping. In *Proc. CHI '03 Extended Abstracts on Human Factors in Computing Systems* (pp. 778–779). New York, NY: ACM Press. doi:10.1145/765891.765986

Telesalud. (2013). Retrieved March 14, 2014, from http://www.tele-salud.com/en/node/72

Thinyane, M., Dalvit, L., Slay, H., Mapi, T., Terzoli, A., & Clayton, P. (2007). An ontology-based, multi-modal platform for the inclusion of marginalized rural communities into the knowledge society. In *Proc. of the 2007 Annual Research Conference of the South African institute of Computer Scientists and Information Technologists on IT Research in Developing Countries*. Port Elizabeth, South Africa: ACM Press. doi:10.1145/1292491.1292508

Tripodi, A. (2004). Prothrombin time international normalized ratio monitoring by self-testing. *Current Opinion in Hematology*, *11*(3), 141–145. doi:10.1097/01.moh.0000130311.10539.b5 PMID:15257011

Vaishnavi, V. K., & Kuechler, W. L. (2008). *Design science research methods and patterns: Improving and innovating information and communication technology*. New York, NY: Auerbach Publications, Taylor & Francis Group.

Virzi, R. A., Sokolov, J. L., & Karis, D. (1996). Usability problem identification using both low- and high-fidelity prototypes. In *Proc. of the SIGCHI Conference on Human Factors in Computing Systems (CHI '96)* (pp. 236–243). New York, NY: ACM Press. doi:10.1145/238386.238516

Vital Wave Consulting. (2009). mHealth for development: The opportunity of mobile technology for healthcare in the developing world. United Nations Foundation, Vodafone Foundation (pp. 9).

This work was previously published in the International Journal of Sociotechnology and Knowledge Development (IJSKD), 6(1); edited by Constance Kampf and José Abdelnour-Nocera, pages 18-35 copyright year 2014 by IGI Publishing (an imprint of IGI Global).

Chapter 32

Integrating Social and Health Services in Greece:
Implementation of Three Pilot CIP–PSP–ICT Programs (ISISEMD, INDEPENDENT, RENEWING HEALTH)

George E. Dafoulas
Independent Researcher, Greece

Lamprini Ch. Oikonomou
Independent Researcher, Greece

Christina N. Karaberi
Independent Researcher, Greece

Kalliopi P. Liatou
Independent Researcher, Greece

ABSTRACT

The integration of e-health services in the Greek Healthcare System is expected to be a challenging task. To this end, three EU co-funded projects (ISISEMD, INDEPENDENT, and RENEWING HEALTH) are tested under realistic conditions integrating e-health and e-care services to the existing health services offered to people that suffer from chronic diseases as well as to their formal and informal caregivers. This chapter aims to give an analytic report of those three European programs in terms of service description, implementation, evaluation, and exploitation. The authors introduce the main characteristics of the Greek healthcare system and the risks that it faces in regards to the major reformation and cut offs due to the economic recession. Then they explain how those risks could become opportunities to promote integrated services.

INTRODUCTION

Short Description of ESY (Greek National Healthcare System)

According to the OECD classification (OECD 1992), the Greek Healthcare System is a mixture of the public integrated, public contract and public reimbursement systems, incorporating principles of different organizational patterns. In relation to the public sector, elements of the Bismarck and the Beveridge model co-exist (Economou, 2010).

Before the establishment of ESY (National Health System) in 1983 the provision of health care in Greece followed the Bismarck model of compulsory social health insurance. Nowadays,

DOI: 10.4018/978-1-4666-8756-1.ch032

health insurance funds continue to play a significant role in the provision and financing of healthcare, especially in ambulatory services and follow two patterns (Economou, 2010, p.16).

The first includes funds that have their own medical facilities and cover primary healthcare needs. The second pattern of provision concerns funds that do not own any medical facilities directly but enter into contracts with medical practitioners who are compensated via a defined fee-for-service on a retrospective basis. The level of compensation is subject to approval by the Ministries of Health and Social Solidarity, of Finance and Economics and of Employment of Social Protection (Economou, 2010).

The social insurance system in Greece comprises a large number of funds and a wide variety of schemes under the jurisdiction of the Ministry of Employment and social Protection. There are approximately 30 different health insurance organizations which provide coverage against the risk of illness. Most of them are administrated as public entities and operate under state control and legislation. However, in many cases there are differences in contribution rates, coverage, benefits and the conditions for granting these benefits resulting in inequalities in access to and financing of services (Economou, 2010).

The unstable and many times unfavorable political, financial and social conditions that took place in Greece during the 20th century had a bad influence and eventually slowed down the development of the Greek national health care system (Theodorou and Mitrosilli, 1999, p.32).

Although nowadays the Greek Public Sector has made a substantial progress, there are still many organizational, management, efficiency and effectiveness problems to be addressed (Theodorou and Mitrosilli, 1999, p.32).

When trying to describe the Greek National Healthcare System, one can focus on a number of characteristics, peculiarities and problems (Theodorou and Mitrosilli, 1999, p.45-52):

- Mixed system of public character with many peculiarities.
- Different subsystems: a fragmented health sector.
- Overlaps and inequalities in healthcare.
- Weak and inadequate public health and primary care.
- Incomplete building and technological infrastructure (although the situation has improved significantly the last years).
- Multitude of physicians and nursing staff shortages.
- Low productivity, uneconomic function, lack of motivation.
- Lack of reliable funding mechanisms and large black economy.
- Centralization and bureaucracy.
- Lack of involvement of the patient in the planning and implementation of health policy.
- Low system reliability and poor user satisfaction.

During the last years there have been many reformation approaches so as to address those weaknesses and improve resource efficiency and quality of health service.

Those weaknesses are the main focus of ICT programs implemented in Greece. To be precise, social and health services fragmentation, incomplete technological infrastructure, low productivity and bureaucracy that lead to the users lack of involvement and low satisfaction level can be handled sufficiently via services like the electronic health record, nurse monitoring systems, tele-monitoring of implantable cardiac, diabetes health motivation systems, home hospitalization programs etc. that are implemented and tested under realistic conditions in ICT programs like those described in this chapter.

Table 1. "Health care reform laws 2001-2007" (Economou, 2010, p.136)

Law	Content	Implementation Status
2889/2001	Decentralization of the health care system and the introduction of autonomous hospital management	Implemented (but hospital reforms later reversed)
2920/2001	Creation of SEYYP (Body of Inspectors for Health and Welfare Services)	Implemented
2955/2001	Creation of a new legislative framework for hospital procurements	Partial Implemented
3029/2002	Reform of the social security system.	Implemented
3106/2003	Reorganization of welfare services with decentralization and better management	Implemented
3172/2003	Reorganization and modernization of services relating to public health	Not implemented
3235/2004	Changes to primary health care services, (family doctor, polyclinics, home care post hospital care, rehabilitation)	Not implemented
3329/2005	Changes to the regional administration of the ESY and to hospital management,	Implemented
3370/2005	Reorganization of public health services: establishment at the Ministry of Health and Social Solidarity	Implemented
3457/2006	Reform of pharmaceutical care, abolishing the positive list and introducing recovery prices	Implemented
3580/2007	Centralization of procurement procedures for public hospitals	In process of implementation

BACKGROUND

The last decade the Greek health care system was put at the centre of political debate and a number of reforms were introduced. Those initiatives can be categorized into two reform processes: the first reform includes legislations passed during 2001-04 and the second during 2005-06. However, as one can see in table.1 many of those changes were contradictory and many times not fully implemented (Economou, 2010, p.136-137).

In 2000 the Minister for Health put forward a plan of 200 measures and initiated a public discussion on reforms. These interventions included: the decentralization and development of regional health structures, the establishment of new managerial structures within public hospitals, the modification of terms of employment for ESY doctors, the merging and coordination of health care funding agencies, the development of public health services, the reorganization of primary health care and the development of structures for the accreditation of services and quality assurance (Economou, 2010, p.137-138).

The first strand of reforms adopted, starting with Law 2889/2001 on the improvement and modernization of the ESY, provided the establishment of regional health authorities, new management structures and prospective reimbursement for public hospitals, (private) afternoon hospital services in public facilities and new employment relations for public hospital doctors. Later, Law 3106/2003 on the reorganization of welfare services decentralized all social care responsibilities to the PeSYs, and renamed them to regional health and welfare authorities (PeSYPs) (Economou, 2010, p.137).

The Stability and Growth Programme 2004–2007 concerning health reformation submitted to the European Commission emphasized to securing the system's financial viability in the short term and its sustainability in the long run. The reform effort attempted to address three issues (Economou, 2010, p140-141):

- The accumulation of debt by hospital suppliers via the establishment of a centralized administrative system for public procurement procedures, a new management system for public hospitals based on operational devolution to the local hospital level and a new computerized accounting system for all ESY hospitals and health centers.
- Cost-containment via the use of information technologies (IT) and enterprise resource planning systems throughout the ESY, the application of modern management methods in ESY hospitals, the introduction of new pricing and costing mechanisms and the establishment of auditing procedures.
- PPPs (Public–private partnerships) for the construction of public hospitals so as to ease the financial burden on the public investment budget (Economou, 2010, p140-141).

However, only a small part of these measures actually materialized and the initiatives undertaken during the period 2005–2008 were rather controversial. Moreover, cost-containment policies, new pricing and costing mechanisms, auditing procedures and the introduction of computerized accounting systems were totally neglected (Economou, 2010, p.140-141).

The most recent reformation (law: 3918/2011) was the coordination of health care funding agencies and the creation of a single financial institution, which acts as a unified health insurance fund. It was envisaged that the new ODIPY (Organization for the Management of Health Care Financial Resources) would manage the revenues of the biggest social insurance organizations, which cover more than 95% of the Greek population (IKA, OGA, OAEE, OPAD), and optionally of other smaller funds. The unification of financing would be combined with the formulation of a basic package of benefits common to all insurance funds and resource allocation according to demographic criteria (Economou, 2010, p.137-138).

CURRENT STATUS

The international experience of implementing health care reforms suggests that a big-bang approach based on the top-down imposition of a grand plan is not the most appropriate way to introduce change (Figueras, Saltman & Mossialos, 1997).

What is more, given the problems of the Greek health care sector, it will be necessary to adopt an incremental approach to future reform, focusing on certain areas of high priority: (a) restructuring of primary health care; (b) pooling of financial resources; (c) changing the payment system of providers; (d) introducing new managerial and administrative methods;(e) adopting cost–effectiveness and monitoring mechanisms; and (f) developing policies for better allocation of resources (Economou, 2010, p.144-145).

The issues raised in primary health care are not new and several reform plans have been proposed (Souliotis & Lionis, 2005). The establishment of primary care groups, consisting of GP (General practitioner) and specialist practices could be a viable solution. The primary care groups should assume responsibility for referring patients to hospitals and other health services, and for maintaining medical records. Systematic review and improvement of the quality and outcomes of primary care groups should be achieved by the introduction of clinical protocols, clinical audit and electronic clinical information systems. Payment by capitation or a combination of capitation and salary instead of fee-for-service could restrict the incentives for physicians to increase health expenditure (Mossialos, Allin and Davaki, 2005).

In addition, rural health centers should be upgraded and used as mechanisms for the enhancement of public health and prevention policies mainly via the establishment of a referral system, the introduction of personal electronic health cards and the adoption of clinical and pharmaceutical protocols (Economou, 2010, p.144-145).

In 2010, Greek economy entered a deep structural and multi-faceted crisis, the main features of which are a large fiscal deficit, huge public debt and a continuous erosion of the country's competitive position. The deficit in 2009 reached 13,6%of GDP (Gross domestic product) and has continued to rise (Economou, 2010, p.16).

Meanwhile many social benefits were dismissed, pensions cut down, whereas the ODIPY reformation made the access to medical care difficult and expensive by increasing the contribution rate of the insured person both from medical care and medication and by establishing a ceiling number of monthly patients of an ODIPY doctor.

CIP-PSP-ICT programs that test under realistic conditions integrated services like Electronic Health files, tele-counseling and remote doctors control have been proven to increase a patients quality of life, decrease the financial and every day care burden and even delay hospitalization, offering a useful alternative to an already financially overloaded household. Integrated tele-care services seems to be in consent with the Health Systems reformation procedure and offer useful services to a number of people who suffer from chronic diseases and helps promote reforms such as the pharmaceutical protocols and electronic health cards. Isisemd, Independent and Renewing Health are only three examples of the impact of the integration of existing health services to a number of people suffering from chronic diseases.

All three programs co-operated with existing public health and social organizations like Open Day Care Centre (KAPI) (a public organizations that offers mostly social and partially health services to the elderly), Help at Home (a public organization that offers social services to chronic patients that are unable to leave home), Trikala's

Public Benefit Municipal Enterprise for Social Development (DEKA) (a public organization that is responsible for the implementation of many social care programs in the region) and lastly the Regional Public Hospital.

MAIN FOCUS

ISISEMD

Background Information

The increasing incidence and prevalence of dementia with the ageing of the Greek population, makes it necessary to offer continuity of care, by linking the formal and informal care sectors in a holistic approach to the management of dementia patients and their families and to bridge the gap between medical practice and the complex and multi-sectorial problems of everyday care of patients. Telecare services attempt to compensate for the gaps in the primary care sector in Greece through facilitating and creating the necessary links and pathways for patients throughout the health care system by developing new support services, addressing the needs of both patients and their informal family carers. There is no approved national dementia strategy in Greece. Furthermore, the impact of the current financial crisis is likely to be seen in increasing numbers of patients and their families unable to pay for private care at home or in Residential Care Units, with a higher burden on informal carers reflected in more dementia patients "abandoned" and dependent on inadequate public Long Term Care services. At the same time, the social and family structure in Greece is undergoing a substantial and irreversible change. Family size is shrinking, very often the elderly live at home alone or in groups consisting of only elderly people. In addition, women's role within the family is changing: now the vast majority of women have a job outside the home, so there is less internal domestic support provided to the family by women, who were traditionally the family caregivers entrusted with the task of providing informal care to frail or elderly family members. The exponential growth in demand for both social and healthcare services makes it increasingly clear that different approaches are required to secure the economic sustainability of the whole health and welfare system.

Project Description

ISISEMD (intelligent system for independent living and self-care of seniors with cognitive problems or mild dementia) (ISISEMD, 2009-2012) is an ICT Policy Support Programme (ICT-PSP-2008-2 licensed under the Grant agreement No 238914) which has designed, implemented, verified, and assessed an assistive technology platform of personalized home care (telecare) for the elderly with cognitive impairment and their caregivers. To prove wide applicability in Europe, the pilot is validated and tested for a period of 15 months under realistic conditions with a total of 142 test volunteers (71 elderly and 71 informal care-givers) in four countries in Europe – Denmark, Greece, Finland and North Ireland.

This section is devoted to describing important aspects of the controlled study as it was validated and tested in Trikala. These aspects include who the test participants were, inclusion and exclusion criteria, how the test participants were recruited and the services evaluation (ease of use, intelligent functioning, importance for care, etc). Overview of ISISEMD evaluation methodology is also presented in this section together with the results from baseline, intermediate and final evaluation. Trikala is one of the four member state regions in Greece which has extensive experience from existing tele-care-at-home services for elderly. A collaboration of the municipality's care delivery organizations DEKA, KAPI and ASKLIPIOS was made in order to support informal carers and those for whom they care.

Target

The aim of the ISISEMD project was to provide a pilot of innovative ICT services in order to support the independent living of elderly people with cognitive problems or mild dementia and at the same time to support the formal and informal caregivers in their daily interaction with the elderly. More specifically, the aim was to improve the elderly ability for self-care by support for their basic daily activities in way that prevented health risks in their homes. The services also strengthened the daily interaction with their social sphere - partners and relatives, friends and care-givers, giving them the feeling of safety and preventing their social isolation. Their cognitive training and activation was strengthened as well.

Characteristics of the Sample

To work with a representative sample of the primary end-users, the recruitment of ISISEMD trial participants for the pilot services followed strongly defined inclusion and exclusion criteria. The World Health Organization's (2007) International Classification of Diseases (ICD-10) is used to classify dementia type and used in conjunction with the Mini Mental State Examination (MMSE) (M. F. Folstein, 1975) to determine cognitive decline. Montreal Cognitive Assessment (MoCA) (Z. S. Nasreddine et al., 2005) (sensitivity 90%) was also administered by specially trained personnel. The main inclusion criterion for primary users is the stage of disease (level of cognitive decline). The Global Deterioration Scale (GDS) (B. Reisberg et al., 1982) is used as a classification standard. GDS is broken down into 7 different stages. Stages 1-3 are pre-dementia stages and stages 4-7 are dementia stages. People classified as stage 5 or greater are unable to live without assistance. The main inclusion criteria for participants in the controlled study are defined as: elderly over 60 years of age diagnosed with stage two (Age Associated Memory Impairment) to four (Mild Dementia), according to the GDS with corresponding to the Mini Mental State Examination (MMSE) scores of 19–26 and living in their own home. Also, the eligible population of informal caregivers was adults over 18 years, recruited based on their relationship with an elderly test participant.

Shortly speaking, ISISEMD test groups are representatives of:

- **Test Group EP:** Primary end users – elderly people with cognitive problems or mild dementia.
- **Test Group (ICG):** Secondary end users – informal care-givers. This includes closest family members who take care of the senior or in some cases neighbors and friends.
- **Test Group FCG:** Secondary end users – formal care-givers. This test group includes care personnel that has contact with the elderly in one or other way.

The Control Group

The control EP group was as characteristically similar to EP group as possible. They were community dwelling, some living alone, with assessment of their cognitive decline based on MMSE/Moca scores. The control group was also administered all rating instruments as the test group (at baseline and final), except questionnaires for user acceptance and user satisfaction because they were not given any technological intervention.

Number of participants: 10 elderly patients with Mild Cognitive Impairment (MCI) or mild dementia (MD) - 20 per trial site (10 intervention and 10 control) with 5 formal caregivers per site and respective number of informal caregivers. The selection of subjects in the group of EP was random.

Equipment Used

There are two categories of equipment in the ISISEMD system: interactive devices and non-interactive devices. The majority of the devices in the ISISEMD platform is non-interactive and include temperature and flood sensors, smoke alarms, electricity monitors for cooking activity, pressure sensors to determine sleeping patterns, and front and fridge door sensors.

In particular, the devices that the older adult with cognitive impairment operates require minimal interaction or no interaction at all. These include the Carebox (HP Touch Screen computer), Lommy (simple GPS device) with only one button which sends and receives phone calls, and internet connection, which is provided to the end users through the project funds. The interactive devices are those which exchange contents when prompted by the user and are under the user's control. Examples of interactive devices for the informal care givers are: -mobile phone, web portal access on a computer and for the elderly people with cognitive problems: a GPS device and a touch screen.

The computer of the Carebox collects data from the sensors installed in the home and the data is sent over the Internet to the ISISEMD web portal. Following the required ethical, privacy, and security requirements, elderly person designate the caregiver that is allowed access to the web portal, where he or she can view only the information that is related to that elderly person. Depending on the user's preferences, the system can automatically send notifications, alerts, and alarms to informal care givers and formal care givers via SMS text messaging or email. Almost all possible aspects of the services are easy to be personalized, based on the individual, current needs of both elderly person and informal care giver. It also notifies elderly person via the Carebox Touch screen if there is a dangerous situation in the home.

Methodology

The following research hypotheses were defined:

1. If the personalized services offered by the ISISEMD platform are based on each client's specific needs, then the feeling of safety, ability for independent living in their home environment, hobbies, and lifestyle will have a positive impact on quality of life;

2. If the services supporting the informal carers will reduce care-related stress then a positive impact on their quality of life, in particular increased feeling of safety, and reduced rates of stress levels, will occur;

3. If the regional care providers will be able to offer social services to these groups of clients which are currently not included in the traditional care model, then there will be an increase in the access to and quality of social care.

Measures

The MoCA was used in conjunction with the MMSE to determine cognitive status. MoCA is designed to screen for MCI and considers attention, concentration, executive functions, memory, language, visual-constructional skills, conceptual thinking, calculations, and orientation in around 10 minutes. In this case, the MoCA score for inclusion would be less than or equal to 26 following the same cognitive functioning parameters as for the MMSE.

In ISISEMD, user acceptance and satisfaction was evaluated by the end user's assessment of the multiple aspects of the service, such as the extent to which they find the technology easy to use, accurate and functional. To collect data, a triangulation of methods was used, consisting of questionnaires, interviews, and structured observations with the users to determine their acceptance and satisfaction with the ISISEMD services. ISISEMD questionnaires for user ac-

ceptance and satisfaction have been inspired by The Quebec User Evaluation of Satisfaction with Assistive Technology (QUEST 2.0) (L. Demers and C. Vincent, 2001) and ETUQ–Everyday Technology Use Questionnaire (L. Demers et al. 2002)–and were administered to both Elderly and Informal Care givers.

A more recent and advanced assessing tool for measuring Quality of Life (QOL) for Informal Caregivers, specifically designed for carers of patients with cognitive problems, is the Scale of Quality of Life of Caregivers (SQLC) (J. M. Glozman, 1998). This tool was used in the controlled study, covering 3 domains: professional activities, social and leisure activities and responsibilities of caregivers to help patients in everyday living.).

Assessing caregiving stress involves an evaluation of how the caregiver experiences the caregiving task to be, involving objective parameters (e.g., number of tasks, time per task) and caregiving capacity (e.g., amount of available time, proximity to care receiving residence), among others. To measure caregiver stress as well as effects from interventions aimed at reducing it, the Zarit Burden Interview (ZBI) short version (M. Bédard et al., 2001) was used in ISISEMD. Questions are on caregiver's health, psychological wellbeing, finances, social life, relationship between carer and patient, and a lower score indicates lower perceived stress.

Data Collection Methods

Collection of the study data was carried out at three stages–at baseline, at intermediate, and at final stages. The pilot started in May, 2010 and final data collection took place in June, 2011.

The intervention and the control groups of EPs and ICG were administered the same ratings scales and questionnaires except the user satisfaction and acceptance. The rating scales for Senior Quality Lifestyles Corporation (SQLC) and ZBI for ICG were administered at baseline, intermediate and final stage for the intervention group, while for the control group–the same rating scales but only at baseline and final stage.

Dissemination Activities

Trikala region was responsible to disseminate the project locally, regionally, nationally and even internationally. For this reason, lots of interviews were conducted (both live and recorded on TV or radio), articles were posted in newspapers, e-magazines, blogs, fora and news sites, and brochures were printed and circulated to institutions, potential users, Alzheimer clinics. A TV live show took place in February 2011 inside the studios of a local TV channel in Trikala, which broadcasts in the Prefecture of Thessaly in Greece, where project's psychologists presented ISISEMD project and displayed a demo of most of the system's capabilities. Additionally, there was a live TV connection in the home of a test EP and a Greek national wide public TV channel, dedicated part of its live "news-broadcasting" and educational show in order to present ISISEMD services. Finally, another public national wide TV channel visited Trikala's premises in February 2011 and had a reportage about ISISEMD project. The two psychologists from Trikala region who were involved in the ISISEMD project had the opportunity to participate in the 7th Panhellenic Conference on Alzheimer's Disease and Related Disorders, which was held in Thessaloniki – Greece from 16 to 20 of February 2011 (http://www.alzheimer-conference. gr/congress_information.html).

Members from E-Trikala, D.E.K.A., Converge ICT Solutions & Services, Aalborg University, Athen's Company of Alzheimer Disease & Related Disorders and Institute of communication & computer Systems (ICCS) of NTUA, worked for a poster which presented the results of the interim evaluation of the ISISEMD project and received award for the best poster by the award selection committee of the conference. Finally, Trikala region attended as many consortium meetings and workshops was possible, in order to monitor the overall progress and locate any further actions might be needed to take in order to adjust the platform for any upcoming user requirements.

Results

During the whole process of piloting the services in real life, it was observed that even when Elderly Participants and Informal Caregivers were skeptical in the beginning, after giving them time to get used to the technology, the elderly and their relatives accept the technology and can see the opportunities for positive impact.

Comments on the combined scores:

- **Cognition (MoCA and MMSE):** Average duration of cognitive decline stage 4 according to GDS is 2 years and in some cases, the illness may progress fast (Reisberg et al., 1982) During the 12 month testing period there was no significant cognitive decline for both the test and the control group. However there was no positive impact to the test person's cognitive state either.
- **Functioning (ADL and IADL):** Both scales measure the elderly level of independency on everyday skills and functions like bathing, shopping, using the phone, taking medicines etc. According to combined scores as they are presented in the above table, Trikala (4,00-4,30) show positive results after the 12 month testing period meaning that the ISISEMD services increased those elderly level of functionality making them more independent on their everyday lives.
- **Quality of the EPs Life (QOL-AD):** Similarly after the 12 moth testing there was an increase of the quality of life for the elderly (30,33-30,90).
- **Quality of the ICG Life (SQLC):** The ICG had a significant increase of their quality of life (70,80-76,00) after the 12

Table 2. Combined scores

Relationship	TEST GROUP Baseline-Final	CONTROL GROUP Baseline-Final	COMBINED Baseline-Final
COGNITION			
MMSE	19,50-19,00	18-16,6	18,75-17,80
MOCA	14,80-14,70	14,2-13,4	14,50-14,05
FUNCTIONING			
ADL	4,30-4,20	5,2-4,8	4,75-4,50
IADL	4,00-4,30	5,6-5	4,80-4,65
QUALITY OF LIFE EP weighted			
QOL-AD	30,33-30,90	37,47-33,47	33,90-32,18
QUALITY OF LIFE ICG			
SQLC	70,80-76,00	82,60-82,60	76,70-79,30
CARE BURDEN ICG			
ZBI	20,40-16,50	21,20-23,20	20,80-19,85

month testing, meaning that the ISISEMD services helped them deal with their everyday chores while taking care of their elderly in a more sufficient way.

- **ICGs Care Burden (ZBI):** According to the test groups final evaluation, there is a significant decrease of the ICGs level of care burden (20,40-16,50) after the 12 months use of the ISISEMD services whereas as far as control group is concerned the ICGs burden was increased (21,20-23,20) after 12 months of care.

Results from users' evaluation for satisfaction and acceptance of the services in Trikala region are displayed in the table below.

Summary of the final evaluations for acceptance of the services and added value:

- **Elderly Persons:** the elderly users felt safer and more independent in their home environment thanks to the ISISEMD services and were therefore very satisfied using them. This also had a positive impact to their quality of life as well. All of them expressed their wish to continue using the services in the future.

- **Informal Carers:** Most of them were very satisfied with using the services. They all believed that their quality of life had increased whereas the everyday care burden had decreased significantly. Lastly they all expressed their wish to continue using them in the future.

Summary of the final evaluations for technical acceptance of the services and ease of use:

- **Elderly Persons:** the elderly people had some difficulty understanding and using the services. However they fully understood the importance of them and were partial or more satisfied using them.

- **Informal Carers:** Informal carers had much less difficulty in comparison to the elderly in using the services and found them very flexible, quite important, and easy to integrate with a positive contribution to their lives.

Table 3. Overall acceptance and satisfaction of the services in the region of Trikala (average score)

EP	Scale	Trikala
Safety about the home environment	3 I feel significantly safer. 2 I feel safer. 1 I do not feel safer. 0 I feel less safe.	2.1
Satisfaction about the system	3 I am more satisfied than I thought I'll be. 2 I am satisfied. 1 I am not satisfied. 0 I am disappointed.	2.0
Change in feeling of quality of life	3 it increases more than I thought I would be. 2 it increases. 1 no change, no influence. 0 it decreases.	2.0
Change in feeling of quality of life for your relative	3 it increases more than I thought I would be. 2 it increases. 1 no change, no influence. 0 it decreases.	2.1
Support in independent living	3 it increases more than I thought I would be. 2 it increases. 1 no change, no influence. 0 it decreases.	2.0
Would you want to use a system like this?	3 I definitely would use a system like this. 2 I would consider using a system like this. 1 I would not consider using a system like this. 0 I would not use a system like this.	2.1
ICG	**Scale**	**Trikala**
Overall feeling of safety	3 I feel significantly safer. 2 I feel safer. 1 I do not feel safer. 0 I feel less safe.	2.4
Overall feeling of satisfaction	3 I am more satisfied than I thought I'll be. 2 I am satisfied. 1 I am not satisfied. 0 I am disappointed.	2.3
Would you want to use a system like this?	3 I definitely would use a system like this. 2 I would consider using a system like this. 1 I would not consider using a system like this. 0 I would not use a system like this.	2.3
Overall change in feeling of quality of life	3 it increases more than I thought I would be. 2 it increases. 1 no change, no influence. 0 it decreases.	1.9
Overall change in feeling of quality of life for EP	3 it increases more than I thought I would be. 2 it increases. 1 no change, no influence. 0 it decreases.	1.9
Overall support in independent living for EP	3 it increases more than I thought I would be. 2 it increases. 1 no change, no influence. 0 it decreases.	2.0
Overall feeling of care	3 it decreases more than I thought I would be. 2 it decreases. 1 no change, no influence. 0 it increases.	2.0

Table 4. Willingness to pay for ISISEMD services and amount in euro

EP	
NO	50%
YES	50%
Amount in euro	per month 100-250
DID NOT GIVE ANSWER	0%
ICG	
NO	30%
YES	70%
Amount in euro	per month 100-300
DID NOT GIVE ANSWER	0%

Willingness to Pay

During the interviews some Informal Care givers expressed their willingness to pay for ISISEMD services depending on the costs. The view of ICG was that the system could prove to be economically feasible. If ICG had money, they would be willing to pay for it.

Results from the questionnaires show that some of the elderly would be willing to pay for the services because they highly appreciate their independence and personal safety.

The table below shows results for the willingness to pay for the services and is illustrated for EP and ICG. The amount they are willing to pay is revealed too.

To conclude with, the results presented in the tables 5 and 6 below are highlighting the impact of the services to both the elderly and the caregivers everyday life on a level of independency, usefulness, importance and quality, giving a clear idea about the real benefits that this kind of integrated services can have to the population.

Sustainability of the Project

The Municipality of Trikala intended to run the ISISEMD services after the end of the project. However, due to recent debt crisis in Greece,

Table 5. Domain results comparison

EP	N= 10
Activities of Daily Living: Maintain former status	80% maintained their basic Activities of Daily Living
Instrumental Activities of Daily Living: Maintaining former status	40% improved their Instrumental Activities of Daily Living
Ability to make phone calls	50% showed mixed maintenance and improvement in ability to make phone calls
Ability to manage meals	30% had maintained ability to manage meals and another 40% showed a mix of maintaining and declining meal management
Medication management	40% showed improvement in medication management
Manage transportation	60% maintained their former ability to take transportation
Manage shopping	50% maintained, improved or had a mixture of the two for their ability to shop
Maintain relationships	30% of EP's maintained their relationships to the original status, with another 30% showing a mix of maintenance and improvement; however 40% had a mix of maintenance and decline
Maintain their social life status	40% of EP's maintained their social life status
Maintain memory status (MMSE/MOCA)	50% of EP's had maintained memory status and another 20% showed a mix of maintenance and improvement
Maintain living situation (independent living – QoLAD)	50% of EP's felt a mix of maintenance and decline in their living situation and 40% felt they maintained their original living situation
Maintain quality of life (QOLAD)	70% of EP's had improvement in their QOL-AD

the Greek government has planned an austerity program, supported by the European Central Bank (ECB), International Monetary Fund (IMF) and the European Commission (EC). Within this framework, the Perfecture of the Region of Thessaly and/or the Greek Ministry of Internal

Table 6. Domain results comparison 2

ICG	N= 10
Maintain their initial employment status – ZBI	At least 50%, but possibly up to 70% of Care-givers were able to maintain their initial employment status, with another 30% showing a mix of maintenance and improvement. Between 80-100% of Care-givers maintained or improved their employment status after using the ISISEMD system
Reduction of care-related stress (care-giver burden) - ZBI	80% of Care-givers had a reduction of care-related stress (care-giver burden) and 0% had an increase in care-related stress; Burden was decreased by 21.8% in all TR ICGs combined
Maintained their relationships to the original status	
Maintained their social life Status	30% of Care-givers had improvement in their social life and another 30% had a mix of maintenance and improvement
Maintain quality of life (SQLC)	80% of Care-givers had improvement in their QOL
TRANSFER OF TASKS (ZBI)	ICG reports maintained level of stress in meeting responsibilities and maintained that they have more to do, yet IADL shows that EP has improved ability from never participating in housekeeping to now performs light daily tasks. EP shows decline in laundry chores from all laundry must be done by others to never participates. ICG reports overall feeling of care responsibilities has decreased

Decentralization and e-Government, overruled DEKA's Executive Board decision, to keep the formal caregivers of the ISISEMD project services after the pilot phase. Therefore, the Municipality of Trikala was not allowed to run the ISISEMD services after the end of the project.

Regarding the added-value that ISISEMD may offer in the future, it varies regarding the different stages of implementation. First of all, the way the product is presented to a potential customer is very important. When a full demonstration of the platform takes place for instance, then it is quite possible for the users to be recruited to the project, which is equivalent to the fact of gaining more clients for the commercial version of the product. So, the way of approaching the 'user/client' is of utmost importance and requires competent diplomacy. This relationship between the end-user and the technical partner responsible for the installation of the product is a factor that ISISEMD has established in depth and can be considered as a thorough basis for similar future implementations.

INDEPENDENT

Point of Departure

The initial focus of the service innovation that was achieved in Trikala was based on both continued wellness of end users and organizational cooperation, with a view to achieving easier coordination of current services and provision of new integrated service components. The implemented INDEPENDENT services were built on existing services that have yet been provided in rather uncoordinated manner.

One is the so called "Help at Home" program which is directed toward senior citizens who suffer from chronic diseases, mobility restrictions and loneliness. The program aims at improving quality of life of the target population by assisting individuals and their family environment.

Moreover, an existing Telecare centre serves elderly people who were equipped with lightweight handheld medical appliances and take measurements of their vital signs which are then transferred (via the telecare centre) to the municipality hospital over PSTN or GPRS for review and feedback by the experts.

Target

With the development of the pilot site for INDEPENDENT, users of "Help at Home" service were recorded to become registered in a common ICT database which includes all care and health records. The psychologists along with the social workers that participate in "Help at Home" program were authorized to advice the end users through teleconsultation. Multilevel access to the care and medical personnel had to be achieved. Operationally speaking, this means for each back-end user different access rights to the information system had to be preserved according to his/her specific role. Integrated and coordinated services were enabled by this new system operating through a more productive and cost-effective service delivery. Additionally, the major problem of mild dementia and depression was addressed as well. Before entering into specific details the identification of fundamental roles that have a key role to play in the framework of INDEPENDENT had to be defined, namely:

- Elderly citizens consist the key user group at the front end level ('external users').
- Health psychologists worked alongside other medical professionals in clinical settings, work towards behavioral change through public health promotion, teach at universities, and conduct research.
- Doctors represented a 'back end' user group who provided ancillary assistance to the psychologists in urgent occasions.
- Computer programmers and engineers were responsible for the maintenance, the support and the debugging of the system and configured the set up for the Electronic Health Record - EHR platform.
- Informal caregivers were the end users of the tele-counseling service to whom the psychological support is offered in order to decrease care burden of the everyday life.

Characteristics: Project Description

INDEPENDENT (ICT Enabled Service Integration for Independent Living) project is Competitiveness and Innovation Framework Pro-gramme project included in THEME [CIP-ICT-PSP.2009.1.3] [ICT for ageing well / independent living] licensed under the Grant agreement no: 250521. Trikala is the Greek pilot site which had ran among the six pilot sites which operated in total. On the Greek part, e-Trikala SA, Trikala's Public Benefit Municipal Enterprise for Social Development (DEKA) and ASKLEPIOS has participated in the project. e-Trikala is the Development company of the Municipality of Trikala. Since 2004, the e-Trikala office is acting in the fields of new broadband technologies, successfully implementing municipal projects. In 2008 it was transformed into e-Trikala SA and until recently it has participated in several eHealth and eCare European projects gaining in this way a remarkable experience in these sectors not in Greek but also in European standards. DEKA is a public provider for the Municipality of Trikala. The aims of this Municipal Enterprise are the Economic, Cultural and Social Development of the Municipality of Trikala and the county in general, through its active participation in the developing procedure for the exploitation of the European and local resources, the undertaking of productive initiatives, the rendering of upgraded services and the development of manpower. After the municipal restructure it is now called ASKLIPIOS. DEKA is responsible for providing the tele-care centre as well as the two psychologists responsible for recruitment, evaluation and psychological support of the end-users. It will also be responsible for the helpdesk receiving the first queries for psychological help. Last but not least, ASKLEPIOS Centre for Open Protection of the Elderly of the Municipality of Trikala (KAPI http://www.deka-trikala.gr/el/koinonikes-domes): KAPI is a public provider for the Municipality of Trikala responsible for the inclusion of the elderly in the society and their participation in various social activities.

Three of the Open Day Care Centers are involved in INDEPENDENT. IP phones are installed in their premises providing users with a private tele - counseling room. The KAPIs and their staff may also act as operators, when they receive calls regarding the project, which they forward either to psychologists or to the technicians etc.

Description: Service Workflow

The main topic of the initiative was to psychologically support the informal caregivers through the conduction of remote counseling. The core components included the local telecare centre infrastructure; a web based electronic health record accessible by different stake holders, video telephony home equipment and broadband connection to the assisted person's home.

The following key roles best describe the functionality of the provided services:

- Telecare operator sets-up joint client folder, handles emergency phone calls and requests by informal care givers.
- Telecare field staff installs and maintains equipment at client's home.
- Psychologist provides video-based counseling to assisted person's informal care giver.
- Psychologists update specific fields of the electronic health record when video telephony session ends.
- Physician receives email alert by telecare operator in need for home visit.
- Physician populates joint client folder with health related data.
- Physician receives automatic alert to look-up joint client folder for data entered in by psychologist after video counseling session.
- Assisted person's family care giver calls telecare centre in case of crisis by telephone.
- Assisted person's family care giver attends video-based tele-counseling sessions.
- Assisted person's children look-up assisted person's client folder remotely.

The digital support infrastructure for all the users of KAPI, DEKA and eTrikala who were registered with common ICT based extended care records, enabled cross-sectoral and multilevel access to the social care and medical personnel. This led to easier coordination of the services hence rendering them more integrated, productive and cost-effective. In addition this platform empowered services like advanced tele-video counseling for psychological support, compared to the present telephone based support line, since tele-psychiatry services require a complete record of the social profile of the patient.

The pilot in Trikala region aimed at the remote help both to the patient and to the family of the assisted person. The system components were the IP video phone for tele-counseling, an ADSL internet line and an EHR accessible to all participants in the pilot. After the installation of such equipment to the patient's home, the informal care giver could start a teleconference by phone with the dedicated telecare centre at scheduled or unscheduled counsels and get help and guidance from professional care givers.

The proposed service also included the completion of an Electronic Health Record (EHR). All concerning parties were given the appropriate credentials and made any changes according to their access level, wherever applicable. The idea is that any family carer may have a view about the status of their relative all the time, as every professional is to upload instructions, alternation in medication, proposed exercises or even comments about the status of the patient.

Pilot User Characteristics

Pilot users can be distinguished in the following categories;

- Older people with mild cognitive problems or mild depression who may benefit from the pilot are mainly identified by KAPI staff, with the support of psychologists of

DEKA. If they qualify according to specified criteria (mild cognitive impairment or mild depression patients that are not institutionalized), they could join the project. Although they were not the main service beneficiaries they were allowed to have limited access (counseling information is not included) to the EHR concerning their medical status. Their main benefit was the opportunity to have a better family care through the psychological support of their care giver.

- Family carers, mostly relatives, potentially qualifying for the pilot were identified by KAPI staff as well, assisted by social workers involved in a dedicated program entitled "Help at Home."
- Professional users consist of staff (psychologists, social care workers, KAPI's doctor) employed by ASKLEPIOS. The KAPI centers apart from all the social services mentioned above also have a medical professional that visits the centers on a weekly basis conducting basic medical procedures such as prescriptions etc. The doctor who visits the KAPI centers on a weekly basis also had some limited access to the EHR.

Inclusion Criteria

The main scope of INDEPENDENT pilot site was to offer integrated services (EHR and tele - counseling) to care givers of people that suffer from mild cognitive impairment or mild depression and to the assisted persons as well. People to be recruited to the service were predefined according to the following criteria:

- People with mild cognitive impairment were initially assessed for cognitive status and present co-morbidities. The MoCA and the MMSE has been used to assess cognitive status.
- People with mild depression were initially assessed for their psychological health status by using the Greek translation of the Geriatric Depression Scale.
- All the participants have being asked to sign this consent form at the beginning of the pilot.
- The collection, processing and management of sensitive personal data hold threats to the patients who have the legal right to be protected according to the 9th Article of the Greek Constitution.

User Distribution

The INDEPENDENT project as implemented in Trikala consists of two case scenarios.

- Providing video phone services to the relatives at home.
- Providing video phone counseling services to the relatives at the KAPI centre.

As far as it concerns the first category, caregivers who approved to have a video phone service in their home should set this device on a private and remote room of the house so as to prevent any disturbances during the tele-psychotherapy session. These sessions took place via video phones or other devices e.g. a PC. Each session lasted 45 minutes maximum on a weekly base.

Secondly, the provision of the service in the KAPI centers specified that the caregivers of the patients would have been able to attend video counseling sessions in a private office, so that the conditions required for conducting a session appropriately, such as an anonymity and quiet would be in place.

In more concrete words, the users recruited during pilot operation were:

- 62 users from home (31 assisted persons and 31 caregivers).

- 200 users from the KAPIs (100 assisted persons and 100 caregivers) while finally there were 182 users from the KAPIs (91 assisted persons and 91 caregivers).

Methodology

INDEPENDENT, as an eCare project consist a combination of social and care services with the use of ICT. For this reason, in first place ICT services having the social profile had to be developed. Nevertheless, computers programmers had to cooperate with social care providers and general practitioners in order to set the requirements of the services (both the Electronic Health Record – EHR and the Video – counseling sessions) and satisfy the appropriate compatibility standards. When the requirements were set, developers proceeded in the software development and hardware selection phase. In the meanwhile, feedback was also provided by social and health care providers in the intermediate. When the software development was completed, functionality was demonstrated and also tested by end users in order for the major comments and remarks to be extracted and be also incorporated. All adequate adaptations and changes were implemented and software was released.

The service implementation in Trikala had also to be thoroughly described in order for the pilot preparation to be completed. In a descriptive way, psychologists were to provide remote video – counseling to informal caregivers of mild dementia or mild depression patients. In other words, the end users of the psychological support via video – phones were informal caregivers, as it was previously mentioned. Informal caregivers could access the service either through their homes or through the Open Day Care Centers for the elderly (KAPI centers). Psychologists, who resided in the Telecare center of the Municipality, could enter the Electronic Health Record before and after the counseling session in order to look up and fill data relevant to counseling. On the other side, the social worker, the nurse and/or the general practitioner who provided social and health care in the KAPI centers looked up client data relevant to medical treatment. A challenging issue was the recruitment of such a large number of users that had specific inclusion criteria only from the 3 KAPI centers, which was solved by expanding the recruitment strategy to all 6 KAPIs and by organizing 6 workshops – daily seminars in order to present INDEPENDENT services to a wider audience.

One of the most important activities carried out through the pilot was evaluation which was structured in three different phases. It was really essential for evaluation activities to be applied in the aforementioned manner in order to define and assess the impact of the service upon the discrete user categories. For practical reasons, the first, the second and the third evaluation stage is accordingly mentioned as T0, T1 and T2.

- T0 measurement took place from May to June 2012 - 262 people were evaluated.
- T1 measurement at October 2012 and finished in November 2012 - 262 people were evaluated.
- T2 measurement from March to April 2013.
- Partners involved and therefore evaluated for user acceptance and satisfaction:
- The psychologist who were responsible for carrying out the users' counseling sessions for the tele-care centre via video-phones.
- The relative (caregiver) who was the main end user.

Apart from these, evaluation data were also documented and reported in order to achieve a more accurate data analysis. Moreover, it was important, during user acceptance and satisfaction evaluation, to document and differentiate the equipment used for the video-phone sessions e.g. the usage of a, IP phone will differ from the usage of a pc or Skype. Therefore such a clarifying question was also included during evaluation. Constantly increasing needs of the ageing population which is engravated both from financial and social reasons will become increasingly stretched which means that the results and findings of the specific pilot project could be extremely important to be analyzed. In the most of the European countries, especially in Southern Europe countries, the funding for health and care is decreased which means that alternative resources should be researched. Thus, it is quite essential to present the results of INDEPENDENT in terms of effects on the users as well as level of satisfaction. In this direction, positive results and levels of satisfaction to both users are outlined in the following points:

- According to Zarit Burden Interview (ZBI) scale that evaluates the caregivers level of everyday burden there were a significant decrease of the burden from T0 evaluation to T2 evaluation (T0:38,9 > T2:32,54)
- According to the World Health Organization Quality of Life - The Brief edition (WHOQOL-BREF) that measures person's that suffers from depression quality of life, there were a significant increase in all four major domains of everyday life (WHOQOL-BREF.,1998):
  - Domain 1 T0: 18 < T2: 19,3.
  - Domain 2 T0: 13,6 < T2: 16,8.
  - Domain 3 T0: 6,4 < T2: 7,3.
  - Domain 4 T0: 20,7 < T2: 21,4.

According to the GDS that measures a person's level of depression, it is proved that there were a significant decrease on the level of depression (T0: 8,57 > T2: 7,27)As far as it concerns the Satisfaction levels of caregivers and the assisted persons, following points can be summed up.

- The satisfaction questionnaires that were administered to both the caregivers and the assisted persons during the second period give a better idea of the services

impact.98% of the Caregivers and 85% of the Assisted persons agreed that the Tele-psychotherapy service resulted in any positive benefits in relation to the quality of life and wellbeing.

- 87% of the Caregivers and 83% of the Assisted persons stated their health conditions management had been improved in a great deal in favor of the Tele-psychotherapy service.
- 60% of the Caregivers and 58% of the Assisted persons think that Tele-psychotherapy service equipment easy to use. Moreover, 57% of the Caregivers stated that the level of their anxiety was decreased in a great deal as a result of using the Tele-counseling service.

Moreover, it should be also mentioned that Staff focus group was also evaluated assessing the impact of the INDEPENDENT project on clients. More specifically, psychologists note that family cares quality of life has increased, while decreasing the everyday care burden has helped most cases improve their psychological health status. The INDEPENDENT services support the users both psychologically and socially. Additionally, both services were useful as the Electronic Health Record offered an integrated communication bridge whereas as the tele-sessions supported them psychologically, decreasing the care burden and increasing the quality of life for both users. Psychologists have also assessed the usability and reliability of the technology noting that the services were simple enough and user friendly while all the information is at the same time easy to use and confidential although a larger screen on the IP phone could improve the tele-sessions quality.

Scales

For assisted persons, cognitive status, psychological health status, quality of life and independence was recorded at baseline along with previous use of information and communication technology as well as demographic information such as age, sex, SES, living arrangement, and relationship to carer. Cognitive status involved administration of the MoCA and the MMSE, and psychological health status using the GDS. Quality of life included administration of the QOL-AD for people with dementia, and the WHO-QOL 100 for people with depression, Assessment of older people: self-maintaining and instrumental activities of daily living (The Gerontologist. 1969;9(3):179-86.). For carers, quality of life, carer burden, and family distress along with previous use of information and communication technology, as well as demographic information such as age, sex, SES, living arrangement, and relationship to the person cared for. Quality of life was measured using the SF-12, while carer burden was measured with the ZBI.

For both assisted persons and end users, satisfaction was assessed using a bespoke satisfaction questionnaire.

Dissemination

In order to recruit the required 400 users for the pilot, the applied strategy included targeted seminars to the KAPI centers of the city and other 'Open Day Workshops' open to public, where the scope of the project had been thoroughly explained. Along with regular press releases and the distribution of leaflets concerning the project, it had been disseminated in local media with live interviews in TV and radio.

In May 2012, 6 workshops-daily seminars were conducted to all of the regional KAPIs titled "Problems during Mild Cognitive Impairment and Mild Depression. The power of counseling". Around 200 people in total attended the meetings and were informed on the INDEPENDENT services.

An exploitation workshop was also organized in Trikala in April 2013 which was attended by stakeholders from various categories like ICT providers, Public Organization that provides social health services, user representatives, Mobile Health Unit which provides mental health services to remote areas of Trikala as well as public sector-provider of health services. The exploitation workshop involved presentation of the elderly main problems by the representative of the Open Day Care Centers in Trikala, INDEPENDENT services and benefits as well as the possibilities for further exploitation with the use of concrete examples. Enough time was given to the participants in order to have a further discussion with the stakeholders

During May 2013, Trikala pilot site representatives participated at the 3rd Mental Health Innovation Forum "Telecare & Patient Compliance, Help Lines – Telecare - TelePsychiatry - Internet Consultation –e-Learning - – Virtual Reality - Games – e-Health - mobile Health" which was organized upon international level with the participation of major Public and Private Health Organizations. In the same direction, a day conference "Technophobia in middle and Third age" took place in Trikala which was also broadcasted by the local media.

The deployment of the 2 different services in combination was a constructive chance to specify the challenges that have been appearing in order for recording and avoid making those in the exploitation phase as well as in the next eCare services framework. First of all, a very common drawback in integrated care that was observed in INDEPENDENT project is the rather uncoordinated way of involvement of several actors. Telecare services can be accordingly designed to cope with such problems. Nevertheless, it was a great implementation challenge for different care providers to get in touch with older people and transfer the incentives to them. Another challenge was to persuade older people who have no previous experience using ICT the value of incorporating such services in their daily life. A significant advantage was the fact that through INDEPENDENT services patients and their informal caregivers were given access to the Electronic Health Record which consists an important step in the sense of making relatives and patients feel less left out of the actual care process.

In this direction relatives should be generally involved in the care process as they can be efficiently informed about the medical status of their relative on a daily basis. On the other hand, it is undeniable that patients had some difficulties in accessing the EHR whereas their relatives could use the EHR in an efficient way. One other challenge is the fact that elderly people need to feel that the provided service would be to their benefit or else they are reluctant to be involved. For this reason a connecting liaison to their basic daily needs had to be clearly stated. Especially in Greece, people over 55 are quite unfamiliar with ICT and for this reason there was insufficient number of users during recruitment, for this reason open days and scheduled visits to the KAPI centers were organized. Another conclusion concerning the exploitation plan of INDEPENDENT was to define a balanced subscription amount upon which the service would be provided under the given financial recession crisis or even adjust to the needs of each user wherever applicable. Some problems were also appeared in the video counseling session's appointments as caregiver forgot their appointments or rescheduled them too often. Consequently, psychologists "trained" their users to be consistent with the time schedule with the use of reminding alerts at their cell phones.

Renewing Health

Project Description

Healthcare services around the world are under pressure to increase the quality of care to patients at a time when the global population is aging, the burden of chronic disease is rising and the economic conditions are challenging. Telehealth has been proposed as one of the solutions to the challenges faced by healthcare systems with aging populations, increasing numbers of patients with chronic conditions and decreasing supply of human resources.(Gartner., 2006)).

Telehealth is the remote exchange of physiological data between a patient at home and medical staff at hospital to assist in diagnosis and monitoring. It comprises home units to measure and monitor temperature, blood pressure and other vital signs for clinical review at a remote location (for example, a hospital site) using phone lines or wireless technology. (COM/2008/689final. http://eur-lex.europa.eu/LexUriServ/LexUriServ. do?uri=COM:2008:0689:FIN:EN:PD, 2011).

However the digital innovation in healthcare has been slow to take hold, due to regulatory complexity, issues related with the accreditation of health professionals who provide telemedicine applications and liability issues, interoperability issues, cost effectiveness and reimbursement for telemedicine services, poor integration of telehealth services in existing health services (http://mhealth.vodafone.com/home.,2012) (Legaly E-health, 2008).

Telemedicine services have been piloted in many clinical areas during the last two decades, but have only exceptionally been integrated into routine clinical practice. There is at the moment, however, insufficient clinical and economic evidence to advocate the large-scale use of tele-monitoring and IT supported health coaching interventions. Similarly, several literature reviews on the effectiveness of telemedicine demonstrate lack of evidence for a comprehensive evaluation of the various aspects of telehealth services (Polisena et al., 2008).

To this direction large public funded RCT studies are under development for the evaluation of tele-health application on clinical, economic, organizational and users-acceptance level in the European Union. (www.kingsfund.org.uk/current_projects/whole_systems_demonstrator_action_research_network/index.html\ 2011), (www.renewinghealth.eu, 2013). One of them, RENEWING HEALTH (www.renewinghealth.eu, 2013) aims at implementing large-scale real-life test beds for the validation and evaluation of innovative telemedicine services trying to use a patient-centered approach and a common rigorous assessment methodology. In 9 regions with advanced telehealth services, belonging to 9 different EU Member States or Associated Countries, service solutions are already operational at local level for the telemonitoring and the treatment of chronic patients suffering from diabetes, COPD or CVD diseases. The focus on Diabetes mellitus, cardiovascular diseases, and chronic obstructive pulmonary disease (COPD) is based due to the fact these conditions are common and long-standing illnesses with a major burden on public health budgets. The services are designed to give patients a central role in the management of their diseases, optimization of the treatment, promoting compliance to treatment, and helping healthcare professionals to detect early signs of worsening. These services will be scaled up, integrated with mainstream Health Information Systems, grouped into a limited number of clusters bringing together services showing similar features, trialled and assessed with a common assessment methodology, and using a common set of primary indicators for pilots belonging to a same cluster. The methodology used for the assessment was based on MAST - A Model for assessment of Telemedicine applications (Kidholm et al., 2012).

Objectives

RENEWING HEALTH addresses clinical outcome, patient/user, economic and organizational objectives.

Clinical Objectives

RENEWING HEALTH aims evaluate the effect of telehealth at the quality of life of the type of chronic patients addressed in the project. Quality of life is expected to be affected by reducing the need for the patient to use emergency services and/or hospital stays. Impact on quality of life will be measured using a validated and reliable generic instrument e.g. SF-36®. The project aim

to provide healthcare institutions and professionals with a way of offering citizens suffering from chronic diseases more timely and appropriate care wherever they are, inside or outside healthcare premises, reducing the incidence of potential complications.

The project also aims to evaluate if a telemedicine-based delivery network can supply healthcare services at least of the same clinical quality and reliability as those supplied through a traditional healthcare delivery network.

Patient/User Perspective Objectives

RENEWING HEALTH aims to evaluate the whether the provision of clinical services through telemedicine that take into proper consideration patients' and professional users' needs and expectations. The level of patients' empowerment and patients' satisfaction using telehealth service will be measured, together with the level of the health professionals satisfaction involved. With regard to patients' satisfaction, collaboration is established with the Whole Systems Demonstrators project in England, to converge towards a single patient's questionnaire.

Economic Objectives

The economic benefits of the telehealth services will be measured by identifying a set of primary and secondary indicators which have an impact on the healthcare expenditure (e.g. number of hospital admissions and average length of stay) and measuring these in the Intervention and in the Control Group. The implementation of the new healthcare model will be evaluated, in order to identify the impact on cost reduction of chronic patients care to the society.

Organizational Objectives

By implementing telemedicine solutions for the care of chronic patients, RENEWING HEALTH faces the challenges of change management creating an organizational model for telemedicine services that ensures a safe and efficient pathway for patients in their journey through the healthcare system. The organizational impact will be measured in a qualitative manner through questionnaires to health care professionals and by description of the organizational setting in which the telemedicine application is used.

Methodology

The evaluation of the large scale pilots in all the 9 participating regions will be carried out using as a basis the MethoTelemed methodology and the MAST (8) assessment model, possibly adjusted to the specific requirements of RENEWING HEALTH if needed. MethoTelemed was (February 2009 – January 2010) a study based on an EC tender which aimed at producing a benchmark document (the "MethoTelemed Guidance") which provides:

- A systematic documentation of the type and extent of telemedicine applications in healthcare systems; and
- A structured framework for assessing the effectiveness and contribution to quality of care of telemedicine applications. The purpose was to develop an academically rigorous and practically useful guidance for a methodology to assess telemedicine applications in Europe.

The evaluation will produce a systematic and multidisciplinary assessment of the impact of the integrated telemedicine services, aiming to serve the objectives of the project. (table.7)

The evaluation of the project will include the following elements:

- A scientific trial protocol for each cluster of projects that includes, among others, a detailed description of objectives, design, methodology, outcomes, statistical considerations.
- The selection/elaboration of questionnaires for collecting the opinion of the various categories of stakeholders.
- Evaluation of outcome taking into account the primary outcomes agreed for each of the clusters and the secondary ones agreed for individual pilots.
- Scaling-up and further uptake of conclusion/ outcomes from the evaluation of telemedicine services, for further exploitation in the participating region, country and across Europe.

The trial protocols were produced in the initial stages of the project included the primary outcomes and relative indicators for each cluster of pilots and secondary outcomes and relative indicators for each pilot. By using the MAST model, the results from the real life project will give decision

Table 7. "Multi-disciplinary assessment"

Patients and Clinical Outcomes	**Organization**
• Quality of life. • Health condition. • Compliance. • Medication. • Self-management. • Pilot related indicators.	• Task distribution. • Personnel satisfaction. • Co-operation relations within the organization or with external part. • Workflow. • Education and knowledge sharing. • Pilot related indicators.
Technology	**Economy**
• User friendliness. • Stability. • Security. • Inclusiveness. • Integration. • Pilot related indicators.	• Hospitalization and readmissions (number and length). • Consultations with GP etc. • Medication costs. • Personal resources. • Technology and maintenance costs. • Pilot related indicators.

makers in other European countries a description of the critical success factors in the implementation of the different types of telemedicine.

The recruitment of patients per pathology is presented in table 8, and per cluster (type of intervention) in table 9. The end of the pilots of Renewing Health is expected in the summer of 2013 and the outcomes of the evaluation in autumn 2013.

Engagement of Stakeholders

Patients suffering from chronic disease and specialists of these diseases are represented at local level through their local associations which will be invited to have a close look at the trials. In the case of the patients, they are also represented

Table 8. "Pathologies and patients basis"

Pathology	Patient Basis
Diabetes	2.269
COPD	1.487
Cardiovascular disease	3.670
Multi-pathologies	152
Total	7.578

in the Consortium by their European Associations in an advisory role (User Advisory Board). Industry too is represented through associations which bring together on a voluntary basis the main eHealth players at world level and form an Industry Advisory Board. These Associations are invited to support the Regional Health Authorities in the technical design of the service solutions.

Interoperability Issues and Integration Issues Tackled in the Project

The issue of interoperability among Personal Health Systems is a major issue for the integration of the telemedicine in every health care services. The RENEWING HEALTH Consortium closely follows the most significant initiative at European level which addresses this problem by introducing new methods of work, with Continua Health Alliance as a member.

Fragmentation is not however present only on technical level in the e-health sector, but in addition in the organizational and policy aspects required to integrate

Care provision across healthcare and social care, by deploying multidisciplinary teams in

Table 9. "Projects in relation to Pathology"

Pathology Projects in Renewing Health	Diabetes	COPD	CVD Diseases	Non Disease Specific Tele-Monitoring
Nurse monitoring program (IT)		X		
Tele-care and tele-health service for elderly and frail people (IT)	X	X	X	
Tele-monitoring of implantable cardiac device (IT)			X	
Better breathing (DK & E)		X		
Telemedicine Ulcer Treatment (DK)	X			
Myhealth@Age (S)	X		X	
The diabetes health Motivation Project (NO)	X			
Health Coaching (F)	X		X	
Home Hospitalization Program (E)		X		
Tele-care service for chronic patients (GR)	X	X	X	X
Optimized treatment of chronic patients (A)	X	X		

operation incorporating social care staff and addressing both clinical and non-clinical, social care related conditions. Therefore special emphasis is given to the evaluation of the organization aspects within Renewing Health pilot interventions.

Use of Results

The RENEWING HEALTH is funded mostly with public money. This allows them to license the technologies free of charge to other Regional Health Authorities willing to adopt them and the European Commission to ensure the availability of the outcomes outside the Consortium.

Dissemination

The dissemination strategy of the Consortium intends to carry out to achieve a wide and well-targeted dissemination of the project results.

The dissemination strategy will be broken down into local and regional, national and international activities, including coverage by local, regional, national and international media, organization or participation in events dedicated to telehealth, preparation of a promotional material and articles in peer reviewed scientific journals, and organization of high-profile Interim Workshop and Final Conference of the project.

CONCLUSION

Lately there has been a lot of discussion on the implementation of alternatives care services such as home care services especially for those patients that suffer from chronic diseases such as cancer, cardiovascular, cognitive impairment etc. The main benefits of such a care approach is considered to be the fact that the patient has the luxury to live in his/her home, surrounded by his/her family and therefore minimize the problems and complications that follow long-term hospitalization such as stress depression etc. What is more, home care is considered to be less expensive: in many cases 10-20% less expensive whereas in some cases it ranges to almost 50% less that the hospitalization costs. Last, the ability of a chronic patient to stay home leads to hospital bed releases and cost saving (Ioannidis, Lopatzidis and Mantis, 1999, p.35).

All three programs have proven to be easy to use with a high level of user satisfaction. What is more evaluation outcomes indicate a positive feedback (decrease of everyday stress, increase of quality of live and level of independency) to the users lives. Those impacts are consistent with the key objectives of the Public Social and Health reformation that is taking place in Greece and can be considered as the answer to the main peculiarities and problems mentioned at the beginning of this chapter.

To conclude with, we firmly believe that the integration of existing services such as public health lines and health files via those programs have proven to be of great value via the establishment of referral systems, the introduction of personal electronic health cards and the adoption of clinical and pharmaceutical protocols.

REFERENCES

Bedard, M., Molloy, D. W., Squire, L., Dubois, S., Lever, J. A., & O'Donnel, M. L. (2001). The Zarit Burden Interview: A new short version and screening version. *The Gerontologist*, *41*(5), 65. doi:10.1093/geront/41.5.652 PMID:11574710

Burckhardt, C. S., & Anderson, K. L. (2003). The Quality of Life Scale (QOLS), Reliability, validity, and utilization. *Health and Quality of Life Outcomes*, *1*, 60. doi:10.1186/1477-7525-1-60 PMID:14613562

Commission Communication. (n.d.). *Telemedicine for the benefit of patients, healthcare systems and societies*. Retrieved December 1, 2001 from http://eurlex.europa.eu/LexUriServ/LexUriServ.do?uri=COM:2008:0689:FIN:EN:PDF

Demers, L., & Vincent, C. (2001). The Quebec User Evaluation of Satisfaction with Assistive Technology (QUEST 2.0). *Assistive Technology, 10*, 600–601.

Demers, L., Weiss-Lambrou, R., & Ska, B. (2002). The Quebec User Evaluation of Satisfaction with Assistive Technology (QUEST 2.0), an overview and recent progress. *Technology and Disability, 14*(3), 101–105.

Development of the World Health Organization. (1998). WHOQOL-BREF quality of life assessment: The WHOQOL Group. *Psychological Medicine, 28*(3), 551–558. doi:10.1017/S0033291798006667 PMID:9626712

Economou, C. (2010). Health Systems in Transition. *Greece Health System Review, 12*(7).

Evaluating mHealth Adoption Barriers. (n.d.). *Human Behaviour Vodafone mHealth Solutions Insights Guide.* Retrieved December 1, 2012, from http://mhealth.vodafone.com/home/

Figueras, J., Saltman, R., & Mossialos, E. (1997). *Challenges in evaluating health sector reform: An overview.* London: London School of Economics and Political Science.

Folstein, M. F., Folstein, S. E., & McHugh, P. R. (1975). Mini mental state: A practical method for grading the cognitive state of patients for the clinician. *Journal of Psychiatric Research, 12*(3), 189–198. doi:10.1016/0022-3956(75)90026-6 PMID:1202204

Gartner. (2006, October). *The potential of telemedicine applications.* Gartner.

Gauthier, S., Reisberg, B., Zaudig, M., Petersen, R. C., Ritchie, K., & Broich, K. et al. (2006). Mild Cognitive Impairment. *Lancet, 367*(9518), 1262–1270. doi:10.1016/S0140-6736(06)68542-5 PMID:16631882

Glozman, J. M., Bicheva, K. G., & Fedorova, N. V. (1998). Scale of quality of life of care-givers (SQLC). *Journal of Neurology. Supplement, 245*(1), S39–S41.

Ioannidis, E., Lopatzidis, A., & Mantis, P. (1999). Υπηρεσίες Υγείας/Νοσοκομείο, Ιδιοτυπίες και Προκλήσεις. Ελληνικό Ανοιχτό Πανεπιστήμιο, vol. A.

Kidholm, K. et al. (2012). A Model for Assessment of Telemedicine applications (MAST). *International Journal of Technology Assessment in Health Care, 28*(1), 44–51. doi:10.1017/S0266462311000638 PMID:22617736

Lawton, M. P., & Brody, E. M. (1969). Assessment of older people: Self-maintaining and instrumental activities of daily living. *The Gerontologist, 9*(3), 179–186. doi:10.1093/geront/9.3_Part_1.179 PMID:5349366

Legaly E-Health. (2008). *A study on the legal and Regulatory Aspects of eHealth (Contract 30-CE-0041734/00-55).* Author.

Logsdon, R. G., Gibbons, L. E., McCurry, S. M., & Teri, L. (1999). Quality of life in Alzheimer's disease: Patient and caregiver reports. *Journal of Mental Health and Aging, 5*(1), 21–32.

Logsdon, R. G., Gibbons, L. E., McCurry, S. M., & Teri, L. (2002). Assessing quality of life in older adults with cognitive impairment. *Psychosomatic Medicine, 64*, 510–519. doi:10.1097/00006842-200205000-00016 PMID:12021425

Lorr, M., Sonn, T. M., & Katz, M. M. (1967). Towards the Definition of Depression. *Archives of General Psychiatry, 17*(2), 183–186. doi:10.1001/archpsyc.1967.01730260055008 PMID:4952175

Mossialos, E., Allin, S., & Davaki, K. (2005). Analysing the Greek health system: A tale of fragmentation and inertia. *Health Economics, 14*, 151–168. doi:10.1002/hec.1033 PMID:16161195

Nasreddine, Z. S., Phillips, N. A., & B'edirian, V. et al. (2005). The Montreal Cognitive Assessment, MoCA: A brief screening tool for mild cognitive impairment. *Journal of the American Geriatrics Society*, *53*(4), 695–699. doi:10.1111/j.1532-5415.2005.53221.x PMID:15817019

Regions of Europe Working Together for Health -RENEWING HEALTH. (n.d.). Retrieved March 1, 2013, from www.renewinghealth.eu

Reisberg, B., Ferris, S. H., de Leon, M. J., & Crook, T. (1982). The global deterioration scale for assessment of primary degenerative dementia. *The American Journal of Psychiatry*, *139*, 1136–1139. PMID:7114305

Souliotis, K., & Lionis, C. (2005). Creating an integrated health care system in Greece: A primary care perspective. *Journal of Medical Systems*, *29*(2), 187–196. doi:10.1007/s10916-005-3006-6 PMID:15931804

Tarricone, R., & Tsouros, A. (2008). *Home care in Europe, an overview*. World Health Organization. Retrieved from http://www.euro.who.int/document/E91884.pdf

Theodorou, M., & Mitrosilli, M. (1999). Υπηρεσίες Υγείας/ Νοσοκομείο, Ιδιοτυπίες και προκλήσεις. Ελληνικό Ανοιχτό Πανεπιστήμιο, vol.C.

Tran, K., Polisena, J., Coyle, D., Coyle, K., Kluge, E.-H. W., Cimon, K., & Scott, R. (2008). *Home telehealth for chronic disease management*. Ottawa, Canada: Canadian Agency for Drugs and Technologies in Health.

Whole Systems Demonstrator Action Research Network (WSDAN). (n.d.). Retrieved December 1, 2011, from http://www.kingsfund.org.uk/current_projects/whole_systems_demonstrator_action_research_network/index.html\

This work was previously published in Achieving Effective Integrated E-Care Beyond the Silos edited by Ingo Meyer, Sonja Müller, and Lutz Kubitschke, pages 240-265 copyright year 2014 by Medical Information Science Reference (an imprint of IGI Global).

Chapter 33
A System for the Semi-Automatic Evaluation of Clinical Practice Guideline Indicators

Alexandra Pomares Quimbaya
Pontificia Universidad Javeriana, Colombia

María Patricia Amórtegui
Pontificia Universidad Javeriana, Colombia

Rafael A. González
Pontificia Universidad Javeriana, Colombia

Oscar Muñoz
*Pontificia Universidad Javeriana, Colombia &
Hospital Universitario San Ignacio, Colombia*

Wilson Ricardo Bohórquez
Pontificia Universidad Javeriana, Colombia

Olga Milena García
Pontificia Universidad Javeriana, Colombia

Melany Montagut Ascanio
Hospital Universitario San Ignacio, Colombia

ABSTRACT

This paper presents EXEMED v2, a system that allows the evaluation of clinical practice guideline indicators. EXEMED v2 includes a knowledge base that supports the definition of executable rules applied over Electronic Health Records (EHR) in order to measure its compliance with a specific clinical guideline. Taking into account that an EHR may include structured attributes and narrative text attributes, EXEMED v2 analyzes both types. The process of evaluation in EXEMED v2 is to define the rules; once the rules are defined EXEMED v2 extracts from the EHR the facts that allow evaluating whether each one of them was accomplished or not. This evaluation includes different levels of certainty, allowing in some cases the interaction of a human evaluator to confirm (or not) automatic evaluation decisions. The functionality of EXEMED v2 was validated applying it in a case study of Acute Myocardial Infarction.

INTRODUCTION

In order to assure high quality in the provision of health services, the use of clinical practice guidelines is very important. Such guidelines are defined as a set of "systematically developed statements to assist practitioner and patient decisions about appropriate health care for clinical circumstances" (Field & Lohr, 1990, p.8). Clinical practice guidelines are primarily used to increase

DOI: 10.4018/978-1-4666-8756-1.ch033

the quality of patient care, to promote the efficient use of resources (Jovell, 1999), and to generate systematic recommendations for doctors. The definition of clinical practice guidelines can be done either by health regulatory agencies (Ministerio de Salud y Protección Social, 2012) or hospitals (Bassand et al., 2007), often based on NICE and SIGN type descriptions (Dunkley & Cross, 2006). This means that the use of clinical practice guidelines may be adapted according to circumstances or different environmental conditions. (Álvarez et al., 2010).

The evaluation of compliance with a clinical practice guideline is performed by evaluating a set of indicators related to hospital follow-up, interventions and behaviors, training, background, and diagnostic criteria, among others. These indicators allow health professionals to compare the quality of health care services with the parameters given in the guidelines, in order to take appropriate actions towards providing a better service to users.

The definition of clinical practice guidelines generally includes information related to: objectives, disease indicators, general considerations, interpretations, recommendations, methodology, implementations and development guide (Ministerio de Salud y Protección Social, 2012). These guides include many variables and relevant information for the proper tracing of the process. However, current guideline documents are very long and do not allow the extraction of this information in a concise and simple way, making it difficult to assess adherence to these guidelines by medical and administrative staff. As a consequence, there has been some research aimed at structuring these guidelines. For example, there are proposals for frameworks that are used to achieve interoperability of content between the Health Level Seven (HL7) and Semantic Web technologies in order to develop clinical guidelines (Casteleiro et al., 2009). Another project proposes a methodology and a software tool to mark-up clinical guidelines using a tree structure and a language called OCML (Svátek & Růžička, 2003). Similarly, languages

like PROforma are specifically designed to capture clinical practice guidelines (Sutton, Taylor, & Earle, 2006) and certain conditionals are explained to select a specific language (Shalom et al., 2009). Furthermore, Open Clinical© shows some methods for the computerization of clinical practice guidelines (OpenClinical 2002-2011). Although these proposals are very relevant for the definition of a clinical guideline, they have not been aimed at representing rules that can be executed or validated in an automatic way on a set of electronic health records,. Although there are frameworks for the compliance evaluation of a set of rules versus specific medical records, they are focused on specific diseases (Toussi et al., 2008) or only evaluate a particular type of conditional (Rao, Krishnan & Niculescu, 2006).

The purpose of this paper is to present EXEMED v2, a system that allows structuring the rules related to clinical guidelines and evaluating them over a set of EHR; EXEMED v2 is an interactive system able to evaluate structured attributes of EHR as well as narrative text attributes. This paper is organized as follows: Section 2 presents some previous research. Section 3, describes the components of EXEMED v2. Section 4 presents the elements used to describe a clinical practice guideline. Section 5, shows the application of the proposal considering a particular disease taken as a case study. Finally, Section 6 describes conclusions and future work.

BACKGROUND

Clinical practice guidelines research has been primarily oriented to: the methodology for defining a guideline, the extraction of narrative text found in a guideline, and indicator assessment of adherence to the guideline (extracted from electronic medical records). This section analyzes the main research initiatives related to the definition of languages or models to express rules and indicators for evaluating the adherence to clinical guidelines.

PROforma, Arden and Gem are compared based on their ability to express rules about clinical guidelines. Basically, PROforma is defined as a process-modeling language that supports the definition of clinical guidelines and protocols as long as a well-defined set of tasks and logical constructs are already in place (Sutton, Taylor, & Earle, 2006). PROforma uses schemas with decision tasks. Arden, a standard from HL7, is an organized structure of MLM - Medical Logic Module - that can be triggered. The syntax has categories and slots; within each category there is a set of slots (Health Level Seven International, 1999), these slots are used for MLM knowledge base maintenance and change control. Arden is useful in many areas, but in terms of clinical guidelines it does not have a standard vocabulary to compare the rules with electronic health records. GEM uses XML schema to describe a comprehensive set of attributes and it can be depicted as a direct graph with indicators from a guideline (Shiffman et al., 2000). Something relevant from GEM is that rules can be categorized as conditional or imperative statements. GEM applies a set of constructs derived from a decision table mode, which offers considerable capabilities for representing and manipulating guideline logic.

In PROforma, Arden and Gem the terminology is different, but they support a basic set of guideline tasks, including: decisions, actions and entry criteria (Ten Teije, Miksch & Lucas, 2008). They have similar components in their syntaxes, as can be seen in Table 1:

As shown in Table 1, PROforma has a different condition statement due to the complexity of languages and the ability to be used by a programming tool.

In addition to the previous comparison, it is also considered important to analyze what rules these languages can describe. Table 2 compares the ability of each one of the proposals to describe precisely a rule considering the elements included in column one.

As can be seen in Table 2, none of the proposals considers all the concepts required for defining the executable rules of clinical guideline. Even though Arden is the most comprehensive proposal, it is more focused on sharing any kind of medical knowledge and due to that its direct evaluation for the analysis of clinical practice guidelines is not straightforward.

From the point of view of the automatic evaluation of clinical guidelines there are not so many proposals, as far as we know. The first work

Table 1. Syntax comparison between: PROforma, Arden and GEM

PROforma (Fox, Patkar & Thomson, 2006), (Zur Muehlen & Shapiro, 2010)	Arden (Fehre, & Adlassnig, 2011), (Samwald et al., 2012)	Gem (Shiffman et al., 2010), (Shiffman,1997)
Unambiguously transitions between states of a task, four conditions has to be used: Start (x), Discarded (x), Cycle (x) and Completed (x)	Call '.....' If .... Conclude ...	IF... THEN clause can be replaced by IF... THEN...BECAUSE.
Allows PROforma specification, defined the value of any expression. The classes that are used to instantiate these objects are arranged in an inheritance hierarchy. The value of the precondition property of a task must be a truth-valued expression.	**For example:** Call causes the MLM named "hyperkalemia" to be executed and this concludes "true" if the potassium is greater than 5 call `hyperkalemia` if potassium > 5.0 then conclude true end if	**For example:** in a child with minor closed head trauma, IF there was no loss of consciousness, THEN skull radiographs are not recommended BECAUSE the substantial rate of false positive radiographs and the low prevalence of intracranial injury among this specific subset of patients lead to a low predictive value of serious injury.

Table 2. Indicators used by PROforma, Arden and GEM

General Indicators	PROforma	Arden	GEM
Phase		x	
Diagnosis	x	x	x
Time	x	x	x
Risk Factor	x	x	
Antecedents	x	x	x
Severity Level			
Location		x	x
Medical interventions	x	x	x
Adverse event		x	

Where:

Phase: It is defined as the possible stages where the patient can be. Such as: Triage, Hospitalization, and Outpatient.

Diagnosis: Defined as ICD10 Code (World Health Organization, 2010).

Time: Defined as the periodicity of an event: years, months, weeks, days, hours, minutes, and seconds.

Risk Factor: It includes variables such as: age, sex, ethnicity and weight.

Antecedents: It is the background related to the pathological, pharmacological, surgical, allergy, toxic, obstetrics and gynecology aspects.

Severity Level: It defines the level into which the patient is with respect to a specific diagnosis: Stable, Crisis, risk grading.

Location: It describes where the patient is located. Examples are General Hospitalization or Intensive Care Unit

Behaviors and interventions: It includes prescribed medicines, prescribed exams, delivered medicine, delivered exams, procedures.

Adverse event: Unexpected events detected after a medicine prescription or procedure.

proposes a framework for analyzing the adherence to clinical practice guidelines on diabetes. This proposal includes a rule-based engine that allows the definition of the type, class and doses for each one of the drugs that are to be evaluated for the treatment of a patient with diabetes. Once these rules are defined, they are compared with the information included in a set of prescriptions given by medical doctors (Toussi et al., 2008). The second work allows in first place structuring medical records using Bayesian techniques and then verifies the adherence to clinical practice guidelines comparing them with the list of suggested drugs in the guideline (Rao, Krishnan & Niculescu, 2006).

As can be seen in previous proposals, frameworks are focused on a single diagnosis or are specialized in a particular type of rule, as the ones related to the prescription of drugs. The aim of this paper is to present a system that allows the definition of rules for a clinical practice guideline and its evaluation using the facts contained in electronic health records.

EXEMED V2: A SYSTEM FOR THE EVALUATION OF CLINICAL PRACTICE GUIDELINE RULES

This section presents EXEMED v2, a system that allows the definition of executable rules that can be applied over EHRs in order to determine its compliance with respect to a specific clinical practice guideline. EXEMED v2 defines the concepts and roles that can be used to define rules derived from a specific clinical guideline. These rules can be evaluated using the facts contained in the medical repository where the EHRs are stored. The evaluation of a rule enables us to identify whether or not the EHR satisfies it.

EXEMED v2 is composed of a set of modules that allow structuring a clinical practice guideline and evaluating the compliance of a set of EHR to it. Figure 1 presents the main modules. The Evaluation Instrument module, which is used to define the rules related to the clinical practice guideline; the Compliance Evaluation module that executes the evaluation of the rules over a set of EHRs; the

Figure 1. EXEMED components

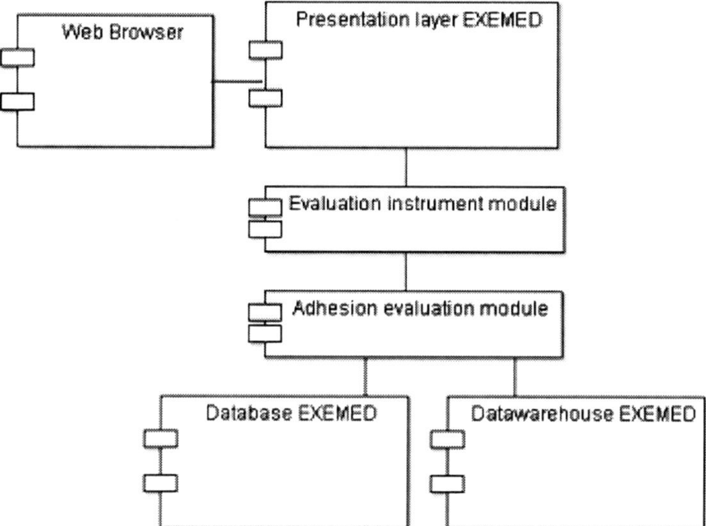

Extraction module in charge of extracting the facts from the medical repository and stores them in a data warehouse; and the Storage module that stores the rules and the results of EXEMED v2. In the following each one of the modules is going to be explained.

Evaluation Instrument Module

The definition of a clinical practice guideline on EXEMED v2 is made using this module. An evaluation instrument is created for each clinical practice guideline that wanted to be evaluated. This instrument represents the set of conditionals that must be accomplished by the EHRs. Each conditional is expressed using a Precedent and a Consequent. Section 4 presents the way these conditionals are defined.

When a user wants to define a clinical practice guideline on EXEMED, he or she has to create a new evaluation instrument for the particular diagnosis; including a header with the name of the instrument, the author, the related diagnosis, etc., and the set of conditionals that describe the guide. Finally, the defined guideline is represented using ARDEN notation.

Extraction Module

For the evaluation of compliance EXEMED v2 must obtain the facts related to patient treatments or characteristics that are typically contained in an EHR system. This module contains the logic required to extract the facts and store them incrementally in a data warehouse. The data warehouse was designed using a star schema with a main fact table that represents the Attention that a patient receives. It also includes a set of dimensions that includes all the details around this attention. The main dimensions are Patient, Time, Diagnosis, Medications, Procedures and Text Notes.

It is important to note that in order to use EXEMED with a specific EHR system this module should be parameterized according to the characteristics of the system database structure.

Compliance Evaluation Module

Using the facts contained in the data warehouse and the rules defined in the evaluation instrument, this module evaluates the compliance of each patient and generates an adherence report. The input to generate this report is a list of patient's identifiers, a range of dates and the identifier of an evaluation instrument. The report consolidates the level of coincidence of the evaluation instrument on the events registered in the EHR system.

In order to evaluate the compliance this module uses structured and non-structured information contained in the data warehouse. Depending on the variables involved in each rule, the system classifies it as a rule that can be automatically evaluated or semi-automatically evaluated. Automatic rules correspond to those that include concepts that can be compared only with structured attributes in the data warehouse. Semiautomatic rules are those that include concepts that should be evaluated in at least one attribute that contains narrative texts.

For the evaluation of automatic rules the system creates dynamically a query that is executed in the data warehouse. In the case of semiautomatic rules, the system applies techniques of natural language processing to search the terms involved in the rule. The following sections explain these processes.

Evaluation of Automatic Rules

In order to assess the compliance of a condition over a patient's related fact, it is necessary to know where a specific concept of a conditional can be evaluated in the data warehouse. This information is included in a knowledge base contained in the Compliance Evaluation Module. However, this information can be modified in case it is necessary.

Given a variable v1 that is structured, EXEMED retrieves information from the knowledge base and dynamically creates the query. It finds for each patient the events in a specified range of dates; for these events the dynamic query is applied. If associated information exists, the system will mark the event as adherent; on the contrary, the system will mark the event as non-adherent.

Evaluation of Semi-Automatic Rules

In the case of unstructured information, the system creates a set of lists containing the entities defined in the conditional. EXEMED uses a natural language processing framework and creates a corpus of documents with each one of the texts related to each patient. Besides, it includes dynamically the lists into the logic of the entity recognition module of the framework. Then, the system runs a task pipeline to search the entities previously defined. If the system finds entities, it will mark the event as adherent. In case semiautomatic conditionals cannot be evaluated, the system shows the narrative texts related to the patient attention to the user; with these texts the user can interact with EXEMED v2 to manually establish if the attention is compliant with the rule. That is the reason why the evaluation in EXEMED v2 is considered semi-automatic.

Storage Module

This module manages the storage of the evaluation instruments, the results of the evaluations and some parametric data about drugs, procedure, diagnoses, etc.

EXEMED CONDITIONAL DEFINITION

As it was presented in Section 3 EXEMED v2 allows defining the type of patients that are relevant for a medical guideline using conditionals. Each conditional represents a characteristic that a patient should have in order to match the guideline.

The objective of EXEMED v2 is to identify the sets of patient records that effectively accomplish the conditionals. Figure 2 presents an example of this. The set A contains all the patients with a specific disease: type 1 Diabetes. The set B represents patients that are located in a specific place in the medical institution; for example, in the intensive care unit. Finally, set C represents all the patients with a medical intervention; for example glycated hemoglobin. The intention of these sets definition is to identify the set D that includes the patients that satisfy the characteristics of the three sets, because they are the ones who satisfy the rule of the guideline that declares that all the patients with diabetes in the intensive care unit should have glycated hemoglobin measured.

The conditionals are defined through concepts; these were identified through the analysis and evaluation of the rules and indicators derived from a sample of clinical guidelines and from sessions with medical doctors with four different medical specializations. Each concept can be used to define the characteristics of a set of patients. A set may be related to one concept or to several concepts. The concepts are explained in the following list.

Conduct or Medical Intervention is the act, fact or method of interfering with the outcome or course of a medical condition. These concepts are specialized in Laboratory Test, Medical Education, Medicine Supply and Procedure.

Location is the place where a medical act, fact or method occurs. The values of location may vary, but typically they include intensive care unit, patient room, pediatric unit and surgical area, among others.

Risk Factor represents all the elements that can increase the likelihood of developing a disease. There are specializations of this concept like biological factor, race, unhealthy behavior, absence of protective behavior and age. (World Health Organization, 2014).

Severity Level describes the categories that measure the relative impact of a disease on a patient. The level may vary according to the diagnosis, but in general they can be specialized in mild, moderate and severe level.

Adverse Event is an injury related to medical management. Medical management includes all aspects of care, including diagnosis and treatment,

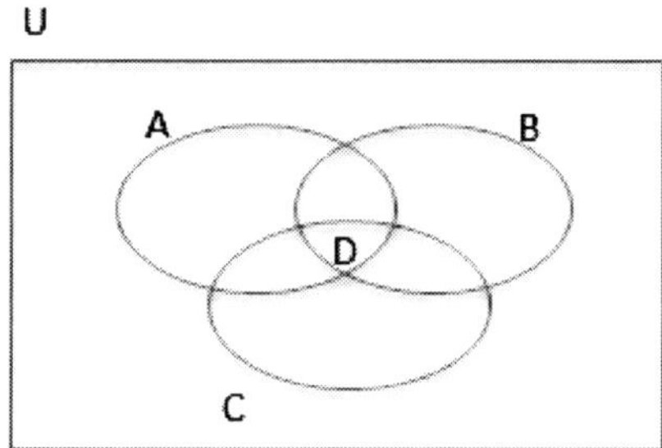

Figure 2. Patient sets

$$A = \text{Patient} \cap hasDiagnosis.T$$
$$B = \text{Patient} \cap inLocation.T$$
$$C = \text{Patient} \cap hasMedicalIntervention.T$$
$$D = A \cap B \cap C$$

failure to diagnose or treat, and the systems and equipment used to deliver care. The concept can be specialized in different concepts like pain, fatigue, convulsion, altered mood, nausea and flushing, among others. (World Health Organization, 2005), (Adverse Events Inc., 2014).

Diagnosis is the identification of the possible patient disease or disorder. It was included because several clinical guidelines include rules associated with a secondary diagnosis; for example diabetes guidelines include rules related to hypertensive patients.

Moment during the attention of the patient. For example admission, hospitalization, hospital discharge, etc.

Antecedent is a relevant patient fact that occurs before and may be linked to subsequent events.

Besides these concepts we define the concept Time that allows describing frequencies related to another concept.

EXEMED APPLICATION IN A CASE STUDY

In order to define rules derived from clinical practice guidelines, as described above, a case study was carried out in a Hospital of Bogotá, Colombia.

This case was implemented through a prototype built using Java, MySQL database and GATE NLP framework; different iterations were executed with the stakeholders who analyzed different cases associated with different specializations. A group of medical doctors provided the rules in narrative texts, based on a specific guideline. Another group of medical doctors defined the rules using the concepts provided by EXEMED.

The case study was aimed at the creation of the evaluation instrument of the clinical practice guideline of Acute Myocardial Infarction (AMI). Hospital staff parameterized the conditionals using the EXEMED prototype. These conditionals are:

1. Any patient suspected of IAMCSST should receive dual antiplatelet therapy unless there any contraindications, at the doses indicated in the guidelines, with bolus of ASA and clopidogrel in patients older than 75 years, Prasugrel and Ticagrelor according to choosing the emergency physician and in accordance with the instructions given in the guidelines.

Which is expressed as:

IF (MOMENT (URGENCY)) AND (RISK FACTORS (AGE YEARS between 1 and 75))

THEN (CONDUCT AND INTERVENTION (DRUGS MADE ACETIL salicylic acid)) AND (CONDUCT AND INTERVENTION (DRUGS MADE CLOPIDOGREL TABLETS 300 MG) OR CONDUCT AND INTERVENTION (DRUGS MADE PRASUGEL 60 MG))

2. Any patient with presumptive Dx AMI must first EKG in the first 10 minutes of arrival at the emergency department performed by qualified and trained personnel.

Which is expressed as:

IF (MOMENT(URGENCY)) AND (TIME (MINUTES [between] 1 [and] 10)) THEN (CONDUCT AND INTERVENTION (STANDARD PROCEDURES EKG))

3. Any patient suspected of IAMCSST admission to the emergency room should have a blood sample for measurement of biomarkers in the first 30 minutes of arrival at the service.

Which is expressed as:

IF (MOMENT (URGENCY)) AND (TIME (MINUTES [between] 1 [and] 30))

THEN (CONDUCT AND INTERVENTION (PROCEDURES CREATINA)) AND (CONDUCT AND INTERVENTION (PROCEDURES TROPONIN I QUANTITATIVE))

The application of EXEMED using this case study allows us to validate its usefulness in describing different kinds of rules derived from different types of diseases. It is important to highlight that during the initial execution of this case it was necessary to assist the medical doctors who create the rules using the prototype; however, once they received the initial training, they improved their ability to create rules by themselves considerably. Moreover, it is important to note that the definition of the evaluation instrument must differentiate whether the conditional corresponds to a conditional related to an acute condition or a chronic diagnosis. This distinction is very important to decide whether to assess compliance in all attentions of the patient during a period of time, or at each attention of the patient during the period of time, respectively.

CONCLUSION

This paper presents EXEMED v2, a system that allows the evaluation of clinical practice guideline indicators using the information contained in Electronic Health Records (EHR). EXEMED v2 provides the concepts and roles needed to express the sets of elements relevant for the definition of rules based on a clinical guideline. The main concepts included in EXEMED v2 are Medical Intervention, Location, Risk Factor, Severity Level, Adverse Event, Diagnosis, Moment, Antecedent and Time.

The implementation of EXEMED v2 provides flexibility to create any kind of rule and to extend it as needed. Moreover, it is useful to evaluate these rules over structured as well as non-structured attributes of EHR.

One of the lessons learned when the compliance evaluation strategy of EXEMED v2 was designed is that it is important to distinguish between different types of conditionals according to the type of concepts they contain. If the concepts can be evaluated using only structured information, it can be classified as an automatic conditional; if it requires the analysis of narrative texts, it would be classified as semi-automatic. In addition, in order to obtain a consistent evaluation, it is mandatory to establish for each conditional if it corresponds to an acute condition or a chronic disease. This fact was very important to establish the way the conditionals should be evaluated.

For future work, it is very important to continue testing the system with different types of diagnosis or conditions. In addition, it is necessary to improve the analysis of natural language to be able to represent more knowledge around the defined conditionals.

REFERENCES

Adverse Events Inc. (2014). *Adverse Events redefining drug safet*. Retrieved from https://www.adverseevents.com/. [Last consulted: Thursday, 10th April 2014]

Álvarez, C. A., Cortés, J. A., Gómez, C. H., Fernández, J. A., Sossa, M. P., Beltrán, F., & Padilla, A. et al. (2010). Guías de práctica clínica para la prevención de infecciones intrahospitalarias asociadas al uso de dispositivos médicos. *Infectio*, *14*(4), 292–308. doi:10.1016/S0123-9392(10)70123-5

Bassand, J. P., Hamm, C. W., Ardissino, D., Boersma, E., Budaj, A., & Fernández-Avilés, F. et al.. (2007). Guía de Práctica Clínica para el diagnóstico y tratamiento del síndrome coronario agudo sin elevación del segmento ST. *Revista Espanola de Cardiologia*, *60*(10), 1070–1080.

Casteleiro, M. A., Des, J., Prieto, M. J. F., Perez, R., & Paniagua, H. (2009). Executing medical guidelines on the web: Towards next generation healthcare. *Knowledge-Based Systems*, *22*(7), 545–551. doi:10.1016/j.knosys.2008.10.003

Dunkley, C., & Cross, J. H. (2006). NICE guidelines and the epilepsies: How should practice change? *Archives of Disease in Childhood*, *91*(6), 525–528. doi:10.1136/adc.2005.080036 PMID:16714728

Fehre, K., & Adlassnig, K. P. (2011). *Service-oriented Arden-syntax-based clinical decision support. Proceedings of eHealth2011* (pp. 123–128). Vienna: Austrian Computer Society.

Field, M. J., & Lohr, K. N. (Eds.). (1990). Clinical Practice Guidelines: Directions for a New Program (Vol. 90, No. 8). National Academies Press.

Fox, J., Patkar, V., & Thomson, R. (2006). Decision support for health care: The PROforma evidence base. *Informatics in Primary Care, 14*(1), 49–54. PMID:16848966

Health Level Seven International (HL7) (1999), *The Arden Syntax for Medical Logic Systems*, v.2.1.

Jovell, A. J. (1999). Metodología de diseño de guías de práctica clínica.*Mapfre Med, 10*(sIII).

Ministerio de Salud y Protección Social. (2012). *Guías de práctica clínica GPC*. Bogotá, Colombia. Retrieved from http://gpc.minsalud.gov.co/Pages/Default.aspx

OPEN Clinical Knowledge management for medical care. *Methods and tools to support the computerisation of clinical practice guidelines: a short introduction.* Copyright OpenClinical. Retrieved from http://www.openclinical.org/gmmintro.html [Last consulted: Thursday, 10th April 2014]

Rao, R. B., Krishnan, S., & Niculescu, R. S. (2006). Data mining for improved cardiac care. *ACM SIGKDD Explorations Newsletter, 8*(1), 3–10. doi:10.1145/1147234.1147236

Samwald, M., Fehre, K., De Bruin, J., & Adlassnig, K. P. (2012). The Arden Syntax standard for clinical decision support: Experiences and directions. *Journal of Biomedical Informatics, 45*(4), 711–718. doi:10.1016/j.jbi.2012.02.001 PMID:22342733

Shalom, E., Shahar, Y., Taieb-Maimon, M., Bar, G., Martins, S. B., & Young, O. et al.. (2009). Can physicians structure clinical guidelines? Experiments with a mark-up-process methodology. In *Knowledge Management for Health Care Procedures* (pp. 67–80). Springer Berlin Heidelberg. doi:10.1007/978-3-642-03262-2_6

Shiffman, R. N. (1997). Representation of clinical practice guidelines in conventional and augmented decision tables. *Journal of the American Medical Informatics Association, 4*(5), 382–393. doi:10.1136/jamia.1997.0040382 PMID:9292844

Shiffman, R. N., Karras, B. T., Agrawal, A., Chen, R., Marenco, L., & Nath, S. (2000). GEM: A proposal for a more comprehensive guideline document model using XML. *Journal of the American Medical Informatics Association, 7*(5), 488–498. doi:10.1136/jamia.2000.0070488 PMID:10984468

Sutton, D. R., Taylor, P., & Earle, K. (2006). Evaluation of PROforma as a language for implementing medical guidelines in a practical context. *BMC Medical Informatics and Decision Making, 6*(1), 20. doi:10.1186/1472-6947-6-20 PMID:16597341

Svátek, V., & Růžička, M. (2003). Step-by-step mark-up of medical guideline documents. *International Journal of Medical Informatics, 70*(2), 329–335. doi:10.1016/S1386-5056(03)00041-8 PMID:12909185

Ten Teije, A., Miksch, S., & Lucas, P. (Eds.). (2008). *Computer-based medical guidelines and protocols: a primer and current trends* (Vol. 139). Ios Press.

Toussi, M., Ebrahiminia, V., Le Toumelin, P., Cohen, R., & Venot, A. (2008). An automated method for analyzing adherence to therapeutic guidelines: Application in diabetes. *Studies in Health Technology and Informatics, 136*, 339. PMID:18487754

World Health Organization. (2005). Draft guidelines for adverse event reporting and learning systems. Geneva, Switzerland: Author. Retrieved March, 16, 2010.

World Health Organization. (2010). *International statistical classification of diseases and related health problems* (Vol. 1). World Health Organization. Retrieved from http://www.who.int/classifications/icd/ICD10Volume2_en_2010.pdf, [Last consulted: Thursday, 10th January 2015]

World Health Organization. (2014), *Health Topics, Risk Factors*. Retrieved from http://www.who.int/topics/risk_factors/en/ [Last consulted: Thursday, 10th April 2014]

Zur Muehlen, M., & Shapiro, R. (2010). Business process analytics. In *Handbook on Business Process Management 2* (pp. 137–157). Springer Berlin Heidelberg. doi:10.1007/978-3-642-01982-1_7

Chapter 34
LiveCity:
The Impact of Video Communication on Emergency Medicine

Camilla Metelmann
Universitätsmedizin Greifswald, Germany

Michael Wendt
Universitätsmedizin Greifswald, Germany

Bibiana Metelmann
Universitätsmedizin Greifswald, Germany

Konrad Meissner
Universitätsmedizin Greifswald, Germany

Martin von der Heyden
Universitätsmedizin Greifswald, Germany

ABSTRACT

The goal of emergency medicine is to treat time-critical diseases and conditions to reduce morbidity and mortality. The improvement of emergency medicine is an important topic for governments worldwide. A common problem is the inevitable lack of support by emergency doctors, when paramedics need their assistance at the emergency site but are without an emergency doctor. Video-communication in real time from the emergency site to an emergency doctor, offers an opportunity to enhance the quality of emergency medicine. The core piece of this study is a video camera system called "LiveCity camera", enabling real-time high quality video connection of paramedics and emergency doctors. The impact of video communication on emergency medicine is clearly appreciated among providers, based upon the extent of agreement that has been stated in this study´s questionnaire by doctors and paramedics. This study is part of the FP7-European Union funded research project "LiveCity" (Grant Agreement No. 297291).

DOI: 10.4018/978-1-4666-8756-1.ch034

INTRODUCTION

Emergency medicine is a crucial part of all health care systems worldwide. The goal of emergency medicine is to treat time-critical diseases or conditions and thus reduce preventable disabilities and deaths. Citizens often judge their government by the quality of critical infrastructure regarding for instance security and emergency medicine (Hsia, Razzak, Tsai, & Hirshon, 2010; Razzak & Kellermann, 2002). One approach to further improve emergency medicine is to balance existing healthcare disparities by using telemedicine. Telemedicine are ICTs (information and communication technologies) in medicine enabling diagnostics and treatment of diseases over geographical distances (Kazley, McLeod, & Wager, 2012; WHO, 2011). Telemedicine is an important future topic as described in the "Global Observatory for eHealth" by the World Health Organization, and the implementation of telemedicine is one of the goals of the European Union (Economic and Social Committee, 2008; WHO, 2011). Telemedicine devices, using a high-definition video communication in real time, offer the highest amount of information-transfer currently available.

This study is an integral part of the FP7- European Union funded research project LiveCity (Grant Agreement No. 297291). The LiveCity Project studies how high-definition video communication in real time can positively contribute to the quality of life of citizens or communities within the European Union in many different areas (Chochliouros, Stephanakis, Spiliopoulou, Sfakianakis, & Ladid, 2012; Weerakkody, El-Haddadeh, Chochliouros, & Morris, 2012). A special video camera, called "LiveCity camera" was developed to connect the different providers of emergency medicine in the European Union - the paramedics at the emergency site and a (remote) emergency doctor.

This study aims to analyze the impact of video communication on emergency medicine. First the medical emergency systems worldwide and in Germany in particular are introduced, followed by a paragraph on the use of telemedicine in emergency medicine and the concept of a tele emergency doctor. In the next section the methodology of the study is described with information regarding the "LiveCity camera". A selection of results is presented and afterwards discussed. Finally conclusions are drawn concerning the impact of video communication on emergency medicine.

BACKGROUND OF STUDY

Medical Emergency System Worldwide

Medical emergency systems are different constitutively or to some extent in every country worldwide. Sometimes even within one country there are different emergency systems, for example China had seven different emergency systems in 2007 (Huiyi, 2007). In some countries the urban areas can provide a higher developed system than rural areas (Vaitkaitis, 2008).

To categorize the variety of systems four different types might be differentiated: (1) no organized structure, (2) basic life support, (3) advanced life support with paramedics and (4) advanced life support with physicians (Roudsari et al., 2007):

1. Many developing countries in Sub-Saharan Africa or parts of Asia have no organized prehospital emergency system (Ali, Miyoshi, & Ushijima, 2006). However in line with population growth, urbanization and industrialization there is an ongoing shift from infectious diseases towards medical conditions like cardiovascular diseases and vehicle accidents. Due to

medical reasons this calls for a higher need of medical emergency systems (Kirsch et al., 1995; VanRooyen, Thomas, & Clem, 1999; WHO, 1996). One approach to improve the quality of emergency medicine in those countries is to teach volunteers of the community high quality first aid (Kobusingye OC, 2006);

2. Basic life support works without trained medical professionals at the emergency site and focuses on fast transport to a hospital and keeping the patient alive during transport, which is for instance the case in Zimbabwe (Thomson, 2005). Advanced life support systems in comparison work on a more sophisticated level of care at the emergency site and during the transport to a hospital, but depend upon well-educated and medically qualified providers (Roudsari et al., 2007);

3. Advanced life support with paramedics as single providers at the emergency site is also called the Anglo-American model. It was developed in the United States of America (Pozner, Zane, Nelson, & Levine, 2004) and is also used e.g. in Ireland (Cummins et al., 2013), the United Kingdom (Black & Davies, 2005), Canada (Symons & Shuster, 2004), Australia (Trevithick, Flabouris, Tall, & Webber, 2003), New Zealand (Hay, 2000), Singapore (Lateef, 2006), South Africa (MacFarlane, Loggerenberg, & Kloeck, 2005) and the Netherlands (Dib, Naderi, Sheridan, & Alagappan, 2006);

4. Advanced life support with paramedics working together with physicians at the emergency site is called Franco-German model (Al-Shaqsi, 2010). It is for example used in France (Adnet & Lapostolle, 2004), Germany (Roessler & Zuzan, 2006), Denmark (Langhelle et al., 2004), Israel (Ellis & Sorene, 2008), Brazil (Timerman, Gonzalez, Zaroni, & Ramires, 2006) and Greece (Papaspyrou et al., 2004) and in the urban areas of Portugal (Gomes, Araújo, Soares-Oliveira, & Pereira, 2004) and Lithuania (Vaitkaitis, 2008).

The main difference between the two advanced life support models is that the Anglo-American model brings the patient to the doctor and in the Franco-German model the doctor is brought to the patient (Dick, 2003).

Medical Emergency System in Germany

The German Medical Emergency System as an example of the Franco-German model is a dual system with two partners, i.e. paramedics and emergency doctors (Harding et al., 2013). Paramedics receive a one- to three-year education in handling emergency situations (Becker, Hündorf, Kill, & Lipp, 2006). Emergency doctors are medical doctors with a special training in intensive care medicine and qualification in emergency medicine (Bundesärztekammer, 2011b).

Figure 1 shows the pathway of a patient, who experiences an emergency and alerts the medical emergency system. The first and prerequisite step is that either the patient or a first-aider, which might be a relative, friend or bystander observing the situation, calls for help. The number to call is 112, the European emergency number, which can be dialed free of charge in case of a medical emergency in all EU countries, Switzerland, Montenegro, Turkey and South Africa (EuropeanComission, 2014).

The 112 call is answered by the emergency dispatcher, who is a paramedic with a special training. The emergency dispatcher will assess all relevant details and will ask the caller for further information, if necessary. The emergency dispatcher will rank with aid of a so-called "Notarztindikationskatalog", an index of urgent necessity, the emergency into the categories "emergency doctor required" or "no emergency doctor required" (Bundesärztekammer, 2013).

Figure 1. Pathway of medical emergency system in Germany

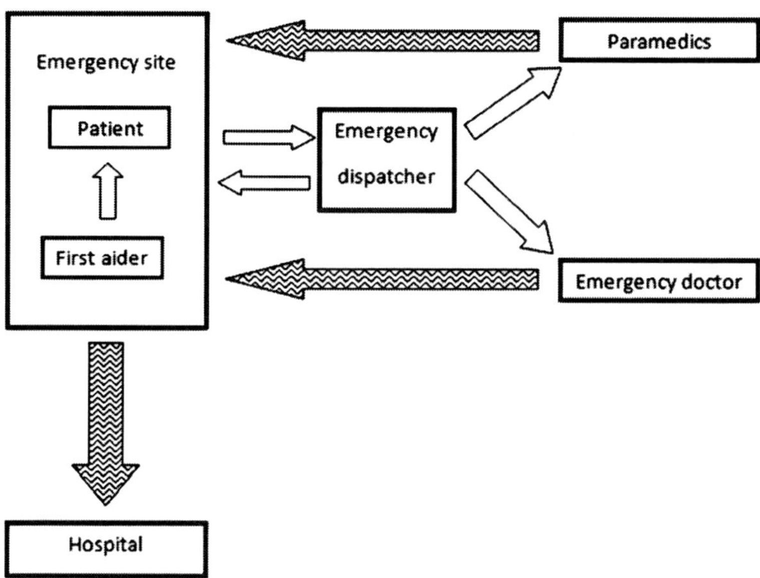

In either case a team of two paramedics will be sent to the emergency site. If the emergency seems to be life-threatening or potentially life-threatening, an emergency doctor is required in addition (Schilling et al., 2012). Hence in this case the emergency dispatcher will alert both the paramedics and the emergency doctor. Approximately only one out of three to one out of four emergency situations require an emergency doctor (Roessler & Zuzan, 2006).

Because the paramedics are alerted in every emergency, there are more paramedics than emergency doctors. This allows a wider geographical spread of paramedics, which places the paramedics closer to potential sites of emergencies.

To bring paramedics and emergency doctors together to meet at the site of emergency, the rendezvous system has been established as the main procedure, that is used in 99.1% (Schmiedel & Behrendt, 2011). The paramedics and the emergency doctors approach the emergency with different cars and meet only at the emergency site (DeutscherBundestag17.Wahlperiode, 2010; Schmiedel & Behrendt, 2011). The rendezvous system allows a high flexibility and leads to a

substantial decrease in the time it takes for the first team of emergency personnel to arrive at the emergency site (Ellinger, 2011). Every federal state government in Germany is obliged by law to organize the required infrastructure for the emergency personnel to arrive within a predefined time (Becker et al., 2006; Binder, 1993). On average the paramedics in Germany arrive at the emergency site after 8.7 minutes and the emergency doctor after 12.3 minutes (Schmiedel & Behrendt, 2011).

At the emergency site doctor and paramedics establish a preliminary diagnosis and start the treatment. The treatment could be either completed at the emergency site, so that the patient can be left at home, which is the case in approximately 5% (Schmiedel & Behrendt, 2011). Or the patient has to be brought to the hospital. The transport of the patient to the hospital is done by the paramedics together with the emergency doctor. Once the patient is in the hospital, the hospital staff will continue the diagnostics and treatment and the paramedics and emergency doctor return to their different bases becoming available for the next emergency patient.

Tele Emergency Doctor

There are special situations, when the rendezvous system could benefit from support by telemedicine, e.g. by a tele emergency doctor. Figure 2 is introducing a tele emergency doctor as an auxiliary partner. The tele emergency doctor is an emergency doctor with special training, who works from a central dispatch place distant from the emergency site. The paramedics can get in contact with the doctor via telemedicine and ask for help.

Telemedicine offers an opportunity to balance uneven allocation of infrastructure and resources including human resources (Sood et al., 2007). Therefore it is used in many different medical disciplines and areas. For example it has huge advantages in emergency medicine, where the transfer of knowledge in short time is critical and potentially lifesaving (Amadi-Obi, Gilligan, Owens, & O'Donnell, 2014).

Telemedicine looks especially promising and supportive, when paramedics are without an emergency doctor at the emergency site but would like to consult one. The absence of the emergency doctor could have several reasons. For example, as mentioned above, in general the emergency doctor arrives at the emergency site some minutes after the paramedics. Although in most cases, this is just a short time, in life-threatening situations, these early minutes are especially crucial. Another reason might be that in the initial assessment the severe extent of the emergency was not identifiable, so that the emergency dispatcher only alerted the paramedics. And in some emergencies the situation can worsen very quickly and unexpectedly, so that it develops into a situation, where an emergency doctor would be needed. Additionally there are emergencies, which are not life-threatening, but in which paramedics would like to have guidance by an emergency doctor. Those situations might be, for example, rare diseases or special circumstances, e.g. difficulties during pregnancy.

In all situations, in which paramedics are without an emergency doctor at the emergency site, but would like to consult one, telemedicine might be the solution. The prerequisite for that is that there is a real time connection for live communication between the paramedics and the tele emergency doctor.

For this contact to be efficient, helpful and according to legal regulations in medicine, the distant consultation has to transport more information than a mere telephone call can perform. The "Model Professional Code for Physicians in

Figure 2. Pathway of medical emergency system in Germany with addition of a tele emergency doctor

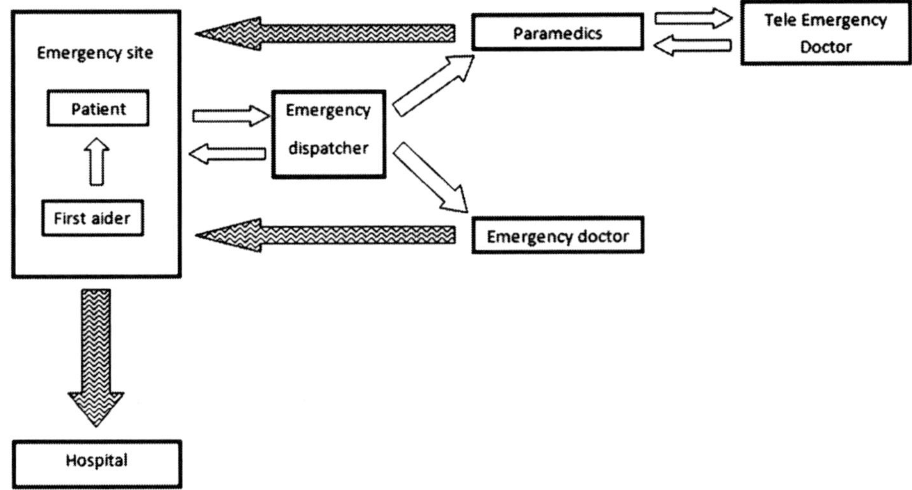

Germany" obligates physicians to an individual and direct treatment of patients also in telemedicine (Bundesärztekammer, 2011a; Katzenmeier & Schrag-Slavu, 2010). This could be achieved for instance by transmission of the patient's vital signs. Vital signs include blood pressure, heart rate and oxygen saturation and allow a dynamic evaluation of the current status of the patient. On the basis of the vital signs and the description of the situation and further information by the paramedics, the tele emergency doctor is now able to assist the paramedics in diagnostics and therapy.

Several different concepts of tele emergency doctors are currently under study or already implemented. One example is TemRas in Aachen, Germany, where an ambulance car is equipped with a video camera, which sends high-definition videos in real-time to the tele emergency doctor. This concept was implemented as part of the medical emergency system in the city of Aachen in April 2014 (Buscher et al., 2014; Kippnich, 2014; Rortgen et al., 2013; Skorning et al., 2009).

METHODOLOGY

LiveCity Camera

The central communicational device in this study is a special video camera with software and hardware newly developed by LiveCity Project-partners in Greece, Portugal and Ireland (Goncalves, Cordeiro, Batista, & Monteiro, 2012; Palma et al., 2013). This camera enables by a microPC a video connection via internet in real time. One of the essentials of good telemedical practice in emergency consultation is a real time connection. Even a small time lag leads to a disturbance in the communication between the paramedics and emergency doctor. The emergency doctor gives instructions based on all the information he got, observes the realization of the instructions, evaluates the actions and improves them, if needed. Hence a time lag is a huge hindrance and can result in such a poor communication, that no meaningful assistance by the emergency doctor is possible. At the same time the high legal standards regarding data security have to be met.

The LiveCity camera as shown in Figure 3 consists of the video-camera itself, worn with a headband above the right ear, a headphone with mouthpiece to enable audio connection in both ways and the microPC, which builds the internet connection. The position of the camera above the right ear was chosen to transmit the same perspective the paramedic has to the emergency doctor. Because the emergency doctor sees the emergency "through the eyes" of the paramedic, he is able to assess all relevant information he needs to evaluate the situation and can then guide even manual activities. The transmitted video is dynamic and follows the head movements of the paramedics. One major advantage of the position of the camera is also, that the paramedic still has both hands free to work, which is of great importance in emergency medicine. Since the work of paramedics requires a lot of bending and kneeling, the microPC is placed in a backpack.

Figure 3. The LiveCity camera worn by a paramedic

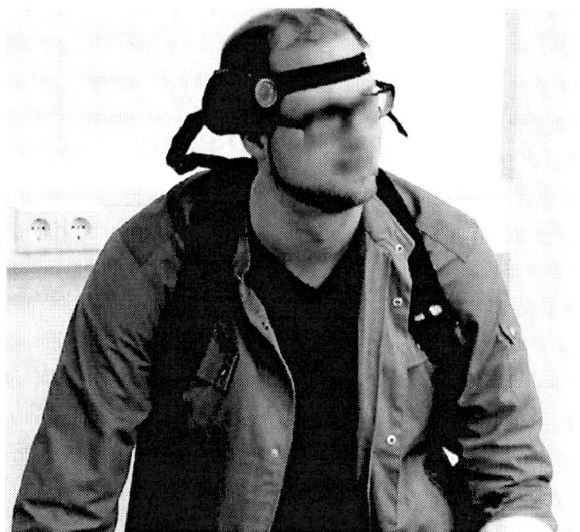

Software of the LiveCity Camera

The transmitted video is received by the remote emergency doctor at a laptop provided with special software (Figure 4). This software allows the emergency doctor to adapt the transmitted video according to the particular needs, e.g. regarding light, contrast and sound level. Another notable function is a snapshot feature. A snapshot can be taken by the emergency doctor at any time and is a high definition photo transmitted independently from the video. Because of the high pixel count it allows the emergency doctor to analyze certain aspects in detail. This is for example very useful for the interpretation of a 12-lead-ECG, where tiny elevations of lines can indicate a myocardial infarction. Because the interpretation of 12-lead-ECG is sometimes very challenging and needs a lot of experience, some authors state, that physicians have a higher success rate in detecting e.g. a heart attack than paramedics have (D. P. Davis et al., 2007). Therefore the snapshot feature was an integral part of the camera development.

Study Design

The aim of the study was to assess the impact of video communication on emergency medicine. The benefit of paramedics consulting a tele emergency doctor by use of the LiveCity camera was investigated in terms of professional work flow and outcome. To prevent potential harm for individuals the study was performed in the fully equipped medical simulation center of the Department of Anesthesiology and Intensive Care Medicine at Greifswald University Medicine (Figure 5). A medical simulation center creates dynamic realistic routine or emergency scenarios with aid of computer-operated mannequins (Johannsson, Ayida, & Sadler, 2005). It is widely used in medicine for educational and research purposes (Cannon-Diehl, 2009; Kyle & Murray, 2010; Levine, DeMaria, Schwartz, & Sim, 2013).

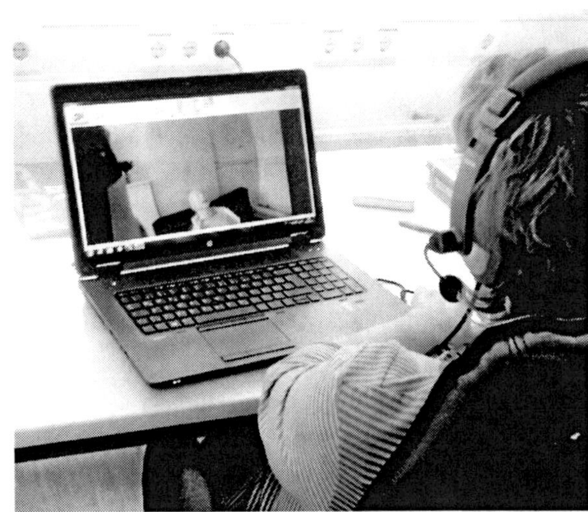

Figure 4. Tele emergency doctor observing emergency site via LiveCity camera

To evaluate the co-operation of paramedics and doctors close to reality, ten typical emergency scenarios from five different categories were standardized and structured for a randomized two-armed protocol. These categories are: "Trauma", "Heart attack", "Stroke", "Rare diseases" and "Complications during pregnancy". For each category two cases with

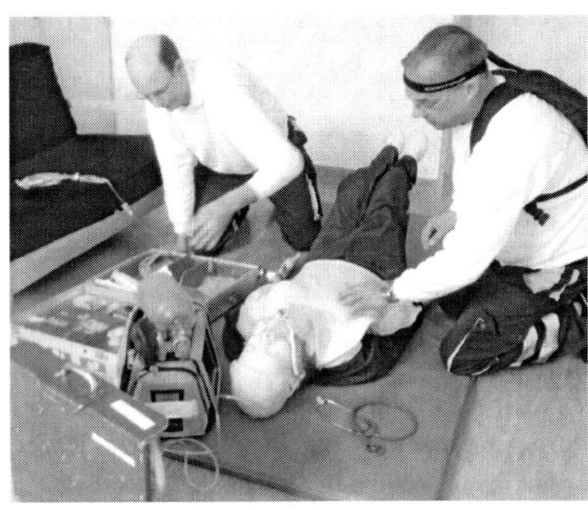

Figure 5. Paramedics at the emergency site treating a "patient" in the simulation center by use of LiveCity camera

similar level of difficulty in terms of diagnosis and treatment were created to allow a cross-over design. Cross-over design was achieved by comparing the results and opinions of paramedics in action at the simulated emergency site: (a) *without* doctor´s support and (b) the same paramedics in corresponding cases another time *with* video-based consultation and contact to a tele emergency doctor. According to usual guidelines in German emergency medicine two paramedics worked together as a team. The sequence of the case scenarios and the assignment to the two cross-over categories was randomized.

To assess the outcome in practical, technical and psychological aspects, paramedics and doctors were interviewed by use of structured questionnaires developed together with the Department for Medical Psychology, Greifswald University Medicine.

RESULTS

10 emergency doctors and 21 paramedics took part in a total of 110 simulated emergency scenarios. All participants (n =31) accomplished every scenario and completed all questionnaires. These are the results of the investigation in terms of "disagree", "partly disagree", "partly agree" or "agree" (ranked on a 4-point Likert scale) or concerning "yes" or "no" questions in the following sentences of the questionnaires:

- **"The scenarios were realistic"**: Considering the total number of 10 emergency doctors, 1 partly disagreed, 5 partly agreed, 4 agreed. Considering the total number of 21 paramedics, 1 partly disagreed, 11 partly agreed and 9 agreed. No emergency doctor or paramedic disagreed (See Table 1);
- **"The scenarios were relevant"**: Considering the total number of 10 emergency doctors, 3 partly agreed, 7 agreed. Considering the total number of 21 paramedics, 7 partly agreed, 14 agreed. No emergency doctor or paramedic disagreed or partly disagreed (See Table 2);
- **"What kind of support would you especially like to get in an emergency situation"**: The paramedics were asked to choose between "help with practical and manual skills" or "help with diagnostics and treatment". 6 of 21 paramedics wished for practical or manual help. 13 of 21 paramedics wished for help with diagnostics and treatment. 2 paramedics could not decide (See Table 3);
- **"I consider the tele emergency doctor as helpful"**: Considering the total number of 21 paramedics, 6 partly agreed and 15 agreed. No paramedic disagreed or partly disagreed (See Table 4);

Table 1. The scenarios were realistic

	Agree	Partly Agree	Partly Disagree	Disagree
Doctors (10)	4	5	1	0
Paramedics (21)	9	11	1	0

Table 2. The scenarios were relevant

	Agree	Partly Agree	Partly Disagree	Disagree
Doctors (10)	7	3	0	0
Paramedics (21)	14	7	0	0

Table 3. What kind of support would you especially like to get in an emergency situation?

	Diagnostics/ Treatment	Practical/ Manual	Undecided
Paramedics (21)	13	6	2

- **"Would you call a tele emergency doctor in cases you wouldn't normally call an emergency doctor"**: Considering the total number of 21 paramedics, 14 answered "yes" and 7 answered "no" (See Table 5);
- **"A tele emergency doctor improves the quality of patient care"**: Considering the total number of 10 emergency doctors, 7 partly agreed and 3 agreed. Considering the total number of 21 paramedics, 8 partly agreed and 13 agreed. No emergency doctor or paramedic disagreed or partly disagreed (See Table 6);
- **"I perceive that the tele emergency doctor leads to a faster start of the therapy"**: Considering the total number of 10 emergency doctors, 9 agreed (3 fully and 6 partly). 1 doctor disagreed partly, but no one to full extent. Of the paramedics, 20 of 21 agreed, in comparison more fully (11) than partly (9). 1 paramedic partly disagreed (See Table 7);
- **"Is transmission of the vital signs without audio or video connection sufficient"**: Only emergency doctors were asked, 8 of 10 answered "no" and 2 of 10 "yes" (See Table 8);
- **"Is transmission of the vital signs with additional audio connection sufficient"**: Again only emergency doctors were asked, and again 8 of 10 answered "no" and 2 of 10 "yes" (See Table 9);
- **"I can imagine working in a tele emergency doctor system"**: Of the emergency doctors 9 of 10 agreed to the summarizing sentence of the study, 4 to full extent and 5 partly. Among the paramedics 16 of 21 agreed and 4 of 21 partly agreed. 1 paramedic and 1 emergency doctor partly disagreed (See Table 10).

Table 4. I consider the tele emergency doctor as helpful

	Agree	Partly Agree	Partly Disagree	Disagree
Paramedics (21)	15	6	0	0

Table 5. Would you call a tele emergency doctor in cases you wouldn't normally call an emergency doctor?

	Yes	No
Paramedics (21)	14	7

Table 6. A tele emergency doctor improves the quality of patient care

	Agree	Partly Agree	Partly Disagree	Disagree
Doctors (10)	3	7	0	0
Paramedics (21)	13	8	0	0

Table 7. I perceive that the tele emergency doctor leads to faster start of the therapy

	Agree	Partly Agree	Partly Disagree	Disagree
Doctors (10)	3	6	1	0
Paramedics (21)	9	11	1	0

Table 8. Is transmission of the vital signs without audio or video connection sufficient?

	Yes	No
Doctors (10)	2	8

Table 9. Is transmission of the vital signs with additional audio connection sufficient?

	Yes	No
Doctors (10)	2	8

DISCUSSION

The impact of video communication on emergency medicine is very welcome among providers, based upon the amount of agreement of paramedics and emergency doctors in this study to a video-based consultation at the emergency site. This is an approach to increase quality of emergency treatment by applying telemedicine. The core piece of the concept is a special video camera, called LiveCity camera.

As Ammenwerth and coworkers have explained, there are three ways of testing a new health information technology. The first way is to evaluate it in a laboratory. But the results are limited by a low external validity. The second way is a field evaluation test, but for this both software and hardware have to be sufficiently mature to not possibly harm any person. So the solution is often the middle way: a simulation study, which combines good internal and external validity (Ammenwerth et al., 2012).

Simulation studies offer the opportunity to conduct experimental cross-over trials with high internal validity. The external validity depends on how realistic the simulated scenarios are. The perception of how realistic a scenario in a simulation center is, is influenced by three different aspects: the equipment fidelity, the environment fidelity and the psychological fidelity (Fritz, Gray, & Flanagan, 2008). The equipment fidelity is characterized by the used hard- and software. In the LiveCity Project the Laerdal mannequin Resusci Anne was used and the vital signs were dynamically simulated with the monitor iSimulate. The environment fidelity is mostly created by the appropriate surrounding for every scenario.

Table 10. I can imagine working in a tele emergency doctor system

	Agree	Partly Agree	Partly Disagree	Disagree
Doctors (10)	4	5	1	0
Paramedics (21)	16	4	1	0

In the LiveCity Project every scenario had different characteristic accessories, e.g. in one case of simulated heart attack a patient was watching sports sitting on a sofa with a football flag while eating potato crisps. Psychological fidelity is the ability of the individual participant to immerse into the simulated situation. Psychological fidelity can be increased by enhancing equipment and environment fidelity (Bauman, 2013).

After finishing all scenarios all participants were asked, if they perceived the simulated cases as realistic. The majority of both emergency doctors and paramedics rated the scenarios as realistic. Thus the possibility of the participants behaving in the study environment similar to their normal behavior is high. This implies a good external validity.

Furthermore all emergency doctors and paramedics partly agreed or agreed that the chosen scenarios were relevant. This is also an indicator for a good external validity. To reflect the broad spectrum of emergencies, different scenarios were developed. The categories "Trauma", "Heart attack" and "Stroke" were chosen, because they belong to the "First Hour Quintet". This term was coined by the sixth European Resuscitation Council Meeting in Florence, Italy in 2002 and describes five emergencies, which are life-threatening diseases in which a fast treatment reduces morbidity and mortality (Krafft et al., 2003; Nilsen, 2012). Worldwide they belonged to the group of top 10 leading causes of death in 2004 and prognosis for 2030 predict them to be within the top 5 leading causes of death worldwide

(WHO, 2010). Thus there are many approaches to improve the therapy, e.g. by telemedicine. The implementation of telemedicine in stroke treatment was recommended by the American Heart Association and American Stroke Association in 2009 (Schwamm et al., 2009). "Rare diseases" and "Complications during pregnancy" are a special challenge in medicine. Often there are no standard operating procedures and the paramedics might not have encountered a similar situation before, which increases the stress level. Another aspect in pregnancy is that the unborn child has to be considered, too e.g. in the application of drugs to manage the emergency. Therefore a video consultation of a tele emergency doctor might be helpful.

Since all paramedics and emergency doctors confirmed that the chosen scenarios were realistic and relevant, the simulation appears to be a suitable model and the findings of the LiveCity study might – at least partly – be transmitted from the simulation center into the existing medical emergency system.

To further assess the need for a tele emergency doctor, the paramedics, were asked, what kind of support they usually would like to get in a "normal" emergency. More than 2/3 of all paramedics answered, that they would want assistance in diagnostics and therapy. Because telemedicine enables the transfer of knowledge, this is the main area, where the tele emergency doctor can support.

One of the main purposes of the tele emergency doctor concept is that the emergency doctor supports and helps the paramedics at the emergency site by providing expertise (Czaplik et al., 2014). After completing all 10 scenarios in the LiveCity Project, all paramedics rated the tele emergency doctor as helpful. Hence they confirmed that knowledge can be transferred via telemedicine to the emergency site. This concept of the teleconsultation via video might be also expanded into other fields of emergency medicine. For example emergency doctors with limited experience, who are at the emergency site, might want to get support by a more experienced emergency doctor. Since some emergencies only occur rarely, the young emergency doctor might not have encountered a similar situation before (Gries, Zink, Bernhard, Messelken, & Schlechtriemen, 2006). And young emergency doctors often have a huge awareness of the responsibility they have and feel the difference between working in a hospital, where help by senior doctors is within reach and being the only doctor at the emergency site (Groos, 2011). Thus the young emergency doctor might also perceive an experienced tele emergency doctor as helpful.

Another advantage of the tele emergency doctor is that support by an emergency doctor is easily accessible without the expensive mobilization of many resources. Additionally this tele emergency support starts without time delay the moment the telemedicine connection is built. In the current German medical emergency system, the paramedic calls the emergency dispatcher, who then alerts the emergency doctor. The "normal" emergency doctor would now start to travel to the emergency site. This whole procedure takes some time, which directly leads to a later start of transport to the hospital. As explained earlier, this time difference could be crucial. Thus paramedics are more likely, to call an emergency doctor. This would presumable lead to a higher quality of emergency medicine.

Paramedics and emergency doctors were asked to rank the impact of a tele emergency doctor on the quality of patient care. All participants agreed or partly agreed that the tele emergency doctor improves the quality of patient care. Bashshur stated in 2002, that telemedicine has the potential to solve the existing problems in geographical differences in access to high standard medical care and might balance the uneven quality of care (Bashshur, 2002). So the improvement of patient care by the tele emergency doctor might be also used to enhance quality of diagnostics and therapies in geographical areas, where a high standard couldn't be achieved before. It would be very interesting to test the concept of a tele emergency doctor in countries outside of the European Union as well, which have not the medical emergency system of "advanced life support", but "basic life support" or "no organized structure". In these systems the transfer of expertise is even more important and can increase the quality of patient care immensely. Roughly 90% of all trauma-related death worldwide occur in developing countries (Gosselin, Spiegel, Coughlin, & Zirkle, 2009). In these countries most trauma-related fatalities happen in the prehospital phase and some could be preventable through appropriate prehospital care (Anand, Singh, & Kapoor, 2013; Mock, Jurkovich, nii-Amon-Kotei, Arreola-Risa, & Maier, 1998). The World Health Organization has published a manual in 2005 how prehospital trauma care management worldwide could be improved (Sasser, Varghese, Kellermann, & Lormand, 2005). One concept for countries without an organized medical emergency system or with a low-grade medical emergency system was to teach volunteer citizens principles of basic life support. These volunteers could then work together to improve the prehospital care. One of the problems in teaching laypersons, who had not received a medical education before, is the low level of literacy (Callese et al., 2014). Therefore there is a need for special curricula, which uses the existing resources. A review by Callese and coworkers showed that trained volunteers can reduce the mortality after trauma. If the volunteers could get help by a remote emergency doctor via telemedicine, this could lead to an even higher increase in quality of care. This telemedicine connection could, for instance, be easily achieved with the LiveCity camera.

As mentioned above, rapid start of treatment in an emergency is crucial. It is also often used as an indicator for the quality of the medical emergency system (DeutscherBundestag17.Wahlperiode, 2010). One demand on telemedicine therefore is to not delay the therapy. In the development of the LiveCity camera huge emphasis was put on reducing the time needed to build the connectivity. One approach was to enhance the capability of the hardware and software. And another one was to develop an easy-to-use and intuitive software,

so that the video camera can be operated while working with the patient. After working with the LiveCity camera the majority of paramedics and emergency doctors partly agreed or agreed that they perceived, that this tele emergency doctor concept leads to an earlier start of therapy. It can be concluded for the LiveCity camera that the early availability of medical expertise regarding diagnostics and therapy leads to such an early start of therapy, that it can outbalance any delay due to technical reasons.

As a consequence, one might argue, that reducing the technical complexity to a minimum might lead to a faster data transmission and thus to an earlier start of therapy. Additionally a complex system is often more failure-prone and requires a more stable and superior internet connection. To assess the possibility to eliminate expandable features, the emergency doctors were consulted, what information was necessary to evaluate the specific emergency situation. 80% of emergency doctors stated, that the sole transmission of vital signs (blood pressure, heart rate, oxygen saturation) would not have been enough. And even the addition of an audio connection would have not been enough for 80% of the emergency doctors to sufficiently treat the emergency patient. This means, that the telemedicine devise also needs to transmit video to enable the tele emergency doctor to successfully support the paramedics.

Despite great promises of telemedicine, the implementation of telemedicine projects into the existing medical systems is a huge challenge (Iakovidis, Maglavera, & Trakatellis, 2000; Zailani, Gilani, Nikbin, & Iranmanesh, 2014). Some very promising telemedicine projects were not as widely implemented as expected. The reason for that is studied worldwide and several "enablers", e.g. well-working technology and training of the users, as well as "barriers", e.g. technical problems and lack of technical support, were discussed (Wade, Eliott, & Hiller, 2014). One main factor for successful implementation of telemedicine is a good acceptance of the idea and device by the users, e.g.

doctors (Rho, Choi, & Lee, 2014). Wade and coworkers stated that acceptance by clinicians is the most important key factor and that if clinicians supported the telemedicine project, various technical problems were tolerated (Wade et al., 2014). The technology acceptance model (TAM) by Davis was applied to telemedicine and it could be shown that both the perceived usefulness and the perceived ease of use are significantly associated with the intention to use the system (F. D. Davis, 1989; Dünnebeil, Sunyaev, Blohm, Leimeister, & Krcmar, 2012; Kowitlawakul, 2011; Rho et al., 2014). In the LiveCity Project an impressive majority of emergency doctors and paramedics agreed, that they could imagine working in a tele emergency doctor system. Therefore the impact of video communication on emergency medicine seems to be as convincing today as promising for the future.

This concept to transfer knowledge in real time through video communication to distant places can improve the quality of medical emergency systems. With the arrival of the first members of the medical emergency team at the emergency site, a high quality in diagnostics and treatment can be achieved. This leads to an earlier beginning of high quality medicine. Polls among citizens showed that the timely access to high quality medical care was rated as the most important quality feature of a health care system (Soroka, 2007). The perceived achievement of this goal, influences the appraisal of the current government and the wish for political change (Soroka, 2007). To achieve the highest benefit of a video consultation in emergency medicine, policy makers worldwide should implement and adapt the idea into the existing medical emergency system of their specific country.

CONCLUSION

A common problem in emergency medicine is the lack of support by emergency doctors, when paramedics reach the site of emergency before the arrival of doctors or even without them arriving, but need their assistance or back up. The aim of this study is an approach to increase quality of emergency treatment in these situations by applying telemedicine. The core piece of the study concept is a special video camera system called LiveCity camera, enabling real time connection of paramedics and emergency doctors by high quality video. Emergency doctors and paramedics tested the work flow and outcome of this kind of communication in a medical simulation center with aid of computer-operated mannequins.

A structured questionnaire confirmed that, the majority of paramedics and emergency doctors considered the tele emergency doctor system (i) as helpful and (ii) an improvement regarding quality of patient care and could (iii) imagine working in a tele emergency doctor system. The impact of video communication on emergency medicine is clearly appreciated among providers, based upon the extent of agreement that has been stated in this study by doctors and paramedics. Thus the concept of a video consultation of an emergency doctor is a good addition to the existing medical emergency system in Germany and the idea could be integrated into other medical emergency systems worldwide as well to enhance the quality of emergency medicine.

ACKNOWLEDGMENT

The present article has been structured in the context of the LiveCity ("Live Video-to-Video Supporting Interactive City Infrastructure") European Research Project and has been supported by the Commission of the European Communities - DG CONNECT (FP7-ICT-PSP, Grant Agreement No.297291).

The authors would like to thank Dr. Ioannis Chochliouros for his continuous support and as a representative of the LiveCity project partners and PD Dr. Dr. Wolfgang Hannöver for inspiring ideas and help with the study design.

REFERENCES

Adnet, F., & Lapostolle, F. (2004). International EMS systems: France. *Resuscitation*, *63*(1), 7–9. doi:10.1016/j.resuscitation.2004.04.001 PMID:15451580

Al-Shaqsi, S. (2010). Models of International Emergency Medical Service (EMS) Systems. *Oman Medical Journal*, *25*(4), 320–323. doi:10.5001/omj.2010.92 PMID:22043368

Ali, M., Miyoshi, C., & Ushijima, H. (2006). Emergency medical services in Islamabad, Pakistan: A public–private partnership. *Public Health*, *120*(1), 50–57. doi:10.1016/j.puhe.2005.03.009 PMID:16198384

Amadi-Obi, A., Gilligan, P., Owens, N., & O'Donnell, C. (2014). Telemedicine in pre-hospital care: A review of telemedicine applications in the pre-hospital environment. *International Journal of Emergency Medicine*, *7*(1), 29. doi:10.1186/s12245-014-0029-0

Ammenwerth, E., Hackl, W. O., Binzer, K., Christoffersen, T. E., Jensen, S., & Lawton, K. et al. (2012). Simulation studies for the evaluation of health information technologies: Experiences and results. *The HIM Journal*, *41*(2), 14–21. PMID:22700558

Anand, L. K., Singh, M., & Kapoor, D. (2013). Prehospital trauma care services in developing countries. *Anaesthesia, Pain & Intensive Care*, *17*(1), 65.

Bashshur, R. L. (2002). Chapter 1: Telemedicine and healthcare. *Telemedicine Journal and e-Health*, *8*(1), 5–12. doi:10.1089/15305620252933365 PMID:12020402

Bauman, E. B. (2013). *Game-based Teaching and Simulation in Nursing and Healthcare*. Springer Publishing Company.

Becker, Johannes, Hündorf, Hans-Peter, Kill, Clemens, & Lipp, Roland. (2006). *Lexikon Rettungsdienst*. Stumpf + Kossendey Verlag.

Binder, G. (1993). *Hilfsfrist Rechtsbegriffe in der Notfallmedizin* (pp. 38–38). Springer Berlin Heidelberg. doi:10.1007/978-3-642-52350-2_38

Black, J. J. M., & Davies, G. D. (2005). International EMS Systems: United Kingdom. *Resuscitation*, *64*(1), 21–29. doi:10.1016/j.resuscitation.2004.10.004 PMID:15629551

Bundesärztekammer. (2011b). Übersicht Notarztqualifikation in Deutschland. www.bundesaerztekammer.de

Bundesärztekammer. (2013). Indikationskatalog für den Notarzteinsatz: Handreichung für Telefondisponenten in Notdienstzentralen und Rettungsleitstellen. *Deutsches Ärzteblatt International*, *110*, 521.

Buscher, C., Elsner, J., Schneiders, M. T., Thelen, S., Brodziak, T., & Seidenberg, P. et al. (2014). The Telemedical Rescue Assistance System "TemRas"--development, first results, and impact. *Biomedizinische Technik. Biomedical Engineering*, *59*(2), 113–123. doi:10.1515/bmt-2013-0025 PMID:24445230

Callese, T. E., Richards, C. T., Shaw, P., Schuetz, S. J., Issa, N., Paladino, L., & Swaroop, M. (2014). Layperson trauma training in low- and middle-income countries: A review. *The Journal of Surgical Research*, *190*(1), 104–110. doi:10.1016/j.jss.2014.03.029 PMID:24746252

Cannon-Diehl, M. R. (2009). Simulation in healthcare and nursing: State of the science. *Critical Care Nursing Quarterly*, *32*(2), 128–136. doi:10.1097/CNQ.0b013e3181a27e0f PMID:19300077

Chochliouros, I. P., Stephanakis, I. M., Spiliopoulou, A. S., Sfakianakis, E., & Ladid, L. (2012). Developing Innovative Live Video-to-Video Communications for Smarter European Cities. In L. Iliadis, I. Maglogiannis, H. Papadopoulos, K. Karatzas, & S. Sioutas (Eds.), *Artificial Intelligence Applications and Innovations* (Vol. 382, pp. 279–289). Springer Berlin Heidelberg. doi:10.1007/978-3-642-33412-2_29

Cummins, N. M., Garavan, C., Dixon, M., Landymore, E., Mulligan, N., & O'Donnell, C. (2013). The Advanced Paramedic Clinical Activity Study (APCAS): An insight into the work of advanced paramedics in the mid-west of Ireland. *Irish Journal of Medical Science, 182*(3), 469–475. doi:10.1007/s11845-013-0915-0 PMID:23370974

Czaplik, M., Bergrath, S., Rossaint, R., Thelen, S., Brodziak, T., & Valentin, B. et al. (2014). Employment of telemedicine in emergency medicine. Clinical requirement analysis, system development and first test results. *Methods of Information in Medicine, 53*(2), 99–107. doi:10.3414/ME13-01-0022 PMID:24477815

Davis, D. P., Graydon, C., Stein, R., Wilson, S., Buesch, B., & Berthiaume, S. et al. (2007). The positive predictive value of paramedic versus emergency physician interpretation of the prehospital 12-lead electrocardiogram. *Prehospital Emergency Care, 11*(4), 399–402. doi:10.1080/10903120701536784 PMID:17907023

Davis, F. D. (1989). Perceived Usefulness, Perceived Ease of Use, and User Acceptance of Information Technology. *Management Information Systems Quarterly, 13*(3), 319–340. doi:10.2307/249008

Deutscher Bundestag 17. Wahlperiode. (2010). *Bericht über Maßnahmen auf dem Gebiet der Unfallverhütung im Straßenverkehr 2008 und 2009 (Unfallverhütungsbericht Straßenverkehr 2008/2009).*

Dib, J. E., Naderi, S., Sheridan, I. A., & Alagappan, K. (2006). Analysis and applicability of the Dutch EMS system into countries developing EMS systems. *The Journal of Emergency Medicine, 30*(1), 111–115. doi:10.1016/j.jemermed.2005.05.014 PMID:16434351

Dick, W. F. (2003). Anglo-American vs. Franco-German emergency medical services system. *Prehosp Disaster Med, 18*(1), 29-35; discussion 35-27.

Dünnebeil, S., Sunyaev, A., Blohm, I., Leimeister, J. M., & Krcmar, H. (2012). Determinants of physicians' technology acceptance for e-health in ambulatory care. *International Journal of Medical Informatics, 81*(11), 746–760. doi:10.1016/j.ijmedinf.2012.02.002 PMID:22397989

Economic and Social Committee, Section for Transport, Energy, Infrastructure and the Information Society. (98). (2008). Opinion of the European Economic and Social Committee on the Communication from the Commission to the European Parliament, the Council, the European Economic and Social Committee and the Committee of the Regions on telemedicine for the benefit of patients, healthcare systems and society COM(2008) 689 final. Brussels.

Ellinger, K. (2011). *Kursbuch Notfallmedizin: orientiert am bundeseinheitlichen Curriculum Zusatzbezeichnung Notfallmedizin.* Dt. Ärzte-Verlag.

Ellis, D. Y., & Sorene, E. (2008). Magen David Adom–The EMS in Israel. *Resuscitation, 76*(1), 5–10. doi:10.1016/j.resuscitation.2007.07.014 PMID:17767990

EuropeanComission. (2014). *Digital Agenda for Europe - About 112.* Digital Agenda for Europe. European Comission. https://ec.europa.eu/digital-agenda/en/about-112. Retrieved from https://ec.europa.eu/digital-agenda/en/about-112

Fritz, P. Z., Gray, T., & Flanagan, B. (2008). Review of mannequin-based high-fidelity simulation in emergency medicine. *Emergency Medicine Australasia*, *20*(1), 1–9. doi:10.1111/j.1742-6723.2007.01022.x PMID:17999685

Gomes, E., Araújo, R., Soares-Oliveira, M., & Pereira, N. (2004). International EMS systems: Portugal. *Resuscitation*, *62*(3), 257–260. doi:10.1016/j.resuscitation.2004.04.013 PMID:15325443

Goncalves, J., Cordeiro, L., Batista, P., & Monteiro, E. (2012). LiveCity: A Secure Live Video-to-Video Interactive City Infrastructure. In L. Iliadis, I. Maglogiannis, H. Papadopoulos, K. Karatzas, & S. Sioutas (Eds.), *Artificial Intelligence Applications and Innovations* (Vol. 382, pp. 260–267). Springer Berlin Heidelberg. doi:10.1007/978-3-642-33412-2_27

Gosselin, R. A., Spiegel, D. A., Coughlin, R., & Zirkle, L. G. (2009). Injuries: The neglected burden in developing countries. *Bulletin of the World Health Organization*, *87*(4), 246–246a. doi:10.2471/BLT.08.052290 PMID:19551225

Gries, A., Zink, W., Bernhard, M., Messelken, M., & Schlechtriemen, T. (2006). Realistic assessment of the physican-staffed emergency services in Germany. *Der Anaesthesist*, *55*(10), 1080–1086. doi:10.1007/s00101-006-1051-2 PMID:16791544

Groos, H. (2011). *Du musst die Menschen lieben: Als Ärztin im Rettungswagen, auf der Intensivstation und im Krieg*. Fischer E-Books.

Harding, U., Lechleuthner, A., Ritter, M. A., Schilling, M., Kros, M., Ohms, M., & Bohn, A. (2013). „Schlaganfall immer mit Notarzt?" – „Pro". *Medizinische Klinik -. Intensivmedizin und Notfallmedizin*, *108*(5), 408–411. doi:10.1007/s00063-012-0137-7

Hay, H. I. (2000). EMS in New Zealand. *Emergency Medical Services*, *29*(7), 95–97, 109. PMID:11183102

Hsia, R., Razzak, J., Tsai, A. C., & Hirshon, J. M. (2010). Placing emergency care on the global agenda. *Annals of Emergency Medicine*, *56*(2), 142–149. doi:10.1016/j.annemergmed.2010.01.013 PMID:20138398

Huiyi, T. (2007). *A Study on Prehospital Emergency Medical Service System Status in Guangzhou*. Hong Kong: University of Hong Kong.

Iakovidis, I., Maglavera, S., & Trakatellis, A. (2000). *User Acceptance of Health Telematics Applications: Education and Training in Health Telematics*. IOS Press.

Johannsson, H., Ayida, G., & Sadler, C. (2005). Faking it? Simulation in the training of obstetricians and gynaecologists. *Current Opinion in Obstetrics & Gynecology*, *17*(6), 557–561. doi:10.1097/01.gco.0000188726.45998.97 PMID:16258334

Katzenmeier, C., & Schrag-Slavu, S. (2010). *Einführung Rechtsfragen des Einsatzes der Telemedizin im Rettungsdienst* (Vol. 2, pp. 1–22). Springer Berlin Heidelberg. doi:10.1007/978-3-540-85132-5_1

Kazley, A. S., McLeod, A. C., & Wager, K. A. (2012). Telemedicine in an international context: Definition, use, and future. *Adv Health Care Manag*, *12*, 143–169. doi:10.1108/S1474-8231(2012)0000012011 PMID:22894049

Kippnich, Uwe. (2014). Mit dem Tablet-PC zum Patienten. *Rettungs-Magazin*(4 Juli/ August 2014).

Kirsch, T. D., Hilwig, W. K., Holder, Y., Smith, G. S., Pooran, S., & Edwards, R. (1995). Epidemiology and Practice of Emergency Medicine in a Developing Country. *Annals of Emergency Medicine*, *26*(3), 361–367. doi:10.1016/S0196-0644(95)70087-0 PMID:7661430

Kobusingye, O. C., Hyder, A. A., Bishai, D., et al. (2006). Chapter 68 Emergency Medical Services Disease Control Priorities in Developing Countries (2nd edition ed.). Washington (DC): World Bank.

Kowitlawakul, Y. (2011). The technology acceptance model: Predicting nurses' intention to use telemedicine technology (eICU). *Computers, Informatics, Nursing, 29*(7), 411–418. doi:10.1097/NCN.0b013e3181f9dd4a PMID:20975536

Krafft, T., Garcia Castrillo-Riesgo, L., Edwards, S., Fischer, M., Overton, J., Robertson-Steel, I., & Konig, A. (2003). European Emergency Data Project (EED Project): EMS data-based health surveillance system. *European Journal of Public Health, 13*(3Suppl), 85–90. doi:10.1093/eurpub/13.suppl_3.85 PMID:14533755

Kyle, R., & Murray, W. B. (2010). *Clinical Simulation*. Elsevier Science.

Langhelle, A., Lossius, H. M., Silfvast, T., Björnsson, H. M., Lippert, F. K., Ersson, A., & Søreide, E. (2004). International EMS Systems: The Nordic countries. *Resuscitation, 61*(1), 9–21. doi:10.1016/j.resuscitation.2003.12.008 PMID:15081176

Lateef, F. (2006). The emergency medical services in Singapore. *Resuscitation, 68*(3), 323–328. doi:10.1016/j.resuscitation.2005.12.007 PMID:16503277

Levine, A. I., DeMaria, S., Schwartz, A. D., & Sim, A. J. (2013). *The Comprehensive Textbook of Healthcare Simulation*. Springer. doi:10.1007/978-1-4614-5993-4

MacFarlane, C., van Loggerenberg, C., & Kloeck, W. (2005). International EMS systems in South Africa: Past, present, and future. *Resuscitation, 64*(2), 145–148. doi:10.1016/j.resuscitation.2004.11.003 PMID:15680521

Mock, C. N., Jurkovich, G. J., nii-Amon-Kotei, D., Arreola-Risa, C., & Maier, R. V. (1998). Trauma mortality patterns in three nations at different economic levels: implications for global trauma system development. *J Trauma, 44*(5), 804-812; discussion 812-804.

Model Professional Code for Physicians in Germany (Berufsordnung) (2011a).

Nilsen, J. E. (2012). *Improving quality of care in the Emergency Medical Communication Centres (EMCC)* Paper presented at the Konferanse for medisinsk nødmeldetjeneste 7. - 8.nov. 2012, Sola, Norway.

Palma, D., Goncalves, J., Cordeiro, L., Simoes, P., Monteiro, E., Magdalinos, P., & Chochliouros, I. (2013). Tutamen: An Integrated Personal Mobile and Adaptable Video Platform for Health and Protection. In H. Papadopoulos, A. Andreou, L. Iliadis, & I. Maglogiannis (Eds.), *Artificial Intelligence Applications and Innovations* (Vol. 412, pp. 442–451). Springer Berlin Heidelberg. doi:10.1007/978-3-642-41142-7_45

Papaspyrou, E., Setzis, D., Grosomanidis, V., Manikis, D., Boutlis, D., & Ressos, C. (2004). International EMS systems: Greece. *Resuscitation, 63*(3), 255–259. doi:10.1016/j.resuscitation.2004.06.009 PMID:15582759

Pozner, C. N., Zane, R., Nelson, S. J., & Levine, M. (2004). International EMS systems: The United States: past, present, and future. *Resuscitation, 60*(3), 239–244. doi:10.1016/j.resuscitation.2003.11.004 PMID:15050754

Razzak, J. A., & Kellermann, A. L. (2002). Emergency medical care in developing countries: Is it worthwhile? *Bulletin of the World Health Organization, 80*(11), 900–905. PMID:12481213

Rho, M. J., Choi, I. Y., & Lee, J. (2014). Predictive factors of telemedicine service acceptance and behavioral intention of physicians. *International Journal of Medical Informatics, 83*(8), 559–571. doi:10.1016/j.ijmedinf.2014.05.005 PMID:24961820

Roessler, M., & Zuzan, O. (2006). EMS systems in Germany. *Resuscitation, 68*(1), 45–49. doi:10.1016/j.resuscitation.2005.08.004 PMID:16401522

Rortgen, D., Bergrath, S., Rossaint, R., Beckers, S. K., Fischermann, H., & Na, I. S. et al. (2013). Comparison of physician staffed emergency teams with paramedic teams assisted by telemedicine--a randomized, controlled simulation study. *Resuscitation, 84*(1), 85–92. doi:10.1016/j.resuscitation.2012.06.012 PMID:22750663

Roudsari, B. S., Nathens, A. B., Cameron, P., Civil, I., Gruen, R. L., & Koepsell, T. D. et al. (2007). International comparison of prehospital trauma care systems. *Injury, 38*(9), 993–1000. doi:10.1016/j.injury.2007.03.028 PMID:17640641

Sasser, S., Varghese, M., Kellermann, A., & Lormand, J. D. (2005). *Prehospital trauma care systems*. Geneva: World Health Organization.

Schilling, M., Kros, M., Ritter, M., Ohms, M., Schäbitz, W. R., & Kusch, W. et al. (2012). Zuweisungskonzept bei akutem Schlaganfall. *Der Nervenarzt, 83*(6), 759–765. doi:10.1007/s00115-011-3448-7 PMID:22278124

Schmiedel, R., & Behrendt, H. (2011). *Leistungen des Rettungsdienstes 2008/09*. Bonn: Dr. Schmiedel GmbH.

Schwamm, L. H., Holloway, R. G., Amarenco, P., Audebert, H. J., Bakas, T., & Chumbler, N. R. et al. (2009). A review of the evidence for the use of telemedicine within stroke systems of care: A scientific statement from the American Heart Association/American Stroke Association. *Stroke, 40*(7), 2616–2634. doi:10.1161/STROKEAHA.109.192360 PMID:19423852

Skorning, M., Bergrath, S., Rortgen, D., Brokmann, J. C., Beckers, S. K., & Protogerakis, M. et al. (2009). „E-Health" in der Notfallmedizin – das Forschungsprojekt Med-on-@ix. *Der Anaesthesist, 58*(3), 285–292. doi:10.1007/s00101-008-1502-z PMID:19221700

Sood, S., Mbarika, V., Jugoo, S., Dookhy, R., Doarn, C. R., Prakash, N., & Merrell, R. C. (2007). What is telemedicine? A collection of 104 peer-reviewed perspectives and theoretical underpinnings. *Telemedicine Journal and e-Health, 13*(5), 573–590. doi:10.1089/tmj.2006.0073 PMID:17999619

Soroka, S. N. (2007). *Canadian perceptions of the health care system*. Toronto.

Symons, P., & Shuster, M. (2004). International EMS Systems: Canada. *Resuscitation, 63*(2), 119–122. doi:10.1016/j.resuscitation.2004.06.010 PMID:15531061

Thomson, N. (2005). Emergency medical services in Zimbabwe. *Resuscitation, 65*(1), 15–19. doi:10.1016/j.resuscitation.2005.01.008 PMID:15797271

Timerman, S., Gonzalez, M. M. C., Zaroni, A. C., & Ramires, J. A. F. (2006). Emergency medical services: Brazil. *Resuscitation, 70*(3), 356–359. doi:10.1016/j.resuscitation.2006.05.010 PMID:16901612

Trevithick, S., Flabouris, A., Tall, G., & Webber, C. F. (2003). International EMS systems: New South Wales, Australia. *Resuscitation, 59*(2), 165–170. doi:10.1016/S0300-9572(03)00343-5 PMID:14625106

Vaitkaitis, D. (2008). EMS systems in Lithuania. *Resuscitation, 76*(3), 329–332. doi:10.1016/j.resuscitation.2007.07.028 PMID:17822828

VanRooyen, M. J., Thomas, T. L., & Clem, K. J. (1999). International emergency medical services: Assessment of developing prehospital systems abroad. *The Journal of Emergency Medicine, 17*(4), 691–696. doi:10.1016/S0736-4679(99)00065-7 PMID:10431962

Wade, V. A., Eliott, J. A., & Hiller, J. E. (2014). Clinician Acceptance is the Key Factor for Sustainable Telehealth Services. *Qualitative Health Research, 24*(5), 682–694. doi:10.1177/1049732314528809 PMID:24685708

Weerakkody, V., El-Haddadeh, R., Chochliouros, I. P., & Morris, D. (2012). Utilizing a High Definition Live Video Platform to Facilitate Public Service Delivery. In L. Iliadis, I. Maglogiannis, H. Papadopoulos, K. Karatzas, & S. Sioutas (Eds.), *Artificial Intelligence Applications and Innovations* (Vol. 382, pp. 290–299). Springer Berlin Heidelberg. doi:10.1007/978-3-642-33412-2_30

WHO. (1996). Report: Investing in health research and development; WHO reference number: TDR/Gen/96.1. Geneva: World Health Organization: Ad Hoc Committee on Health Research Relating to Future Intervention Options.

WHO. (2010). *Injuries and violence: the facts.* Geneva.

WHO. (2011). *Telemedicine – Opportunities and developments in Member States: report on the second global survey on eHealth 2009 Global Observatory for eHealth series* (Vol. 2). World Health Oragnization.

Zailani, S., Gilani, M. S., Nikbin, D., & Iranmanesh, M. (2014). Determinants of Telemedicine Acceptance in Selected Public Hospitals in Malaysia: Clinical Perspective. *Journal of Medical Systems, 38*(9), 1–12. doi:10.1007/s10916-014-0111-4 PMID:25038891

This work was previously published in the International Journal of Electronic Government Research (IJEGR), 10(3); edited by Vishanth Weerakkody, pages 47-65 copyright year 2014 by IGI Publishing (an imprint of IGI Global).

Chapter 35

An Autonomous Intelligent System for the Private Outdoors Monitoring of People with Mild Cognitive Impairments

Antoni Martínez-Ballesté
Universitat Rovira i Virgili, Spain

Frederic Borràs Budesca
Universitat Rovira i Virgili, Spain

Agustí Solanas
Universitat Rovira i Virgili, Spain

ABSTRACT

The aim of this chapter is to describe a system for the private outdoor monitoring of patients with Mild Cognitive Impairments (MCI) and dementia. The system has been designed for patients suffering from early stages of Alzheimer's disease and people suffering from MCI and dementia. Virtually, the system may be applied to any person capable of living autonomously but might get lost whilst doing his/her everyday activities, due to a decrease in their cognitive function. The system uses off-the-shelf smartphones carried by patients to detect abnormal situations and to raise alarms accordingly. The authors describe the system, detail its features, and discuss its utility and relevance both technically and socially.

BACKGROUND

The average age of the world population has increased progressively over the last 50 years as a result of the decrease of fertility and the increase in life expectancy. It is believed that life expectancy will grow in about 10 years by 2050. The ageing of the population is one of the most important challenges for public healthcare systems since they have to face the rise of an aged and very demanding population and their associated health conditions, namely chronic illnesses, injuries and disabilities.

DOI: 10.4018/978-1-4666-8756-1.ch035

According to the Organisation for Economic Co-operation and Development:

In most OECD countries the population is ageing. Due to higher life expectancy and low fertility rates, the elderly population (those aged 65 years and over), accounts for almost 15% of OECD population in 2010, up from just over 12% 15 years earlier. The proportion of elderly population is remarkably lower in the emerging economies (India, South Africa, Brazil and China) and Mexico, Turkey and Chile. (OECD, 2013)

This demographic shift (cf. Figure 1) will result in a huge impact on society and actions have to be taken in the years to come to cope with it. The aforementioned ageing of the population leads to an increase in the cases of cognitive disorders like Mild Cognitive Impairment (MCI), Parkinson's disease (PD) and Alzheimer's disease (AD).

We pay special attention to MCI because it can be seen as a precursor of the early stages of AD and PD and other types of dementia that imply impaired memory function whilst the cognitive function is generally preserved (Petersen, 2001). MCI is a brain function syndrome involving the onset and evolution of cognitive impairments beyond those expected based on the age and education of the individual, but which are not significant enough to interfere with their daily activities (Petersen, 1999). Annual prevalence estimates for MCI in the United States range from 3% to 4% in the eighth decade (Ganguli, 2004) in the general population. Amongst community-dwelling African Americans, the estimated prevalence is 19.2% for those aged 65-74 years, 27.6% for those aged 75-84 years, and 38% for those aged 85 years and older (Unverzagt, 2001). The prevalence of mild cognitive impairment increases with age. The prevalence is 10% in those aged 70-79 years and 25% in those aged 80-89 years (Roberts, 2008). Many studies indicate that the risk of Alzheimer disease (AD) is significantly higher in women than in men, and it is therefore presumed that the likelihood of developing MCI is greater in women than in men (Anderson, 2013).

People suffering from MCI and early stages of different types of dementia might experience a decrease in their cognitive capabilities that might affect their mobility patterns but they still have considerably high degrees of autonomy (*i.e.* they can live alone, walk, do exercise). The most appar-

Figure 1. Percentage of elderly population in OECD countries in 2010 and in 1995 (or first available year) Source OECD.

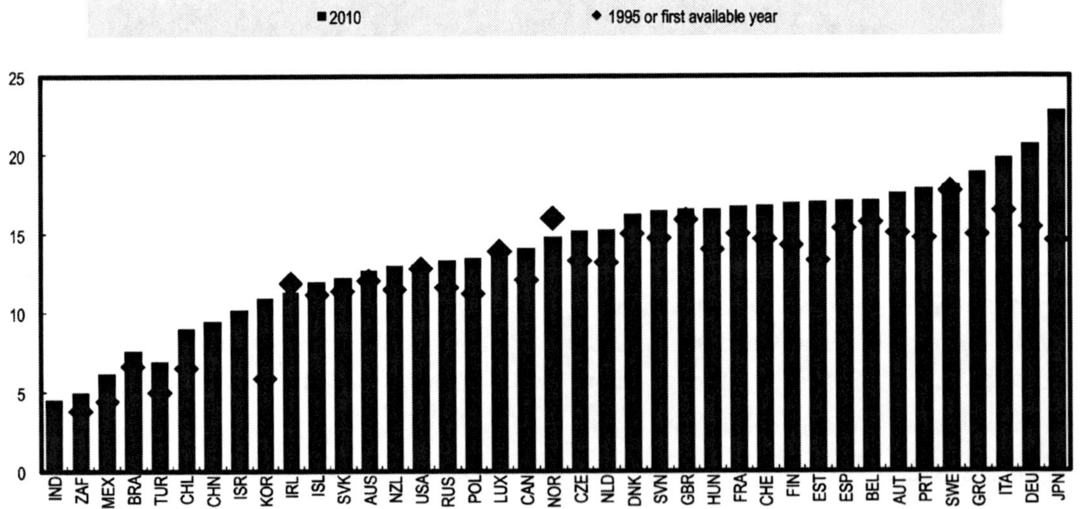

ent impairment is related to their memory function: patients might become spatially and temporally disoriented, and might have problems in finding their way home, or they could forget to accomplish tasks. Note that this problem could translate into abnormal mobility patterns, for example, patients will follow strange paths to reach their homes, or they will go to the supermarket more frequently (because they forget to buy what they need).

THE SIMPATIC PROJECT

This chapter is devoted to the description of a monitoring system that is the result of our research in the SIMPATIC project (Intelligent System for the Private and Autonomous Surveillance based on Information and Communication Technologies, Martínez-Ballesté, 2012. This project has been funded by Fundació La Caixa under the Recercaixa programme.). In this project, we studied the wide deployment of mobile technology and developed a new intelligent system that monitors the localization of users, who suffer from MCI. The proposed system behaves autonomously (*i.e.*, without any user interaction) and also in an intelligent way: thus, it learns from the user and it adapts its reactions to fit his/her requirements, also it detects abnormal users behaviour and a variety of risky situations (namely the user is in a dangerous area such as roads or the edge of a cliff, the user has fallen…) Our proposal detects threats autonomously using an artificial intelligent module. Our tool is suitable for common mobile devices and users and it self-adapts to fulfil their privacy and mobility requirements.

The SIMPATIC project has a clear social component that tries to bring the newest scientific developments to the groups of the society that mostly need them. We do not aim at replacing human carers but to provide them with a powerful tool able to simplify their job, improve their efficiency, reduce costs, and keep the fundamental rights of patients fully guaranteed.

Contribution and Plan of the Chapter

In this chapter we present a system that allows the monitoring of people with MCI. We show the platform in an informative manner. First, in Section 2 we summarize the related work in this field. In Section 3 we describe the properties of the whole system (*i.e.* the mobile application running in the smartphone, the web service and the intelligent system in the server). In Section 4 we address some implementation aspects. Section 5 elaborates on the technical and social validation of the prototype. Finally, Section 6 concludes the chapter.

Mobile Health

With the aim to provide healthcare systems with better tools to cope with the needs of elderly, many efforts have been devoted to their improvement in terms of efficiency, accuracy, and sustainability. Recently, we observed that the healthcare model is shifting towards a patient-centric approach in which patients are not only passive elements of the systems but proactive contributors to their health and that of the others. To this end, Information and Communication Technologies (ICT) play a fundamental role to improve the quality of life of patients and also to reduce the costs of healthcare systems.

The wide adoption of ICT within the healthcare sector led to the concept of electronic health (e-health) (Eysenbach, 2001), which is contributing to the reduction of costs and the increase of efficiency. Following the consolidation of e-health, the generalised use of mobile devices with positioning capabilities (*e.g.*, smartphones) opened the door to the idea of mobile health (m-health), which could be understood as the delivery of healthcare services via mobile communication devices. m-Health has an extraordinary potential since it adds to the advantages of e-health all the benefits related to the ubiquity of mobile devices (*i.e.*, global monitoring capabilities, wide availability and immediacy).

ICT might be used for a variety of health-related tasks, namely communication between patients, doctors and carers, distant provision of care, remote support to diagnostic, electronic medical records, medication adherence control, etc. The use of ICT in the healthcare sector has significantly contributed to the reduction of management costs and to the increase of efficiency. In this line, e-health substantially reduces the displacements of professionals and patients, globally brings down the cost of medical resources, and makes treatments and health watchfulness more comfortable to patients. All in all, e-health might be considered a revolution in this area. However, a probably more important revolution is taking place due to the use of mobile devices (*e.g.*, smartphones): mobile health (m-health) that could be defined as the discipline founded on the use of mobile communication devices in medicine, or more specifically, the delivery of healthcare services via mobile communication devices, or "Emerging mobile communications and network technologies for healthcare systems" (Istepanian, 2006). The use of mobile devices helps to perform tasks more efficiently. Especially the remote monitoring of patients and the communication between professionals, relatives and patients will highly benefit from m-health. In this sense, it could be said that m-Health redefines healthcare services in three main aspects:

1. It allows easy access to an unprecedented number of services and knowledge,
2. It can be user-oriented, and
3. It can be personalised.

m-Health clearly extends the capabilities of indoor monitoring environments and it is a powerful tool that allows the advance of several lines of research, namely the continuous assessment of the state of patients, the early detection of emergency situations, the detection of changes in health con-

ditions, the detection of abnormal situations, the early detection of fragile situations, etc. For the most recent advances on e-health and m-health the interested reader can refer to (Solanas, 2013).

There are commercial products that have approached the problem of monitoring people by using ICT. However, to the best of our knowledge the proposed solutions are not entirely autonomous and require the active intervention of the patient (by pressing a button) or the carer (actively monitoring the location of the patient). Also, most solutions require the use of specific hardware that might increase acquisition costs and refrain patients from using them.

THE PROPOSED APPROACH

The core of the system developed in the SIMPATIC project consists of an intelligent module that uses the location of patients to detect anomalies (cf. Figure 2). In a nutshell, each patient carries a smartphone with a mobile application running in the background. The patient's location is sent at specific time intervals to the server, which will raise alarms upon certain simple conditions related to the patient (e.g., entering a dangerous area, being outside home at midnight, etc.). In turn, the patient's mobile application is linked to that of one or more carers. This application will show alarms related to the patient (a carer could be a relative of the patient, a nurse, etc.).

The proposed system also has a website in which carers might check a log of alarms of patients, set up alarm conditions and other aspects of the system.

In the following section we describe the main actors and functioning of our system.

Main Actors

In our system we distinguish between patients and carers.

Figure 2. Scheme of our proposed approach, with one patient and two carers

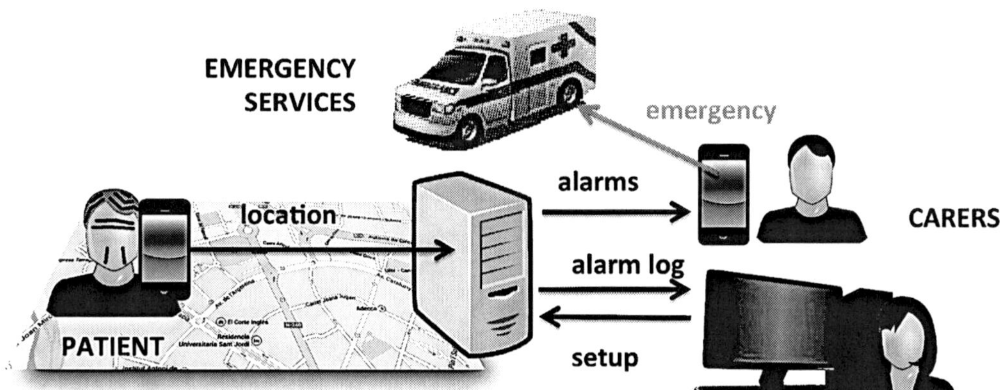

1. **Patients:** These are people who suffer from MCI. They are able to live autonomously: they perform their everyday activities without risks. They can go shopping, have a walk, etc., but due to their cognitive impairments they might get lost and require assistance. Affected people cannot predict where and when they might be lost, they even might not be aware they are getting lost. Moreover, patients can live on their own, or at their relative's homes. However, it is common that patients live in retirement homes. In this scenario, patients are allowed to have some outdoors activities but they must return at a certain time. Moreover, especially during weekends and holiday periods, relatives can take patients outside the house to spending some days together.

2. **Carers:** Carers are people that are closely related to patients due to a variety of reasons. In the case of patients that live on their own, carers could be relatives. In the case of retirement homes, one or more carers usually are in charge of looking after a set of patients. All in all, in our system, a carer is the one that will receive the alarms generated by the mobile application of one or more patients. Hence, we devise three scenarios:

   a. One patient has only one carer assigned in the system. In this scenario, only one person will receive the alarms from that patient. Hence, the carer has to pay special attention to the messages generated by the system and, in consequence, alarms must be notified to the carer in a reliable manner (e.g. via his/her smartphone, an SMS message, an automatic call, etc.).

   b. One patient has more than one carer. In this case, the chances of successfully notifying someone of an alarm are greater than in scenario (a). However, the procedure is the same and repeats for as many carers as necessary.

   c. One or more carers are assigned to a set of patients. This is the general case of retirement homes, for instance. But we could also think of a specialist or a group of specialists in cognitive disorders that use our system to record the behaviours of their patients aiming at improving their diagnoses.

Carers communicate with the system using two interfaces:

- **A Web Frontend:** Carers log into a website to setup the system and alarm conditions (this aspect is later detailed in the chapter), and also to review a log of alarms of their patient or patients.

- **A Mobile Application Installed in Their Smartphone:** This is used to receive alarms in real time, but due to the web browsing capabilities of the smartphone, virtually any function offered by the website frontend could be operated from the mobile device.

In addition, there is a third actor that might take part in the system: the emergency services. These are actors that ensure public safety by addressing emergencies (e.g. firemen and rescue services, medical emergencies, etc.). In normal conditions, these emergency services do not play an active role in the system (i.e. they do not directly interact with the system). However, their help could be required when an emergency situation that cannot be hold by carers arises.

Alarms

By using the aforementioned website frontend, carers can configure and activate several kinds of alarms. In this section we describe the situations that raise alarms. There are four kinds of alarms:

1. Zone alarms,
2. Movement alarms,
3. Device alarms, and
4. Panic alarms.

Zone Alarms

Zone alarms are defined using a map tool in the web frontend of the system. This tool enables the creation of points and polygons to configure the home zone and the secure/dangerous zones.

- **Home Zone:** The home zone is the location in which the patient lives. Carers describe the periods of time in which the patient is "at home". For instance, an alarm

might be raised if the patient is not in the "home zone" from 9 PM to 9 AM. As it can be observed in Figure 3, a house icon represents home zones.

- **Secure Zones:** Carers can define a set of secure zones, by drawing polygons on a map. They can choose whether an alarm is raised if patients abandon these secure zones. In Figure 3, secure zones are represented by green polygon.

- **Dangerous Zones:** Some carers may prefer to define dangerous zones so as to give patients more freedom during their walks. Hence, dangerous zones where patients should not go can be defined. In Figure 3 a highway is seen as a dangerous zone, and represented using a red polygon.

The home zone is related to the situation of "being at home": if the location of the patient (i.e. his/her smartphone) matches the home zone and the GPS precision decreases, with a high probability it indicates that the patient has arrived home. In this case, the smartphone application proceeds with a "home checking" routine: the patient will receive a message requesting if he/she is really at home; Also, under this circumstances, if the battery level is under a certain value, the mobile application will request the mobile phone to be plugged into the power.

Movement Alarms

The main goal of movement alarms is to detect abnormal situations related to the movement of patients. On the one hand, there are situations that are easy to detect:

- **No Movement:** In this case, the carer can select a period of time (e.g. 10 minutes). The server will raise an alarm if it detects that the smartphone did not move for this period of time. Naturally, this alarm is disabled if the patient is at home (i.e. the

Figure 3. Map in which the home zone, a secure zone (green polygon) and an insecure zone (red polygon) are defined; inside the secure zone there is a park.

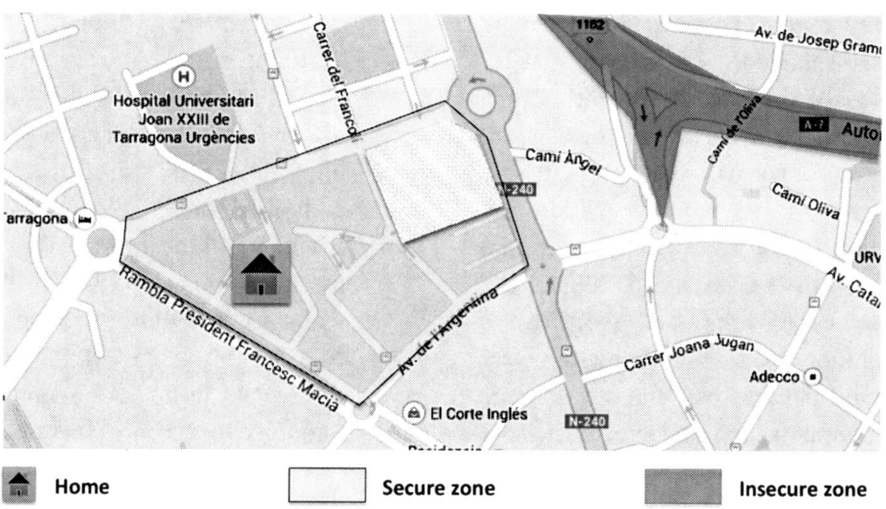

aforementioned "being at home" situation has been confirmed).

- **Speed:** The aim of this alarm is to detect whether the patient has boarded a transportation system such as a train, a car, etc. The carer can select amongst a set of speeds and if the system detects that the average speed of the patient matches these speeds it will raise an alarm. The smartphone application sends the location at specific time intervals and, hence, selecting these kinds of alarms might imply increasing the sampling frequency, in order to compute speeds in a precise manner.

On the other hand, there are situations related to the movement of patients that are not so easy to detect. As it was previously mentioned, artificial intelligence is a core component of the system: besides detecting alarm situations, our system learns from patient's movements and behaviours. In this sense, the system considers two complex alarm situations, in which artificial intelligence plays a key role:

- **Wandering:** Patients with MCI tend to get lost. This can be controlled by the system by using a set of the previously described alarms (the patient is not moving, is not at home, etc.). However, most systems simply control that patients are not in dangerous zones. Unfortunately, people that suffer from cognitive impairments might start wandering around inside secure zones. In Figure 3, we can observe that inside the secure zone there is a park. Naturally, the patient will enjoy walking inside this secure zone. However, it is possible that he/she cannot find the way out. In this situation, patients tend to describe micro-routes that should be analysed to detect wandering situations. If these situations were not considered, the system would not raise any alarm because, in the park example, the patient is inside a secure zone.

- **Abnormal Situation:** Most retired people tend to follow a pattern (daily, weekly) whilst they perform their everyday activities. The intelligent component of our system studies these patterns of movement. We consider the utilization of the data acquired for both discovering routine patterns and detecting anomalous situations. Consequently, after some usage of the system, some abnormal situations can be detected and the system could arise an abnormal situation alarm.

The detection of wandering and abnormal behaviours represents a clear added value of our system. To the best of our knowledge, there is no commercial tool able to automatically detect these behavioural patterns associated to people with MCI and dementia and, in fact, this is a hot research topic.

Device Alarms

Device alarms are related to the technical functioning of the device, and they aim at improving the reliability of the whole system.

- **Battery:** As we mentioned before, the home checking routine asks the patient to plug the smartphone if necessary. Certainly, running out of battery when patients are outside their homes endangers the functioning of the system. Hence, we consider essential that the server raises an alarm in case of low battery level.
- **No GPS Coverage:** If the device loses its GPS coverage, or the GPS precision is too low, the server might arise an alarm (only if the carer activated it). Usually, the reduction of GPS precision is due to the fact that the patient has entered into a building (as in the case of entering the home zone). However walking through narrow streets might also entail a reduction of GPS precision. Hence, it is very useful for the system to have previous knowledge about the GPS precision at any point of the city. In fact our system makes use of such information: it allows the server to improve the

location information received from the device. Figure 4 shows an example of a GPS precision map for a quarter in the city of Tarragona.

- **No Connection:** Although high speed and reliable data connections are quite common, there are some places in which telecom operators do not have high quality 3G coverage. In these cases, the data link used by smartphones could downgrade to 2G technologies. Our communication protocols feasibly work with such connections. With this alarm, the server would communicate to the carer that no data has been received for a period of time. In most situations the lack of data reception will be due to lack of connectivity, but other scenarios are devised (for instance, the smartphone has fallen down and broken into pieces...).
- **Device Falling:** Smartphones use to have accelerometers and other components that might be used to detect abrupt movements, such as falls. In that sense, if a fall is detected, the mobile application produces a sound (aiming at attracting the attention of the patient, in the case of accidental fall from a coat's pocket). Moreover, it urgently sends an alarm to the server.

Finally, we believe that off-the-shelf wearable devices, such as "smart watches" can easily be integrated into our system. For instance, some models could replace the smartphone.

Panic Alarm

The last kind of alarm that we have considered is the panic alarm. It merely consists on urgently informing the carer that the patient has pressed a panic button in the smartphone. Note that some smartphones targeted to elderly are equipped with such buttons. However, we could think of a button on the application interface.

Figure 4. Example of a heat map of the GPS precision in a quarter of the city of Tarrgona; the darker, the better

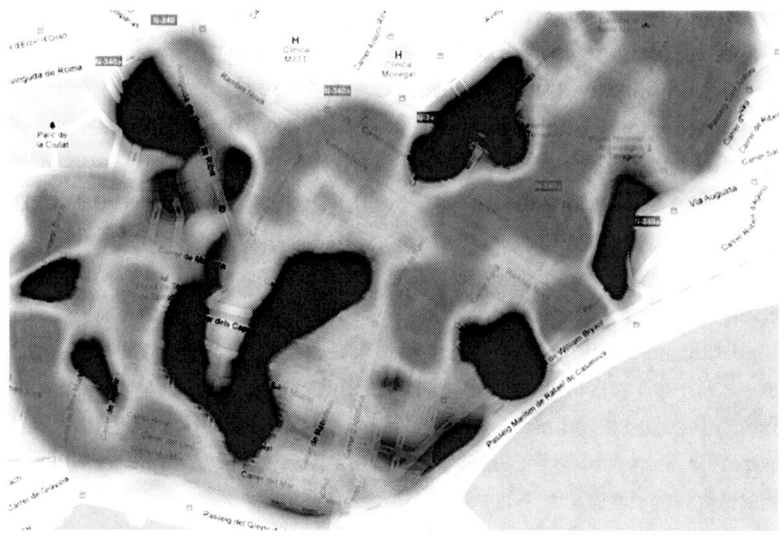

Enrolment Procedure

Before a patient is allowed to use our system, a carer should execute the enrolment procedure, that consists of four steps:

- **Website Sign-Up:** Once in the website, the carer presses a register button. He/she introduces some contact information and his/her password. Once the registration is finished, the carer receives two "binding tokens" (alphanumeric strings): the patient mobile application code and the carer mobile app code. The carer can add additional carers for this patient.
- **Application Downloading:** The mobile applications (the one for the patient's device and the one for the carer's device) are freely installed from the digital distribution platforms of mobile applications (e.g. Android Market, Apple Store).
- **Application Linking:** After initiating the mobile applications, they will request the binding tokens, so that the applications could be linked to the server.

- **Patient Information:** The enrolment process entails introducing some information on the patient: fields such as name, surname, age, etc. Additionally, some other relevant information must be introduced, namely blood type, language, whether the patient suffers from diabetes, Parkinson's disease or blood pressure issues, vision and hearing impairments, etc. In case of alarm, this information will be sent to emergency services if necessary.

Once the enrolment procedure is finished, the carer can define alarm zones, and activate predefined movement and device-related alarms. Additionally, carers can select whether alarms must be sent to their mobile applications or simply stored in the alarms log of the system (note that most frequently, carers chose to receive the alarms in their smartphones). Finally, in order to activate the system, the carer presses an on/off button on the website and the server starts logging and analysing information sent from the smartphone of the patient.

Receiving and Checking Alarms

Once the system is up and running, the server receives locations and information from the mobile application of the patient, evaluates them according to the alarm rules, etc. Locations are stored so that the artificial intelligence module can use them to learn the movement patterns of the patient and analyse possible deviations from usual behaviours.

If an alarm situation is detected, the server will notify carers via their mobile application. Moreover, the alarm will be logged in the server's database. Some other information is also stored along with the alarm, for instance the location of the device when the alarm situation was detected. All these data can be accessed through the web frontend.

However, upon receiving an alarm the carer should assess the significance of the alarm. For instance, if the patient has entered a dangerous zone (e.g. is walking along a railway track) and the carer is far from this place, an emergency situation arises. In this case, by pressing a button on the carer's mobile application the emergency services will receive the details of the alarm, together with the data related to the patient (i.e. hearing problems, language, etc.).

Our system also considers the case in which the carer wants to know about the state of the patient, even if no alarm has been raised by the system. Naturally, carers can use their smartphone to call the patient and check whether the latter has any problem and everything goes as usual. Our system offers the carer the option to send an "are-you-ok" message from his/her mobile application. In turn, the patient's application will emit a sound and open a simple interface in which the patient can choose between "yes" and "no".

Adding Privacy and Security

Our tool is designed as a non-invasive technology. With this aim, our system works on a plain smartphone that could be used for other activities.

Moreover, carrying a smartphone is natural, whilst other "assistance devices" somehow stigmatises the patient (i.e. everyone will notice that the patient suffers from some disease if he/she wears a necklace with a red button).

Notwithstanding, we want to focus on security. Since our proposal plays a crucial role with respect to the physical security of patients and the wellbeing of carers, we must pay attention to the security aspects of the information involved in the system. In this sense, the messages generated and sent during the functioning (locations, alarms, etc.) are cryptographically signed in order to avoid alterations by attackers. In addition, what we have called "the server" is in fact a set of redundant servers aiming at providing the service in a reliable and resilient way.

However, the main ethical concern might be related to the location privacy of the patient. In principle, carers can check whenever they want which is the current location of the patient. We believe that the supervision should be private to avert any hindrance from the patient. Avoiding the "big brother" effect is paramount to guarantee the acceptance of patients with a high degree of autonomy. Hence, we assume that if alarm conditions are not met, the location of patients should be kept secret. To that end, we could use classical cryptographic tools to implement encryption of the location of the patient: when the server receives the location of the patient's smartphone, this datum is momentarily used for evaluating alarm situations and for feeding the artificial intelligence modules. Afterwards, the location is encrypted and stored in the server's databases. This would prevent the administrators of the service from accessing the location data and use it dishonestly, for instance, selling them to third parties with marketing purposes. At least and, according to legislation (European Parliament, 1995) since location could be considered data related to an individual (the patient) it should not be released to these third parties without the explicit consent of patients.

Regardless the location is stored encrypted or not, the fact is that the web frontend could easily prevent carers from "watching in real time" the current location of patients (if they are not meant to). Nevertheless, we could imagine a specific situation in which:

1. No alarm has been raised, and
2. The patient is missing.

Certainly, this situation is infrequent, due to the wide set of alarms that our system can manage. However, in this scenario, let us imagine that the carer needs to know where is the patient. This situation is addressed by using a new actor of the system: the official carer.

An official carer is a person that is legally related to the patient and, somehow responsible for the wellbeing and safety of patients (e.g. civil servants such as social workers, doctors, nurses, or public human carers). If carers want to know where the patient is, they might use their mobile app to request the disclosure of locations to these official carers. In turn, if official carers (such as caregivers in a retirement home) want to disclose the current location of a patient, they could use their mobile application or the web frontend to request such permission to carers. This scenario of requesting the patient's location during no-alarm situations is addressed in (Solanas, 2013).

Note that our system has been designed with privacy protection in mind. However, patients might decide to grant complete data access to their carers and all these privacy-preserving functions are disabled. We have learnt from experience that in most situations patients and carers prefer to have complete access to the data at any time, mainly for the sake of the physical security of the patient. In this sense, security is regarded as much more important than privacy.

IMPLEMENTATION

In this section, we describe our prototype implementation of the proposed system. We have developed the server, the web frontend and the mobile applications for the Android platform. We have implemented a set of the aforementioned functionalities: zone alarms, movement alarms and some of the device alarms. The aim of this prototype is to proceed with a pilot test on a controlled population in the area of Tarragona. The pilot test is later described in this chapter.

In the next lines we provide the reader with some details about the mobile applications and the web frontend.

Mobile Applications

- The mobile apps have been implemented natively, i.e. they are specifically programmed for each smartphone platform, aiming at gaining complete control over the components of the smartphone.
- The mobile application running on the patient's smartphone periodically obtains the location of the device together with the precision of the GPS. Also, it obtains the battery level. All these data are packed into a signed message that is sent to the server, which will evaluate whether an alarm situation occurs. In parallel, any abrupt movement of the device will activate the fall detection routine, which checks the physical stability of the device and sends a message to the server if necessary. The patient's mobile application runs in the background, but we have considered three situations that require the interaction of the patient with the application in foreground:
- The "being at home" situation.

- The "panic" situation, in which a panic alarm is sent
- The "are-you-ok" situation. For the sake of simplicity and clarity, instead of using textual buttons, patients can choose between a smiling face and a serious face to communicate their state.

The carer's mobile application is focused on alarm reporting. Figure 5 shows a screenshot of the carer's mobile application for the Android platforms, in which some alarms are listed. If the carer taps on an alarm message, a map showing the description of the alarm and the location of the patient's smartphone pops up.

Web Frontend

The server has been implemented using the Apache-PHP-MySQL tool stack and is currently running on a dedicated server.

Figure 5. The carer application showing some alarms (text is in Catalan): two zone alarms and one speed alarm (in red) and a battery level message (in green)

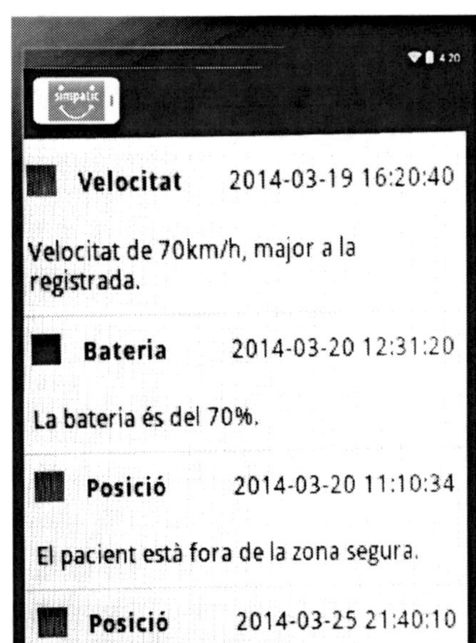

The web frontend comprises two parts: the patient management part and the alarm log part. First, we describe some relevant aspects of the patient management part (cf. Figure 6).

The web frontend allows registering a patient (cf. Figure 6-A) and specifying some additional data (that will be sent to emergency services in case of certain alarms, cf. Figure 6-B). It also provides access to the zone alarm edition tool (Figure 6-C) in which carers can locate the home zone, the secure zones and the dangerous zones. This part uses the Google Maps API and some polygon drawing tools.

Finally, there is a part focused on the configuration and switching of movement and device alarms.

The alarm log section lists the most recent alarms received from the patient's mobile application (see Figure 7). From this list, carers can access the locations where alarms have been detected. Alarms can be managed (i.e. deleted and sorted) according to their categories.

EVALUATION

In order to perform a holistic evaluation of the system, we distinguish between two different dimensions: technical validation and social validation.

Technical Validation

The technology has been validated through experimentation with different mobile phones and platforms. Specifically, the system has been tested in two high performance Android smartphone (a Google's Nexus 4 and a Samsung Galaxy S), and a constrained resource Android smartphone (a Samsung Galaxy Pocket).

We have obtained results on battery duration, GPS precision in the city of Tarragona (refer to the map in Figure 4) and feasibility of the whole system. For instance, using the patient's application running on a Samsung Galaxy S, the battery lasts up to 62.5 hours (sending a location

Figure 6. The web frontend part related to patient management

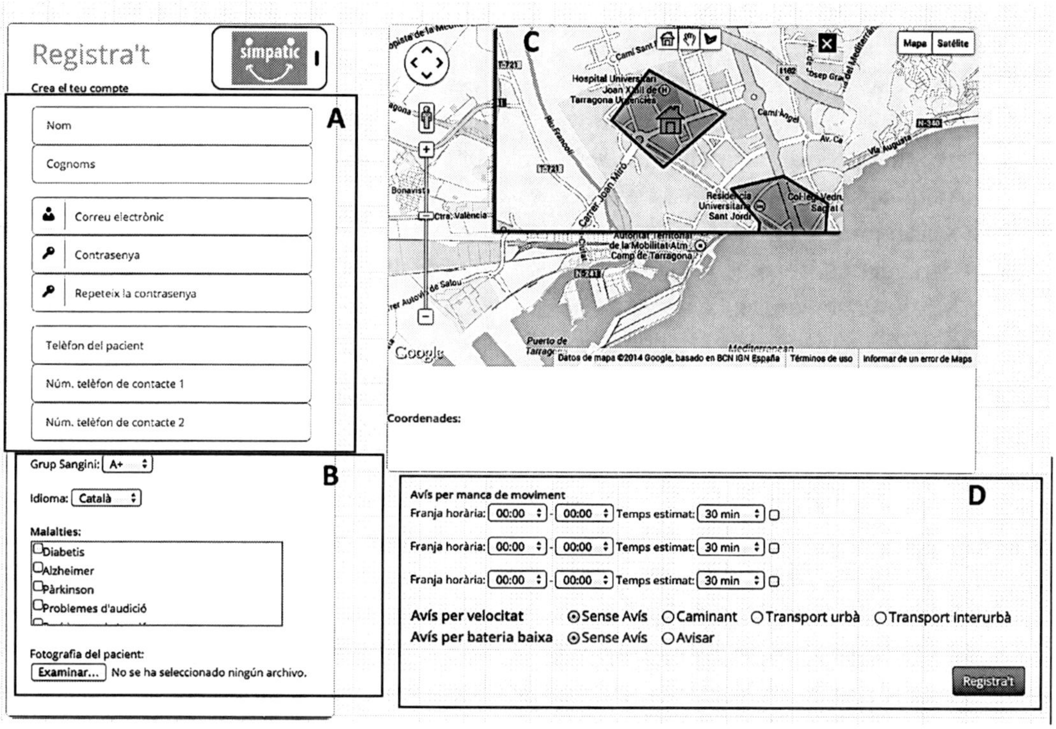

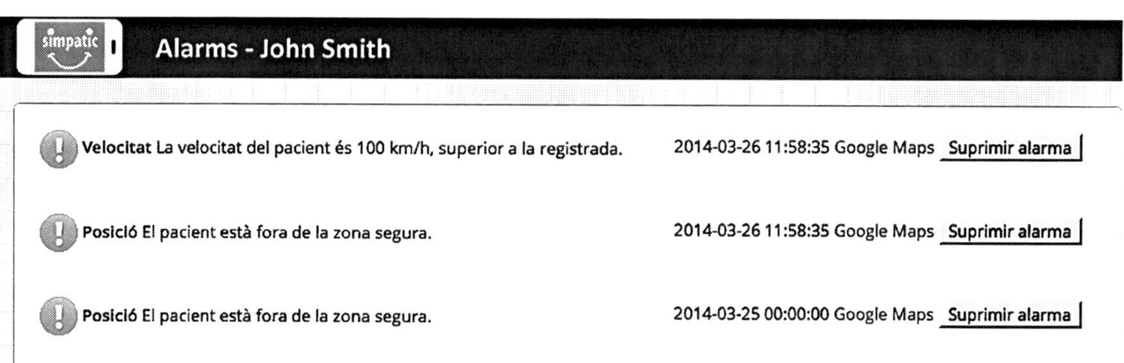

Figure 7. List of the most recent alarms in the alarm log of the web frontend

message every 5 minutes). Note that this result is only approximate and might vary depending on the operating system, the GPS chipset, the data network, and the smartphone used. However, all the performed evaluations indicate that the system is feasible and could perform properly in practice.

Social Validation

Social validation refers to the acceptance of the system by the target population (elderly and carers) and also to the usability of the interfaces of the tools we have implemented.

Up to now, we have conducted several preliminary tests on the usability of the web frontend and the carer's mobile application. It is natural that many of the carers, especially in the case of relatives, are middle-aged people or even elderly. Certainly, smartphones are not tools that naturally fit elderly environments (although we believe that this will change in the near future). Current mobile phones that address this target concentrate on simplicity, large keys, etc. Moreover, some manufacturers start to include tools (some of them based on location) aiming at improving the safety of their users. However, although the so-called "knowledge digital divide" (Graham, 2011) tends to disappear if we consider age as the variable, we cannot assume that every carer is able to use the website without difficulty.

Last but not least, before putting the system in production, it must be tested in a little scale real-life scenario. To this end, we have planned a pilot test in the city of Tarragona. This pilot test will involve both patients and their carers, and also health professionals. The process comprises several steps that are described next:

- First, we have to define the target patients. It is interesting that all patients involved in the experiment suffer from a similar degree of impairment. This way, the obtained results could shed light over the specific impairment analysed (e.g. Alzheimer, MCI).
- Second, we have to seek for the active participation of carers. Both patients and carers must have a smartphone to run their mobile applications.
- Third, we have to make some demonstrations on the functioning of the system. Moreover, we are considering offering some assistance services for carers and patients, in order to help them with the usage of the system.
- Finally, we have to count on the doctors that are in charge of the patients. They play a key role in finding candidates for the pilot test, and analysing their evolution throughout the process.

The aim of the pilot test is both technical and social. The first goal of the pilot test is to re-validate the technical aspects of our solution. Additionally, the pilot test will allow us to do more exhaustive tests on the usability of the mobile application and the web frontend.

A third goal of the pilot test is to acquire information on the locations, movements and behaviours of people that suffer from MCI. Also, we are thinking of piloting with a group of elderly without any impairment affectation (in the sort of a ground truth control set). This could be useful to extract knowledge and to compare the results between the two sets of users. The aim of these acquired data is to help with the development of more advanced alarms (e.g. the aforementioned wandering detection).

CONCLUSION

In this chapter we have presented some of the results of the SIMPATIC Project: a framework that allows the remote monitoring of people with MCI by means of mobile phones and a proper ICT infrastructure.

After discussing the issues related to the ageing of our society, we have described a system that allows the private and intelligent monitoring of people with MCI and dementia. The proposed system takes into consideration two main actors: patients and carers, and allow that the latter supervise the former by using off-the-shelf ICT.

We have analysed our proposal in detail and we described the set of alarms and processes that take place during its normal operation. Also, we have shown the main challenges (i.e. technical and social) that have been faced and we have described the pilot test that is going to be carried in the city of Tarragona.

Although the proposed system has very interesting properties and functionalities, it is still to be improved in a variety of ways. Our future research will concentrate on the following lines:

- Analyse the data obtained during the pilot test.
- Test a wandering detection tool specially designed to analyse micro-routes of MCI and dementia patients.
- Test the abnormal behaviour detection module.
- Seamlessly integrate our system with that of the emergency services in a smart city scenario that uses a "smart city operating system".
- Extend the system to cover other disabilities and mental disorders.

REFERENCES

Solanas, A., Patsakis, C., Conti, M., Vlachos, I. S., Ramos, V., Falcone, F., & Martínez-Ballesté, A. et al. (2014). Smart health: A context-aware health paradigm within smart cities. *IEEE Communications Magazine, 52*(8), 74–81.

Anderson, H. S. (2013). Mild cognitive impairments. *Medscape.* Retrieved March 12, 2014, from http://emedicine.medscape.com/article/1136393-overview

European Parliament. (1995). *European Parliament and the Council: Directive 95/46/EC of 24 October 1995 on the protection of individuals with regard to the processing of personal data and on the free movement of such data.* Retrieved March 12, 2014, from http://www.dataprotection.ie/docs/EU-Directive-95-46-EC/89.htm

Eysenbach, G. (2001). What is e-health? *Journal of Medical Internet Research, 3*(2), e20. doi:10.2196/jmir.3.2.e20 PMID:11720962

Ganguli, M., Dodge, H. H., Shen, C., & DeKosky, S. T. (2004). Mild cognitive impairment, amnestic type: An epidemiologic study. *Neurology, 63*(1), 115–121. doi:10.1212/01.WNL.0000132523.27540.81 PMID:15249620

Graham, M. (2011). Time machines and virtual portals: The spatialities of the digital divide. *Progress in Development Studies, 11*(3), 211–227. doi:10.1177/1464993410001100303

Istepanian, R., Laxminarayan, S., & Pattichis, S. S. (2006). *M-health: Emerging mobile health systems.* Springer. doi:10.1007/b137697

Martínez-Ballesté, A., & Solanas, A. (2012). *Research project "SIMPATIC: Sistema inteligente de monitorización privada autónoma basado en TIC".* [Intelligent System for Private and Autonomous Monitoring based on ICT]. Retrieved June 1, 2014, from http://projecte-simpatic.cat

OECD. (2013). *Organisation for economic co-operation and development factbook 2013: Economic, environmental and social statistics: Population and migration: Elderly population by region.* Retrieved June 1, 2014, from http://www.oecd-ilibrary.org/sites/factbook-2011-en/02/01/04/index.html?itemId=/content/chapter/factbook-2011-12-en

Petersen, R., Doody, R., Kurz, A., Mohs, R. C., Morris, J. C., Rabins, P. V., & Winblad, B. et al. (2001). Current concepts in mild cognitive impairment. *Archives of Neurology, 58*(12), 1985–1992. doi:10.1001/archneur.58.12.1985 PMID:11735772

Petersen, R. C., Smith, G. E., Waring, S. C., Ivnik, R. J., Tangalos, E. G., & Kokmen, E. (1999). Mild cognitive impairment: Clinical characterization and outcome. *Archives of Neurology, 56*(3), 303–308. doi:10.1001/archneur.56.3.303 PMID:10190820

Roberts, R. O., Geda, Y. E., Knopman, D. S., Cha, R. H., Pankratz, V. S., Boeve, B. F., & Rocca, W. A. et al. (2008). The Mayo Clinic study of aging: Design and sampling, participation, baseline measures and sample characteristics. *Neuroepidemiology, 30*(1), 58–69. doi:10.1159/000115751 PMID:18259084

Solanas, A., Martinez-Balleste, A., Perez-Martinez, P. A., Pena, A. F., & Ramos, J. (2013). m-Carer: Privacy-aware monitoring for people with mild cognitive impairment and dementia. *IEEE Journal on Selected Areas in Communications, 31*(9), 19–27. doi:10.1109/JSAC.2013.SUP.0513002

Unverzagt, F. W., Gao, S., Baiyewu, O., Ogunniyi, A. O., Gureje, O., Perkins, A., & Hendrie, H. C. et al. (2001). Prevalence of cognitive impairment: Data from the Indianapolis study of health and aging. *Neurology, 57*(9), 1655–1662. doi:10.1212/WNL.57.9.1655 PMID:11706107

Wilson, J. M. G., & Jungner, G. (1968). Principles and practice of screening for disease. *Chronicle Geneva: World Health Organization, 22*(11), 473. PMID:4234760

KEY TERMS AND DEFINITIONS

E-Health (Electronic Health): The use of computer systems and telecommunications networks to improve the processes involved in medicine, both for diagnosis and relationship between professionals and users.

MCI (Mild Cognitive Impairments): Sensorial or memory slight failures, usually associated to initial stages of dementia and mental or cognitive diseases.

M-Health (Mobile Health): The use of mobile smartphones and mobile networks to improve the processes involved in medicine, both for diagnosis and relationship between professionals and users.

S-Health (Smart Health): The use of the technology to interact with the smart city and offer to the citizens a plethora of smart services related with health.

This work was previously published in Advanced Technological Solutions for E-Health and Dementia Patient Monitoring edited by Fatos Xhafa, Philip Moore, and George Tadros, pages 137-152 copyright year 2015 by Medical Information Science Reference (an imprint of IGI Global).

Chapter 36
Cloud Services for Healthcare:
Insights from a Multidisciplinary Integration Project

Konstantinos Koumaditis
University of Piraeus, Greece

George Vassilacopoulos
University of Piraeus, Greece

George Pittas
University of Piraeus, Greece

Andriana Prentza
University of Piraeus, Greece

Marinos Themistocleous
University of Piraeus, Greece

Dimosthenis Kyriazis
University of Piraeus, Greece

Flora Malamateniou
University of Piraeus, Greece

ABSTRACT

Healthcare organisations are forced to reconsider their current business practices and embark on a cloud adoption journey. Cloud-Computing offers important benefits that make it attractive for healthcare (e.g. cost effective model, big data management etc.). Large Information Technology (IT) companies are investing big sums in building infrastructure, services, tools and applications to facilitate Cloud-Computing for healthcare organisations, practitioners and patients. Yet, many challenges that such integration projects contain are still in the e-health research agenda like design and technology requirements to handle big volume of data, ensure scalability and user satisfaction to name a few. The purpose of this chapter is (a) to address the Cloud-Computing services for healthcare in the form of a Personal Healthcare record (PHR) and (b) demonstrate a multidisciplinary project. In doing so, the authors aim at increasing the awareness of this important endeavour and provide insights on Cloud-Computing e-health services for healthcare organisations.

DOI: 10.4018/978-1-4666-8756-1.ch036

INTRODUCTION

The introduction of Cloud-Computing and its business models have been some of the biggest changes impacting not only the IT sector but also several others including healthcare. The impact of Cloud-Computing on healthcare can be characterized as a positive change as it provides integration at a manageable cost and it introduces a new market of services. These two issues will be analyzed in the following paragraphs.

Doctor's clinics, hospitals, and healthcare organisations (e.g., insurance bodies) require fast access to medical data, computing and large storage facilities which are not provided in the traditional settings (e.g., legacy systems). Additionally, in today's fast communication world medical data needs to be shared across various settings and geographical locations in a fast secure way without limitations (e.g., errors, cost) that might cause significant delay in treatment and loss of time. Recently, cloud technology has started replacing legacy healthcare systems and offers easier and faster access to medical data (e.g., exam results, patients history, etc.) as defined by the way it is stored (e.g., public, private or hybrid). Literature depicts that Cloud-Computing offers significant benefits to the healthcare sector with its business (e.g., pay-as-you-go) model and integration capability (Kuo, 2011). Renowned global IT players like Microsoft, Oracle, Amazon have already heavily invested in more powerful, reliable and cost-efficient cloud platforms, extending their new offerings for e-health services, such as Microsoft's HealthVault, Oracle's Exalogic Elastic Cloud, and Amazon Web Services (AWS) (Zhang, Cheng, & Boutaba, 2010).

The integration that can be achieved from such Cloud-Computing healthcare services is conceptualized under the term integrated patient centered care (Leventhal, Taliaferro, Wong, Hughes, & Mun, 2012). Integrated patient centered care reflects on integrated Healthcare Information Systems (HIS) (with elements as e-health cloud services) requiring coordination across professionals, facilities, support systems that is continuous over time and between patient visits (Singer et al., 2011). This approach is observed on national healthcare strategies that encourage patient involvement in their healthcare treatment. For example, the American Recovery and Reinvestment Act of 2009 (ARRA) laid down by the U.S. government is encouraging businesses in the healthcare industry to utilize certain applications of electronic records (Black et al., 2011). Following similar legislative opportunities worldwide, patients increase their involvement with cloud healthcare services (Axelsson, Melin, & Söderström, 2011). This is a growing involvement, seen in parallel with mechanisms for the collection of information (obtained by mobile and other sources) in order to develop an enhanced, complete and integrated view of citizens health status.

This is an emerging area of e-health and a new market segment for contemporary organizations, given the term m-health (Chatterjee, Chakraborty, Sarker, Sarker, & Lau, 2009). According to a recent report m-health applications that are published on the two leading platforms, iOS and Android, has more than doubled in only 2.5 years to reach more than 100,000 apps (e.g., 1st quarter of 2014) with a market revenue of USD 2.4bn in 2013 and projections to grow to USD 26bn by the end of 2017 (Research2guidance, 2014). The major source of income for m-health application publishers will come from services (69%). These services typically involve backend structures of servers and/or teams of medical staff which monitor and consult with doctors, patients and general healthcare-interested individuals. Sarasohn-Kahn (2010), identified that a major mobile application vendor provides 5,805 health, medical and fitness applications with 73% of them used by patients and 27% by healthcare professionals (Sarasohn-Kahn, 2010). A big advantage to the growth of this market is the parallel advance of the smartphones. Evidently, the latest generation of smartphones is increasingly viewed as handheld computers rather than as phones, due to their powerful on-board computing capability, capacious memories, large screens and open operating systems that encourage application development (Boulos, Wheeler, Tavares, & Jones, 2011). Additionally, another promising area that allows people to be constantly monitored regarding their physical condition is the integration of sensing and consumer electronics. Market experts forecast that monitoring services will correspond to about US$ 15 billion market pool in 2017 (Chowdhury, Krishnan, & Vishwanath, 2012). These services either as m-health and/or via the internet in-home networks, can aid residents and their caregivers by providing continuous medical monitoring, memory enhancement, control of home appliances, medical data access, and emergency communication (Alemdar & Ersoy, 2010).

The aforementioned approaches empower the patients and allow them to take their own measurements, and provide verbal and written inputs (Clemensen, Rasmussen, Denning, & Craggs, 2011). In a technological respect the empowerment happens through information-sharing, offering the patients a visual overview of their course of treatment, letting the patients take their own measurements, and letting them provide verbal and written inputs (Clemensen et al., 2011). Many of these applications are based on Service Oriented Architecture (SOA) as e-health services can be easily delivered to both desktop and mobile computer devices using, for instance, JavaScript and HyperText Markup Language (HTML). Based on the SOA paradigm e-health services can be exposed and run over cloud (in the form of SaaS) (Poulymenopoulou, Malamateniou, & Vassilacopoulos, 2012).

Therefore, it is evident that Cloud-Computing can be used to provide efficient, scalable, portable, interoperable and integrated IT infrastructures that are cost effective and maintainable. Yet, despite the significant importance of these technologies, the healthcare sector has not paid much attention on these technologies. The healthcare industry is a laggard in the adoption of cloud services and this is mainly due to the challenges (e.g., financial, security, interoperability etc.) that such shift holds. As a result, many standalone applications exist in the area of healthcare providing services and supporting the activities of all actors involved such as patients, healthcare professionals, laboratories, hospitals.

At this point emphasis must be placed in past failures of IT systems in industry in general and healthcare in particular and have cost millions of Euros and even the death of patients (Avison & Young, 2007; Dwivedi et al., 2013). For that reason, it is of high importance to research the Cloud Services for Healthcare from a multidiscipline perspective (e.g., technological, medical, business and academic).

PERSONAL HEALTHCARE RECORDS (PHR)

Most developed countries are facing important overall problems regarding health care services, such as:

1. Aging population with increased demand on specialized health care services (e.g., chronic diseases),
2. Need for increased efficiency with limited financial resources (e.g., staff/bed reduction),
3. Requirements for increased accessibility of care outside hospitals (e.g., home care) to name a few.

To these problems, advances in information and communication technologies have provided considerable assistance in the form of Electronic Healthcare Records (EHRs). Yet, it seems that traditional EHRs, which are based on the 'fetch and show' model, provide limited functionality that does not cover the spectrum of the patients' needs. Therefore, new solutions as the PHRs appeared to narrow this gap. In more detail, PHRs' data can come from various sources like EHRs, health providers (e.g., e-Prescibing, e-Referal), and/or directly from the patient him/herself – including non-clinical information (e.g., exercise habits, food and dieting statistics, etc.) (Koufi, Malamateniou, & Vassilacopoulos, 2013). The PHR concept is a new multidiscipline area of research, with crucial aspects as it deals with the wellbeing of patients.

Three general PHR models have been proposed (Detmer, Bloomrosen, Raymond, & Tang, 2008):

1. The stand-alone model,
2. Electronic Health Record (EHR) system, and
3. The integrated one, which is an interoperable system providing linkage with a variety of patient information sources such as EHRs, home diagnostics, insurance claims etc.

The main types of health information supported by PHRs are problem lists, procedures, major illnesses, provider lists, allergy data, home-monitored data, family history, social history and lifestyle, immunizations, medications and laboratory tests (Halamka, Mandl, & Tang, 2008; Tang, Ash, Bates, Overhage, & Sands, 2006). Widely known PHR platforms in terms of centralized web-based portals include Dossia (www.dossia.org) and Microsoft Health Vault (www.healthvault.com) platforms. Many systems presented in literature offer integration with already established PHRs platforms (Reti, Feldman, & Safran, 2009; Zhou, Yang, Álamo, Wong, & Chang, 2010). Early experiences from the adoption of PHR-based systems have been found to be positive, showing that such systems can be feasible, secure, and well accepted by patients (Jennett & Watanabe, 2006). Nonetheless, today's EHRs and PHRs are far from being what the citizens consider as of value to their health, since for the public view, health means more than being disease-free.

Following this trend for patients' empowerment, academics, practitioners and patients advocate in favor of the patient centered healthcare systems. Still the aforementioned advocates have not yet reached a concise definition of Patient-Centered e-health (PCEH) that is shared across the research disciplines that focus on health and Information Technology (IT) (Wilson & Strong, 2014). The lack of consensus can be attributed, amongst other,

1. On the number of challenges that are involved in transitioning healthcare delivery to a more patient-centered system, and
2. The lack of proof-of-concept through well-documented and effective PCEH projects.

Thus, the challenge to integrate and redesign existing healthcare systems towards a more patient-centered exists (Leventhal et al., 2012).

To this end, the authors introduce in this chapter a list of PHR/EHR approaches and provide a brief introduction for each in the following section.

CURRENT PHR/EHR CLOUD-COMPUTING PROJECTS

Literature includes various examples of PHR and EHR approaches with different themes, addressing various aspects and produced in diverse settings (e.g., industry, academia etc.). This composes a mosaic of different examples that individual researchers of the field and/or developers need to consider before embarking in the Cloud-Computing e-health journey. Studying past endeavors one may learn from the successes and diverge from the mistakes of others. Therefore, our intentions for presenting such examples extend from providing a helpful list of recent PHR/EHR projects to illustrate unique techniques to implement Cloud services, describe ways to resolve the integration challenges faced, provide recent advances from academia and industry and highlight lessons learned and recommendations. The authors acknowledge that this is not an exhaustive list of examples but a suitable one for the theme and audience of this book.

To provide a better illustration and help the reader understand this important integration issue, the authors researched the literature and depict herein a twofold categorization of the findings, such as:

1. PHR/EHR solutions and/or
2. PHR/EHR components.

This provides a useful categorization in the current ongoing PHR issues discussion. Starting with the PHR/EHR below the identified projects are presented in an alphabetical list.

- **CareCloud:** Offers several approaches ranging from SaaS, to data analytics and IaaS. It offers healthcare practices a way to manage their practice with a plethora of tools. CareCloud allows the management of patient records, appointments, billing and reporting. Charts solution provides an easy to use EHR system. CareCloud also has solutions for doctor – patient virtual interaction (SUCRE, 2014).

- **ClearHealth Office:** A solution for small practices (fewer than ten physicians or 20,000 encounters per year) that can be distributed in two forms. The one is on premises and the second is cloud based. The first one (on premise), requires hardware and detailed setup processes. The second one is a cloud solution that removes the need for hardware and the problems with detailed setup. It is called HealthCloud and promises to deliver ready-to-go installations of ClearHealth Office on fully managed and secured datacenters owned by Amazon. This service is suitable for US practitioners, interested in self-serving their installations (ClearHealth, 2013).

- **EMC Electronic Health Record Infrastructure Solutions:** Consist of integrated, validated solutions with industry-leading healthcare ISV partners, clinical applications, and best-in-class hardware, software, and services to help caregivers to move forward with their EHR deployment. EMC provides the supporting IT infrastructure aligned with clinical services needs for the highest levels of performance, availability, security, virtualization, and integration (EMC, 2014).

- **Healthcare Trustworthy Platform:** A multilevel Personal Health Record (PHR) platform based on the Trustworthy Cloud Technology that allows people to share health data while guaranteeing security and privacy. It aims to integrate of third party applications and give them access to user's health data (e.g., view, add and update). It also provides a high security model which allows the patients to decide how and with whom to share data (Tclouds, 2014).

- **HealthVault:** The most popular solution in our list is the well-known HealthVault. It is being distributed through Windows Azure cloud server, which is already widely implemented in business environments and in some public administrations. Microsoft HealthVault provides one place to store and access of health information online. It supports interoperability with other healthcare providers. There is a growing list of devices such as pedometers, blood pressure monitors, blood glucose monitors, and even weight scales which work with HealthVault. In that way the users, don't have to enter anything by hand, just upload their data directly to HealthVault from compatible devices (Microsoft, 2014).

- **Medscribler:** A SaaS solution for recording patient data. It uses mobile technologies such as tablets and smartphones and handwriting recognition software to allow ease submission of patient data. It is an EMR solution that provides a quick and intuitive way to update medical records of patients. These records can be stored in a cloud. This solution provides an innovative approach to the problems of mobile practicing of medicine. The doctor is able to update patient records via a network connection and thus has no need for bulkier equipment than a tablet computer (Medscribbler, 2014).

- **OpenEMR:** A free and open source Electronic Health Records (EMR) and medical practice management application that can run on multiple platforms. OpenEMR is supported by a community of volunteers and professionals. This software can be implemented into a cloud as SaaS. It supports cloud structures, encryption, remote access and web browser access (OpenEMR, 2014).
- **SOFTCARE:** A multi-cloud-enabled platform which has developed a prototype of a monitoring system for seniors that allow caregivers (formal and informal) and senior users to get real-time alarms in dangerous or potentially dangerous situations and warnings on long-term trends that could indicate a future problem. It is based on Artificial Intelligence techniques that allow the recognition of daily activities based on the data obtained from an accelerometer (bracelet device) and location information (AAL-Europe, 2013).
- **X1.V1:** Another integration platform is X1.V1. It offers effective tools to generate reports about
  - The general healthcare status of the population,
  - The quality of healthcare performance, and
  - The financial costs. In that way, it facilitates the cooperation among the different caregivers in the provision

of diagnosis and treatment. Another intuitive feature is that it enhances epidemic diseases and cancer detection rate (Deadalus, 2014).

- **Zappa:** An open source, extensible, scalable and customizable cloud platform for the development of e-Health/m-Health systems. It aims at delivering resources as services over Internet (Cloud-Computing). Moreover, the platform is intended to provide uninterrupted monitoring with the goal of obtaining some information that can be subsequently analyzed by physicians for diagnosing. It has also been developed two e-Health applications based on that platform:
  - Zappa App,
  - Cloud Rehab (Ruiz-Zafra, Benghazi, Noguera, & Garrido, 2013).

Having described the PHR/EHR solutions, the second part of list, the PHR/EHR components are depicted.

- **Cloud Rehab:** is a full m-Health system that is used to monitor the daily activities of patients with severe brain damage. It is a component to the Zappa cloud platform mentioned above. Cloud Rehab consists of two applications
  - Web application, and
  - Android application. Web application is being used by the medical staff to manage patients' medical information. Whereas, android application is being used by the patient. The mobile application monitors heart rate and sends the data to the cloud (Ruiz-Zafra et al., 2013).
- **DAPHNE:** A Data as a Service (DaaS) platform for collecting, managing and analyzing wellness data in order to provide healthy lifestyle and preventive medicine (Daphne, 2013). DAPHNE platform is

open to hardware and software developers, providing data for different personalised health services, both for the citizen and the service provider.

- **EMC Collaborative Healthcare Solutions:** Provides a patient-centric infrastructure to "content-enable" Picture Archiving and Communication System, Hospital Information System, and Electronic Medical Record applications for accessing all relevant clinical, financial, and operational data. Based on open standards, the solution is in accordance with the Integrating the Healthcare Enterprise initiative that promotes the coordinated use of established standards. Their solution enhances operational agility through the abstraction of applications and infrastructure, improves financial performance by managing physical and virtual assets with highly automated tools, and secures access to and prevents loss of protected health information (SUCRE, 2014).
- **VIGOR++:** An international research project that aims to create a personalised gastrointestinal tract model, which facilitates accurate detection and grading of Crohn's disease. VIGOR++ processes multiscale information from patients, including laboratory, MRI, colonoscopy and microscopy (histopathology) data. Its techniques are integrated in the 3DNetMedical.com medical imaging cloud service, to make them immediately available in a clinically usable environment (Vodera, 2014).
- **Zappa App:** An m-Health system used to monitor the heart rate, temperature and blood pressure of the patient. It is a component to the Zappa cloud platform which is mentioned above. In addition, Zappa App is able to save the vital sign values, detect health problems and share information with a doctor or medical staff that are in the same place as the patient (Bluetooth) (Ruiz-Zafra et al., 2013).

The aforementioned categorized list is presented in Table 1. The first column is an arithmetic count of the projects, the second the name, the third the type based on our categorization, the fourth the description and the last column the reference for each.

The aforementioned PHR/EHR solutions utilize the Cloud-Computing advances to achieve common goals, therefore they hold similarities such as:

1. Integration,
2. Interoperability, and
3. Lower business expenses.

All of the aforementioned approaches try to integrate different systems to manage medical information based on a centralized system hosted on cloud. Furthermore, they try to provide users with the ability to access the systems through different type of operating systems (e.g., Windows, Linux, and MAC OS) and devices (e.g., desktop, laptop, tablet, smartphones, and medical sensors). The solutions presented in Table 1 leverage Cloud-Computing benefits to lower expenses both on Operating Expenditure (OPEX) and Capital Expenditure (CAPEX) at the health section. For example, solution number [7] can run in different systems, while [1,4,9] support integration of different type of systems resulting to lower business expenses.

Apart from the similarities, the above mentioned solutions also have differences between them, such as:

1. Different type of users,
2. Different target territories, and
3. Different type of devices.

For example, solution number [8] is designed for senior people, [2] for small practices and [11] for patients with severe brain damage, [2] targets USA practitioners and [11, 15] address mobile devices implementations.

Table 1. Requirements: proposed technologies

	Name	Type	Description	Reference
1.	CareCloud	EHR	An easy to use EHR system which provides solutions for doctor – patient virtual interaction.	(SUCRE, 2014)
2.	ClearHealth Office	EHR	Provides an open source solution for running a small practice.	(ClearHealth, 2013)
3.	EMC Electronic Health Record Infrastructure Solutions	PHR/ EHR	Provides clinical applications, hardware, software, and services.	(EMC, 2014)
4.	Healthcare Trustworthy Platform	PHR	PHR platform for sharing securely health data and providing integration with 3rd party applications.	(Tclouds, 2014)
5.	HealthVault	PHR	Provides one place to store and access all health information online.	(Microsoft, 2014)
6.	Medscribler	EHR	SaaS solution providing intuitive way to solve the mobile's practicing issues of medicine.	(Medscribbler, 2014)
7.	OpenEMR	EHR	Free and open source Electronic Health Records (EHR) and medical practice management application that can on multiple platforms.	(OpenEMR, 2014)
8.	SOFTCARE	PHR	Multi-cloud-enabled platform monitoring senior people.	(AAL, 2013)
9.	X1.V1	PHR/ EHR	Integrated platform with intuitive features statistical reports about patients, caregivers and financial costs)	(Deadalus, 2014)
10.	Zappa	PHR/ EHR	Extensible, scalable and customizable cloud platform for the development of e-Health/m-Health systems.	(Ruiz-Zafra et al., 2013)
11.	Cloud Rehab	COM/ NT	M-health system monitor daily activities of patients with severe brain damage	(Ruiz-Zafra et al., 2013)
12.	DAPHNE	COM/ NT	Data as a Service (DaaS) platform for collecting, managing and analyzing wellness data in order to provide healthy lifestyle and preventive medicine	(Daphne, 2013)
13.	EMC Collaborative Healthcare Solutions	PHR/ EHR	Provides a patient-centric infrastructure to "content-enable" Picture Archiving and Communication System, Hospital Information System, and Electronic Medical Record applications.	(SUCRE, 2014)
14.	VIGOR++	COM/ NT	Personalised gastrointestinal tract model, which facilitates accurate detection and grading of Crohn's disease.	(Vodera, 2014)
15.	Zappa App	COM/ NT	M-health system for monitoring the heart rate, temperature, blood pressure of patient	(Ruiz-Zafra et al., 2013)

The aforementioned Cloud-Computing solutions hold several merits and aim at the same goal, provide better e-health services. Yet, due to the critical nature of healthcare and the importance of successful implementation of such endeavors, there is still need for rigorous research that can carefully examine the development steps and provide "best-fit" technologies. To accommodate this need the authors' involvement in a multidiscipline e-health integration project that utilizes Cloud-Computing. This endeavor is analyzed in the following section.

PROVIDING INTEGRATED E-HEALTH SERVICES FOR PERSONALIZED MEDICINE UTILIZING CLOUD INFRASTRUCTURE (PINCLOUD)

The proposed project *Providing INtegrated e-health services for personalized medicine utilizing CLOUD* infrastructure (PINCLOUD), seeks to integrate different application components, leading to the provision of an end-to-end personalized disease monitoring and medical data service "anytime, anywhere", which ensures an independent living regardless of age (Koumaditis et al., 2014). Additionally, from a managerial and research perspective it can be emphasized that the multidiscipline nature of this project provided a multidiscipline R&D team. The authors of this chapter are part of this team covering a wide range of disciplines from healthcare professionals, IT experts, researchers from both academia and business.

Introduction

The scenario upon which PINCLOUD is developed, as seen in Figure 1, plays as such: a patient governs his\her PHR that can be remotely monitored by a doctor located either at a hospital or at an individual medical office. Complementary to the PHR's stored information the doctor monitors the patient using a home-care platform that receives and analyses patient's medical data. The proposed home-care platform will include among others the following services:

1. Asthma or COPD disease management;
2. Hyper-tension disease management;
3. Diabetes monitoring;
4. ECG monitoring;
5. Video/Audio Access to physicians for remote consultation;
6. Remote picture and text archiving and communication service (back-up/long term

Figure 1. Providing integrated e-health services for personalized medicine utilizing cloud infrastructure

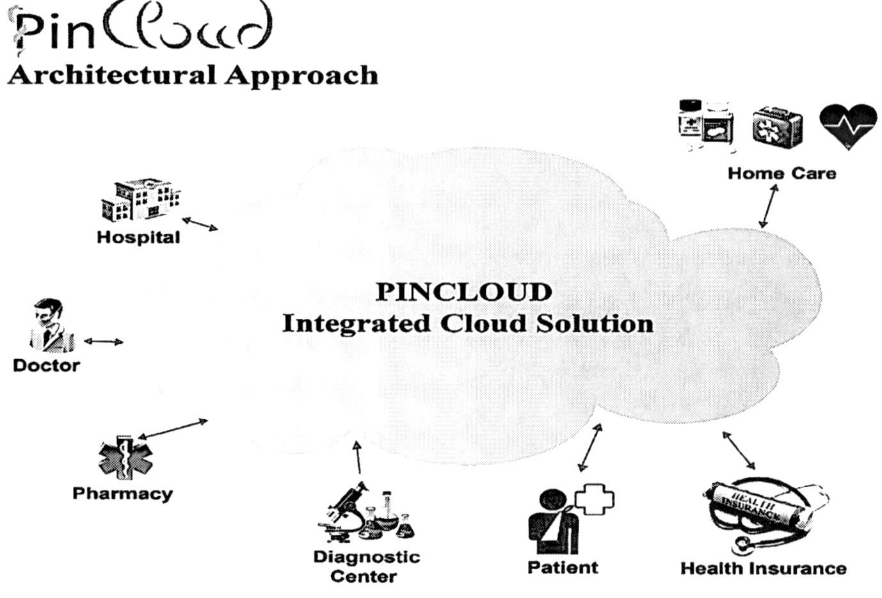

archiving complementary to infrastructure operated by hospitals); and

7. Fall Prevention and Detection Services.

The doctor can access the patient's PHR online through the PINCLOUD Integrated Cloud Solution. The latter can support the doctor in decision making and results in better quality of health service. In more detail, the doctor retrieves and updates the patient's medical data and can also use the proposed on-line system to:

1. Prescribe a new medicine;
2. Fill in an e-referral for specific exams (e.g., blood test);
3. Inform and advise his/her patient; or
4. Ask the patient to visit the hospital.

Following the doctor's advice, the patient visits a pharmacy, or a diagnostic center or a hospital. At the final stage, the healthcare service providers (doctors, hospitals, diagnostic centers) and pharmacies interact with the health insurance organisation to compensate all outstanding orders and medical actions.

MAIN IDEAS AND REQUIREMENTS

Service and data availability is crucial for healthcare providers who cannot effectively operate unless their applications are functioning properly and patients' data are available in a consistent manner. This is also the case for PINCLOUD. PINCLOUD's services (e.g., E-Prescription, E-Referral, Home-Care and PHR) ought to be available continuously with no interruptions or performance degradation since they will be used for decision making regarding the patients wellbeing.

New development projects, as PINCLOUD need to reinsure service availability to the participating healthcare providers and other organizations. In addition, hardware and software instal-

lations, upgrades, and reconfigurations have to be managed and maintained without any service interruptions that may cause problems. In order to achieve the availability in a cost efficient way the use of Cloud-Computing seemed to be the appropriate solution and thus the PINCLOUD was designed based on its features. Features such as cost-saving, agility, efficiency, resource consolidation, business opportunities and Green-IT are relevant and applicable to the healthcare sector (Chang et al, 2011; Chang, 2013b; Chang 2014).

Moreover, PINCLOUD potentially will be responsible for the governance of a big volume of medical and thus sensitive data. The protection of such data is paramount. At this stage of the project the protection of these data is achieved with a Private Cloud delivery model. A Private Cloud model is operated by a single organization. In the private cloud, the technology resides within an organization's own data centre and the resources are deployed as needed to the different departments. In our project, a private IT company which is part of the consortium has provided the Private Cloud's infrastructure. In that way, the developers can overcome the challenges associated with other Cloud models (e.g., Public, Hybrid) since the ability to manage and control sensitive patient data remains within the organization.

As mentioned above, PINCLOUD is based on the well-known Cloud-Computing three service models' structure, namely:

1. Software as a Service (SaaS),
2. Platform as a Service (PaaS), and
3. Infrastructure as a Service (IaaS).

The way that PINCLOUD is decoded in the three models is depicted in Figure 2 and it is explained in the following paragraphs.

Respectively, PINCLOUD provides the user interaction through SaaS. In theory, SaaS is the capability provided to the consumer to use the provider's applications running on a cloud infrastructure (Mell & Grance, 2009). The applications

Figure 2. PINCLOUD's services and actors

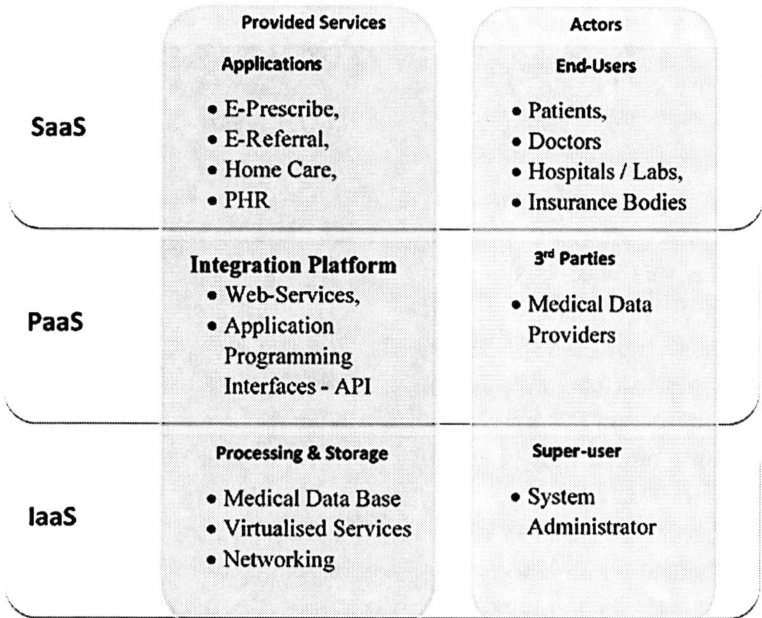

are accessible from various client devices through either a thin client interface, such as a web browser (e.g., web-based email), or a program interface. PINCLOUD as depicted in Figure 2, offers four applications:

1. E-prescription,
2. E-referral,
3. Home-Care, and
4. PHR.

These applications provide the main functionality required and are being consumed by End-Users (e.g., Patients, Doctors, Hospitals/Labs and Insurance Bodies). All these users access the PINCLOUD through user-interface provided as a service. For example, a PINCLOUD registered user can have access to his/her medical record online.

In addition, PINCLOUD takes advantage of PaaS service model. Literature presents PaaS as the capability provided to the consumer to use and or deploy into the cloud infrastructure consumer-created or acquired applications created using programming languages and tools supported by the provider (Mell & Grance, 2009). Accordingly, the R&D team takes advantage of the PaaS model and provides open source components as Web-Services and Application Programming Interfaces (APIs) that facilitate the integration with third parties (e.g., Medical Data Providers, Hospitals). For example, when a hospital decides to be integrated in the PINCLOUD system, it can allocate and consume the Web-services' API that the R&D team have created.

The processing and storage capability of PINCLOUD is based on IaaS model. IaaS is the capability provided to the consumer to provide processing, storage, networks, and other fundamental computing resources while the consumer can deploy and run arbitrary software, which can include operating systems and applications (Mell & Grance, 2009). PINCLOUD takes advantage of the IaaS and provides data processing and storage of medical data. IaaS consists of multiple Virtual Machines (VM), Medical Data Base and Network Infrastructure. In the given case, multiple VMs are utilized with each one dedicated to a specific service (e.g., Database, Access Control, Backup). The Medical Data Base handles the data processing and storage while network infrastructure handles the connectivity between the different VMs. The only user who is responsible for the smooth operation of the VMs and the services running on them is the PINCLOUD's administrator.

What is more, the proposed architecture encompasses a mechanism that aims at dynamic deployment of application services in cloud infrastructures. The mechanism incorporates a monitoring framework that collects information, both on infrastructure and on application levels. With respect to the infrastructure metrics, CPU and memory are monitored on different time intervals, while number of users, response time, and location of requests are collected on the application level. Based on the aforementioned information, different deployment policies are put in place (e.g., deployment of additional VMs or deployment in different locations) so as to enable provision of quality of service guarantees for the presented cloud healthcare application.

To this end, one of the first responsibilities assigned to the R&D team was to list the requirements of the blueprint architecture. Counting several meetings and long brainstorming sessions with the cooperating partners and their project teams, various requirements were highlighted. In this section, the authors present the most relevant to the theme of this publication (e.g., relating to Cloud-Computing issues), such as:

- Virtualization,
- Healthcare Interoperability,
- Security,
- Big Volume of Data,
- Scalability,
- Responsive,
- Content Management,
- Dynamic and Scalable User Interface.

Based on the above aforementioned requirements the R&D team embarked on the design and implementation of the PINCLOUD application and technologies. The conceptualization, development steps and direction taken to accommodate the project requirements are depicted in the following section.

DESIGN AND IMPLEMENTATION

'Virtualization' is at the core of most cloud architectures. The concept of virtualization allows an abstract representation of logical and physical resources including servers, storage devices, networks and software. The basic idea behind it is to pool all physical resources and their management as a whole, meeting the individual demands from these shared resources (Lupse, Vida, & Stoicu-Tivadar, 2012). In our case, we used multiple Virtual Machines (VM) each one running one service. For example, Data storage, Data processing, interconnectivity with 3rd parties' medical providers and user interface were placed in Individual VMs. Using Virtualization has many benefits including:

1. Easier replication and cloning a VM than physical server,
2. Lower down time in case of failure,
3. Lower power consumption and saving resources by running multiple Virtual Machines (VM) within the same physical server (Chang, 2013a).

Another requirement is the interoperability which is the ability of two or more systems or components (e.g., two or more HIS) to exchange data and use the information that has been exchanged (Lupse et al., 2012). Legislation surrounding e-Health communications promote a standardized communication process with standards and protocols. For example, the Integrating the Healthcare Enterprise (IHE) organization provides standards (e.g., HL7, DICOM, etc.) to enhance the interoperability and information sharing (IHE, 2012). An enabler of these standards is the SOA paradigm. An example of this is the recognised Healthcare Services Specification Program (HSSP) program, which is a collaborative effort between standards groups HL7 and OMG to address interoperability challenges within the healthcare sector, operating on SOA (HSSP, 2013). To ensure interoperability with 3rd parties, PINCLOUD adopts HL7 CDA (Clinical Document Architecture). The HL7 CDA standard is a document markup standard that specifies the structure and semantics of "clinical documents" for the purpose of data exchange (Lupse et al., 2012). In that way, PINCLOUD achieves integration with the providers' HIS and also data integrity.

Another important requirement that was taken under consideration is the security and protection of information against unauthorized access. As different users including:

1. Patients,
2. Doctors,
3. Hospitals,
4. Insurance companies, and
5. Pharmacies access the system, sensitive information may be provided only to authorized users (Narayanan & Giine, 2011).

In our case, Access Control is a critical part of PINCLOUD due to the large amount of sensitive medical data and the multiple users who interact with it. Access rights to resources must be granted at the right time to the right users in order to avoid unauthorized access to medical data. For example, a doctor should be given access to medical history of a patient only after patient's approval. In that way, we can reinsure protection against unauthorized access and distribution of medical data.

PINCLOUD is a multidiscipline e-health integration project. The need for this integrated approach to handle big volume of medical data is critical. Big data is high-volume, high-velocity and high-variety information assets that demand

cost-effective, innovative forms of information processing for enhanced insight and decision making (Altman, Nagle, & Tushman, 2013). The systems need to handle and store these big amounts of medical data in a secure and consistent manner. A plateau of well-known database systems exists, most of them based on SQL, yet those cannot handle big data since they are not scalable (Cuzzocrea, Song, & Davis, 2011). Thus, one of the early motivation was to research and examine contemporary systems to handle large volume of data appropriate for the purpose of this project. Our research surfaced several interesting results like:

1. The current trend for big data is document based databases, and
2. Two of the most prominent database systems are Couchbase and MongoDB (COUCHBASE, 2014; MongoDB, 2013).

The latter are open source document based databases and from the on-going examination seem promising and fit for the purpose of this project.

Another important feature that was taken under consideration is the scalability. Due to the type (e.g., numerous different users and real time data streaming) of the application the developers needed to ensure its availability regardless of the number of concurrent connections. The only way to achieve this is through technologies which support scalability and take advantage of Cloud-Computing features. Due to the familiarization of the R&D team with SOA it was considered as the best practice available. Yet, the challenging part was to select the appropriate technologies to implement SOA. In a process to scan the spectrum of available "best-fit" solutions the R&D team examined various technologies, but dropped most of them since they are not compatible with the big data paradigm. From the examination process, the most prominent ones are nodejs and scala. These are highlighted since both

1. Support the aforementioned document based databases,
2. Provide high flexibility, and
3. Offer high availability (;).

As stated, it is important for the PINCLOUD integrated service users to access the web from their mobile devices. Thus, it was essential to provide the ability to the users to have access to the application through multiple devices such as:

1. Desktops,
2. Laptops,
3. Tablets, and
4. Smartphones.

One of the important tasks was to insure that the system will provide the best user experience on all the aforementioned devices. This may provide higher adoption rates of the applications. The responsiveness was insured by adopting responsive interface which is the optimal viewing experience (e.g., easy reading and navigation with a minimum of resizing, panning, and scrolling) across a wide range of devices (Marcotte, 2011). After analyzing various frameworks that support responsive design at the moment on top of our list is bootstrap (Bootstrap, 2014). Bootstrap is developed and distributed free by Twitter Company and allows easy and quick responsive design implementation.

Another consideration taken was the dynamic User Interface (UI). Many cases in healthcare emphasize the correlation of a good UI with the high adoption rates and vise-versa. Therefore the need to make sure that the best practices and state of the art technologies will be followed for this issue, was ever-present. HTML5 is the latest version of the well-known HyperText Markup Language (HTML) and provides features which facilitate not only the user interaction but also the developing phase (Pilgrim, 2010). PINCLOUD is set to adhere to a healthy adoption percentage and thus a user friendly web interface to the end-users was a requirement. Therefore, the HTML5

which provides portability across different mobile platforms was utilized (Preuveneers, Berbers, & Joosen, 2013).

Additionally an issue the R&D team had to tackle was how to consume the web-services (e.g., different options exist like server-side and client-side consumption). For consuming the web services various options of JavaScript frameworks had to be considered (e.g., AngularJS, Backbone.js, CanJS and Ember.js). Through an evaluation of these frameworks and promoting the client-side consumption two were selected:

1. AngularJS, and
2. ember.js.

The more promising one is AngularJS, developed by Google which is widely used lately as it provides dynamic and scalable User Interface (UI) (Google, 2014; Tilde, 2014).

In order to facilitate the administration of the web application's content, several Content Management Systems (CMS) that provide state of the art features such as

1. Extensibility,
2. Remote access,
3. Users management, were considered.

Currently, top of our list are Liferay and Drupal (Drupal, 2014; Liferay, 2014). Liferay is the most widely known java based CMS, while Drupal is based on PHP Hypertext Preprocessor. Both of them are open source solutions having very large communities which provide support and security updates. In that way, the R&D team can focus on the improvement of the core features of PINCLOUD and not at the updates (e.g., security updates). For our needs, Liferay approach was a favorite due to the familiarization of the R&D team with Java.

An illustrative view of the aforementioned requirements alongside the proposed solutions are depict in Table 2.

Table 2. Requirements: proposed technologies

Requirements	Proposed Solutions
Virtualization	Virtual Machines (VM)
Healthcare Interoperability	HL7 CDA Standard, DICOM
Security	Private Cloud, Role Based Access Control
Big volume of data	Document Based Databases (Mongodb, Couchdb)
Scalability	SOA, nodejs, Scala
Responsive User Interface	Twitter Bootstrap, Foundation, Skeleton
Dynamic and scalable User Interface	AngularJS, ember.js, HTML5
Content Management	Liferay CMS, Drupal

Currently PINCLOUD is in its implementation phase, upon which the various components such as:

1. PHR platform,
2. E-prescribing and e-referral, and
3. Homecare applications, are being developed and tested (Lab of Medical Informatics, 2014).

The implementation is based on the technologies addressed in this section. In the next Section an example of the E-Prescribing Analysis is highlighted.

E-PRESCRIBING BUSINESS PROCESS

In this section the authors provide an analysis of the E-Prescription Service. This analysis is highlighted as to offer a suitable example of a complex business process addressed in our work. This close examination aids the reader to understand the configuration of E-Prescribing throughout the different Cloud-Computing models (SaaS, PaaS and IaaS). The analysis id presented with the aid of two Figures:

1. Figure 3 that depicts the business process, and
2. Figure 4 that illustrates the configuration of the E-Prescription through the different Cloud-Computing models.

Analysis

After a patient examination the doctor (e.g., general practitioner) prescribes medicines to a patient using the PINCLOUD application. Yet, before the doctor gain access to the E-Prescription service, he/she needs to be authenticated using his credentials through the web interface (Login) of the PINCLOUD. This step is the first step of the sequence depicted in Figure 3. After a successful user authentication, he/she is prompted four options to select, such as:

Figure 3. E-prescription process

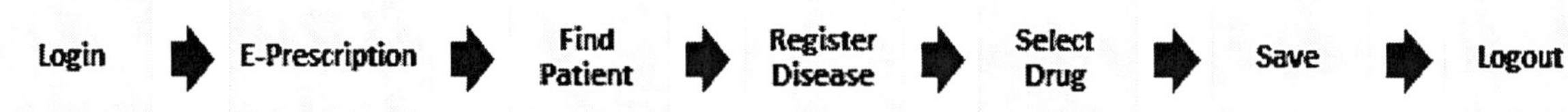

Figure 4. E-prescription analysis

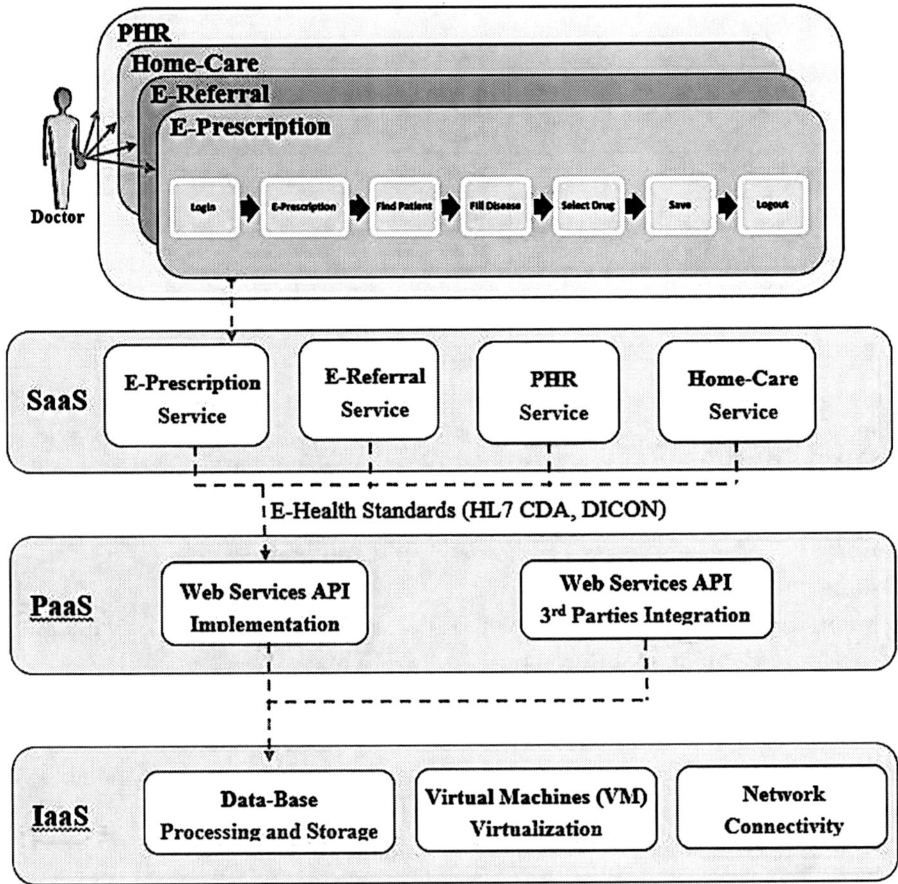

1. PHR,
2. Home-Care,
3. E-Referral, and
4. E-Prescription.

These four options are the main services provided through the PINCLOUD platform.

In the scenario presented in this sub-section the doctor selects E-Prescription. Subsequently, he/she locates the patient using the patient's Social Security Number (S.S.N.) which is unique for each patient. Before the doctor can prescribe the medicine, it is required by the system to register the diagnosed disease and any relevant treatment comments (e.g., free text) that he/she feels is applicable. The patient's disease is encoded based on the Worlds Healthcare Organization International Statistical Classification of Diseases and Related Health Problems that is now at its 10th Revision (e.g., ICD 10). ICD10 standard is considered as a best practice and therefore applicable in PINCLOUD. The next sequence in the business process, allows the doctor to select the drugs through a suggested drugs' list. The suggested list corresponds to the diagnosed disease and the patient's medical history which is stored in PINCLOUD storage infrastructure. The doctor is not limited to the listed drugs but he/she can also choose other drugs beyond the listed ones based on his professional judgment. The doctor can also fill the dosage (e.g., number of pills) and other information of usage (e.g., frequency, oral etc.) for each selected drug. After filing all the information for the prescribed drugs, the system validates the selection of drugs based on their interaction on issues such as:

1. Other drugs,
2. Patient's allergies, and
3. Medication history.

Consequently, if the cross-checking produces no alerts, the prescription is stored waiting to be processed in Pharmacies.

As mentioned in the introduction, PINCLOUD is divided into three service models (e.g., SaaS, PaaS and IaaS). To be more specific, SaaS provides all the PINCLOUD's services such as:

1. PHR,
2. Home-Care,
3. E-referral, and
4. E-Prescribe.

The SaaS connects users to aforementioned services while providing basic functions such as

1. Web interface,
2. A secure communication, and
3. Authentication control.

In order to support the scalability, the application can be installed on multiple machines which are clustered. The use of HTTPS protocol guaranties a lightweight security and makes the application compliant with HIPAA security regulations.

Additionally, PINCLOUD takes advantage of PaaS by providing two kinds of APIs, the first one is for the interconnectivity between the different provided services and the storage, while the second one provides the ability to 3rd parties to connect with PINCLOUD.

The R&D team used Representational state transfer (REST) architectural style to develop the web services APIs. With REST it is feasible to design unique URLs dynamically to represent remote health records objects as needed. The frontend sends HTTP requests over Secure Sockets Layer (SSL) to obtain a JavaScript Object Notation (JSON) of the desired medical data. With REST, the identification of the resources (doctor, patient, lab results, drugs, medical exams) is straightforward. There is no need for the client to create complex requests to query the server. To be compliant with HIPAA security regulations, a POST method is used and the sensitive information (e.g., a query on a patient name) is passed in the body of the request as a JSON object over an SSL connection. All request and response headers have a content type "application/json" which means that complex queries and responses are in the form of JSON arrays or JSON objects. In addition to this, each time the user logs in, the server provides a security token which is mediatory each time the user is calling any API operation. This installment is placed for authentication reasons.

As the Figure 4 depicts, APIs run on PaaS and they handle the communication between the SaaS and IaaS. The exchanged information between those two services follows the E-health standards such as

1. Health Level 7 (HL7) for transferring clinical and administrative data,
2. Clinical Document Architecture (CDA) for encoding, structure and semantics of clinical documents, and
3. Digital Imaging and Communications in Medicine (DICOM) standard for handling, storing, printing, and transmitting information in medical imaging.

The First API includes operations for the aforementioned SaaS services. More specificly, it includes all the required operations as they are depicted in Table 3 below, like:

1. Login of user,
2. Retrieve patient's profile,
3. Creation of a new prescription, and
4. Specific prescription retrieval.

Table 3. Examples API operations

POST /users/login	Login of user
GET /users/{userId}/patient/{SSN}	Retrieve patient profile
POST /users/{userID}/patient/{SSN}/ prescription/add	Create a new prescription
GET /users/{userID}/patient/{SSN}/ prescription/{prescriptionId}	Return specific prescription

The API operations were designed to be versatile, secure and easy to use.

The second API is designed for 3rd parties (e.g., medical providers) which interact with PINCLOUD. Currently, it is under development. These providers already use their own solutions which have different architecture. This makes the integration difficult. The aim of the API is to facilitate the integration with 3rd parties' solutions. Additionally, the integration can be facilitated using e-health standards like HL7 CDA.

In Figure 4, the IaaS back-end functions are depicted, including amongst others:

1. The storage servers with their database system,
2. The virtual machines, and
3. Networking functions.

In more detail, the IaaS in our case, consists of three different kinds of servers:

- **Primary Servers:** Virtual Machines (VM) running the PINCLOUD applications. These servers are responsible for performing most of the computation.
- **Specific Servers:** Virtual Machines (VM) whose main task is to manage the communication with the database and with other servers.
- **Control Server:** Virtual Machine (VM) which monitors the overall PINCLOUD status. This server is responsible for creating

and removing virtual machines dynamically based on dynamically changed requirements (e.g., too many concurrent users).

Moreover, IaaS provides a network which interconnects all the VMs by establishing a secure connection between them in order to complete all the requests between PINCLOUD application services.

User Interface

The aim of the R&D team is also to provide a user friendly web interface. Thus a balance between implementation of the required functionality required to complete a task and how the task is exposed through the user interface is needed. In other words, the user interface should not only be functional but also usable. To achieve this, the R&D team follows the user interface development process which is presented below in three phases, like:

1. Design,
2. Implementation, and
3. Testing.

At the current moment, the project is at the implementation phase.

- The Design Phase includes:
  - Determination of the initial requirements and goals for PINCLOUD,
  - Identification of use cases,
  - Conceptual design,
  - Logical design, and
  - Physical design.
- The Implementation Phase includes:
  - The prototyping of mockups that focus on the interface and user interaction, and

- ○ Building the user interface and preparation for upcoming design changes.
- The Testing Phase is set build test and evaluation scenarios and run those with various users.

To provide a clear view of the implementation phase, an example of the UI screens are presented below. The screens are divided in five main sections, like:

1. Patient's Information (seen in Figure 5),
2. Disease (seen in Figure 6),
3. Reasoning (seen in Figure 6),
4. Featured Prescription Drugs (seen in Figure 6), and
5. Suggested Medical Treatment (seen in Figure 7).

Starting with the 'Patient Information' screen, as seen in Figure 5, based on which the Doctor retrieves the patient's profile information prior to prescribing the drugs. In more detail, he/she needs to query using a unique identifier Social Security Number (SSN) and the PINCLOUD returns the patient's profile details.

Afterwards, as it is depicted in Figure 6 the doctor fills the diagnosed disease and any relevant comments (e.g., free text). The doctor chooses the "add drug" button in order to prescribe a new drug.

After the selection of the "add drug" selection, a modal window appears, as Figure 7 depicts. The doctor fills the drastic ingredients for the suggested treatment based on the diagnosed disease and PINCLOUD returns a list of suggested drugs to let the Doctor select the appropriate one. Afterwards, he/she chooses amongst several characteristics, such as:

1. Package of the selected drug,
2. Way of offer (e.g., oral),
3. Quantity,
4. Frequency (e.g., 1 pill every 6 hours), and
5. Treatment duration (e.g., 10 days).

Additionally, an option to include further instructions exists. In the event of a drastic ingredient interacting with patient's disease then PINCLOUD returns a message (alert) and prevents the doctor from adding the selected drug. Otherwise, the system displays the table of the selected drugs as it is depicted in Figure 6 (bottom half of figure). Finally the Doctor can:

1. Cancel the entered details in case of mistake,
2. Save temporary the prescription to be used later, and
3. Submit the final prescription.

Figure 5. Screen: patients' information

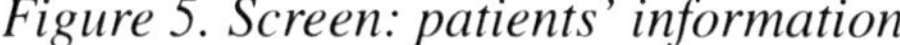

Figure 6. Screen: disease-reasoning-featured prescription drugs

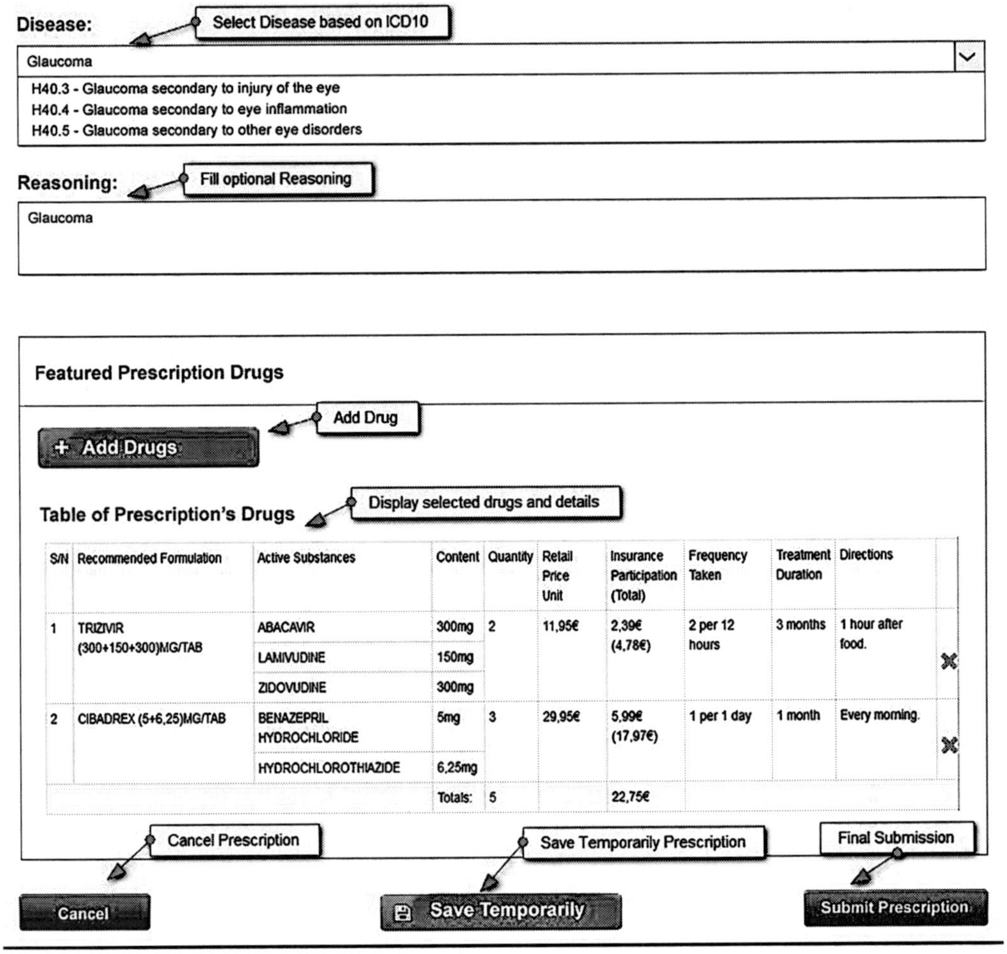

Disease:
Select Disease based on ICD10
Glaucoma
H40.3 - Glaucoma secondary to injury of the eye
H40.4 - Glaucoma secondary to eye inflammation
H40.5 - Glaucoma secondary to other eye disorders
Reasoning:
Fill optional Reasoning
Glaucoma
Featured Prescription Drugs
Add Drug
+ Add Drugs
Table of Prescription's Drugs
Display selected drugs and details
S/N Recommended Formulation Active Substances Content Quantity Retail Price Unit Insurance Participation (Total) Frequency Taken Treatment Duration Directions
1 TRIZIVIR (300+150+300)MG/TAB ABACAVIR 300mg 2 11,95€ 2,39€ (4,78€) 2 per 12 hours 3 months 1 hour after food.
LAMIVUDINE 150mg
ZIDOVUDINE 300mg
2 CIBADREX (5+6,25)MG/TAB BENAZEPRIL HYDROCHLORIDE 5mg 3 29,95€ 5,99€ (17,97€) 1 per 1 day 1 month Every morning.
HYDROCHLOROTHIAZIDE 6,25mg
Totals: 5 22,75€
Cancel Prescription
Save Temporarily Prescription
Final Submission
Cancel
Save Temporarily
Submit Prescription

EXPECTED BENEFITS

PINCLOUD project is set to build a reliable, secure and extensible platform warranting stakeholder collaboration and hopefully enjoying public trust. The expected benefits for all participant organizations include:

1. The development of integrated healthcare services that improve quality of service and reduce costs;
2. Business process reengineering, improvement, simplification and integration;
3. Enhanced decision making for health organizations and significant reductions to medical errors;
4. Standardization, automation, synchronization, better control and communication;
5. Improved coordination, management and scheduling of specific health supply chains and services;
6. Development of monitoring systems that improve quality of care of patients at home;
7. Establishment of an infrastructure that provides up-to-date information;
8. Development of an innovative organizational environment for the participating hospital using horizontal processes instead of the traditional hierarchical organization;
9. Implementation of an extensible and maintainable infrastructure that can be enriched with other medical services;

Figure 7. Screen: suggested medical treatment

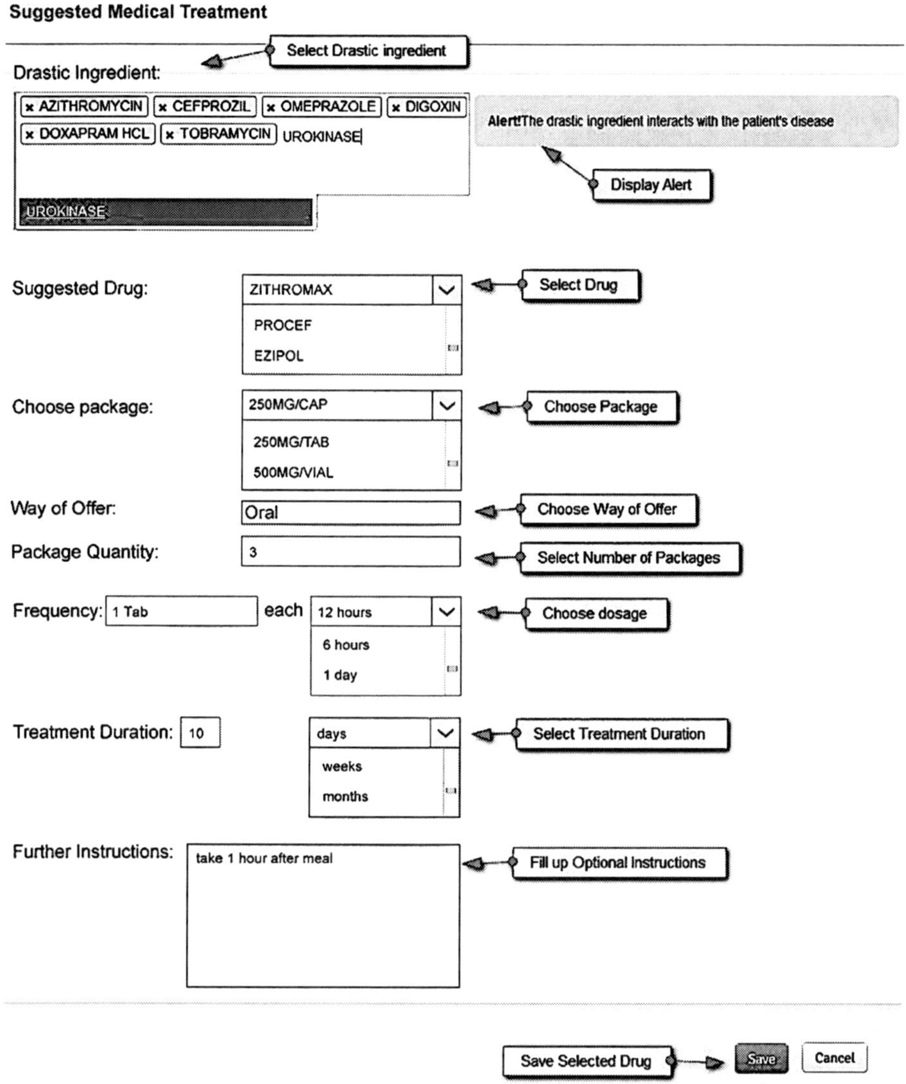

10. Development of an appropriate, sustainable technological framework that can be deployed and applied in other relevant situations and environments;
11. Investigation of state-of-the art technologies and novel research that extends the body of knowledge;
12. Significant research outcomes and publications of excellent quality;
13. Production of new platforms, infrastructures, and solution that can be further exploited;
14. Knowledge and expertise gained can lead to competitive advantage; and
15. Production and export of technical know-how for all the participants.

The results of the proposed project are of great importance for the businesses that deal with the e-health sector as they will gain the potential to achieve competitive advantages through the project. The area of healthcare is significant and the need for advanced and innovative IT solutions in this area is apparent too. Thus, the participant enterprises will have the opportunity to:

1. Develop an integrated platform that can be used by other organizations in the future;
2. Better understand and analyze the complexities of the Greek healthcare environment;
3. Experiment and implement innovative integrated solutions that can be turned into products;
4. Gain expertise and know-how on a complex area;
5. Sell these products and know-how at national and international level since PINCLOUD seeks to develop an innovative solution;
6. Obtain and reinforce experiences that can be used for the development of other network-oriented systems; and
7. Extend their business activities.

The benefits for both healthcare organizations include among others:

1. Specifications of processes for the management of healthcare processes;
2. Simplification and acceleration of business processes;
3. Better management of healthcare tasks;
4. Personalized disease monitoring and cost calculation;
5. More efficient operation; and
6. Economies of scale.

The benefits to the academic institutions participating in the project are equally important and include:

1. Knowledge exchange and transfer;
2. Engagement in innovative research;
3. Investigation of state of the art technologies;
4. Opportunity to publish research articles of high quality;
5. Prospect to conduct applied research and combine theory and practice.

FUTURE RESEARCH

Cloud-Computing has transformed the way many healthcare organizations work and offer healthcare services. In the previous section the benefits of such an endeavor alongside the steps taken so far to realize the implementation of a secure and reliable system, were analyzed. Yet, further research is required both in the testing and evaluation of our design and implementation.

To this end, the R&D team engineered several mechanisms to test and evaluate PINCLOUD and its components. For example, a proof-of-concept test will be implemented to check the communication of various sensors with the main PHR. The results of this test will be examined by healthcare professionals and provide initial evaluation of the technologies used. Additionally, testing mechanisms have been designed for the other components (e.g., e-prescribing and e-referral) as well. Besides, PINCLOUD will be implemented in two different cloud IaaS providers so as to study the interoperability in two different settings. The results of this test will provide insights into the utilized technologies (e.g., Table 2) and if needed reconfigurations and adjustments will be implemented. The authors expect the results of this test to be the subject of our next publication.

CONCLUSION

The current trend of adopting Cloud-Computing in the medical field can tackle several HIS challenges from integration of legacy systems to well needed reduction of cost. Standardized Cloud Services for Healthcare can be beneficial to patients, practitioners, insurance companies, pharmacies, etc.

Yet, as discussed in this chapter, several approaches with similarities and differences are proposing the integration of the Cloud Services for Healthcare in the form of a PHR. This patient centered approach over the cloud is a relative new issue that requires thorough examination with a multidiscipline lens. To aid this discussion the authors presented their involvement in a multidiscipline project and highlighted the steps taken so far from design and implementation, to technology considerations and decisions on current trends. The reader through this presentation has the chance to understand how a complex idea addressed by PINCLOUD as the E-Prescribing correlated through the three Cloud-Computing service models (SaaS, PaaS amd IaaS). Therefore, the authors believe that the issues highlighted in this chapter will provide useful insights and guidance for e-health developers concerned with the integration of Cloud Services in healthcare.

REFERENCES

AAL-Europe. (2013). Ambient assisted living catalogue of projects 2013. Retrieved April 18, 2014, from http://www.aal-europe.eu/

Alemdar, H., & Ersoy, C. (2010). Wireless sensor networks for healthcare: A survey. *Computer Networks*, *54*(15), 2688–2710. doi:10.1016/j.comnet.2010.05.003

Altman, E. J., Nagle, F., & Tushman, M. L. (2013). Innovating without Information Constraints: Organizations, communities, and innovation when information costs approach zero. *Harvard Business School Organizational Behavior Unit Working Paper* (14-043).

Avison, D., & Young, T. (2007). Time to rethink health care and ICT? *Communications of the ACM*, *50*(6), 69–74. doi:10.1145/1247001.1247008

Axelsson, K., Melin, U., & Söderström, F. (2011). *Analyzing best practice and critical success factors in a healthcare information systems case-Are there any shortcuts to succesfull IT implementation?* Paper presented at the 19th European Conference on Information Systems – ICT and Sustainable Service Development, Helsinki, Finland.

Black, A. D., Car, J., Pagliari, C., Anandan, C., Cresswell, K., Bokun, T., & Sheikh, A. et al. (2011). The impact of eHealth on the quality and safety of health care: A Systematic overview. *PLoS Medicine*, *8*(1), e1000387. doi:10.1371/journal.pmed.1000387 PMID:21267058

Bootstrap. (2014). Bootstrap. Retrieved April 18 2014, from http://getbootstrap.com/

Boulos, M. N., Wheeler, S., Tavares, C., & Jones, R. (2011). How smartphones are changing the face of mobile and participatory healthcare: An overview, with example from eCAALYX. *Biomedical Engineering Online*, *10*(1), 24. doi:10.1186/1475-925X-10-24 PMID:21466669

Chang, V. (2013a). A case study for business integration as a service. Trends in e-business, e-services, and e-commerce: impact of technology on goods, services, and business transactions. Hershey, PA: IGI Global.

Chang, V. (2013b). *Cloud computing for brain segmentation technology*. Paper presented at the IEEE CloudCom 2013. http://eprints.soton.ac.uk/357188/

Chang, V. (2014). Cloud computing for brain segmentation–a perspective from the technology and evaluations. *International Journal of Big Data Intelligence*, *1*(3).

Chang, V., De Roure, D., Wills, G., John Walters, R., & Barry, T. (2011). Organisational sustainability modelling for return on investment (ROI): Case studies presented by a National Health Service (NHS) trust UK. CIT. *Journal of Computing and Information Technology*, *19*(3), 177–192. doi:10.2498/cit.1001951

Chatterjee, S., Chakraborty, S., Sarker, S., Sarker, S., & Lau, F. Y. (2009). Examining the success factors for mobile work in healthcare: A deductive study. *Decision Support Systems*, *46*(3), 620–633. doi:10.1016/j.dss.2008.11.003

Chowdhury, M., Krishnan, K., & Vishwanath, S. (2012). *Touching lives through mobile health: Assessment of the global market opportunity.* India: PricewaterhouseCoopers.

ClearHealth. (2013). ClearHealth smart. simple. sustainable. Retrieved April 15, 2014, from http://clear-health.com/

Clemensen, J., Rasmussen, J., Denning, A., & Craggs, M. (2011). *Patient empowerment and new citizen roles through telehealth technologies - The early stage.* Paper presented at the Third International Conference on eHealth, Telemedicine, and Social Medicine Gosier France.

COUCHBASE. (2014). COUCHBASE NoSQL Database. Retrieved April 15, 2014, from http://www.couchbase.com

Cuzzocrea, A., Song, I.-Y., & Davis, K. C. (2011). Analytics over large-scale multidimensional data: the big data revolution! In *Proceedings of the ACM 14th international workshop on Data Warehousing and OLAP*. Glasgow, Scotland, UK. doi:10.1145/2064676.2064695

Daphne. (2013). Daphne data-as-a-service platform for healthy lifestyle and preventive medicine. Retrieved April 15, 2014, from http://www.daphne-fp7.eu/node/21

Deadalus. (2014). Interoperability Platform X1.V1. Retrieved April 17, 2014, from http://dedaluschina.com.cn/products-solutions/interoperability-platform-x1-v1/

Detmer, D., Bloomrosen, M., Raymond, B., & Tang, P. (2008). Integrated personal health records: Transformative tools for consumer-centric care. *BMC Medical Informatics and Decision Making, 8*(1), 45. doi:10.1186/1472-6947-8-45 PMID:18837999

Drupal. (2014). Drupal open source content management platform. Retrieved April 18, 2014, from https://drupal.org/

Dwivedi, Y., Ravichandran, K., Williams, M., Miller, S., Lal, B., Antony, G., & Kartik, M. (2013). IS/IT project failures: A review of the extant literature for deriving a taxonomy of failure factors. In Y. Dwivedi, H. Henriksen, D. Wastell, & R. De' (Eds.), *Grand successes and failures in IT public and private sectors* (Vol. 402, pp. 73–88). Berlin Heidelberg: Springer. doi:10.1007/978-3-642-38862-0_5

EMC. (2014). Electronic health record infrastructure solutions. Retrieved April 17, 2014, from http://greece.emc.com/industry/public-sector/electronic-health-record-infrastructure.htm

Google. (2014). Angularjs. Retrieved April 15, 2014, from https://angularjs.org/

Halamka, J., Mandl, K., & Tang, P. (2008). Early experiences with personal health records. *Journal of the American Medical Informatics Association, 15*(1), 1–7. doi:10.1197/jamia.M2562 PMID:17947615

HSSP. (2013). Healthcare services specification program. Retrieved January 19, 2013, from http://hssp.wikispaces.com/

IHE. (2012). Integrating the healthcare enterprise. Retrieved March 1, 2011, from http://www.ihe.net/

Jennett, P., & Watanabe, M. (2006). Healthcare and telemedicine: Ongoing and evolving challenges. *Disease Management & Health Outcomes, 14*(1).

Koufi, V., Malamateniou, F., & Vassilacopoulos, G. (2013). An Android-enabled PHR-based system for the provision of homecare services. *International Journal of Measurement Technologies and Instrumentation Engineering, 3*(2), 1–18. doi:10.4018/ijmtie.2013040101

Koumaditis, K., Themistocleous, M., Vassilacopoulos, G., Prentza, A., Kyriazis, D., Malamateniou, F., Mourouzis, A. (2014). *Patient-centered e-health record over the cloud*. Paper presented at the International Conference on Informatics, Management and Technology in Healthcare, Attica, Greece.

Kuo, A. M.-H. (2011). Opportunities and challenges of cloud computing to improve health care services. *Journal of Medical Internet Research*, *13*(3), e67. doi:10.2196/jmir.1867 PMID:21937354

Lab of Medical Informatics. (2014). Providing integrated eHealth services for personalized medicine utilizing cloud infrastructure. Retrieved April, 17, 2014, from http://pincloud.med.auth.gr/en

Lausanne, É. P. F. d. (2014). Scala. Retrieved April 18, 2014, from http://www.scala-lang.org/

Leventhal, T., Taliaferro, P., Wong, K., Hughes, C., & Mun, S. (2012). The patient-centered medical home and health information technology. *Telemedicine Journal and e-Health*, *18*(2), 145–149. doi:10.1089/tmj.2011.0130 PMID:22304440

Liferay. (2014). Liferay. Retrieved April 18, 2014, from http://www.liferay.com/

Lupse, O. S., Vida, M. M., & Stoicu-Tivadar, L. (2012). *Cloud computing and interoperability in healthcare information systems*. Paper presented at the The First International Conference on Intelligent Systems and Applications, INTELLI 2012.

Marcotte, E. (2011). *Responsive web design*. Editions Eyrolles.

Medscribbler. (2014). Medscribbler. Retrieved April 16, 2014, from http://www.medscribbler.com/

Mell, P., & Grance, T. (2009). The NIST definition of cloud computing. *National Institute of Standards and Technology*, *53*(6), 50.

Microsoft. (2014). HealthVault. Retrieved April 15, 2014, from https://www.healthvault.com

Mongo, D. B. I. (2013). MongoDB (from "humongous") is an open-source document database, and the leading NoSQL database. Retrieved April 15, 2014, from http://www.mongodb.org/

Narayanan, H. A. J., & Giine, M. (2011). *Ensuring access control in cloud provisioned healthcare systems*. Paper presented at the Consumer Communications and Networking Conference (CCNC), 2011. IEEE. doi:10.1109/CCNC.2011.5766466

Nodejs. (2014). Node.js platform. Retrieved April 15, 2014, from http://nodejs.org/

OpenEMR. (2014). OpenEMR a free and open source electronic health records. Retrieved April 15, 2014, from http://www.open-emr.org

Pilgrim, M. (2010). *HTML5: up and running*. O'Reilly Media, Inc.

Poulymenopoulou, M., Malamateniou, F., & Vassilacopoulos, G. (2012). Emergency healthcare process automation using mobile computing and cloud services. *Journal of Medical Systems*, *36*(5), 3233–3241. doi:10.1007/s10916-011-9814-y PMID:22205383

Preuveneers, D., Berbers, Y., & Joosen, W. (2013). The future of mobile e-health application development: exploring HTML5 for context-aware diabetes monitoring. *Procedia Computer Science*, *21*, 351–359. doi:10.1016/j.procs.2013.09.046

Research2guidance. (2014). *mHealth application developer economics 2014: The state of the art of m-health app publishing* (pp. 43). Retrieved from http://mhealtheconomics.com/mhealth-developer-economics-report/

Reti, S. R., Feldman, H. J., & Safran, C. (2009). Governance for personal health records. *Journal of the American Medical Informatics Association*, *16*(1), 14–17. doi:10.1197/jamia.M2854 PMID:18952939

Ruiz-Zafra, Á., Benghazi, K., Noguera, M., & Garrido, J. L. (2013). *Zappa: An open mobile platform to build cloud-based m-health systems. Ambient Intelligence-Software and Applications* (pp. 87–94). Springer.

Sarasohn-Kahn, J. (2010). *How smartphones are changing health care for consumers and providers* (1st ed., pp. 23). California HealthCare Foundation. Retrieved from http://www.chcf.org/

Singer, S., Burgers, J., Friedberg, M., Rosenthal, M., Leape, L., & Schneider, E. (2011). Defining and measuring integrated patient care: Promoting the next frontier in health care delivery. *Medical Care Research and Review, 68*(1), 112–127. doi:10.1177/1077558710371485 PMID:20555018

SUCRE. (2014). Sucre state of the art report. Retrieved April 13, 2014, from http://www.sucreproject.eu

Tang, P., Ash, J., Bates, D., Overhage, J., & Sands, D. (2006). Personal health records: Definitions, benefits, and strategies for overcoming barriers to adoption. *Journal of the American Medical Informatics Association, 13*(2), 121–126. doi:10.1197/jamia.M2025 PMID:16357345

Tclouds. (2014). TClouds - Trustworthy clouds healthcare scenario. Retrieved April 15, 2014, from http://www.tclouds-project.eu/downloads/factsheets/tclouds-factsheet-15-healthcare.pdf

Tilde. (2014). Emberjs. Retrieved April 15, 2014, from http://emberjs.com/

Vodera. (2014). VIGOR++ virtual gastrointestinal tract. Retrieved April 15, 2014, from http://www.vigorpp.eu/

Wilson, V., & Strong, D. (2014). Editors' introduction to the special section on patient-centered e-health: Research opportunities and challenges. *Communications of the Association for Information Systems, 34*(15).

Zhang, Q., Cheng, L., & Boutaba, R. (2010). Cloud computing: State-of-the-art and research challenges. *Journal of Internet Services and Applications, 1*(1), 7-18.

Zhou, F., Yang, H., Álamo, J., Wong, J., & Chang, C. (2010). Mobile Personal Health Care System for Patients with Diabetes. In Y. Lee, Z. Z. Bien, M. Mokhtari, J. Kim, M. Park, J. Kim, & I. Khalil et al. (Eds.), *Aging friendly technology for health and independence* (Vol. 6159, pp. 94–101). Berlin Heidelberg: Springer. doi:10.1007/978-3-642-13778-5_12

KEY TERMS AND DEFINITIONS

CAPEX: Capital Expenditure.

HIS Integration: The alignment of HIS in an interoperable environment.

HIS Interoperability: The ability of HIS to work together and exchange information.

HIS: Information systems designed to facilitate healthcare services.

IaaS: Infrastructure as a Service.

OPEX: Operational Expenditure.

PaaS: Platform as a Service.

PCEH: Patient Centered e-health.

SaaS: Software as a Service.

SOA: An architectural paradigm to build ecosystems of services.

This work was previously published in Delivery and Adoption of Cloud Computing Services in Contemporary Organizations edited by Victor Chang, Robert John Walters, and Gary Wills, pages 292-317 copyright year 2015 by Information Science Reference (an imprint of IGI Global).

Chapter 37
Identification of Chronic Wound Status under Tele-Wound Network through Smartphone

Chinmay Chakraborty
Birla Institute of Technology, India

Bharat Gupta
Birla Institute of Technology, India

Soumya K. Ghosh
Indian Institute of Technology Kharagpur, India

ABSTRACT

This paper presents a tele-wound framework for monitoring chronic wound status based on color varia-tion over a period of time. This will facilitate patients at remote locations to connect to medical experts through mobile devices. Further this will help medical professionals to monitor and manage the wounds in more timely, accurate and precise manner using the proposed framework. Tele-medical agent (TMA) collects the chronic wound data using smart phone and send it to the Tele-medical hub (TMH). In TMH, the wound image has been segmented using Fuzzy C-Means which gives highest segmented accuracy i.e. 92.60%, then the wound tissue is classified using proposed Bayesian classifier. The smart phone supported prototype system has been demonstrated with snapshots using very compatible and easy to integrate Hypertext preprocessor (PHP) and MySqL. The proposed system may facilitate better wound management and treatment by providing percentage of wound tissues.

1. INTRODUCTION OF CHRONIC WOUND

Management and monitoring of chronic wounds is a major challenge. A tele-wound care comprising transmission of chronic wound (CW) images and a clinical protocol to home bound patients resulted in reductions of emergency visits, hospitalization, hospital utilization and cost [Rees, et al. 2007]. More than $25 billion is spent annually on the treat-ment of CWs [Hopf, H. W. 2006]. In the United States, the percentage of the aged population (age

DOI: 10.4018/978-1-4666-8756-1.ch037

65 and more) is projected to increase from 12.4% in 2000 to 19.6% in 2030 [U.S. Census Bureau. 2013]. The cost-effectiveness analysis is used to measure and compare the relative costs and results associated with various interventions as comprehensively as possible [Weinstein, M. C. et al. 1996]. The CW size can be determined using various methods have been developed and validated including wound depth [Coulomb, B. et al. 1986], surface area [Thomas, A. 2002] [William, P.B et al. 1997] length and width [Herbin, M. et al. 1993] and volume [Thomas, G. 2004]. The authors [Stremitzer, S. et al. 2007] were to investigate the spread and variety in CW judgment. The different tissues like granulation, fibrin, necrosis, CW size, depth, exudate and edges were judged and the therapeutical consequences were determined. Several CW assessment tools have been developed like pressure sore status tool (PSST) [Julien, M. et al. 2008], the sessing scale [Ferrell, B. A. et al. 1995], sussman wound healing tool (SWHT) [Sussman, C. et al. 2007], pressure ulcer scale for healing (PUSH) [Plassmann, P. et al. 2013] and wound healing scale (WHS) [Julien, M. et al., 2008] to monitoring wound healing status.

In prior work, a smart phone app has been developed to take CW images using smart phone or tablets integrated camera [Chakraborty, C. et al. 2014] [Friesen, MR. et al. 2013]. The high resolution camera integrated smart phone used to monitoring and recording apps which contains clinical information (data, wound images) through store-and-forward tele-health platform [Clifford, G. D. et al. 2012]. The high quality wounded portion images can be sent via Internet to a distant centre for advice on management. The remote patient monitoring is one of the type of home tele-health that enables patient monitoring and transfer of patient health related data. The main purpose of electronic health systems are like to improve and increase the accessibility to the health care facilities for rural peoples, provide self treatment facility, improved doctor-patient interaction, provide cost effective health care, increase patient's

access their health record and maintain the health care provider [Das D. et al. 2014]. Telemedicine [Wootton, R. et al. 1999] is an emerging field in advance communication systems and medical informatics, is able to deliver the healthcare data and sharing of medical expertise using wireless technologies GSM/WLAN/SATELLITE/2G/3G/4G) in the span of tele-oncology, tele-pathology, tele-radiology, emergency healthcare and tele-dermatology. Today's remote people's are facing lot of problems on treatment like not available good clinicians and specialty care in rural area, provider shortages, patient can loses a day's wage, to pay for travel expenses, clinicians appointment is not readily guaranteed. Where as many cases are extremely trivial and of non emergency type. Therefore, clinicians charge a lot of money that's why Telemedicine have been taking a major breakthrough by providing fast and efficient diagnosis. And also maintaining e-prescription for referral cases, time and cost saved and clinicians can work from anywhere using smart phone. A handheld computing device like personal digital assistant (PDA) is used to monitoring patient's remotely [Chantelle, G. et al. 2006]. The author [Meum, T. 2012] discussed the implementation and use of an electronic medication management system (EMMS) using new technology to reduce the incidence of serious errors. The large numbers of rural peoples in the world have been suffering with different types wound. However, due to the lack of trained clinicians, this adds up in suffering population. The huge improvement and development in mobile communication throughout the world reduce the problem up to some extent. Our medical experts with Telecommunication engineering are trying to mitigate these problems. The portable, handheld device like smart phone can be used to capturing high quality wound images and acquiring patient's demographic information and send it to TMH through secure [Mukherjee, A. et al. 2015], web based medium. The Telemedicine based wireless body area networks can be used for continuous remote patient monitoring

Figure 1. Ulcer 1

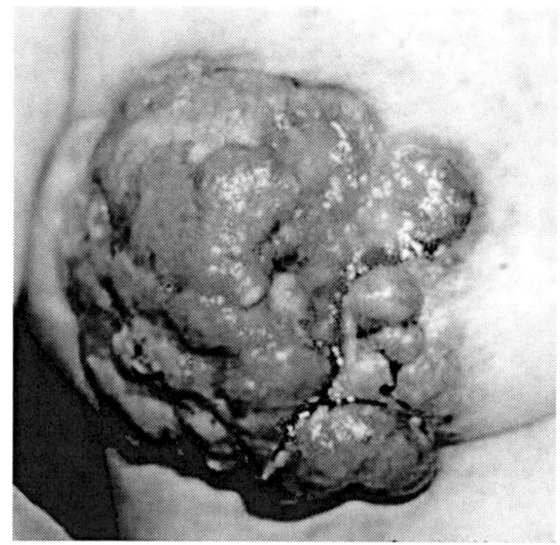

Figure 2. Ulcer 2

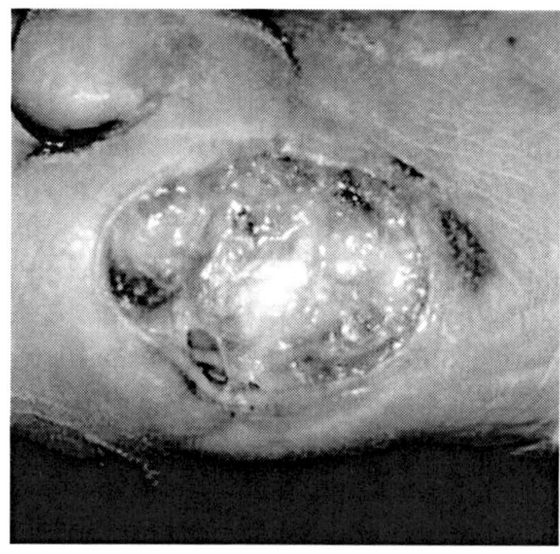

Figure 3. Ulcer 3

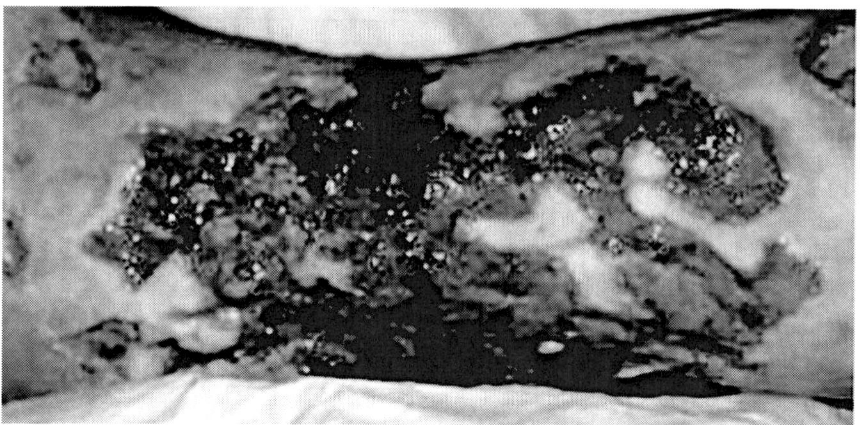

[Chakraborty, C. et al. 2013] where CW image collected by high resolution camera based smart phone through image sensor. This paper also discussed about Electronic health records (EHR) services that are being used form maintain wound database and bridging geographical distances. Wound healing has been taken longer duration and regular check-up with certain interval is one of the big abstract to clinic, the TMA act as a major role on data collection from various telemedicine centre's (TC). Figures 1 through 4 depict the different types of ulcerous cases.

The high featured smart phones like Xolo, APPLE, Nokia, SAMSUNG GALAXY TAB, Windows phone, BlackBerry, iOS, Canon, Adobe, ANDROID platforms can be used for sensing, acquiring the variety of medical data collection and monitoring applications. This paper deals a MySqL/PHP framework for acquiring, processing, analyzing and understanding CW images and gives best treatment facility to the patients in the help of percentage of tissue color. But CW treatment is not only depending on color information and texture information also. The several research articles designed metadata for dermatological imaging using ORACLE, SQL, XML, SAS8, PHPMYADMIN and MS ACCESS platform but these are licensed and cost effective. The Tele-wound application under telemedicine

Figure 4. Ulcer 4

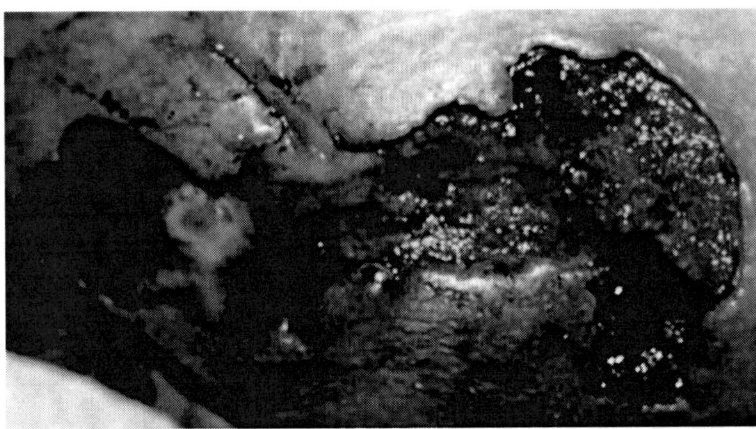

approach should have a good user interface, easy to use, gives fast response, throughput, gives best performance in case of fault and error free. The different ulcerous cases can be transformed using multimedia messaging an email. Metadata can be defined as a structured information system that carries big strength of medical information. The chronic wound is mainly a wound that does not heal in an orderly set of stages and in a predictable amount of time. It mostly affect aged people, delayed skin re-growth, depression, slow older cell proliferation rate, social isolation, long term and costly treatment, they can't visit clinics frequently. There are four main types of chronic wounds like pressure ulcer, diabetic ulcer, venous ulcer and arterial or ischemic ulcer respectively. A wound consists of non-uniform mixture of red granulation (G) tissue, yellow slough (S) tissue and black necrotic (N) tissue.

This paper has been organized is as follows. The importance of tele-wound network and mobile wound health monitoring systems are presented in section 1. In section 2, proposed system model have been introduced, followed by section 3 discussed the operation of this proposed model. In section 4, experimental outcomes with screenshots have been demonstrated. In section 5 gives the advantageous features of clinical decision making systems followed by section 6 on concluding remarks.

2. PROPOSED SYSTEM MODEL

Our proposed scheme provides telemedicine added CW status monitoring system of remote patients with certain interval and also reduce the frequent clinic visits. Smart-phone enabled telemedicine service overcomes the shortcomings of computer based telemedicine like requirement not portable, wired service and constant electricity [Chakraborty, C. et al. 2014]. Tele-monitoring provides to monitor the patient's vital signs regularly for reducing time and cost [Stephane, M. 2005].

The good quality wounded image has been chosen in smart-phone by TMA from various TCs, form metadata and is sent to the TMH and stored in wound database with PIDNUM for monitoring the wound status problem remotely. The metadata can be extracted in TMH and then clinical information saved in global wound database and wound image goes to image processing toolbox for preprocessing, segmentation, feature extraction and classification purpose and gives percentages of wounds. Based on this CW classification results, clinicians can be sent prescribed medication electronically. Figure 5 depicts proposed telemedicine based CW monitoring system configuration. The different necessary attributes of this models has been discussed below:

Figure 5. Proposed wound monitoring system over telemedicine platform

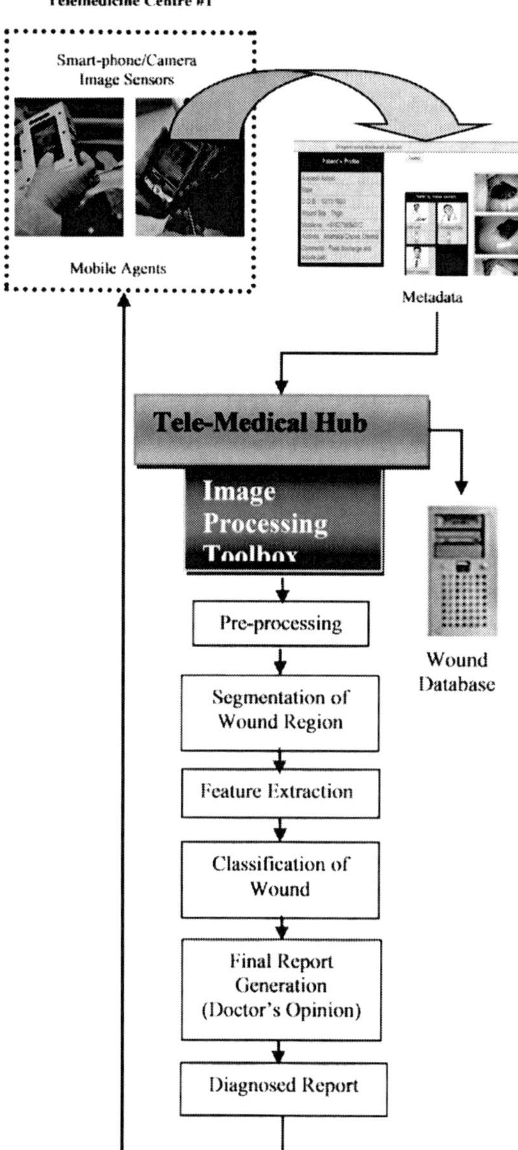

- **Patient's End:** All patients are not conscious about their disease. They will require different treatment related information during and after the assessing and managing the chronic wound. The chronic wound affected patient are not willing to move from home, they needs remote care facility, make contact with TMA who are having inexpensive smart phone;

- **TMA:** Agent is responsible for creating his account in the apps and feeds the form with relevant clinical information. TMA is putting image and clinical information as a metadata format in the apps that shown in Figure 6;

- **Telemedicine Centre:** The several number of TC's have to be set up in every populated rural area for providing specialist care. This centre's consist of preliminary treatment facility, local clinicians, agents, high technology added smart phone and necessary peripherals:

  ○ **Information Transmission Schemes:** The metadata can be sent from rural to best clinics or clinicians through smart phones, the effective transmission schemes are essential. The quick and cost effective solutions like GSM and GPRS (data rate upto 40 kbit/s) is one of the best choices. The GPRS is gives good performance by having direct uploading capability and easily interfaced with modem and controller from patient's end to TMH in medical data transmission;

  ○ **TMH:** This is the mainly centrally received, transmitted, monitored patient's status and managed all TC's. The best clinicians or clinics are associated with this section. The patient's can get optimal treatment from this TMH. The patient information stored in wound database and wound image goes to TMH for further image processing like pre-processing, segmentation, feature extraction and classification respectively;

- **Doctor's End:** The clinicians keep on checking patient's profile for reports from patients. When clinicians logs in the apps and is redirected to patient's profile he finds that he has a case which asks for care and diagnosis. He clicks on the link on the arrived case which says "visit". The clinician having two options like he can go ahead and analyze the wound or can refer the report to other existing clinicians on the apps using PIDNUM. The clinicians regularly keep sending more intelligent and effective e-prescribed medication and wound status related feedback. It helps patients who are in remote areas and do not have access to expert care and advice;

- **Wound Database:** The patient and clinician is to be registered in the database. The database keeps the patients visiting status and clinicians given time and date subject to availability. The Medetec wound image database [Medetec, 2014] consists of different types of wound images. There are no papers available on wound database; the global wound database is developed for particular wound related information storing, sharing and analyzing purpose that shown Table 1. Table 1 present the metadata format for patient profile creation. Now a day's electronic documentation maintaining is essential task because of patient can go through different doctor with unique PIDNUM. Electronic documentation technologies are mostly used at health care services such as electronic health records (EHR), point of care (POC), point of service (POS), health information technology (HIT) and electronic prescribing systems and electronic medication administration records (eMAR) etc.;

- **Image Processing Toolbox:** The image processing toolbox have been associated with TMH. When metadata received by TMH, the clinical information saved with PIDNUM in database and wound image goes to image processing toolbox for pre-

processing, segmentation and classification of wound tissue types;

- **End-to-End Care Unit:** This section started from patient's data acquision to clinician's feedback reception through TMA, TC and TMH. TMA receives patient's image and clinical data by smart phone and send it to via wireless platform. This data stores in wound database.

3. OPERATION

This developed prototype CW monitoring system allows clinicians to diagnose the progress of a wound timely. The wounded portion can be capture by smart phone and also TMA is able to collect patient's demographic information like name, age, PIDNUM, sex, address at time of diagnosis, current medication, occupation, duration of disease, previous case history, diagnosis by doctor's, site of involvement, approximate size of wounds and parental history, finally makes a metadata format. This metadata can be embedded in JPEG format and transmitted globally using web application.

Figure 6. TMA used Smartphone

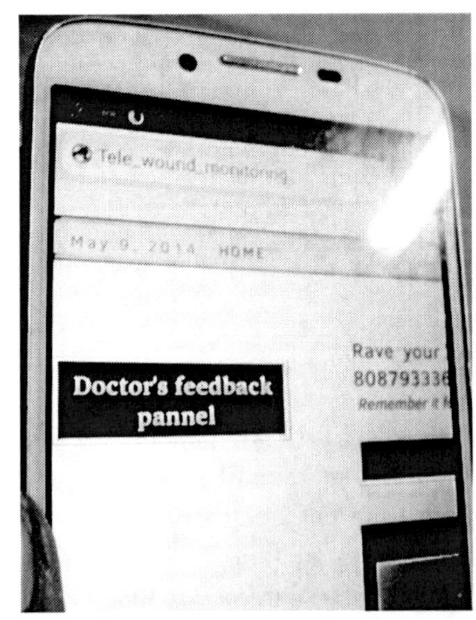

Table 1. Wound database

Name	PID-Num	DoB	Address	Uploaded Image	WoS	Types of Wound	Parents History	Previous Patient History	Contact No.	Clinicians Comment	Clinician Seen
K. Mishra	20978	12.08.1960	Dunka	s.jpg	Ankle	Diabetic, open	No	First time	+919908##	Bad pain	Yes
P. Bansal	66543	07.12.1967	Manisas	p.jpg	Hand	Pressue, open	No	First time	+918909##	Etching	Yes
H. Meena	98523	09.03.1956	Chora	6.jpg	Leg	Venous, open	Yes	First time	+919452##	Pain	No
O. Sheela	96745	12.12.1962	Nikashi	Gt.jpg	Hand	Diabetic, open	No	First time	+919732##	Normal but developing wound	No
N. Kandar	12098	06.09.1970	Haripur	Kl.jpg	Palm	Diabetic, open	No	First time	+919123##	Not healed taken medication 15 days	Yes
S. Reddy	89540	03.04.1952	Kerol	o.jpg	Ankle	Venous, open	Yes	First time	+919956##	Pain and etching	No
T. Jana	89723	01.02.1952	Pinduput	n.jpg	Leg	Diabetic, open	No	First time	+917818##	Severe pain	Yes
H. Trivedi	10056	03.05.1965	Sibtala	t.jpg	Other	Pressure, open	No	First time	+919678##	Malignant wound for 1 month	yes

PIDNUM – Patient ID Number, DOB – Date of Birth, WOS – Wound of Site

This paper attempts very efficient tool using low cost, open source and easy to access MySqL/PHP. The web application server runs on PHP program and metadata stored in MySqL database in TMH. This metadata (clinical information and CW image) goes to TMH via wireless environments then patient clinical information stored in global wound database with unique PIDNUM and CW image processed to image processing toolbox respectively. The image processing toolbox consists of:

1. **Pre-processing Approach:** The main aim of this stage is to eliminate the background noise and improve the CW image quality for the purpose of determining and segmenting the area of interest in the image. Input for pre-processing step is RGB wound image, whereas output is the enhanced image in RGB format with goal of better segmentation of region of interest. This section involves color correction, median filtering, color homogenization and anisotropic diffusion filtering respectively:

    a. **Color Correction:** CW images are filled with improper color casts resulting object represent untrue color. To bring back the true color of the object in image 'color correction' is 'required. The two most effective common techniques used for automatic color correction are Gray world assumption [Ebner, M. 2002] and Retinex theory [Land, E. H. 1974], but their applicability depends on the nature of the images;

    b. **Median Filter:** Considers each pixel in the CW image in turn and looks at its nearby neighbors to decide whether or not it is representative of its surroundings. This filter mostly used to remove the impulse noise;

    c. **Color Homogenization:** Smoothing of the CW image, while preserving the edges is critical task for enhanced segmentation of wound area.

Anisotropic diffusion filter [Pietro, P. et al. 1987] is used in order to reduce noise and homogenize color variations that could have undesirable effects on segmentation;

d. **Anisotropic Diffusion Filtering:** Use in image processing and computer vision applications which aim at reducing image noise by smoothing, while preserves significant parts of the image content, typically edges, lines or other details that are important for the interpretation of the image [Perona, P. 1990];

2. **Segmentation Approach:** CW image segmentation plays major role in computer vision, pattern recognition and disease diagnosing in medical images. Medical wound image segmentation is one of the most attractive areas of research because successfulness of the post-processing techniques highly depends on the accuracy of image segmentation. CWs mostly possess irregular shapes, vague boundaries and very heterogeneous colorations. Wild, T. et al. [2008] discussed elaborately computer based wound healing evaluation using color segmentation. This is an easy-to-use, accurate and cost saving method to investigate the healing status. In this paper Fuzzy C-Means (FCM) and spatial Fuzzy C-Means (SFCM) are applied to the lesion image. The wound affected portion can be extracted from the whole background image using these segmentation techniques. The segmented and computed CW data can be saved in the wound database and can be used in the comparison of the status of the lesion at different intervals. The FCM technique works well compared to SFCM technique. Clustering validity indices are computed and have been compared with FCM and SFCM algorithm. FCM is able to preserve more valuable information from the original CW image but does not incorporate

clinical information about spatial context. SFCM approaches reduce the number of spurious blobs and segmented images are more homogeneous:

a. **Fuzzy C-means (FCM):** It can be seen as the fuzzified version of the K-means algorithm. The segmentation of CW imaging data involves partitioning the image into the different cluster regions with similar intensity values. FCM approach is particularly suitable for segmentation of medical wound images. This technique allows one piece of medical data to belong to two or more clusters, developed by Dunn [Dunn, 1973] and modified version developed by Bezdek [Bezdek, J. C. 1981], generally used in pattern recognition. SFCM and FCM algorithms are implemented in MATLAB environment;

b. **Spatial Fuzzy C-Means (SFCM):** FCM clustering with spatial constraints is an effective algorithm suitable for image segmentation. SFCM contributes fuzziness for belongingness every pixel and explains spatial contextual information. SFCM approach increase the computational time because of highlights of spatial constraints if wound datasets are become large. FCM allows a pixel in more than one cluster depends on degree of membership. The summation of membership function in the neighborhood in every pixel provides the spatial function information [Mark, E. 2003];

3. **Classification Approach:** Clinicians can be diagnose based on three main classes of wound tissues like red for granulation tissue, yellow for slough and black for necrotic escher. The main aim of this approach is to distinguish the CW tissues in granulation, slough and necrotic tissue by making use of extracted features. Such a red-yellow-black

(RYB) model is used by clinicians as a descriptive tool [Ballerini, L. et al. 2010]. The color of CW provides important clues about its status to the clinician. Efficient classifier like Bayesian classifier is used to classify the CW images. The three classes of CW tissues can be identified. Bayesian classification is based on probability theory and more specifically based on Bayes' decision theory [Duda, R. et al. 2007]. This probability value is used to generate a model with a decision rule that always provides a response with an answer to the class that has the highest probability after application of Bayes' theorem [Sebastiani, F. 2002]. Figures 7 through 11 depicts the representation of original image, pre-processing and segmented image output.

4. EXPERIMENTAL RESULT

Experimental results show the effectiveness of the proposed technique. Our prototype system can be evaluate in terms of (a) *Timeliness* – patients can contact TMH in timely manner, (b) *Safety* – constantly getting optimal treatment facility in secure way over wireless communication technologies, (c) *Efficiency* – provide low cost optimal treatment facility over short time, (d) *Smooth Interaction* – effective communication between clinicians and patients are needed, (e) *Interoperability* – transferring medical information like patients records via web application over electronic media, (f) *Reuse* – can be used for other applications, (g) *Reliability* – precisely wound image processing is possible via web application in reliable way,

Figure 7. Original CW image

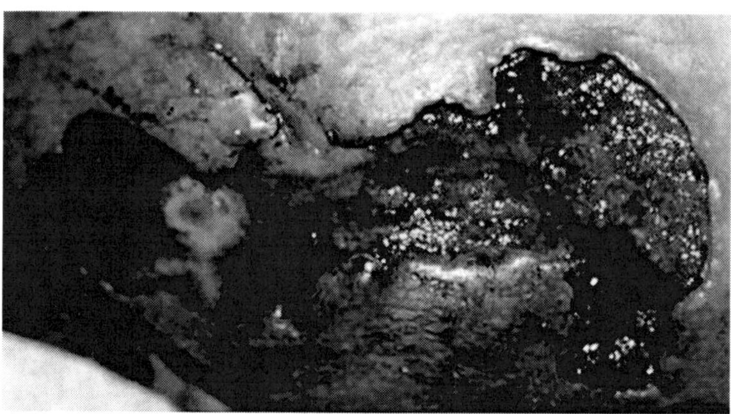

Figure 8. After color correction

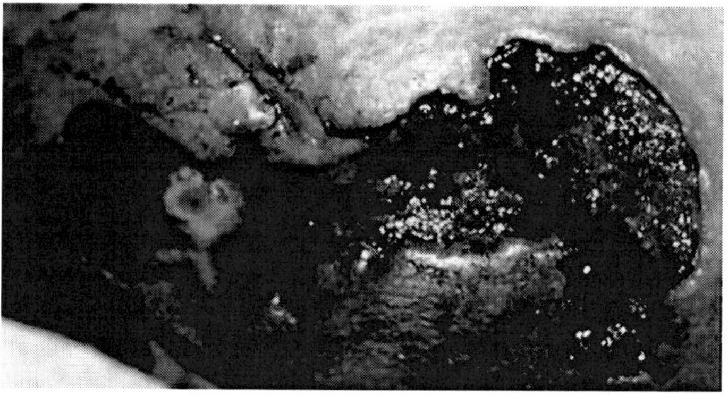

Figure 9. After median filtering

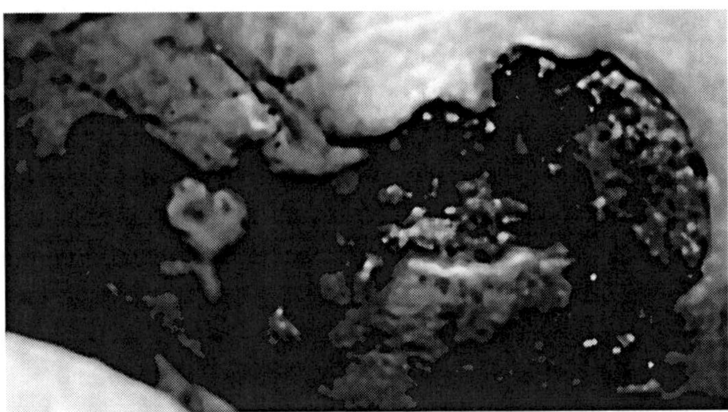

Figure 10. Image after anisotropic diffusion filtering

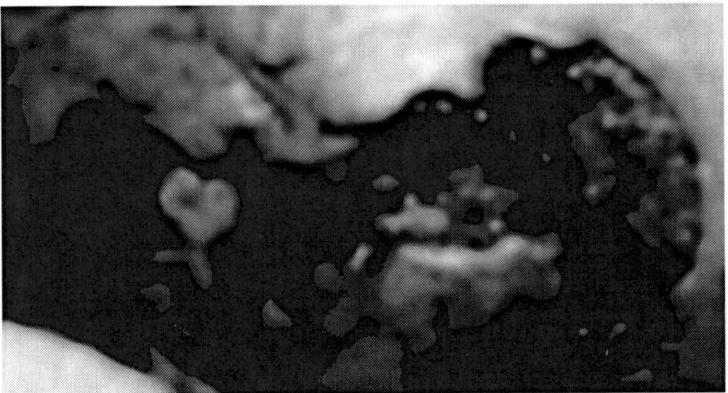

Figure 11. Segmented CW image

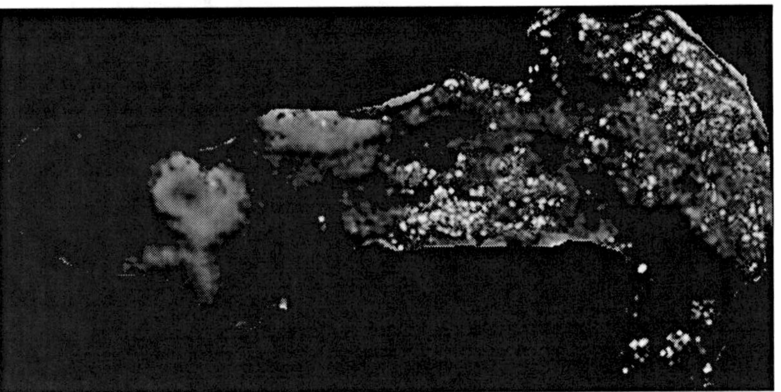

(h) *Usability* – how easy it is for an patients to operate successfully, (i) *Scalability* – medical data can be stored in wound database, (j) *Wound Care Coordination* – provided very good coordination between TMA and TMH, (k) *Information Management* – electronically maintain patient's history with prescribed medication. Image segmentation algorithms were tested on 77 digital photographs of all five different types of CWs. All the CW images were selected and validated by skin specialists. Manual segmentation by the expert has been taken as the segmentation gold standard. Here segmented is done by application of FCM and SFCM clustering algorithms on D_r and D_b channel and then post-processing is done to get precise wound area segmentation with smooth boundaries. The performance of CW area segmentation was further validated by ground truth images labeled by clinical experts. The performance of segmentation algorithms relative to gold standard has been estimated using segmentation accuracy (SA), Jaccard coefficient (JC), Dice coefficient (DC), positive false rate (rfp), negative false rate (rfn), and sensitivity (S). Here SFCM gives segmented accuracy of 89.90 in D_r channel, whereas FCM outperforms with an overall highest segmented accuracy of 92.60. In this case FCM gives better results in terms of SA, DC and S. Table II describe the results. Bayesian classifier is used to classify CW tissue percentage wise like in Figure 12 gives G tissue is 93.42%, S tissue is 4.52% and N tissue is 2.07% respectively. The decision making for the percentage of wound depicts the amount of wound recovery status timely i.e. in this image

red color is dominant so this is initial stage but after certain interval redness is going to convert to yellow color i.e. repairing stage and finally it would be blackish color i.e. repaired tissue. In this work, the following threshold values were used like 255 for G tissue, 200 for N tissue and 100 for S tissue respectively. The Bayesian classifier gives highest overall accuracy of 86.99%. The authors [Hazem, et al. 2011] have been shown the different overall accuracies like 80%, 81% and 68% using K-NN, Fuzzy K-NN and KMs respectively. In this case, CW image can be segmented using FCM approach in D_r channel. This paper identifies the implementation of early state-of-the-art treatment is the key factor to effectively monitoring wounds healing rate. However, this treatment modality must be holistic in its approach and take much time to heal properly. The clinicians could be prescribed medication based on status of the percentage of tissue. This time-to-time updation process is stored in wound database. The result of this paper is very much compatible with international wound database.

The Figure 13 deal with the screenshot of TMA is taking patient's details and put into apps.

In Figure 16, Clinician is visited patient's wound history by giving unique PIDNUM and

Figure 12. Classification of CW image

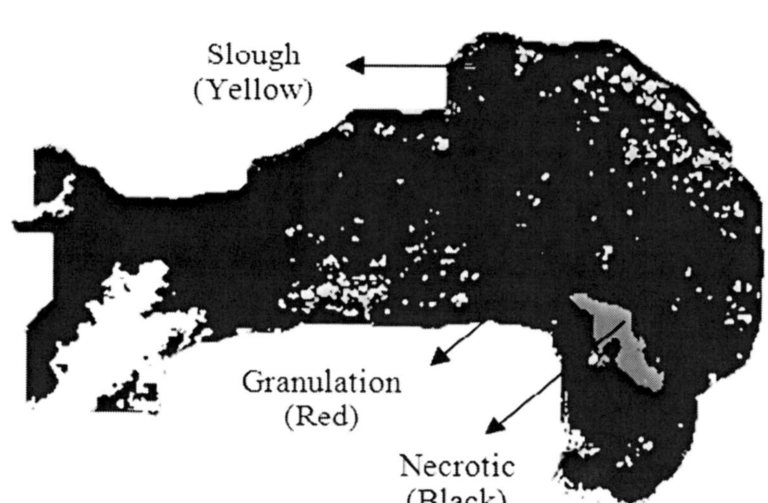

Table 2. Parameters for CW segmentation

	D$_r$ Channel				
	DC (%)	*JC (%)*	*Rfp (%)*	*Rfn (%)*	*S (%)*
SFCM	83.89	72.25	4.76	35.75	88.25
FCM	84.83	73.66	4.37	34.59	90.78

Figure 13. Screenshots of patient's clinical information entry page

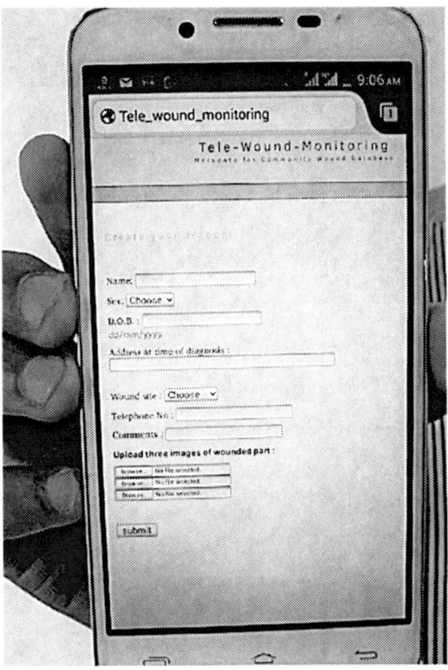

Figure 14. Screenshots of patient's wounded image

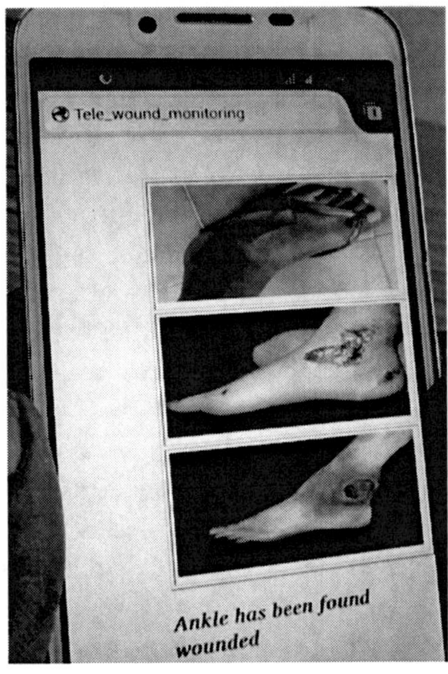

Ankle has been found wounded

Figure 15. Screenshots of list of clinicians

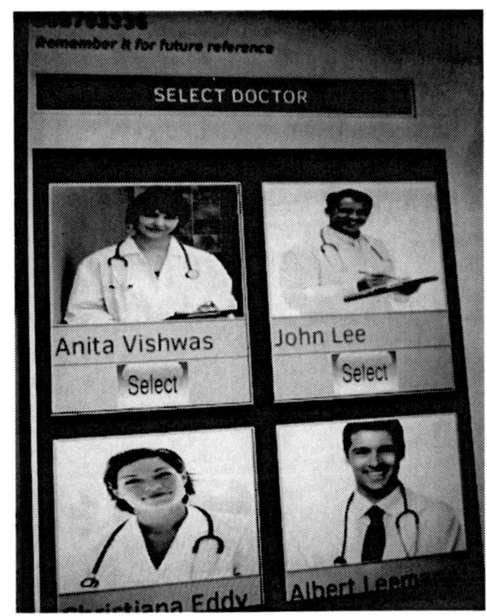

seen the wound status. Actually the redness is there in skin then this is first stage of ulcer or granulation, if yellow colored tissue is there then patient's have taken some medication, slightly repaired then this is known as slough and if wounded portion is mostly black colored then this is repaired necrotic.

Clinicians prescribed based on the percentage of wound tissue. Figure 17 is shown the wound image status with unique PIDNUM and clinician can prescribed.

Figure 16. Screenshots of clinicians visited wound cases

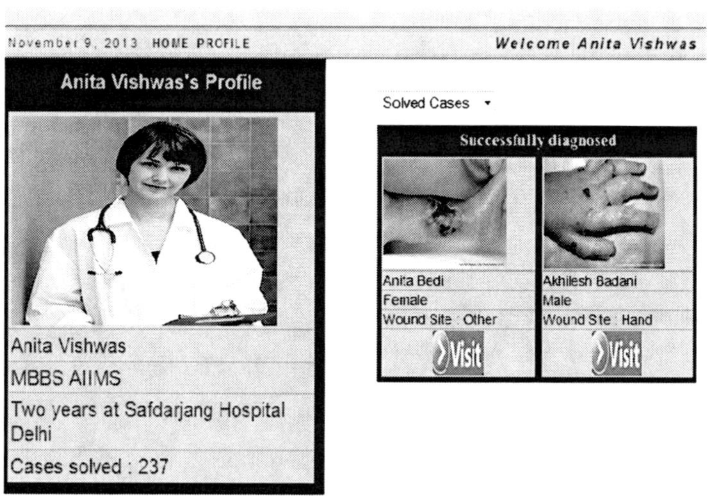

Figure 17. Screenshots of patient treated with PIDNUM

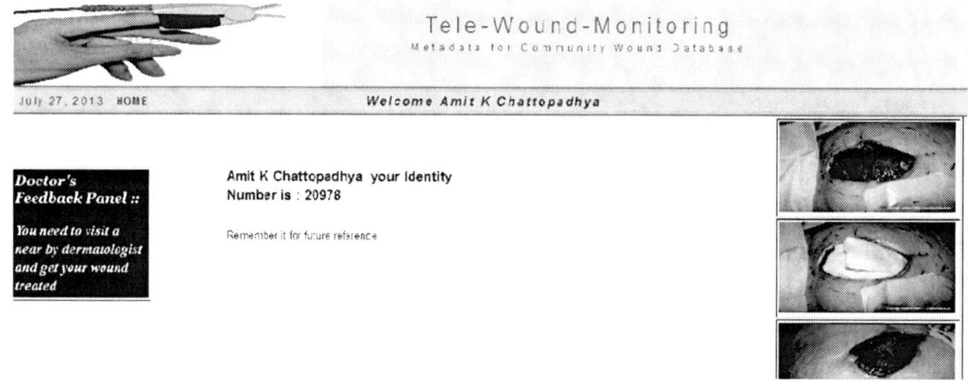

5. CLINICAL DECISION MAKING SYSTEM

The clinical decision making system plays an important role in telemedicine system. This system provides clinicians, staff, patient's with knowledge and person specific information, to enhance health and health care. This system includes computerized alerts and reminders, diagnostic assistance, prescription decision support, information retrieval, clinical guidelines, condition specific order sets, medical image recognition and interpretation, focused patient data reports and summaries and therapy critiquing and planning etc. This healthcare system is designed to assist clinicians and other health professionals on decision making tasks. In this paper TMA captures CW image by smart phone and processed to central control unit like TMH. TMH consist of global wound database system to store the patient clinical information and image processing toolbox receives CW image for further processing like pre-processing, segmentation and classification respectively. Clinicians can take decision based on percentage of wound tissue present on this color image and refers e-prescribed medication to the patient end. So this decision making system gives better treatment results regarding disease recovery. The need of clinical decision making system is to help the clinicians to make treatment decisions (or progress of healing rate) based on percentage of wounds.

6. CONCLUSION

In this paper, we present a remotely access chronic wound monitoring system, using portable and easy management tool like smart phone over a Telemedicine framework. The time and cost can be minimized and maintained e-prescription with respect to unique patient identification number (PIDNUM) in online wound database using this superior user friendly technique. Smart phone is storing metadata and send it to TMH via Internet/2G/3G/4G for diagnosis. The proposed approach gives the possibility of better quality treatment, more effective, scalable and precise evaluation. Wound database is maintaining e-prescription for future assistance. The performance of the FCM provides satisfactory results compared to SFCM algorithm. The main aim of this paper is to develop CW image processing techniques for automated wound area measurement and accurate wound tissue classification through quantitative biomarker identification for automated CW assessment. Clinician's gives valuable feedback after visiting wound image and patient's details through online medical report transfer at their clinic/home and even while on move, henceforth the less movement for patient and minimized costs. In future, the better authentication mechanism is required for sending the multiple numbers of patient's information through the transmission medium which gives the security to the patient. Availability of videoconferencing and tele-wound monitoring in problem give more flexibility and improvement in rural remote care. It may also provide clinical guidance through tele-wound care in remote areas where there is lack of clinical expert in wound care.

REFERENCES

Ballerini, L., Li, X., Fisher, R., & Rees, J. (2010). A query-by-example content-based image retrieval system of non-melanoma skin lesions. *Medical Content-Based Retrieval for Clinical Decision Support, 5853*, 31–38. doi:10.1007/978-3-642-11769-5_3

Bezdek, J. C. (1981). *Pattern recognition with fuzzy objective function algorithms*. Plenum Press. doi:10.1007/978-1-4757-0450-1

Chakraborty, C., Gupta, B., & Ghosh, S. K. (2013). A review on telemedicine-based WBAN framework for patient monitoring, *Telemedicine and e-health*, Marry Ann Liebert. *Inc, 19*(8), 619–626.

Chakraborty, C., Gupta, B., & Ghosh, S. K. (2014). Mobile metadata assisted community database of chronic wound. *Elsevier: Int. Journal of Wound Medicine, 6*, 34–42.

Chakraborty, C., Gupta, B., & Ghosh, S. K. (2014). Tele-wound monitoring through smartphone, IEEE: *Int. Conf. on Medical Imaging, m-Health and Emerging Comm. Syst. (MedCom)*, 197-201.

Chantelle, G., & Khaled, E. E. (2006). Who's using PDAs? Estimates of PDA use by health care providers: A systematic review of surveys. *Journal of Medical Internet Research, 8*(2), e7. doi:10.2196/jmir.8.2.e7 PMID:16867970

Clifford, G. D., & Clifton, D. (2012). Wireless technology in disease management and medicine. *Annual Review of Medicine, 63*(1), 479–492. doi:10.1146/annurev-med-051210-114650 PMID:22053737

Coulomb, B., Saiag, P., Bell, E., Breitburd, F., Lebreton, C., Heslan, M., & Dubertret, L. (1986). A new method for studying epidermalization in vitro. *The British Journal of Dermatology, 114*(1), 91–101. doi:10.1111/j.1365-2133.1986.tb02783.x PMID:2417615

Das, D., Maji, P., Dey, G., & Dey, N. (2014). Ethical E-Health: A possibility of the future or a distant dream? [IJEHMC]. *International Journal of E-Health and Medical Communications*, *5*(3), 17–28. doi:10.4018/ijehmc.2014070102

Duda, R., Hart, P., & Stork, D. (2007). *Pattern classification*. Wiley India.

Dunn (1973). A fuzzy relative of the ISODATA process and its use in detecting compact well-separated clusters, *Journal of Cybernetics*, 3(3), 32-57.

Ebner, M. (2002). A parallel algorithm for color constancy. Technical Report 296, *University at Ẅurzburg, Lehrstuhl f̈ur Informatik II, Ẅurzburg*, Germany.

Ferrell, B. A., Artinian, B. M., & Sessing, D. (1995). The sessing scale for assessment of pressure ulcer healing. *Journal of the American Geriatrics Society*, *43*(1), 37–40. doi:10.1111/j.1532-5415.1995.tb06239.x PMID:7806737

Friesen, M. R., Hamel, C., & McLeod, R. D. (2013). A mHealth application for chronic wound care: Findings of a user trial. *International Journal of Environmental Research and Public Health*, *10*(11), 6199–6214. doi:10.3390/ijerph10116199 PMID:24256739

Hazem, W., Yves, L., & Sylvie, T. (2011). Enhanced assessment of the wound-healing process by accurate multi-view tissue classification. *IEEE Transactions on Medical Imaging*, *30*(2), 315–326. doi:10.1109/TMI.2010.2077739 PMID:20875969

Herbin, M., Bon, F. X., Venot, A., Jenlouis, F., & Dubertret, M. L. (1993). Assessment of healing kinetics through true color image processing. *IEEE Transactions on Medical Imaging*, *12*(1), 39–43. doi:10.1109/42.222664 PMID:18218389

Hopf, H. W. (2006). Wound repair and regeneration. *Wound Healing Society and the European Tissue Repair Society*, *14*(1), 55–60.

Julien, M., Michael, E., & Guillermo, S. (2008). Sparse representation for color image restoration. *IEEE Transactions on Image Processing*, *17*(1), 53–69. doi:10.1109/TIP.2007.911828 PMID:18229804

Land, E. H. (1974). The retinex theory of colour vision. *Proc. Royal Inst. Great Britain*, *47*, 23–58.

Mark, E., Roberts, & Ela, C. (2003). An artificially evolved vision system for segmenting skin lesion images, *MICCAI*, 1, 655-662.

Medetec wound database (2014). Retrieved October 10, from http://www.medetec.co.uk/files/medetec-image-databases.html

Meum, T. (2012). Electronic medication management – a socio-technical change process in clinical practice, *ACM: CSCW, Medical Care and Health Intervention*, 11-15.

Mukherjee, A., Dey, G., Dey, M., & Dey, N. (2015). Web-based intelligent EEG signal authentication and tamper detection system for secure telemonitoring. *Springer International Publishing*, *74*, 295–312.

Perona, P., & Malik, J. (1990). Scale-space and edge detection using anisotropic diffusion Romeny BTH, ed. IEEE Transactions on Pattern Analysis and Machine Intelligence, 12(7), 629-639.

Pietro, P., & Jitendra, M. (1987) Scale-space and edge detection using anisotropic diffusion. *Proc. of IEEE Computer Society Workshop on Computer Vision*, 16–22.

Plassmann, P., Harding, K. G., & Melhuish, J. M. (1994). Methods of measuring wound size - a comparative study. *Ostomy/Wound Management*, *6*(2), 54–61. PMID:7546091

Rees, R. S., & Bashshur, N. (2007). The effects of tele wound management on use of service and financial outcomes. *Telemedicine Journal and e-Health*, *13*(6), 663–674. doi:10.1089/tmj.2007.9971 PMID:18069917

Sebastiani, F. (2002). Machine learning in automated text categorization. *ACM Computing Surveys*, *34*(1), 1–47. doi:10.1145/505282.505283

Stephane, M. (2005). The current state of telemonitoring: a comment on the literature, *Telemedicine and e-Health*, Mary Ann Liebert Inc., 11(1), 63-69.

Stremitzer, S., Wild, T., & Hoelzenbein, T. (2007). How precise is the evaluation of chronic wounds by health care professionals? *International Wound Journal*, *4*(2), 156–161. doi:10.1111/j.1742-481X.2007.00334.x PMID:17651230

Sussman, C., & Bates-Jensen, B. Wound Care (2007). A collaborative practice manual for health professionals. 3rd Ed. Wolters Kluwer/Lippincott Williams & Wilkins, Philidelphia, US.

Thomas, A. Krouskop, Robert, B., Michael, S. & Wilson. (2002). A noncontact wound measurement system. *Journal of Rehabilitation Research and Development*, *39*(3), 337–346. PMID:12173754

Thomas, G. (2004). Wound outcomes: The utility of surface measures. *Lower Extremity Wounds*, *3*(3), 125–132. doi:10.1177/1534734604264419 PMID:15866803

U.S. Census Bureau. International data base. Table 094. Midyear population, by age and sex. Retrieved February 19, 2013, from www.census.gov/population/www/projections/natdet-D1A.html

Weinstein, M. C., Siegel, J. E., Gold, M. R., Kamlet, M. S., & Russell, L. B. (1996). Recommendations of the panel on cost-effectiveness in health and medicine. *Journal of the American Medical Association*, *276*(15), 1253–1258. doi:10.1001/jama.1996.03540150055031 PMID:8849754

Wild, T., Prinz, M., Fortner, N., Krois, W., Sahora, K., Stremitzer, S., & Hoelzenbein, T. (2008). Digital measurement and analysis of wounds based on colour segmentation. *European Surgery*, *40*(1), 325–329. doi:10.1007/s10353-008-0378-0

William, P. B., & Stephen, J. S. (1997). Automatic quantitative analysis of healing skin wounds using colour digital image processing, World Wide Wounds, Ed. 1.1.

Wootton, R., & Craig, J. (1999). *Introduction to telemedicine, Royal Soc.* London: Medicine Press.

This work was previously published in the International Journal of Rough Sets and Data Analysis (IJRSDA), 2(2); edited by Aboul Ella Hassanien, Ahmad Taher Azar, and Nilanjan Dey, pages 58-77 copyright year 2015 by IGI Publishing (an imprint of IGI Global).

Chapter 38
Medical Data Analytics in the Cloud Using Homomorphic Encryption

Övünç Kocabaş
University of Rochester, USA

Tolga Soyata
University of Rochester, USA

ABSTRACT

Transitioning US healthcare into the digital era is necessary to reduce operational costs at Healthcare Organizations (HCO) and provide better diagnostic tools for healthcare professionals by making digital patient data available in a timely fashion. Such a transition requires that the Personal Health Information (PHI) is protected in three different phases of the manipulation of digital patient data: 1) Acquisition, 2) Storage, and 3) Computation. While being able to perform analytics or using such PHI for long-term health monitoring can have significant positive impacts on the quality of healthcare, securing PHI in each one of these phases presents unique challenges in each phase. While established encryption techniques, such as Advanced Encryption Standard (AES), can secure PHI in Phases 1 (acquisition) and 2 (storage), they can only assure secure storage. Assuring the data privacy in Phase 3 (computation) is much more challenging, since there exists no method to perform computations, such as analytics and long-term health monitoring, on encrypted data efficiently. In this chapter, the authors study one emerging encryption technique, called Fully Homomorphic Encryption (FHE), as a candidate to perform secure analytics and monitoring on PHI in Phase 3. While FHE is in its developing stages and a mainstream application of it to general healthcare applications may take years to be established, the authors conduct a feasibility study of its application to long-term patient monitoring via cloud-based ECG data acquisition through existing ECG acquisition devices.

DOI: 10.4018/978-1-4666-8756-1.ch038

INTRODUCTION

Utilizing cloud computing resources such as Amazon EC2 (Amazon, n.d.), Microsoft Azure (Microsoft, n.d.), or Google (Google, n.d.) is commonplace for many corporations, due to its ability to prevent vast infrastructure investments. This concept dates back to the beginning of the Internet boom more than a decade ago with the emergence of the *Application Service Provider (ASP)* model: Rather than making an investment in costly server hardware, software licensing fees, and the personnel to manage this infrastructure, corporations can *rent* computation time, storage space, and licensing fees by running such applications as Salesforce.com (Salesforce, n.d.) over the Internet. The ASP model prevents upfront costs: a monthly subscription fee and a flexible licensing scheme allows smaller corporations to immediately start using such programs and expand with virtually no boundaries, since the computational and storage resources are provided by the application service provider (ASP) and the ASP can pool resources for many other clients. Additionally, this eliminates the need for corporations to have any expertise in setting up such sophisticated server infrastructure and the training on the application is done through online seminars.

Another dramatic example of such an ASP model is Paypal (Paypal, n.d.). The introduction of a merchant Application Programming Interface (API) by Paypal allowed any size corporation to start their business with near-zero investment, accept payments over the Internet by using Paypal as the intermediary, and grow with virtually no boundary. These examples show that, it is natural to shift the responsibility of computing (and storage) infrastructure investments to operators that can deliver their services by using the Internet as the delivery channel (i.e., Cloud Operators). By virtualizing their computational and storage resources, these cloud operators can provide these resources to their customers at a fraction of what the customers can build them for.

While endless examples exist for such generic cloud computing offerings, one area that can benefit significantly from it deserves specific attention: Medical cloud computing. When the data storage is outsourced to a cloud operator over the Internet, an important issue arises: data privacy. Although different applications have different sensitivity levels to this issue, the highest level of sensitivity is clearly in the medical arena (Kocabas et al, 2013). Personal Health Information (PHI) is one of the most scrutinized concepts, protected by laws and regulations of the U.S.A. The Health Insurance Portability and Accountability Act (HIPAA, n.d.) dictates a strict set of rules and regulations to prevent the PHI from being misused. Therefore, to expand the cloud computing into the medical arena, one must clearly formulate the entire concept around these restrictions.

Cloud computing is an active research area for medical applications, partly due to the push by the US government to modernize the US Health system (Lobodzinski & Laks, 2012). The motivations behind this move are: 1) improving the quality of healthcare by using additional cloud-based long-term patient monitoring data that are otherwise unavailable to the healthcare professionals, and 2) reducing the operational costs at healthcare organizations (HCO) by eliminating the datacenters operated by HCOs. Long-term patient monitoring data (e.g., patient vitals such as ECG and blood pressure), obtained by sensors that transmit their patient information over the cloud can be used as an auxiliary diagnostic tool to improve diagnostic accuracy. This expands the boundaries of an HCO to outside the HCO by allowing the patients to use long-term monitoring devices, such as ECG patches.

In this chapter, we study the feasibility of such a cloud-based long-term monitoring system while preserving PHI. Preserving PHI requires ensuring data privacy at three distinct phases: Phase I. Acquisition, is where the medical data is acquired from a patient, whether it is within the HCO, or outside the HCO via disposable devices such as

ECG patches (Leaf, n.d.), Phase II. Storage, where the data is stored in the cloud for future access, and, Phase III. Computation, is where the data is processed, whether during a real-time application execution by a doctor, or by the long-term patient monitoring software.

Existing AES-based encryption techniques (NIST, 2001) can ensure data privacy in phases I and II. However, ensuring data privacy during the application execution (i.e., Phase III) is only possible by transferring the data back and forth between the cloud and the mobile device. During this transfer, data must be in encrypted format while in the cloud, and must be decrypted when it reaches the mobile device. In contrast to this conventional methodology, we investigate an emerging new technique called Fully Homomorphic Encryption (FHE) (Gentry, 2009; Brakerski, Gentry, & Vaikuntanathan, 2012) and the possibility of its utilization in medical data analytics. We specifi-

cally investigate the application of remote health monitoring by using existing commodity ECG patches (Leaf, n.d.) and cloud computing. In our conceptual system, the entire application runs in the cloud, and the data acquisition (Phase I) and the visualization of analytics (Phase III) are achieved by thin devices (i.e., devices with significantly lower computational and storage capability as compared to the cloud resources). Therefore, these end nodes are disposable and the entire functionality of the application execution is outsourced to the cloud.

Our conceptual system, shown in Figure 1, depicts phase I (Acquisition) of the long-term health monitoring through the use of remote sensors, incorporating AES encryption and transmission capability. While we specifically focus on the ECG-based applications in this chapter, expansion of it to other medical applications is straightforward. The System in Figure 1 can be applied to any system containing sensors that have similar capabilities

Figure 1. Proposed cloud-based long term health monitoring system

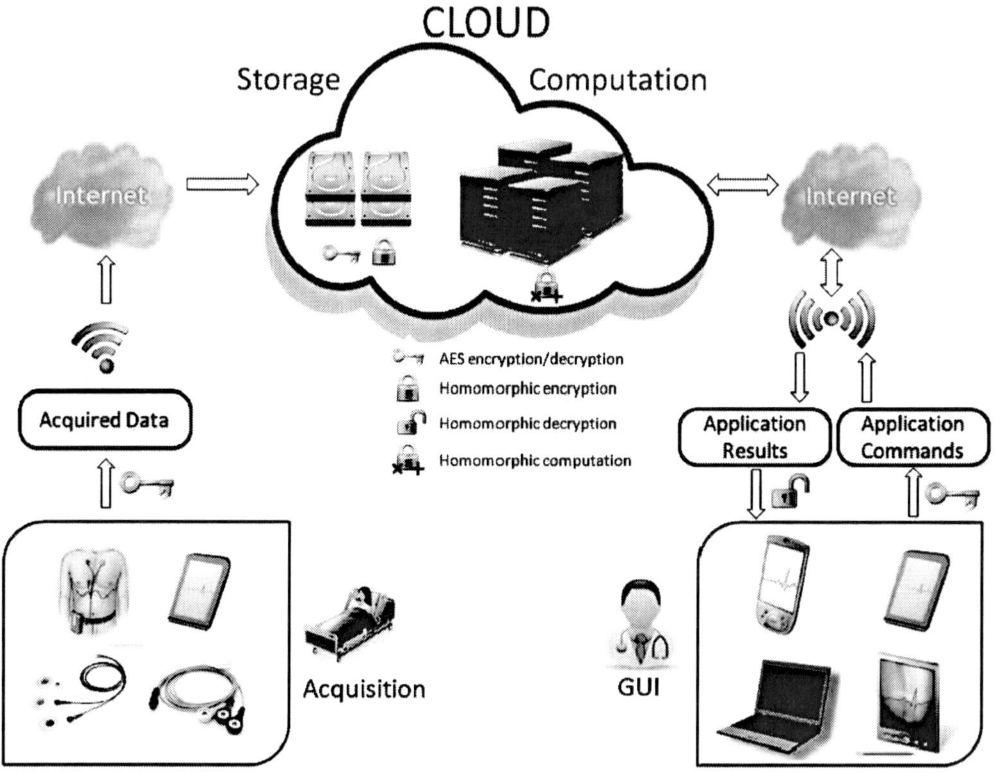

with a backend application that has similar characteristics. Phase II (storage) and III (computation) are strictly in the cloud in this system.

This system is conceptualized to use the end nodes as thin devices, where the loss of a thin device does not necessarily imply compromised PHI, since the device contains almost no information. This is due to the real-time transmission of the PHI right after its acquisition. Since no data are kept in the acquisition devices in the long term, the privacy management responsibility of the data is only relevant in the cloud. A similar argument is true for the display devices (e.g., tablets). Since Phase III is primarily performed in the cloud, and no data is stored in the GUI device, the loss of a GUI device (see Figure 1) presents no privacy issues. The system in Figure 1 pushes the entire workload into the cloud, making the end nodes mere acquisition and display devices. The compromise of acquisition and GUI devices implying the potential compromise of PHI has become an important consideration by the FDA recently (FDA, 2013) and shows the importance of designing a system that doesn't depend on strict security standards on the end nodes to ensure overall system security.

In this chapter, we investigate the feasibility of running medical applications in the cloud by formulating Full Homomorphic Encryption (FHE) as the core of this idea. We identify the challenges in making this possible for the specific remote-ECG monitoring applications, without loss of generality. We provide pointers to the potential of FHE acceleration while it is being widely researched (PROCEED, n.d.) to arrive at conclusions for its practical use in more widespread medical applications. This chapter is organized as follows: We provide background information on Fully Homomorphic Encryption (FHE) and Electrocardiogram (ECG), followed by the introduction of a cloud-based medical application in detail. The challenges related to different parts of this application are determined and the results based on existing ECG-based patient data derived

from the THEW database (Couderc, 2010) are presented. We conclude our chapter with discussions on future research challenges.

BACKGROUND INFORMATION

We will use Electrocardiogram (ECG) data to gain an insight into the challenges in applying FHE into medical applications. In this section, first we will provide background information on Fully Homomorphic Encryption (FHE) and focus on two important FHE schemes. Next, we will provide background information on ECG by using sample data acquired from the THEW worldwide ECG database (Courderc, 2010) and identify operations that are necessary to provide insight for a doctor during the diagnosis of cardiovascular diseases.

Emergence of Fully Homomorphic Encryption (FHE)

Conventional symmetric-key and public-key cryptosystems encrypt the data such that only authorized parties can access the data. In order to perform operations on the data, one needs to decrypt the encrypted data first and then perform the operations. On the other hand, FHE schemes enable computing meaningful operations on the encrypted data without observing the actual data. In other words, an example computation, $c = a + b$, becomes possible using FHE without actually knowing a and b.

To compute arbitrary functions on encrypted data, an FHE scheme should be capable of performing homomorphic additions and homomorphic multiplications over the encrypted text (termed *ciphertext*), which corresponds to addition and multiplication operations on the unencrypted message (termed *plaintext*) respectively when the resulting ciphertext is decrypted. Since any function can be represented as a combination of additions and multiplications, FHE scheme can compute arbitrary functions.

The FHE scheme is very useful in scenarios, where computation is outsourced to a third party and privacy of the data must be preserved at all times. With this scheme one can encrypt the data and store it in a database/cloud, and later ask a third party to perform some operations on the encrypted data. The third party never sees the original data but performs operations on the ciphertexts only, returning the result in encrypted form, which can only be decrypted by the secret key owner.

The idea of the homomorphic encryption was first proposed by Rivest et al. in 1978 (Rivest, Adleman, & Dertouzos, 1978). Since then, many schemes have been proposed (Goldwasser & Micali, 1982; El Gamal, 1985; Cohen & Fischer, 1985; Paillier, 1999; Damgård & Jurik, 2001), but these schemes support the only homomorphic addition or homomorphic multiplication, not both simultaneously within a single scheme. The closest cryptosystem to achieve the FHE scheme was proposed in (Boneh, Goh, & Nissim, 2005), which could perform many additions but only one multiplication. With his breakthrough work in 2009, Gentry (2009) proposed the first mechanism for an FHE scheme which could perform an arbitrary number of additions and multiplications homomorphically.

Gentry's FHE Scheme

Gentry's (2009) proposal for the first FHE scheme is based on ideal lattices. An ideal lattice is a discrete additive and a multiplicative subgroup in n-dimensional space which can be represented by its basis vector. The fact that a lattice can have an infinite number of bases plays a key role for creating a public-key cryptosystem. Similar to other public key cryptosytems (Diffie & Hellman, 1976; Rivest, Shamir, & Adleman, 1978), security of the lattice based cryptosystems is based on an intractable problem which is very hard to solve unless a secret key is known. The hard problem in Gentry (2009) is the Closest Vector Problem (CVP) which states that given a point in n-dimensional

space, it is hard to find the closest lattice point. If a good basis is known for the lattice, one can use Babai's nearest-vector approximation algorithm (Babai, L., 1985) to solve the CVP problem efficiently. The good basis of a lattice consists of almost orthogonal base vectors having a large decryption radius and it is used as the secret key. Figure 2 demonstrates the difference of decrypting a ciphertext with a good (on the left) and a bad (on the right) basis vector, where the result is mapped to an incorrect point on the lattice when a bad basis vector is used.

In Gentry's FHE scheme, encryption is performed by first mapping a message to a lattice point and then adding a small random noise to create the final ciphertext. The decryption can be done only by using a good basis which is only known by the secret-key holder. Homomorphic addition and homomorphic multiplication operations are performed by adding and multiplying lattice points respectively. During the homomorphic operations the noise inside the ciphertext grows with each operation. Specifically, homomorphic addition roughly doubles the noise, while homomorphic multiplication squares the noise. After several operations, the magnitude of the noise in the ciphertext exceeds the threshold at which a successful decryption is no longer possible even with the knowledge of a good basis. This limits the number of operations that can be performed with this scheme and is also referred to as *SomeWhat Homomorphic Encryption (SWHE)* scheme. Gentry proposed a remarkable bootstrapping method (i.e., recryption) to transform SWHE scheme into FHE scheme by evaluating the decryption function homomorphically. The recryption operation resets the noise inside the ciphertext and enables computation of arbitrary functions indefinitely.

Although Gentry's scheme is the first plausible mechanism for an FHE scheme, it has several inefficiencies both in terms of storage and computation. Messages are encrypted bitwise and in order to increase the noise threshold the ciphertext size must be large, which results expansion in storage space: For example, the size of a ciphertext encrypting 1-bit message could be multi-million bits, which presents an unacceptable data expansion ratio for most practical implementations. The homomorphic operations over very large ciphertexts are also compute-intensive and cost of the recryption operation is very high making Gentry's FHE scheme impractical.

Several FHE schemes and implementations have been proposed after Gentry's FHE scheme (Dijk, Gentry, Halevi, & Vaikuntanathan, 2010; Brakerski & Vaikuntanathan, 2011b, 2011a; Coron, Mandal, Naccache, & Tibouchi, 2011; Gentry & Halevi, 2011a; Naehrig, Lauter, & Vaikuntanathan, 2011; Smart & Vercauteren, 2010; Stehle & Steinfeld, 2010; Brakerski et al., 2012; Halevi & Shoup, n.d.; Gentry, Halevi, & Smart, 2012) to address the inefficiencies and make FHE more practical. (see Figure 2)

BGV Scheme

At present the BGV scheme (Brakerski et al, 2012) and its implementation (Halevi & Shoup, n.d.) are one of the most promising works for a practical FHE. The BGV scheme is based on Ring Learning with Errors (RLWE) primitives (Lyubashevsky, Peikert, & Regev, 2010). In the BGV scheme both messages and ciphertexts are defined over polynomial rings.

Several methods are introduced by the BGV scheme to improve the performance of earlier FHE schemes. A ciphertext is partitioned into slots by using the techniques in (Smart & Vercauteren, 2011), where each slot can pack a multi-bit message. Packing multiple messages into one ciphertext also enables computing homomorphic operations in Single Instruction Multiple Data (SIMD) fashion. The expensive recrypt operation can be avoided by using the leveled version of the BGV scheme. In the leveled version of the BGV scheme, homomorphic operations are performed up to L levels. Since each homomorphic addition and multiplication increases the noise in the ciphertext, only a limited number of homomorphic operations can be performed. While homomorphic addition does not increase the noise level significantly, homomorphic multiplication roughly squares the noise amount. Thus the level L is determined by the depth of multiplication operations for the function to be evaluated. The level of the function to be computed can be defined beforehand and then the parameters of the scheme can be adjusted during the key generation.

Figure 2. Homomorphic encryption with good (left) and bad (right) basis vectors mapping to a correct and incorrect result, respectively

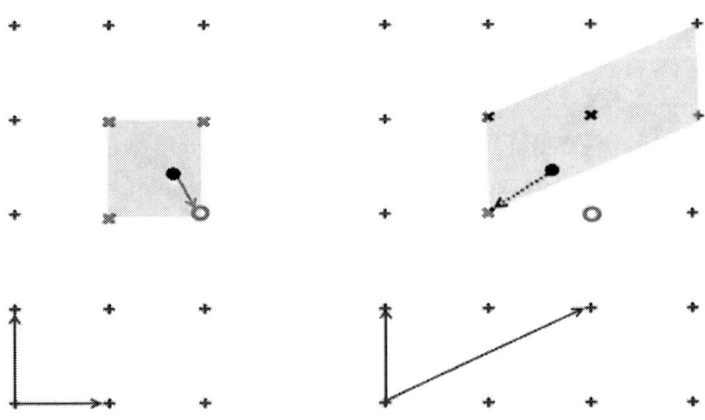

Medical Data Analytics on ECG Data

An exhaustive list of medical data such as echo/MRI imaging data, subject drug treatment, and physiological monitoring signals are routinely acquired and used for assessing a patients' health state by healthcare organizations (HCO). Among the list of medical data, we have opted to limit our feasibility assessment to a simple, yet real, set of data acquired from a subject coming to the Emergency Department (ED) of the University of California San Francisco Hospital for chest pain (Shusterman et al, 2007) and shared by the THEW initiative (Courderc, 2010). This data contain recordings of a patient's heart rhythms for 24-hours, acquired by a 12-lead Holter system. The device was hooked up to the patients when they arrived at the ED. In order to demonstrate the feasibility of our concept, we used information about the patient's heart rate (HR). There are standard ECG measurements that a cardiologist needs to access from this information that require computational tasks. Among these, we selected five measurements to be extracted from ECG tracing as examples, these are: 1) the minimum HR, 2) the maximum HR, 3) the average heart rate, 4) the presence of abnormal cardiac beats, and 5) the frequency of the ectopic beats. These five quantifiers can be extracted from the annotation file of the ECG, i.e., the file containing the vital information about each cardiac beat type and duration as shown on Figure 3. These five ECG measurements provide essential analytic information to the cardiologist about the patient's heart state. First, the cardiologist will evaluate if the average heart rate is in normal ranges, and then the cardiologist will check if the heart rate variation during the recordings are appropriate based on the patient physical activity, finally the frequency of abnormal cardiac beats will be checked. These abnormal beats can be discriminated based on their morphology. They are often present in healthy individuals but they may be associated with some risk if their frequency of occurrence is too high.

Structure of the Captured ECG Data

In general, the electrocardiogram (ECG) annotation file provides information which includes what type of cardiac contraction for each beat and the temporal distance between consecutive beats. The temporal distance is usually measured between two consecutive R peaks which is the peak of positive deflection in the QRS complex. Figure 3 shows the information extracted from a real ECG signal.

In this work, we have planned to assess the feasibility of implementing secure cloud-based monitoring using the ECG annotation file. The

Figure 3. One-lead tracing in which the number on top of each cardiac beat signal represents the time distance in millisecond between the current displayed beats, while the other characters, such as V and S, denote irregular beats corresponding to potential heart conditions.

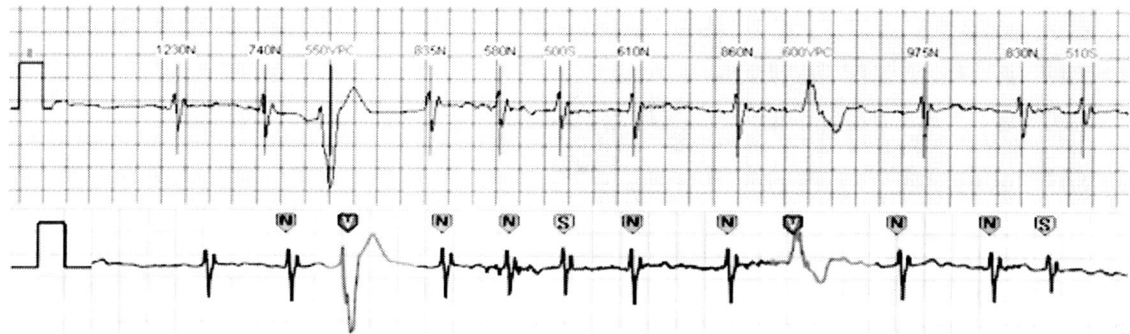

annotation file is a binary file containing two parts: 1) the header information and 2) the beat annotation. The header provides the information related to the original ECG, such as the number of leads, sampling frequency, recording time, and other technical specifications of the digital ECG signal. The header information is followed by the beat annotations, where each beat annotation segment consists of 4 bytes of binary data organized as three fields. First two fields are label information for classifying the recorded ECG beat type. The last field contains 2 bytes of information related to the temporal distance (i.e., *toc*) of the current beat from the last recorded beat. The size of the annotation file depends on the length of the acquired ECG tracings. In our experiments, we will use a sample ECG annotation file from the THEW ECG database (Courderc, 2010), which has a 24-hour ECG tracing record of a patient and contains 87,896 beat annotations.

THE DESIGN OF A CLOUD-BASED MEDICAL APPLICATION

Our proposed cloud-based application is based on offloading almost entire computation to the cloud. Our application is based on mainly three distinct parts: 1) Real-time medical data acquisition devices, 2) Cloud-based storage and computation, 3) GUI (end) node. In the following subsections, we will analyze each part individually.

Data Acquisition through Thin Devices

Acquisition devices are front-end of our cloud based medical application. These devices are capable of acquiring real-time medical data. Examples of such devices are disposable ECG patches attached to a patient or mobile ECG carts used in hospitals. Furthermore, with decades of research and development, current ECG recording technologies have matured enough to allow a patient to self-monitor at home. Figure 4 (left) shows a sample device from Alivecor (2013), which can be attached to a Smartphone and the software that is included with the device is capable of recording ECG samples. A sample ECG recording obtained from the device is shown in Figure 4 (right), which has sufficient accuracy to be useful in clinical diagnostics. To protect the patient's privacy, we assume the acquisition devices are capable of performing AES encryption of patient data and transmitting the encrypted data wirelessly (Fahad et al, 2012; Soyata et al, 2012b; Soyata et al, 2012c; Soyata et al, 2013).

Figure 4. (Left) Commercial ECG screening device from Alivecor. (Right) Recorded ECG data using the Alivecor device

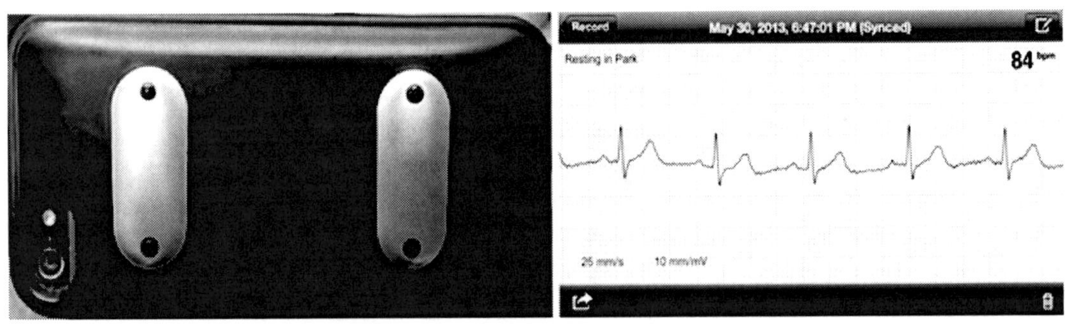

Considering the significant computational difference of encrypting data between AES (National Institute of Standards and Technology, 2001) and FHE, it is unrealistic for an acquisition node to execute real-time FHE encryption, while AES encryption has trivial computational demands and available even in the least expensive devices. Therefore, we formulate the acquisition node is oblivious to FHE encryption and only responsible for encrypting the patient data with AES encryption, while the conversion of AES encrypted data to FHE encrypted data is performed in the cloud.

AES to FHE Conversion Agent

Since homomorphic encryption cannot be performed during the acquisition phase, the data has to be transmitted into the cloud in AES-encrypted format. We propose to store all of the patient data in AES-encrypted format, since AES is a storage-neutral conversion (i.e., the AES-encrypted version of a 128-bit raw data occupies 128-bits also). While this completely solves the privacy of the stored data, conversion of AES-encrypted data to FHE-encrypted data has to be performed at some point, before any computation can be done by using FHE. We will experiment with a background AES to FHE conversion agent, a portion of the cloud software to continuously convert the AES-encrypted data into its FHE counterpart.

Converting AES-encrypted data to FHE-encrypted data requires evaluating AES decryption function homomorphically. To estimate the cost of AES to FHE conversion we refer to (Gentry et al., 2012). In (Gentry et al., 2012), the authors implemented the AES-128 decryption function with the BGV scheme (Brakerski et al., 2012) and provided latency/throughput analysis with different design choices. An AES-128 decryption operates on blocks of 128-bit (i.e. 16B) data, where granularity of the operations is 1 Byte. In the first design, a ciphertext is set to hold 864 plaintext slots where each slot holds information for 1B message. With this setting 16 slots can be used to contain

one AES-encrypted data, thus $\lfloor 864 \div 16 \rfloor = 54$ AES decryption operation can be performed in parallel. The overall evaluation runs in 36 hours; however since 54 AES decryptions have been performed in parallel, throughput is around 40 minutes per one AES decryption. In the second design, 16 ciphertexts are used and each ciphertext is set to hold 720 plaintext slots. Similar to the first design settings each slot holds information for 1B message, but this time each slot associated with different AES-encrypted data, thus 720 AES decryption operation can be performed in parallel. Although with this setting total evaluation time is around 5 days, throughput for one AES decryption is reduced to 5 minutes. Although the second design provided better throughput results than the first design, it requires larger memory to store all variables. Therefore, we will use the first design setting as our reference.

Based on the results were reported in (Gentry et al, 2012) to be around 36 hours for the decryption of 54 AES blocks (16B each), approximately 150 Sec is needed to convert 1B. Using these results as the basis, we calculate that, the AES to FHE conversion agent will need to process 87,896 beat annotations (175,792B assuming 2B per annotated element) to convert a 24-hour patient annotated recording to FHE. Therefore, the computation time for this conversion is approximately 7,324 hours. Using the estimated conversion time, the required speedup is around 305x to compute the results at the rate of arrival (i.e., 24-hours). We will show in the following subsection how, it is possible to parallelize this process to perform AES to FHE conversion at the rate of arrival if sufficient hardware parallelism is available.

Storage and Computation in the Cloud

As previously mentioned, acquisition nodes are assumed to be capable of AES encryption and AES-encrypted version of the medical records permanently stored in the cloud. In order to operate on medical data with FHE, AES-encrypted medical records have to be converted to FHE-encrypted version. Although we note that AES to FHE conversion is compute-intensive, this conversion has to be performed only once.

The AES to FHE conversion can be performed offline while the conversion time will be exposed as a delay in providing the remotely monitored patient data to the doctor. This delay might not be important, since the doctor typically needs these results in a few days after the remote monitoring has been completed. This latency tolerance can be translated into further cost savings for the HCO, by performing AES to FHE conversion when the computation resources are less expensive. For instance, Amazon Web Services (AWS) offers Micro instances which have basic computation capabilities yet they can be rented at no cost.

In addition to the delay in providing AES to FHE conversion, a certain amount of compute-caching can also be performed offline. For example, assume a set of 10,000 results that need to be added to provide the average heart rate to the doctor. These results to add are generally in very predictable intervals, thereby generating predictable patterns in pre-computable results. As an example, to reduce the real-time compute strain in the cloud when the doctor is running the application, every 100 results can be summed, and the results can be cached in the storage area. Such a process can be accelerated using specialized accelerators (Guo et al, 2010; Soyata et al, 2012a) and computation optimization techniques (Soyata et al, 1993; Soyata & Friedman, 1994a; Soyata & Friedman, 1994b; Soyata et al, 1995; Soyata & Friedman, 1997; Soyata, 1999).

In this specific example, which is also demonstrated in Figure 5, a typical operation is to calculate the sum (and, thus, the average) of 10,000 numbers. It is feasible to pre-compute sums for 100-number chunks. Observing that, this will expand the required storage by 100x as compared to storing only the initial 10,000 results, this provides a trade-off between latency and storage by shifting the application execution time from offline to online computation. This idea can be further expanded by building a compute-cache that has a log-tree structure by calculating every 100, and every 10,000, etc., permitting computations to be sped up at the expense of higher storage.

Figure 5. Compute-caching example

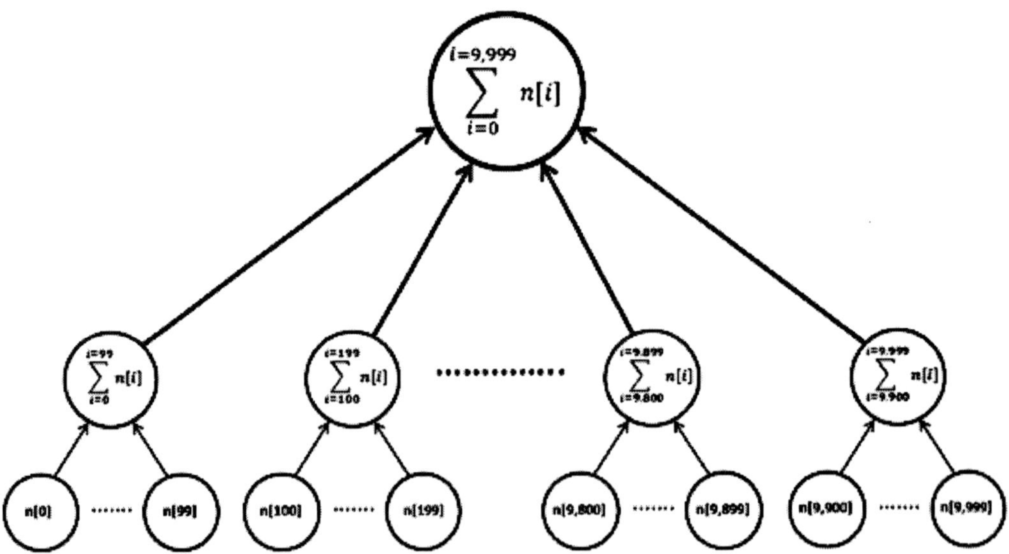

Storage Management in the Cloud

Considering the significant amount of storage that FHE requires, a natural question to ask is the total required amount of storage for each application. We conceptualize the cloud storage that an FHE-enabled application requires as composed of three separate areas: 1) The AES-data area, which is where the medical records are permanently stored in AES-encrypted format, 2) The FHE data-cache area, which is the FHE-encrypted copy of the original AES data, only for certain records, 3) The FHE compute-cache area, which is the pre-computed results for portions of the FHE data-cache.

We assume that, three distinct spaces will be allocated to each one of AES data, FHE data-cache, and FHE-compute cache. This implies a hierarchical storage which resembles closely a computer's memory subsystem, where, AES-data area is analogous to a computer disk, since the conversion from AES to FHE takes a long time, FHE data-cache is analogous to computer memory, since there is a significant penalty in bringing the data in from the memory into the cache, and FHE compute-cache is analogous to L3 cache, where the results in this cache can be converted to useful results significantly faster than the ones in the FHE data-cache.

In this proposed tiered storage scheme, the FHE data-cache and FHE compute-cache are completely disposable, i.e., discarding any information in these caches only hurts performance, but does not cause data loss. This allows the cloud application to dynamically adjust the contents of each cache, thereby modulating the application response time vs. required storage and computation.

Displaying the Application Results through GUI Devices

The backend of our application is the GUI device which runs the GUI portion of the medical application and displays the results to the doctor.

Since the cloud is responsible for performing entire set of computations with FHE, the end result will be in the FHE-encrypted format when it is transferred to the GUI device. This necessitates that the GUI device has to perform decryption of FHE-encrypted ciphertexts. Furthermore, to avoid exposing the medical data at any point, decryption needs to be performed only on the Smartphone of the authorized personnel.

Considering that, within the FHE framework, the decryption has a fairly low compute-intensity as compared to the intermediate computations, this is feasible for the GUI device. Since most current Smartphones have multiple processor cores and are expected to amass an ever increasing computational power, it is reasonable to expect the decryption process to take close to real-time and acceptable to the user. Therefore the GUI end-node has to have minimal capability in 1) running an OS such as Android or iOS to provide a user interface to the doctor, and 2) perform homomorphic decryption.

PERFORMANCE EVALUATION

In this section, we will evaluate calculating the average heart rate of a patient with two FHE schemes: Gentry's FHE scheme (Gentry, 2009) and the BGV scheme (Brakerski et al, 2012). We will use the library in (Gentry & Halevi, 2011b) for the former scheme, while the library in (Halevi & Shoup, n.d.) will be used for the latter.

We run our simulations on a computation node in UR Bluhive cluster (University of Rochester, Center for Integrated Research Computing, n.d.) which has two Intel Xeon E5450 processors, each with four cores running at 3GHz with 16GB RAM in total.

Calculating the Average Heart Rate

In order to demonstrate the feasibility of our concept, we selected finding the average heart rate of the patient as our case study. To compute the average heart rate of a patient, we will use an ECG annotation file from the THEW ECG database (Courderc, 2010). The annotation file consists of 24-hour ECG data of the patient captured with a 12-lead Holter system sampling at 1,000Hz. The file contains 87,896 entries for temporal distance (*toc*) of consecutive heart beats and each *toc* value is represented by 12-bit number.

We calculate average heart rate of a patient during N heart beats in two steps: 1) Accumulate the *toc* values for N heart beats, 2) divide the final sum by N, and then finally multiply with sample acquisition time. The trivial division and multiplication operation for the second step is expensive to perform with the FHE, thus we require performing this step at the Smartphone. The first step will be computed completely in the cloud and the FHE encrypted result will be sent to the Smartphone along with FHE encrypted information related to the second step (i.e. N and acquisition time). The Smartphone can decrypt the result from the first step, and information related to second step then it can perform trivial division and multiplication to find the average heart rate.

Results Based on the Gentry's FHE scheme

In Gentry's FHE scheme (Gentry, 2009), encryption is performed on individual bits. In other words, encrypting a message of m-bits will generate m ciphertexts. Homomorphic operations on the ciphertexts correspond to bit-wise arithmetic. Specifically, homomorphic addition results in XOR operation and homomorphic multiplication results in AND operation of the message bits. Table 1 presents the execution times for each FHE primitive on the cluster node.

In order to perform integer additions with bit-wise operations, we choose to implement Ripple Carry Adder. First, we calculate the sum and carry homomorphically for each bit and then the carry is forwarded to next level computation. The noise inside the ciphertext grows during carry computation which involves homomorphic multiplication. To prevent decryption errors, we need to perform recryption operations for the carry before forwarding to next level computation. Based on the results presented in Table 1, recryption operation takes longer than the rest of the operations and thus 99.9% of the execution time for adding two m-bit number is spent during recryption operation.

To analyze computational and storage requirements of Gentry's FHE scheme, we calculate the average heart rate of the patient during one-hour. The patient record for one-hour consists of approximately 4,096 *toc* values where each *toc* value is a 12-bit number. A 24-bit accumulator is chosen to prevent overflow for adding 4,096 12-bit numbers. Computing one-hour average heart rate finished in approximately 700 hours on the cluster node. Each ciphertext has a size of roughly 0.1MB and storing one-hour of patient record requires $\approx$ 4.8GB of storage space. Since each ciphertext encrypts one-bit, this is equal to storage expansion of 800,000X. Our experiment results indicate that using Gentry's FHE scheme is impractical both in terms of computation and storage.

Results Based on the BGV scheme

In the BGV scheme (Brakerski et al., 2012), messages and ciphertexts are defined over polynomial rings. Homomorphic addition and multiplication

Table 1. Execution time of the operations for the Gentry's FHE scheme

Operation	Execution Time
Encryption	1.45 Sec
Decryption	0.2 Sec
Recryption	24.95 Sec
Addition	< 1 μs
Multiplication	1.79 ms

Table 2. Execution time of the operations for the BGV scheme

Operation	Execution Time
Encryption	1.65 sec
Decryption	0.65 sec
Addition	0.11 ms
Multiplication	0.8 sec

of ciphertexts will correspond to ring additions and multiplications respectively. Table 2 presents the execution times for each FHE primitive on the cluster node.

To perform additions of *toc* values with polynomial rings we use the methods described in (Naehrig, M., et al, 2011) to encode each *toc* value. In (Naehrig et al, 2011), each message is represented by its binary encoding and each bit of the message is set as one of the coefficients of the message polynomial. Homomorphic additions correspond to polynomial additions and as long as the coefficients of the plaintext do not exceed plaintext space *p,* correctness are assured. The final result after computation can be recovered by first decrypting the ciphertext and then evaluating the resulting polynomial at 2.

To analyze computational and storage requirements of the BGV scheme, we calculate the average heart rate of a patient during 24 hours. To represent a 12-bit *toc* value we choose to work with polynomials of degree 12. We set the parameters of the BGV scheme which enable us to pack 200 slots in each ciphertext. Since each ciphertext can pack 200 *toc* values, accumulating the 87,896 *toc* values can be performed by $\lceil 87,896 \div 200 \rceil = 440$ additions. Based on our simulations on the cluster node, computing 24-hour average heart rate takes approximately 70 ms. In terms of storage, one ciphertext has a size of roughly 65KB and storing entire patient records require 28 MB of storage space. Each ciphertext encrypts 200 *toc* values with 12-bit each, which corresponds to a data expansion ratio of $65,000\times8/200\times12 \approx 217$.

While computing the average is slow compared to its no-encryption version, the BGV scheme is very close to providing the result in real-time with a moderate expansion in storage.

We perform following experiment to investigate maximum achievable speedup by utilizing the parallelism in the cloud. We look at the parallelism at the process - level, since the library in (Halevi & Shoup, n.d.) is not thread-safe. We launch multiple concurrent processes and assign each process independent portions of the data. The results of each process can be combined later through OS-level pipes. Table 3 presents the speedup due to process-level parallelism on the cluster node. The speedup column is normalized to the single-thread runtime. The Efficiency column indicates the percentage speedup compared to the ideal speedup due to parallelism (i.e., *N* threads for *N* times speedup).

CONCLUSION AND FUTURE WORK

In this chapter, a long-term health monitoring system is introduced to achieve the end goal of detecting patient health issues by continuously monitoring the ECG data acquired outside the Healthcare Organization (HCO). This system consists of ECG acquisition devices, a cloud-based medical application, and back-end devices that display the monitoring results. While such a system can be trivially implemented by today's technology by using existing ECG devices, cloud computing resources and highly capable Smartphones, one important issue arises when the intended applica-

Table 3. Multi-process runtime using a dual-socket Xeon server

Process	Runtime (ms)	Speedup	Efficiency (%)
1	69.8	1.00	100
2	35.8	1.95	97.4
4	21.5	3.25	81.4
8	11.75	5.96	74.5

tion is a medical application: The protection of Personal Healthcare Information (PHI).

Significant liability is associated with mishandling PHI in the U.S.A., whether intentional or unintentional. The Health Insurance Portability and Accountability Act (HIPAA, n.d.) mandates strict regulations on protection PHI. Due to the unacceptable risks associated with mishandling PHI (due to whatever reason, including hardware or software malfunction or an intentional security breach), cloud operators, such as Amazon (Amazon, n.d.) do not sign a Business Associate Agreement (BAA) which shifts a portion of the liability to the cloud operator. Without a form of a guarantee that the PHI will be safe during cloud based operation, HCO's cannot take the risk and host their medical application in the cloud. This non-starter renders all of the benefits of cloud computing useless to an HCO.

This chapter formulates a system, in which the cloud can execute the medical application without the concern of PHI protection. This is achieved by an encryption system, called, Fully Homomorphic Encryption (FHE), which permits operations on encrypted data. Since the cloud operator can operate on data that it cannot observe, the data is secure even if there is a security breach. Only the parties with a private key can decrypt the data that was initially encrypted with FHE. Therefore, the protection of PHI implies protecting the private keys, which is the same responsibility as protecting passwords when accessing a computer.

We argue that, by providing such a tool for cloud operators to operate on encrypted data, and making the password protection the responsibility of the HCO, cloud operators will be motivated to sign a BAA. In fact, we have observed this at the University of Rochester Medical Center, where a small cloud backup company is willing to sign a BAA as long as the key is not stored in their system and the responsibility of the protection of the private keys lies 100% with the HCO. It is the conclusion of this chapter that, the same concept

will eventually extend to the execution of a medical application when small operators sign a BAA to run a medical application as long as they are not storing the private keys. Managing the privacy of these keys is a significantly easier task for an HCO as compared to managing the privacy of the entire datacenter they are operating. This concept, therefore, holds the key to revolutionizing the US healthcare.

ACKNOWLEDGMENT

This work was supported in part by the National Science Foundation grant CNS-1239423 and a gift from Nvidia corporation.

REFERENCES

Alivecor. (2013). *ECG screening made easy.* Retrieved from http://www.alivecor.com

Amazon. (n.d.). *Amazon web services (AWS).* Retrieved from http://aws.amazon.com

Babai, L. (1985). On Lovász' lattice reduction and the nearest lattice point problem. *STACS, 85,* 13–20.

Boneh, D., Goh, E. J., & Nissim, K. (2005). Evaluating 2-DNF formulas on ciphertexts. In *Theory of cryptography* (pp. 325–341). Berlin: Springer. doi:10.1007/978-3-540-30576-7_18

Brakerski, Z., Gentry, C., & Vaikuntanathan, V. (2012). (Leveled) fully homomorphic encryption without bootstrapping. In *Proceedings of the 3rd Innovations in Theoretical Computer Science Conference* (pp. 309-325). ACM.

Brakerski, Z., & Vaikuntanathan, V. (2011). Efficient fully homomorphic encryption from (standard) LWE. In Proceedings of Foundations of Computer Science (FOCS), (pp. 97-106). IEEE.

Brakerski, Z., & Vaikuntanathan, V. (2011). Fully homomorphic encryption from ring-LWE and security for key dependent messages. In *Proceedings of Advances in Cryptology–CRYPTO 2011* (pp. 505–524). Berlin: Springer. doi:10.1007/978-3-642-22792-9_29

Cohen, J. D., & Fischer, M. J. (1985). A robust and verifiable cryptographically secure election scheme. In *Proceedings of Foundations of Computer Science* (pp. 372–382). IEEE. doi:10.1109/SFCS.1985.2

Coron, J. S., Mandal, A., Naccache, D., & Tibouchi, M. (2011). Fully homomorphic encryption over the integers with shorter public keys. In *Proceedings of Advances in Cryptology–CRYPTO 2011* (pp. 487–504). Berlin: Springer. doi:10.1007/978-3-642-22792-9_28

Couderc, J. P. (2010). The telemetric and holter ECG warehouse initiative (THEW): A data repository for the design, implementation and validation of ECG-related technologies. In Proceedings of Engineering in Medicine and Biology Society (EMBC), (pp. 6252-6255). IEEE.

Damgård, I., & Jurik, M. (2001). A generalisation, a simplification and some applications of Paillier's probabilistic public-key system. In *Proceedings of the 4th International Workshop on Practice and Theory in Public Key Cryptography: Public Key Cryptography* (pp. 119-136). Berlin: Springer-Verlag.

Diffie, W., & Hellman, M. (1976). New directions in cryptography. *IEEE Transactions on Information Theory, 22*(6), 644–654. doi:10.1109/TIT.1976.1055638

ElGamal, T. (1985). A public key cryptosystem and a signature scheme based on discrete logarithms. *IEEE Transactions on Information Theory, 31*(4), 469–472. doi:10.1109/TIT.1985.1057074

Fahad, A., Soyata, T., Wang, T., Sharma, G., Heinzelman, W., & Shen, K. (2012). SOLARCAP: Super capacitor buffering of solar energy for self-sustainable field systems. In *Proceedings of SOC Conference* (SOCC), (pp. 236-241). IEEE.

FDA. (2013). *FDA safety communication: Cybersecurity for medical devices and hospital networks.* Retrieved from http://www.fda.gov/medicaldevices/safety/alertsandnotices/ucm356423.htm

Gentry, C. (2009). *A fully homomorphic encryption scheme.* (Doctoral Dissertation). Stanford University, Palo Alto, CA.

Gentry, C., & Halevi, S. (2011). Fully homomorphic encryption without squashing using depth-3 arithmetic circuits. In Proceedings of Foundations of Computer Science (FOCS), (pp. 107-109). IEEE.

Gentry, C., & Halevi, S. (2011). Implementing Gentry's fully-homomorphic encryption scheme. In *Proceedings of Advances in Cryptology–EUROCRYPT 2011* (pp. 129–148). Berlin: Springer. doi:10.1007/978-3-642-20465-4_9

Gentry, C., Halevi, S., & Smart, N. P. (2012). Homomorphic evaluation of the AES circuit. In *Proceedings of Advances in Cryptology–CRYPTO 2012* (pp. 850–867). Berlin: Springer. doi:10.1007/978-3-642-32009-5_49

Goldwasser, S., & Micali, S. (1982). Probabilistic encryption & how to play mental poker keeping secret all partial information. In *Proceedings of the Fourteenth Annual ACM Symposium on Theory of Computing* (pp. 365-377). ACM.

Google. (n.d.). *Google app. engine.* Retrieved from http://code.google.com/appengine

Guo, X., Ipek, E., & Soyata, T. (2010). Resistive computation: avoiding the power wall with low-leakage, STT-MRAM based computing. *ACM SIGARCH Computer Architecture News, 38*(3), 371–382. doi:10.1145/1816038.1816012

Halevi, S., & Shoup, V. (n.d.). *HElib*. Retrieved from https://github.com/shaih/HElib

HIPAA. (n.d.). *Wikipedia*. Retrieved from http://en.wikipedia.org/wiki/Hipaa

Hoang, D. B., & Chen, L. (2010). Mobile cloud for assistive healthcare (MoCAsH). In *Proceedings of Services Computing Conference* (APSCC), (pp. 325-332). IEEE.

Hoang, D. T., Niyato, D., & Wang, P. (2012). Optimal admission control policy for mobile cloud computing hotspot with cloudlet. In *Proceedings of Wireless Communications and Networking Conference* (WCNC), (pp. 3145-3149). IEEE.

Kocabas, O., Soyata, T., Couderc, J. P., Aktas, M., Xia, J., & Huang, M. (2013). Assessment of cloud-based health monitoring using homomorphic encryption. In *Proceedings of the 31st IEEE International Conference on Computer Design*. IEEE.

Leaf. (n.d). *World's thinnest 3-lead ECG patch*. Retrieved from http://www.clearbridgevitalsigns.com/brochures/CardioLeaf_ULTRA_Brochure.pdf

Lobodzinski, S., & Laks, M. (2012). New devices for every long-term ecg monitoring. *Cardiology Journal*, *19*(2), 210–214. doi:10.5603/CJ.2012.0039 PMID:22461060

Lyubashevsky, V., Peikert, C., & Regev, O. (2010). On ideal lattices and learning with errors over rings. In *Proceedings of Advances in Cryptology–EUROCRYPT 2010* (pp. 1–23). Berlin: Springer. doi:10.1007/978-3-642-13190-5_1

Micciancio, D. (2001). Improving lattice based cryptosystems using the Hermite normal form. In *Cryptography and lattices* (pp. 126–145). Berlin: Springer. doi:10.1007/3-540-44670-2_11

Microsoft. (n.d.). *Windows Azure*. Retrieved from http://www.microsoft.com/windowazure

Naehrig, M., Lauter, K., & Vaikuntanathan, V. (2011). Can homomorphic encryption be practical? In *Proceedings of the 3rd ACM Workshop on Cloud Computing Security Workshop* (pp. 113-124). ACM.

NIST. (2001). Advanced encryption standard (AES) []. Washington, DC: NIST.]. *Federal Information Processing Standard, FIPS-197*, 1.

Paillier, P. (1999). Public-key cryptosystems based on composite degree residuosity classes. In *Proceedings of Advances in Cryptology–EUROCRYPT'99* (pp. 223–238). Berlin: Springer. doi:10.1007/3-540-48910-X_16

Paypal. (n.d). *Paypal*. Retrieved from https://www.paypal.com

PROCEED. (n.d.). *Programming computation on encrypted data*. Retrieved from http://www.darpa.mil/Our_Work/I2O/Programs/PROgramming_Computation_on_EncryptEd_Data_(PROCEED).aspx

Rivest, R. L., Adleman, L., & Dertouzos, M. L. (1978). On data banks and privacy homomorphisms. *Foundations of Secure Computation*, *32*(4), 169–178.

Rivest, R. L., Shamir, A., & Adleman, L. (1978). A method for obtaining digital signatures and public-key cryptosystems. *Communications of the ACM*, *21*(2), 120–126. doi:10.1145/359340.359342

Salesforce. (n.d.). *Salesforce customer relationship management (CRM)*. Retrieved from http://www.salesforce.com

Shusterman, V., Goldberg, A., Schindler, D. M., Fleischmann, K. E., Lux, R. L., & Drew, B. J. (2007). Dynamic tracking of ischemia in the surface electrocardiogram. *Journal of Electrocardiology*, *40*(6), S179–S186. doi:10.1016/j.jelectrocard.2007.06.015 PMID:17993319

Smart, N. P., & Vercauteren, F. (2010). Fully homomorphic encryption with relatively small key and ciphertext sizes. In *Proceedings of Public Key Cryptography–PKC 2010* (pp. 420–443). Berlin: Springer. doi:10.1007/978-3-642-13013-7_25

Smart, N. P., & Vercauteren, F. (2011). Fully homomorphic SIMD operations. In *Proceedings of Designs, Codes and Cryptography*. Academic Press.

Soyata, T. (1999). *Incorporating circuit level information into the retiming process*. (Doctoral Dissertation). University of Rochester, Rochester, NY.

Soyata, T., Ba, H., Heinzelman, W., Kwon, M., & Shi, J. (2013). *Accelerating mobile-cloud computing: A survey*. Academic Press.

Soyata, T., & Friedman, E. G. (1994). Retiming with non-zero clock skew, variable register, and interconnect delay. In *Proceedings of the 1994 IEEE/ACM International Conference on Computer-Aided Design* (pp. 234-241). IEEE.

Soyata, T., & Friedman, E. G. (1994). Synchronous performance and reliability improvement in pipelined ASICs. In *Proceedings of ASIC Conference and Exhibit*, (pp. 383-390). IEEE.

Soyata, T., Friedman, E. G., & Mulligan, J. H. Jr. (1993). Integration of clock skew and register delays into a retiming algorithm. In *Proceedings of Circuits and Systems* (pp. 1483–1486). IEEE. doi:10.1109/ISCAS.1993.394015

Soyata, T., Friedman, E. G., & Mulligan, J. H. Jr. (1995). Monotonicity constraints on path delays for efficient retiming with localized clock skew and variable register delay. [). IEEE.]. *Proceedings of Circuits and Systems*, *3*, 1748–1751.

Soyata, T., Friedman, E. G., & Mulligan, J. H. Jr. (1997). Incorporating interconnect, register, and clock distribution delays into the retiming process. *IEEE Transactions on Computer-Aided Design of Integrated Circuits and Systems*, *16*(1), 105–120. doi:10.1109/43.559335

Soyata, T., & Liobe, J. (2012). pbCAM: Probabilistically-banked content addressable memory. In *Proceedings of SOC Conference* (SOCC), (pp. 27-32). IEEE.

Soyata, T., Muraleedharan, R., Funai, C., Kwon, M., & Heinzelman, W. (2012). Cloud-vision: Real-time face recognition using a mobile-cloudlet-cloud acceleration architecture. In Proceedings of Computers and Communications (ISCC), (pp. 59-66). IEEE.

Soyata, T., Muraleedharana, R., Langdonb, J., Funaia, C., Amesc, S., Kwond, M., & Heinzelmana, W. (2012). COMBAT: Mobile-cloud-based compute/communications infrastructure for battlefield applications. [). SPIE.]. *Proceedings of the Society for Photo-Instrumentation Engineers*, *8403*, 84030K–1. doi:10.1117/12.919146

Stehlé, D., & Steinfeld, R. (2010). Faster fully homomorphic encryption. In *Proceedings of Advances in Cryptology-ASIACRYPT 2010* (pp. 377–394). Berlin: Springer. doi:10.1007/978-3-642-17373-8_22

University of Rochester, Center for Integrated Research Computing. (n.d.). *Bluehive cluster*. Retrieved from http://www.circ.rochester.edu/wiki/index.php/BlueHive_Cluster

Van Dijk, M., Gentry, C., Halevi, S., & Vaikuntanathan, V. (2010). Fully homomorphic encryption over the integers. In *Proceedings of Advances in Cryptology–EUROCRYPT 2010* (pp. 24–43). Berlin: Springer. doi:10.1007/978-3-642-13190-5_2

KEY TERMS AND DEFINITIONS

Advanced Encryption Standard (AES): Widely used symmetric-key cryptography published by National Institute of Standards and Technology (NIST).

Cloud Computing: A distributed computing system that relies on use of shared resources connected by the Internet to manage data and perform computations.

Electrocardiogram (ECG): Recording electrical activity of the heart to measure and diagnose abnormal rhythms of the heart.

Encryption: Encoding the contents of a message such that only authorized parties can access the message.

Graphical User Interface (GUI): An interface that allows visualization of information in graphical format.

Holter System: Portable monitor used for recording electrical activity of a patient continuously during 24-48 hours of daily activity.

Homomorphic Encryption: An encryption system capable of performing meaningful operations on the encrypted messages without accessing the original message.

Lattice-Based Cryptography: Cryptographic systems in which primitives are based on the hardness of lattice problems.

Long Term Health Monitoring: Monitoring patients during extended period of time for diagnosing and treating health issues at an early stage.

Mobile-Cloud Task Partitioning: Partitioning and assigning different subtasks to mobile devices or to cloud based on computational resource requirements of each subtask.

This work was previously published in the Handbook of Research on Cloud Infrastructures for Big Data Analytics edited by Pethuru Raj and Ganesh Chandra Deka, pages 471-488 copyright year 2014 by Information Science Reference (an imprint of IGI Global).

Chapter 39

Ambulance Dispatching System with Integrated Information and Communication Technologies on Cloud Environment

Jian-Wei Li
Chaoyang University of Technology, Taiwan

Yi-Chun Chang
Hungkuang University, Taiwan

Chia-Chi Chang
Chaoyang University of Technology, Taiwan

Yung-Fa Huang
Chaoyang University of Technology, Taiwan

ABSTRACT

The quality of emergency medical services (EMS) prior to a patient's arrival at a hospital is directly affected by the efficiency to dispatch an ambulance for first aid. In this paper, we created an ambulance dispatching system for first aid, which is integrated with Information and Communication Technology (ICT) and performed on a cloud platform. In virtue of ICT, the system can readily monitor the movements of ambulance with Geographic Information System (GIS) and determine any ambulance dispatching task and saves more time spent in transporting an accident victim to a hospital. Furthermore, the system running on a cloud platform is characteristic of integrated medical resources and terminal equipment with or without powerful hardware that is flexibly added into or removed from the system for supporting dispatch.

INTRODUCTION

The booming Internet and communication techniques have driven development of Information and Communication Technology (ICT) (Huang & Chen, 2010). The more effective achievements and better application services than those in the past should be attributed to ICT appropriately integrated into different fields. Currently, the exponentially growing populations suffering from chronic diseases in each country have been inevitably imposing heavy burdens on the social medical system of a rapid ageing society. Against this background, the effective medical resource management and fast physiological information processing in a medical system supplemented by

DOI: 10.4018/978-1-4666-8756-1.ch039

ICT for methodical health care of patients has become an important issue (Gupta, M., 2006; Barmentlo, M., 2007; Masson, Y., 2007; Kiefer, S., 2007; Halford, S., & Lotherington, A. T., 2015; Hilty, L. M., & Aebischer, B., 2015). Moreover, the developed countries have made huge investments in manpower and material resources related to researches, for example, EU's "ICT for Better Healthcare" for research of e-health in Framework Programme 6 (FP6) and Framework Programme 7 (FP7) to which hundreds of millions of Euros have been provided (European Commission, 2009).

In the case of ambulance dispatching for emergency medical service which is intended to give an accident victim first aid prior to further treatment in a hospital, a service center should be responsible for supply of urgent medical resources and ambulance dispatching (History of the Emergency Medical Services, 2014; Medic One began with a basic need and focused vision, 2014). In this regard, a service center that depends on radio to communicate with the ambulance staff for current status and dispatching still fails in proactively detecting movement of an ambulance anytime and performing immediate dispatching for any urgent accidental event. Furthermore, a service center not collecting real-time information for dispatching may delays ambulance dispatching when a case reporter who informs the service center of an accident by telephone does not provide a precise location.

For a patient waiting for first aid, time spent in case report by emergency telephone or a dispatched ambulance arriving at the scene and moving to a hospital is very precious. During decision-making of dispatching an ambulance and transportation of a patient, time is critical to the patient's life because the probability of successful rescue is reduced by 7% to 10% for every one-minute delay of first aid (Cummins, R. O., Eisenberg, M. S., Hallstrom, A. P., & Litwin, P. E., 1985). In this regard, a complete and fast ambulance dispatching system and a vehicle-borne patient physiology monitoring system for time-effectiveness of

rescuing a victim who suffers from an accidental event or the onset of a disease will contribute to rescue of more precious lives. In this paper, we integrate several existing ICT such as smart devices built in Global Position System (GPS) and the third generation (3G) mobile communications systems, Geographic Information System (GIS) (Kenneth E. Foote & Margaret Lynch, 2015), 3G/4G networks, and cloud system to accelerate the process of ambulance dispatching and develop an ambulance dispatching system for emergency medical services. The system constructed on a cloud platform comprises subsystems as follows: (1) case management subsystem; (2) ambulance management subsystem; (3) route planning subsystem; (4) ambulance dispatching subsystem; (5) patient physiology monitoring subsystem.

The system running on a cloud platform is characteristic of integrated medical resources and terminal equipment with or without powerful hardware that is flexibly added into or removed from the system for supporting dispatch. In addition, the movements of ambulances are readily controlled by ICT-based system with GIS and cloud computing supporting a service center's decision-making of any dispatching task, saving time for on-board emergency care, and improving quality of emergency medical services prior to treatment of a hospital.

BACKGROUND

As a brand-new concept for Internet service, cloud computing based on the principles of parallel computing and grid computing for organization of a huge cloud platform provides on-line services accessed by users without powerful hardware facilities. Three service models offered by cloud computing are (Sun Microsystem, 2009):

1. **IaaS (Infrastructure as a Service):** IaaS provides virtualized recourses over the Internet, such computing resource, storage,

and networking services. Users can purchase IaaS services instead of purchasing additional hardware. Well-known IaaS providers are Amazon Web Services (AWS), Windows Azure, Google Compute Engine, and so on.

2. **PaaS (Platform as a Service):** PaaS provides a platform to users and developers who follow rules and constraints of PaaS so that the programs are compiled and executed on the cloud platform. Moreover, PaaS monitors access of application services, deploying resources automatically. Well-known PaaS platforms for software development and management are AWS Elastic Beanstalk, Google App Engine, and so on.

3. **SaaS (Software as a Service):** SaaS directly gives users application services as required. Differing from software widely known, software of SaaS exists in services, helpfully simplifies software deployment and maintenance, and reduces manpower hired in an IT department. Well-known SaaS providers are Google Gmail, Microsoft 365, and so on.

The cloud computing architecture of Hadoop based on open sources is used to manage and distribute tasks to a huge number of servers for running in a cloud system (Apache Hadoop project; Tom Whit, 2012). Hadoop facilitates construction of a cloud platform, PaaS, and even cloud services like IaaS. In Hadoop, MapReduce creates a distributed computing environment and Hadoop Distributed File System (HDFS) offers huge storage space for a distributed database, i.e., HBase (Hadoop database). HBase, which is an open source and a NoSQL (Not Only SQL) database (NoSQL), is constructed in HDFS and provides a distributed storage system for structured data. In our research, the system running on a cloud platform is based on Hadoop and HBase (Apache HBase; Lars George, 2011).

SYSTEM ARCHITECTURE

For integrated medical resources and accelerated operation of a system, the emergency medical service system tested in our research is constructed on a cloud platform on the basis of Hadoop and the cloud database of HBASE. Additionally, the system in the running architecture includes three roles such as case reporter, service center and ambulance, all of which work with the emergency medical service system constructed on the cloud platform, as shown in Figure 1.

- **Case Reporter:** The case reporter carries an Android smart mobile device for accessing 3G networks and GPS. The application for fast case report installed in the mobile device of the case reporter proactively transmits information such as latitude/longitude coordinates detected by the GPS system to the service center.
- **Ambulance:** The ambulance is also equipped with an Android smart mobile device like that held by a case reporter for accessing 3G networks and GPS. The ambulance proactively informs the service center of service status as well as latitude/longitude coordinates and receives tasks assigned by the service center.
- **Service Center:** The service center receives and depends on information from a case reporter such as latitude/longitude coordinates and medical demands to dispatch a proper ambulance and determine a hospital to which a patient is transported. In addition, the service center governing the mechanisms for ambulance management and dispatching can control service status of an ambulance anytime.

The emergency medical service system running on the cloud platform consists of multiple subsystems, that is, ambulance management

Figure 1. The system running on the Hadoop cloud platform

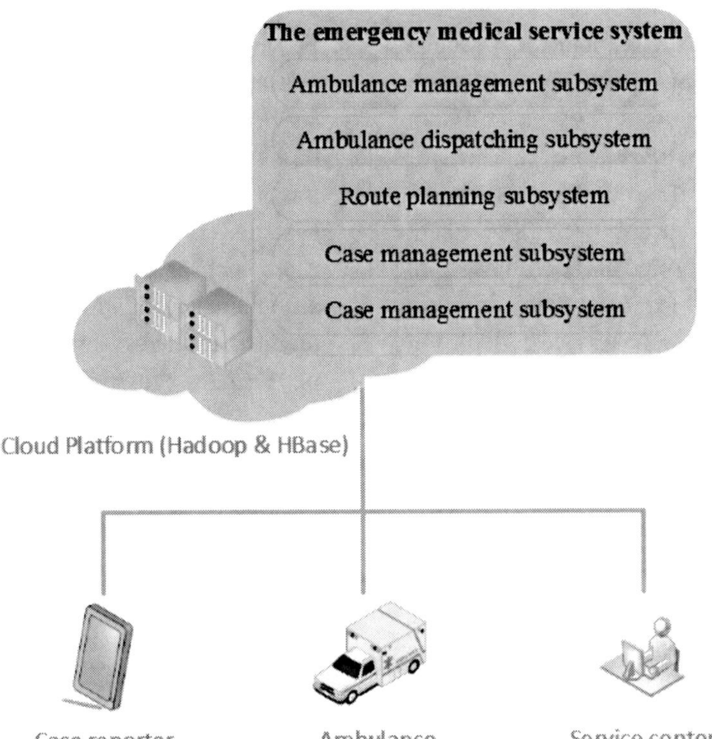

subsystem, case management subsystem, route planning subsystem, ambulance dispatching subsystem, and patient physiology monitoring subsystem, all of which coordinate with each other for completion of a task.

1. **Ambulance Management Subsystem:** The roles involved in the ambulance management subsystem are cloud platform, service center and ambulance ("in service" or "available"). With a task received and verified by an ambulance's vehicle-borne application, the status of the ambulance which is available is transformed to "in service" and updated in the cloud platform. On the other hand, the status of an ambulance that has transported a patient to a hospital is transformed to "available" and updated in the cloud platform. In addition, the service center steadily controls movement of an ambulance and makes a decision of vehicle dispatching by depending on the ambulance's latitude/longitude coordinates proactively uploaded to the cloud platform.

2. **Case Management Subsystem:** The roles involved in the case management subsystem are cloud platform, service center and case reporter. This subsystem demonstrates functions as follows:

a. **Case Acceptance:** The demand for emergency medical service and corresponding latitude/longitude coordinates are uploaded to the cloud platform and received by the service center when a case is reported with the application for case report. At the moment, the service center relies on the ambulance management subsystem and the route planning subsystem to quickly locate an ambulance closest to the scene of a case reported as well as any immediate and available hospital. Then, an ambulance can be dispatched by the service center.

b. **Case Tracking:** The function coordinates with the ambulance management subsystem. (a) an ambulance completing a task: the route of the ambulance is recorded for future references; (b) an ambulance in service: the status of the ambulance driving on roads is immediately tracked

3. **Route Planning Subsystem:** The route planning subsystem is developed with the Google map (Google map API). The roles involved in route planning subsystem are service center and ambulance.

a. When the service center accepts a case, The latitude/longitude coordinates corresponding to the scene of a case and ambulances are proactively acquired by the route planning subsystem for real-time computing and sorting as references of an ambulance to be dispatched by the service center: (1) time for available ambulances arriving at the scene and sorting of ambulances by time; (2) time for an ambulance driving from the scene to a hospital and sorting of hospitals by time.

b. When the dispatching task is determined, the dispatched ambulance acquires the route planning for this task. The route planning is divided into two stages with a task received by an ambulance: Stage 1, an ambulance arriving at the scene of a case reported; Stage 2, an ambulance moving from the scene to a hospital. The route planning for Stage 1 is activated with an ambulance verifying the task, and the route planning for Stage is activated with an ambulance arriving at the scene.

4. **Ambulance Dispatching Subsystem:** The roles involved in the ambulance dispatching subsystem are cloud platform, service center and ambulance. Referring to two types of sorting provided by the route planning subsystem, the service center makes decisions for an ambulance to be dispatched and a hospital available. The selected ambulance is dispatched immediately with the command made via the cloud system.

5. **Patient Physiology Monitoring Subsystem:** The physiological information of a patient who is being transported by an ambulance is transmitted to a hospital for remote group consultation of doctors and preparation of first aid by the patient physiology monitoring subsystem. The physiological information transmitted to a hospital via 3G mobile networks is fulfilled in the patient physiology monitoring subsystem consisting of gadgets like physiological signal sensor, IP Camera and ZigBee.

OPERATING PROCEDURES IN THE SYSTEM

With five subsystems cooperating with each other for one task, the two major operating procedures are shown as follows:

- Service center

As shown in Figure 2-(a), the service center receiving the messages for emergency medical services from a case reporter and the corresponding locations uploaded to the cloud platform will activate the route planning subsystem to proactively access latitude/longitude coordinates of the scene of a case reported from the case management subsystem for (1) computing of time for available ambulances arriving at the scene and sorting of ambulances by time and (2) computing of time for an ambulance driving from the scene to available hospitals and sorting of hospitals by time, both of which are the basis of dispatching an ambulance by the service center. After the ambulance to be dispatched is selected, the ambulance should receive and verify the command of dispatching from the service center via the cloud platform and further latitude/longitude coordinates of the scent of a case reported (the hospital) for pre-arrival routing planning at Stage 1 (post-arrival routing planning at Stage 2). The operating procedure will be completed with the ambulance arriving at the hospital and changed service status updated to and received by the cloud platform.

- Ambulance

As shown in Figure 2-(b), the location of a case reported and the corresponding route are shown on the ambulance which receives and verifies the command for one task issued by the service center. The ambulance arriving at the scene also receives the location of a hospital and the route from the scene to the hospital transmitted by the service center. The operating procedure will be completed with the ambulance arriving at the hospital and changed service status updated to and received by the cloud platform.

SYSTEM DEMONSTRATION AND ROAD TEST

The system test is based on a private car simulating an ambulance and provided with equipment such as Android smart phone built in 3G and GPS. The case reporter also carries an Android smart phone built in 3G and GPS. The service center is a laptop computer as the hardware equipment.

System Demonstration at a Case Reporter

The passive reporting mechanism and the automated reporting mechanism are available to a case reporter: the passive reporting is defined as a case reported by a witness who uses his/her mobile device; the automated case reporting is integrated with the fall detection system for automated reporting.

- Passive reporting

A witness finding an accident victim on the road or outdoors reports the case for an ambulance via the application for case report installed in his/her mobile phone. As shown in Figure 3, the location of a case reported should be positioned by GPS and transmitted to the cloud platform with "Send" on the mobile phone pressed.

- Automated case reporting with the fall detection system integrated

In order to achieve automated case reporting, this paper integrates the fall detection system (Hsien-Chou Liao et al., 2014). Depending on Radio-frequency identification (RFID) (GS1 General Specifications, 2015) and visual tracking technology for positioning and monitoring a patient, the system will upload the name and the location of a patient who stumbled or fell out of bed and was shot by a video camera to the service center via the automated case reporting system. The automated case reporting system also transmits photos of the patient stumbling based on determination of the fall detection system to the cloud platform from which the service center accesses the patient's information and injury conditions for assignment of any medical staff, as shown in Figure 4.

Figure 2. Flow chart for ambulance dispatching: (a) operating procedure at the service center and (b) operating procedure at an ambulance

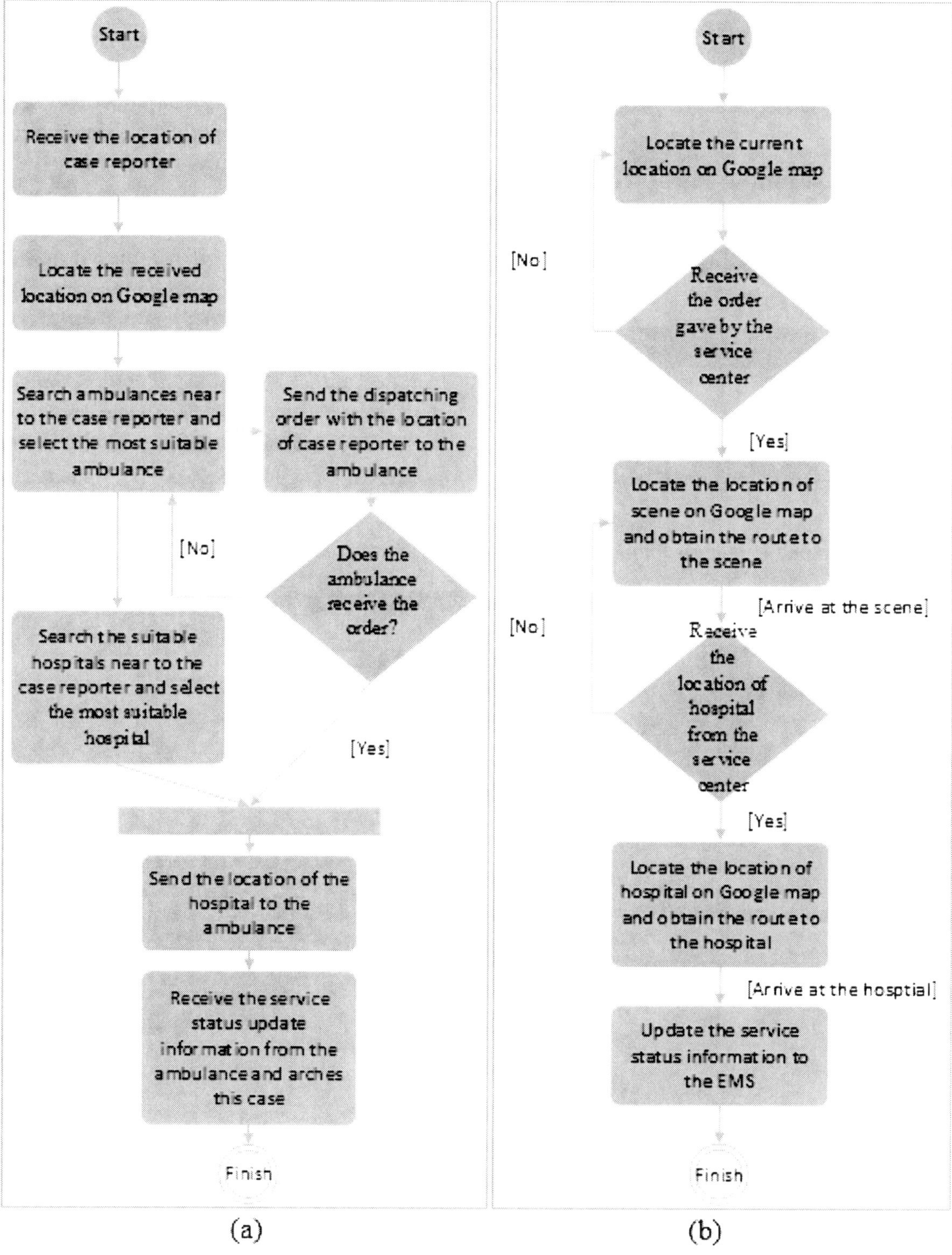

Figure 3. Case report and real-time positioning at a case reporter's mobile device

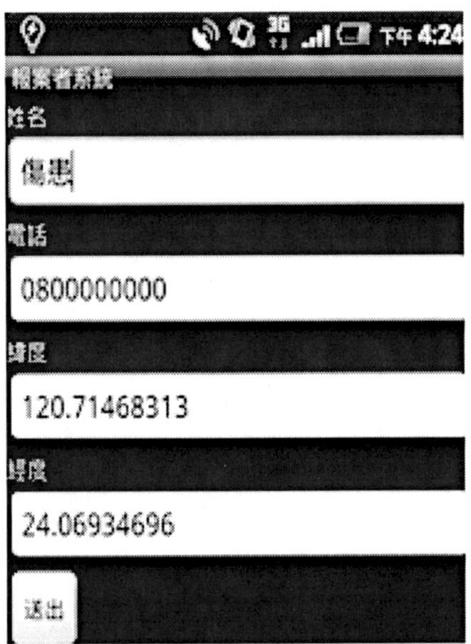

System Demonstration at the Service Center

The service center (system) constructed on the cloud system runs well with or without powerful hardware equipment, particularly with common hardware devices. Figure 5 is the landing page for accessing the service center that is activated with the "Enter System" button pressed by the staff member on duty. Moreover, the hardware devices can be added into or removed from the service center for supporting deployment of the staff member on duty. The functions such as case acceptance, ambulance dispatching, two-stage routing planning, and job logging for completion of a task are designed in the service center.

The case management page monitoring any new case is first displayed to the staff member on

Figure 4. Automated case reporting with the fall detection system integrated

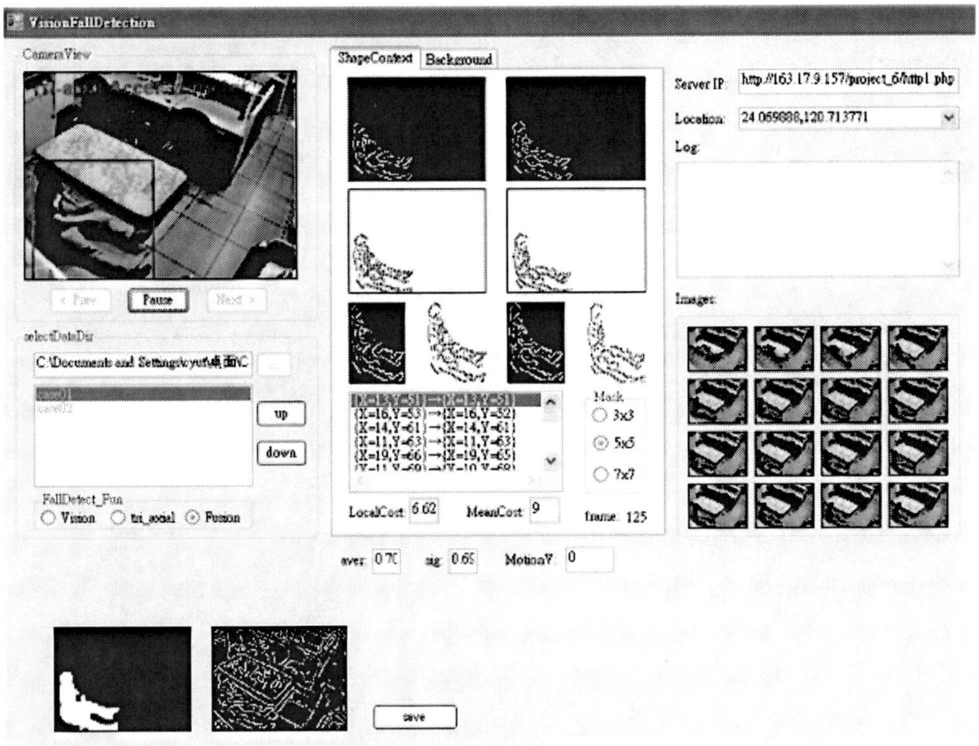

Figure 5. Landing page for the service center

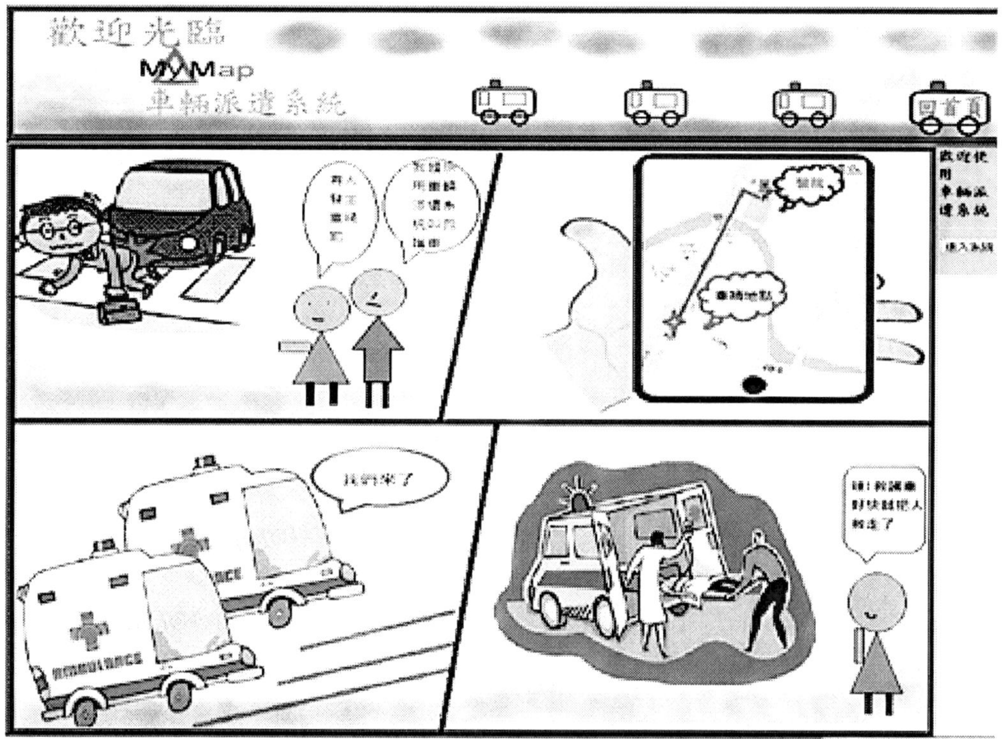

duty who logins the system and possibly observes "no case reported" as shown in Figure 6. Otherwise, the case management page may display a new case along with a voice alarm automatically as shown in Figure 7, which is a passive reporting case. Detailed injury conditions of a patient as well as photos shot by a video camera are indicated on the case management interface of the service center which is integrated with the fall detection

Figure 6. "No case reported" displayed on the case management page

system by turns as shown in Figure 8, which is an automated case reporting case.

For ambulance dispatching, the information of making a decision for dispatching should be obtained first. With the "route planning" button pressed, the information such as estimated time of available ambulances arriving at the scene of a case reported, sorting of ambulances, and locations of ambulances can be immediately displayed on the screen as shown in Figure 9. Moreover, the location of a case reported and the corresponding street views are also displayed on the screen. The service center will dispatch an ambulance to arrive at the scene in the shortest time, displaying the route on the screen as shown in Figure 10, and completing dispatching with the route affirmed and the location of the case reported transmitted to the ambulance. Then, the user will enter the page for selection of a hospital in which the time of an ambulance arriving at an available hospital from the scene and sorting of hospitals by time are displayed. As shown in

Figure 7. Page for a passive reporting case affirmed by the service center

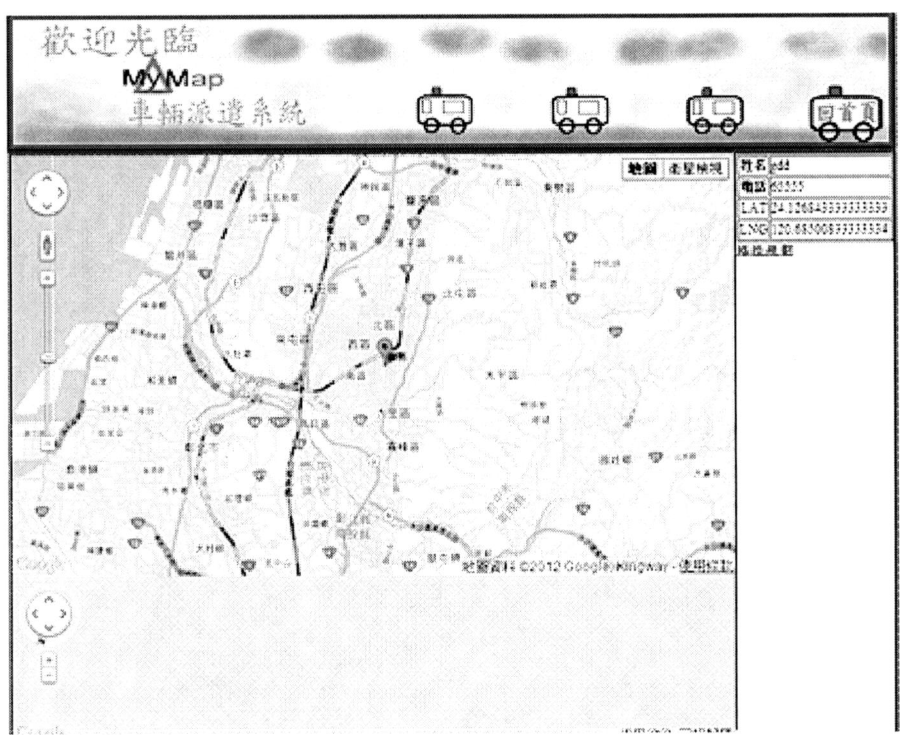

Figure 8. Page for a automated case reported by the fall detection system and displayed on the service center

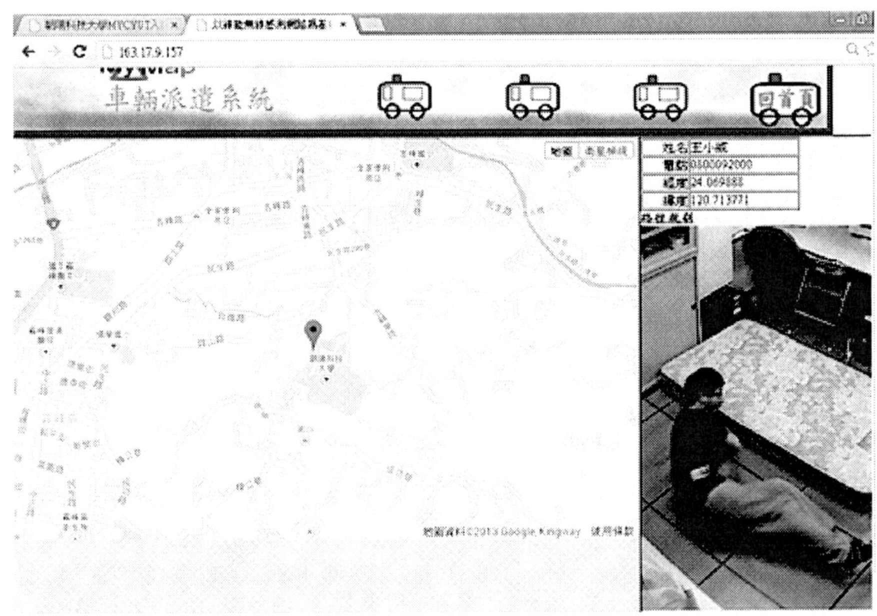

Figure 9. Page for locations of available ambulances, time of ambulances arriving at the scene of a case reported, and sorting of ambulances displayed on the service center

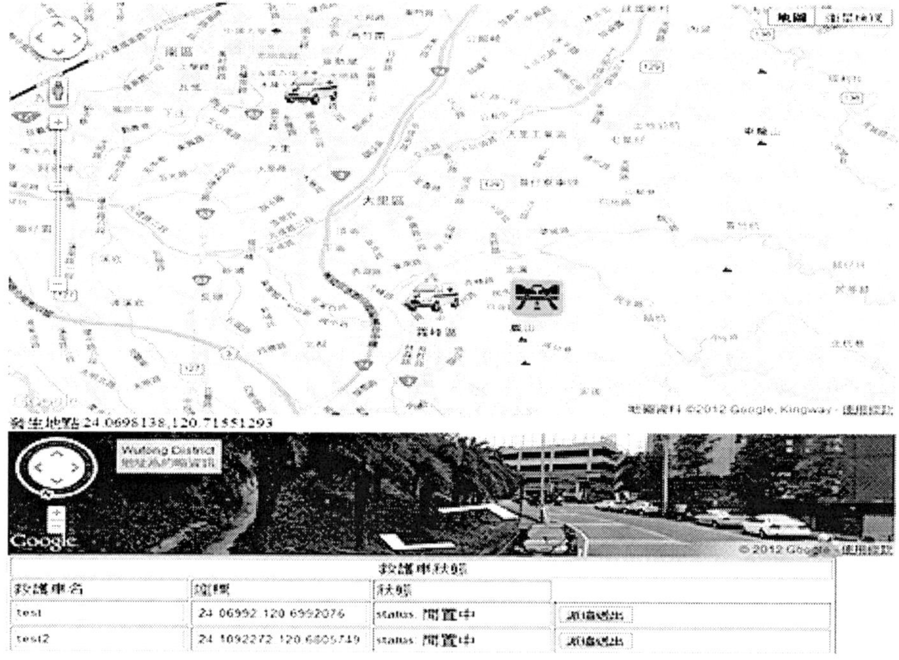

Figure 10. Page for routing planning at Stage 1 and transmission of the command to dispatch an ambulance displayed on the service center

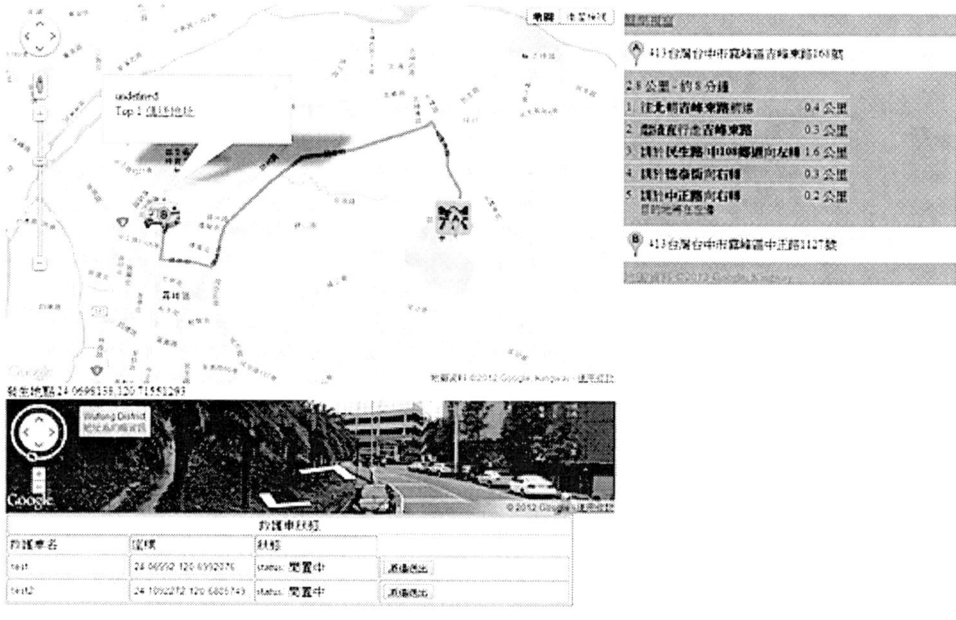

Figure 11. Page for available hospitals and routing planning at Stage 2 displayed on the service center

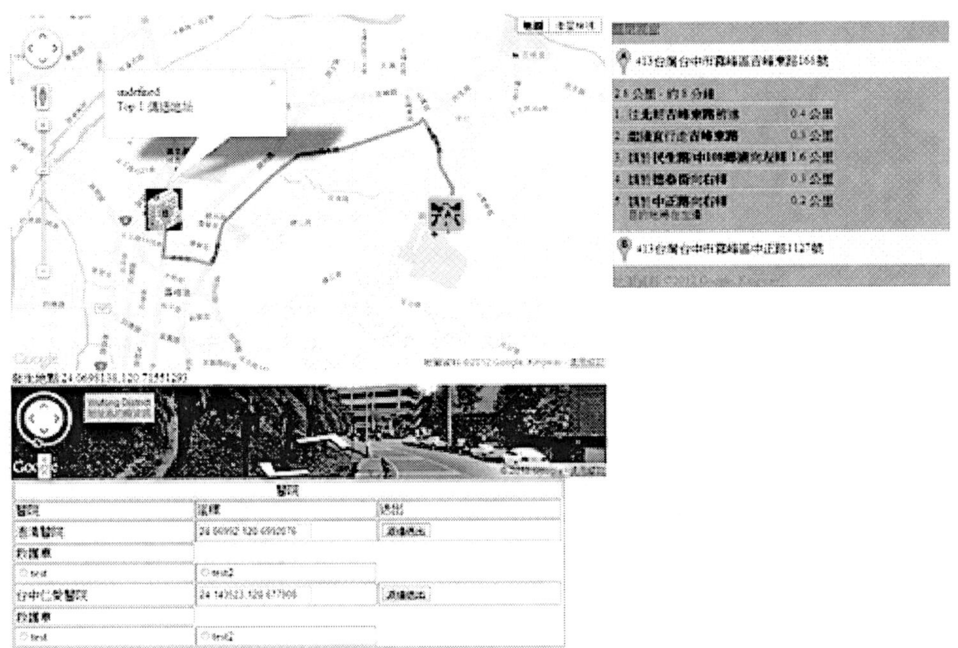

Figure 12. Page for the recorded route of an ambulance dispatched

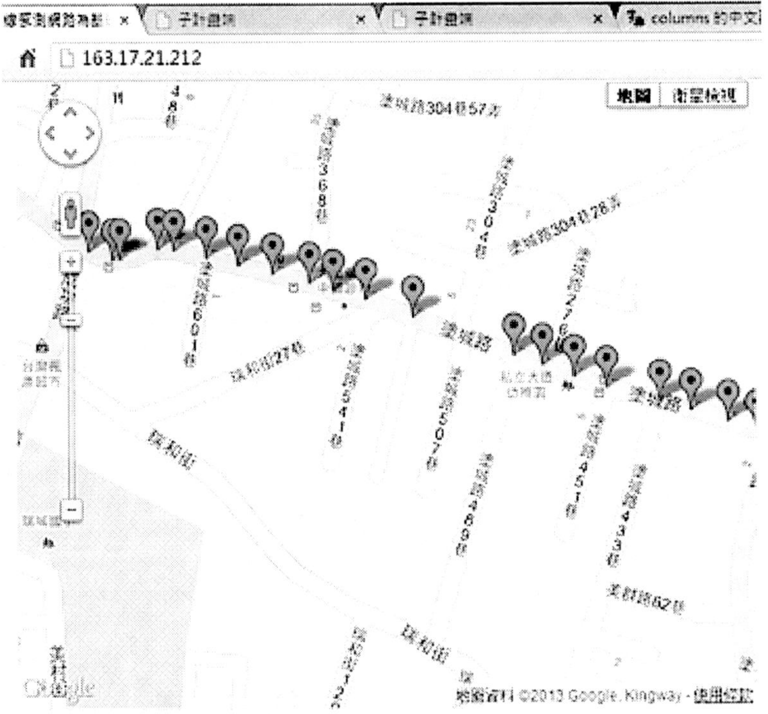

Figure 11, the above information and the locations of hospitals are displayed on the screen and transmitted to the ambulance. With the task completed, the route followed by the ambulance will be stored for future references as shown in Figure 12.

System Demonstration of the Ambulance

As shown in Figure 13, the location of an ambulance positioned by GPS is transmitted to the ambulance's Android smart mobile device and further the ambulance management subsystem in the cloud platform. Moreover, the service status of an ambulance is immediately updated to the ambulance management subsystem such as an "available" ambulance ready to be dispatched and an ambulance "in service" with no task assigned from the service center. The popup message for taking on a task, if any, will be indicated as shown in Figure 14. With "Confirm" pressed, the shortest route in route planning at Stage 1 for an ambulance arriving at the scene of a case reported will be drawn by Google map as shown in Figure 15-(a).

The navigation function of Web View in the Android smart phone automatically plans the shortest route by which an ambulance arrives at the scene of a case reported quickly. With the "Stage 2" button pressed, the ambulance having arrived at the scene informs the cloud platform of a successful rescue and is ready to receive the location of a hospital issued by the service center. At the moment, a dialog box to ask for "task acceptance" is displayed as shown in Figure 15-(a). Then, the ambulance will follow the shortest route drawn by Google map in route planning from the scene to a hospital as shown in Figure 15-(b). Finally, the service status of the ambulance which arrives at the hospital and completes a task is updated to the cloud platform.

Figure 13. Real-time location of an ambulance

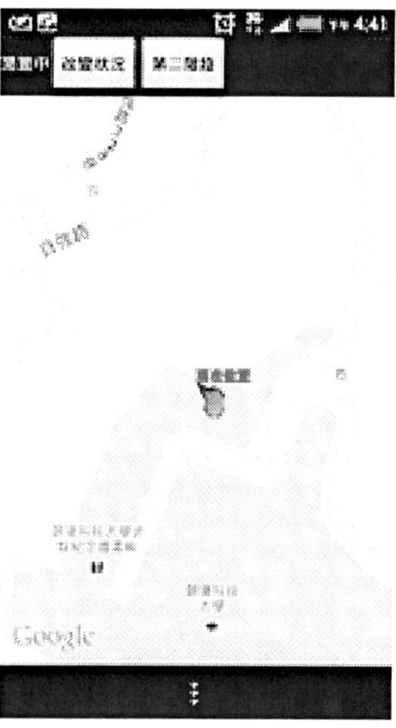

Figure 14. Dialog box for a task issued by the service center and received by an ambulance

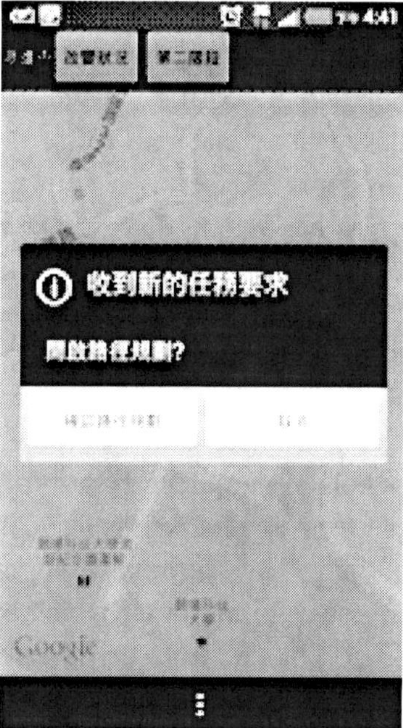

Figure 15. Routing planning for an ambulance: (a) Stage 1; (b) Stage 2

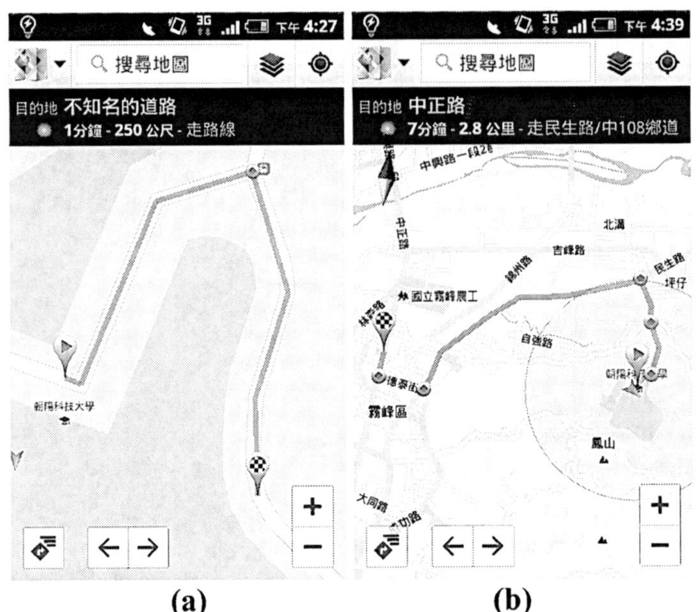

(a)   **(b)**

CONCLUSION

In this research, we create an ambulance dispatching system for emergency medical services with various integrated ICT, which works on a Hadoop-based cloud platform with a distributed database system, HBase, as a storage system. There are five subsystems designed on the cloud platform: (1) case management subsystem, (2) ambulance management system, (3) route planning subsystem, (4) ambulance dispatching subsystem and (5) patient physiology monitoring subsystem, all of which coordinate with each other for running the whole system. The system running on a cloud platform is characteristic of integrated medical resources and terminal equipment with or without powerful hardware which is flexibly added into or removed from the system for supporting dispatch. Meanwhile, the movements of ambulances are readily controlled by the system with GIS and cloud computing which supports a service center to determine any dispatching task and saves more time spent in transporting an accident victim to a hospital.

ACKNOWLEDGMENT

The research is supported by the Ministry of Science and Technology of the Republic of China under the grant number MOST 103-2221-E-324 -012 and MOST 103-2221-E-241 -008.

REFERENCES

Amazon Web Services (AWS) - Cloud Computing Services. from http://aws.amazon.com

Apache Hadoop project, from http://hadoop.apache.org

Apache HBase, from http://hbase.apache.org

Chuang-Ming Huang and Yuh-Shyan Chen. (2010). *Telematics Communication Technologies and Vehicular Networks: Wireless Architectures and Applications, Information Science Reference.* IGI Global.

Cummins, R. O., Eisenberg, M. S., Hallstrom, A. P., & Litwin, P. E. (1985). Survival of out-of-hospital cardiac arrest with early initiation of cardiopulmonary resuscitation. *The American Journal of Emergency Medicine, 3*(2), 114–119. doi:10.1016/0735-6757(85)90032-4 PMID:3970766

European Commission (2009). ICT for better Healthcare in Europe. E-health - Better Healthcare for Europe, European Commission, Information Society and Media Directorate.

GS1 General Specifications, version 15. (2015). GS1, The Global Language of Business.

Google App Engine. Platform as a Service, from https://cloud.google.com/appengine

Google map API, Retrieved July 1, 2013, from https://developers.google.com/maps/

Gupta, M. (2006). ICT and Healthcare – Challenges and Opportunities. *Eurescom*, Helsinki. Barmentlo, M. (2007). The shifting patient paradigm: embedding healthcare in everyday lives. *Personal Health Systems Conference*, Brussels.

History of the Emergency Medical Services. Retrieved May 31, 2014, from http://www.fdmadison.org/public-education/history-of-ems

Hsien-Chou Liao., Yu-Ming CHEN, Wen-Chang CHENG, Jia-Yu JHANG & Jungpil SHIN. (2014) Fall Detection Based on the Fusion of Vision and Tri-axial Accelerometer. International Conference on Advanced Computer Science and Engineering (ACSE2014), Guangzhou, China

Kenneth, E. Foote and Margaret Lynch. Geographic Information Systems as an Integrating Technology: Context, Concepts, and Definitions. Retrieved Feb 1, 2015, from http://www.colorado.edu/geography/gcraft/notes/intro/intro.html

Kiefer, S. (2007). Personal Health Systems (PHS) Overview and Research Trends. Personal Health Systems Conference, Brussels.

Habetha, J. (2007). Wearable and ambient systems for personal healthcare applications - The MyHeart project. Personal Health Systems Conference, Brussels.

Halford, S., & Lotherington, A. T. (2015). Technical change and the untroubling of gendered ageing in healthcare work. Gender, Work and Organization, 1-17.

Hilty, L. M., & Aebischer, B. (2015). ICT Innovations for Sustainability. Springer International.

Lars George. (2011). *HBase: The Definitive Guide.* O'Reilly Media.

Masson, Y. (2007). Health and technology. *Personal Health Systems Conference*, Brussels.

Medic One began with a basic need and focused vision. Medic One Foundation. Retrieved May 31, 2014, from http://www.mediconefoundation.org/who-we-are/history/

Microsoft Azure, from http://azure.microsoft.com/

NoSQL, from http://nosql-database.org

Sun Microsystem. (2009). Introduction to Cloud Computing architecture. White Paper, 1st Edition.

Tom Whit. (2012). *Hadoop: The Definitive Guide* (3rd ed.). O'Reilly Media / Yahoo Press.

This work was previously published in the International Journal of Grid and High Performance Computing (IJGHPC), 6(4); edited by Emmanuel Udoh, Ching-Hsien Hsu, and Mohammad Khan, pages 72-87 copyright year 2014 by IGI Publishing (an imprint of IGI Global).

Chapter 40
Mobile Healthcare Computing in the Cloud

Tae-Gyu Lee
Korea Institute of Industrial Technology, Korea

ABSTRACT

Previous medical services for humans provided healthcare information using the static-based computing of space-constrained hospitals or healthcare centers. In contrast, current mobile health information management computing and services are being provided so that they utilize both the mobility of mobile computing and the scalability of cloud computing to monitor in real-time the health status of patients who are moving. In addition, data capacity has sharply increased with the expansion of the principal data generation cycle from the traditional static computing environment to the dynamic computing environment. This chapter presents mobile cloud healthcare computing systems that simultaneously leverage the portability and scalability of healthcare services. This chapter also presents the wearable computing system as an application of mobile healthcare.

INTRODUCTION

This chapter describes system structure, information flow and application or service scenario in order to build a cloud computing based on mobile healthcare system. In order to implement this system, one must satisfactorily accommodate the characteristics of mobile healthcare device, client, or the special advantages of information system on the mobile computing, ubiquitous computing, wearable computing and cloud computing, etc (Barry, 2006; Gunther, 2006; Monique, 2010).

First, mobile healthcare is rising as an important concept to implement real-time remote medical treatment service. The mobile healthcare

is increasing usage of portable devices such as PDA or Smartphones/Smartpads while guaranteeing mobility of patients, for their free activity. It also identifies the condition of patients on a real-time basis, in other words in order to provide healthcare information service immediately without delay of time. HL7 establishes a standard of supporting messaging interwork and compatibility between existing information system and health & medical treatment information service based on the standard layer of OSI. This can support the scalability of mobile health care (Jim, 2007; Daniel, 1999; Vietanh, 2000; Deborah, 2001; Ian, 2002; Malik, 2003).

DOI: 10.4018/978-1-4666-8756-1.ch040

Second, mobile computing implements multilateral healthcare services through gathering and analyzing various types of healthcare information without setting limitations on the specific medical treatment of mobile users. And it extends the static computing based on wire as a dynamic and flexible computing environment.

Third, ubiquitous computing supports a sensing network, which recognizes user status (place, time, weather and temperature, etc) without limitation of place and time. It also supports freedom of user connection and seamless connectivity.

Fourth, wearable computing is an item which is steadily being studied in various business fields because of its advantages such as clothing-based wearability, portability, and lightness. This is attracting people's interest as a next generation computing item with a composition that has combined the advantages of mobile computing and ubiquitous computing (Rehman, 2012; Polly, 2000; Sungmee, 2003; Peter, 2007; Franz, 2004; Shirley, 2009). Especially, it shows strength as a form of important critical mission applications from the emergence of the cases of applying wearable computing to the field of healthcare (Peter, 2007; Franz, 2004; Shirley, 2009).

Fifth, cloud computing has been proposed based on the distribution of the system in order to consolidate the economic efficiency of existing computing or system flexibility and scalability aspects (Bhaskar, 2009; Hoang, 2011; Sanjit, 2010). The implementation of healthcare-cloud information system based on such cloud system can effectively support large-scale healthcare client as a background computing system located in the back of mobile healthcare user.

Healthcare clients would want to identify their own health condition on a real-time basis at a free daily living environment and receive medical services instantly in case abnormal symptoms are discovered. In order to implement such real-time mobile client healthcare, the following requirements must be supported. First, the body information of mobile user must be gathered on a real-time basis. Second, a seamless wireless mobile network infrastructure must be supported for the satisfactory transmission of health information continuously.

In order to satisfy these requirements, wearable computing and clouding computing must be combined based on the mobile healthcare client, mobile computing and ubiquitous computing as it is described above. Through such various integrated configuration of computing, the mobile healthcare service for mobile client shown as Figure 1 should be implemented.

Mobile healthcare can provide a mobile healthcare solution that makes information available to users (Wikipedia, 2012). Recently, mobile healthcare has been an increasingly important topic because it employs bio-sensing and mobile user information to provide real-time monitoring of a customer's body. The flow of information in embedded bio-sensing systems from the standpoint of the user of mobile healthcare is a series of forwarding processes, which collect sensing data from bio-sensing nodes. First, the sensing node senses the state of the user's body, and collects analogue or digital bio-signal data. Next, it delivers the collected data over wired or wireless communication links. Finally, a backbone-computing node in the Internet receives the filtered data as a relay or a final node. When executed in reverse, a healthcare process may be executed that will control or monitor the bio-sensing nodes on the user's body.

Figure 1 depicts services that monitor the momentum, the electrocardiogram, and the respiration, which are mobile healthcare services. These services check the user's health as the user changes location. Furthermore, the remote healthcare service makes doctor-patient consultation possible, and the emergency healthcare service supports emergency calls and emergency medical services. In addition, the body posture service monitors the body shape in order to observe the acute syncope patients such as the elderly. The body temperature service checks the mobile user's body temperature and provides notification when it is abnormal.

Figure 1. Healthcare services in mobile computing

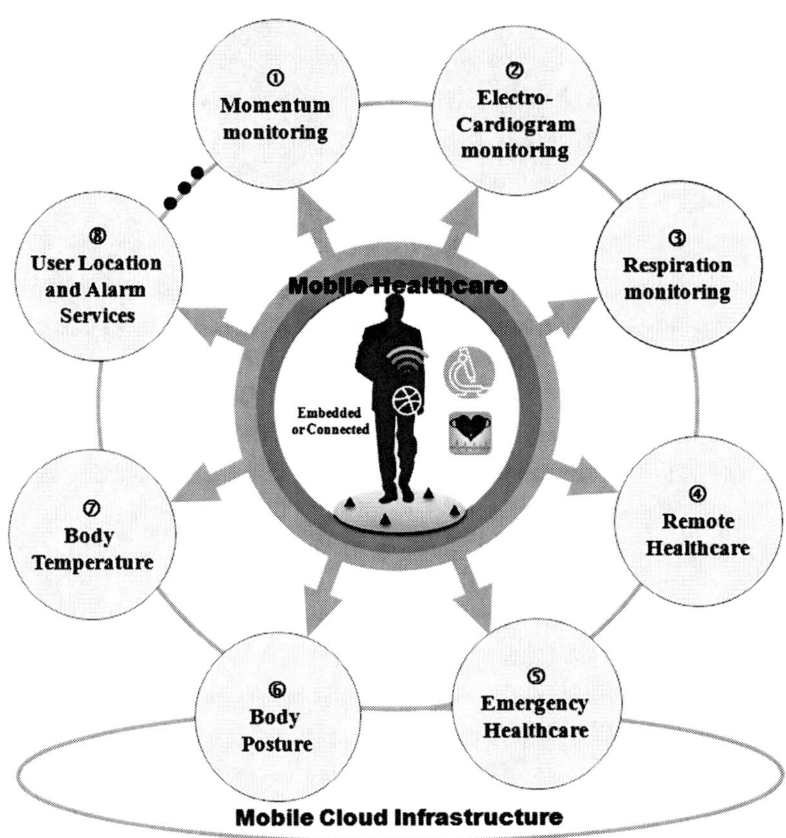

Finally, the user location and alarm services provide the appropriate medical information and notification via alarm about a hazardous area as required depending on the location of the user.

In order to build a mobile healthcare service, the mobile cloud infrastructure is provided various computing to mobile users at the rear including bio-information sensing, transfer, storage, analysis, evaluation, and feedback. The mobile cloud enhances the features of mobile computing such as scalability, portability, compatibility, etc of system resources including the user.

Mobile healthcare is recognized as the best alternative to monitor and to guide the health status of the mobile user. Mobile cloud is recognized as the best alternative to support mobile computing services of mobile or wireless devices, and is recognized as a means to differentiate economy, flexibility and lightweight in the mobile healthcare system (Pat, 2013; Zachary, 2013).

For providing the fast and accurate healthcare of mobile user, the mobile healthcare devices located on the front need lightweight and real-time characteristics. At the same time, the mobile cloud system located on the rear strengthens the system characteristics such as scalability, portability, safety, security, mobility, etc (Logicworks, 2013).

This chapter proposes the following computing service objectives to readers. First, it provides a mobile computing design architecture and organization for healthcare services. Second, it shows the processing and flow of healthcare data in a mobile computing environment. Finally, it provides versatile healthcare applications and healthcare-information services that use real-time cloud computing.

In this chapter, the following details will be described as an alternative plan for reflecting such requirements. First, the mobile healthcare system architecture and components are presented. Next, the mobile healthcare networks and information flows are described. Then the application and service sectors of mobile healthcare including wearable healthcare system are presented. Finally, the conclusion will be presented.

BACKGROUND

Mobile healthcare stands for all healthcare services provided to the user moving freely based on the mobile healthcare information system including mobile devices and remote medical devices. The definition of such mobile healthcare has been defined in the following various fields.

The definition of mHealth of the Global Observatory for eHealth (GOe) of the WHO (World Health Organization) is as follows:

mHealth is a component of eHealth. mHealth or mobile health is the realization of medical and public health supported by mobile devices, such as mobile phones, patient monitoring devices, personal digital assistants (PDAs), and other wireless devices (Misha, 2011, p.6; Guido, 2007).

mHealth involves the utilization of and capitalization on a mobile phone's core utility of voice and short or multimedia messaging service (SMS/MMS) as well as more complex functionalities and applications including mobile web, third and fourth generation mobile telecommunications (3G and 4G systems), global positioning system (GPS), wireless local area network (WLAN), and Bluetooth technology.

According to Wikipedia, the term mHealth was coined by Professor Robert Istepanian and denoted the use of "emerging mobile communications and network technologies for healthcare." The definition used at the 2010 mHealth Summit of the Foundation for the National Institutes of Health (FNIH) was "the delivery of healthcare services via mobile communication devices" (Wikipedia, 2012).

The HL7 Mobile Health Workgroup declared that they want to support the mission of developing standards for mobile health services, data and information interoperability, security and integration in mobile and wireless healthcare and public health systems to reduce costs, improve quality and delivery, guide informed-decisions and promote individual and population health (HL7, 2012).

The existing definition on mobile healthcare or special features, advantages and disadvantages on access are in the following (Misha, 2011; Panagiotis, 2005; Khamish, 2005; Daniela, 2007; Guido, 2007).

As the initial information service of mobile healthcare, simple text, emergency call and voice information are exchanged while providing healthcare services such as medical examination reservation, specialized counseling and treatment management, etc. But it has many shortcomings in disease prevention, real-time health monitoring and implementing diagnostic services. Also, the situation is that latest smart devices and wearable medical services are almost nonexistent.

IT medical information technology supports remote counseling between doctor and patients through remote information exchange. However, this has limitations on new healthcare market of health monitoring, sports guide and healthy life guide, etc. This does not have latest smart device and wearable computing components. Especially, since the healthcare sensing is single module or functional approach products and services, a balanced aspect based on overall healthcare information system is absent.

HL7 supports messaging interwork and compatibility between existing information system and healthcare system based on the standard layer of OSI. But it has structural limitations in real-time, mobility and scalability aspects. This also gets limitations in the interwork of recent smart technology and cloud system technology (Bhaskar, 2009; Hoang, 2011; Sanjit, 2010). This gets restricted as a medical information system limited to application layer such as SaaS in order to building up a cloud medical information system. This becomes difficult to build up platform and infrastructure of medical information system with lower cloud systems such as PaaS or IaaS.

Previous mobile health service remains at a simple medical supplemented information services such as message, emergency call and voice counseling, etc. In order to expand as healthcare real-time monitoring and healthcare diagnosis service, the installation of wireless transmission system for sending medical information such as photo image or video, etc and the installation of cloud information transmission environment for implementing economical large scale real-time information transmission service are required as well as the client device technology.

In order to build up a cloud based mobile healthcare service, the following issues must be solved. First, the mobile client must support lightweight and mobility support for mobile healthcare. Also, it must support seamless healthcare information flows and heterogeneous network integration for mobile healthcare. The components and applications of mobile healthcare (variety/diversification) must support modules and apply products that interwork with existing e-health/health center while providing an exclusive handheld mobile device, supporting interwork module with commercial smart phones and must support new personal healthcare devices such as wearable products.

The features of mobile cloud such as scalability, portability, safety, security, mobility, etc enhances the mobile healthcare service of mobile users. Scalability should ensure the continued scalability of the system resources, due to the increase in the number of users of mobile healthcare. Portability is to support the user's devices replacement, the program transplant, etc using the mobile agent technique. For safe information transmission, the safety enforces the safe network and information

system by the fault-tolerant network configuration. Mobile cloud security supports the security cloud configuration, which is required for supporting dynamic security based on context-awareness. Mobility cloud supports to ensure a seamless user-mobility. Mobile cloud computing can improve the performance of healthcare organization, but mobile cloud infrastructures require a highly secure and auditable computing platform to meet statutory and regulatory requirements governing the handling of protected health information (Chris, 2013; Shams, 2013).

HEALTHCARE APPLICATION SCENARIOS AND SERVICES

In this section, we present mobile healthcare scenarios and describe the issues related to mobile computing components working in real-time.

Mobile healthcare applications include applications related to health/medicine, social network/life, and human-to-human services. These mobile healthcare applications may be applied to all aspects of our lives.

In mobile healthcare services, information scenarios are provided to optimize computing performance and resource efficiency. Especially event scenarios that occur in mobile healthcare can be divided according to the logic of the components that make up the network topology of mobile computing. This study generally assumes that the following stepped (or partial) processes are present, across the entire process from the bio-sensing node to the application servers as shown in Figure 2. Moreover, these scenarios can be used to evaluate the optimal methods for processing real-time event-scenarios for the entire process.

It first monitors the patent's status and detects the abnormal states of the patient. It captures the developing state of a patient's body. Finally, it informs a patient about dangerous environmental information.

Figure 2. Mobile healthcare application scenarios

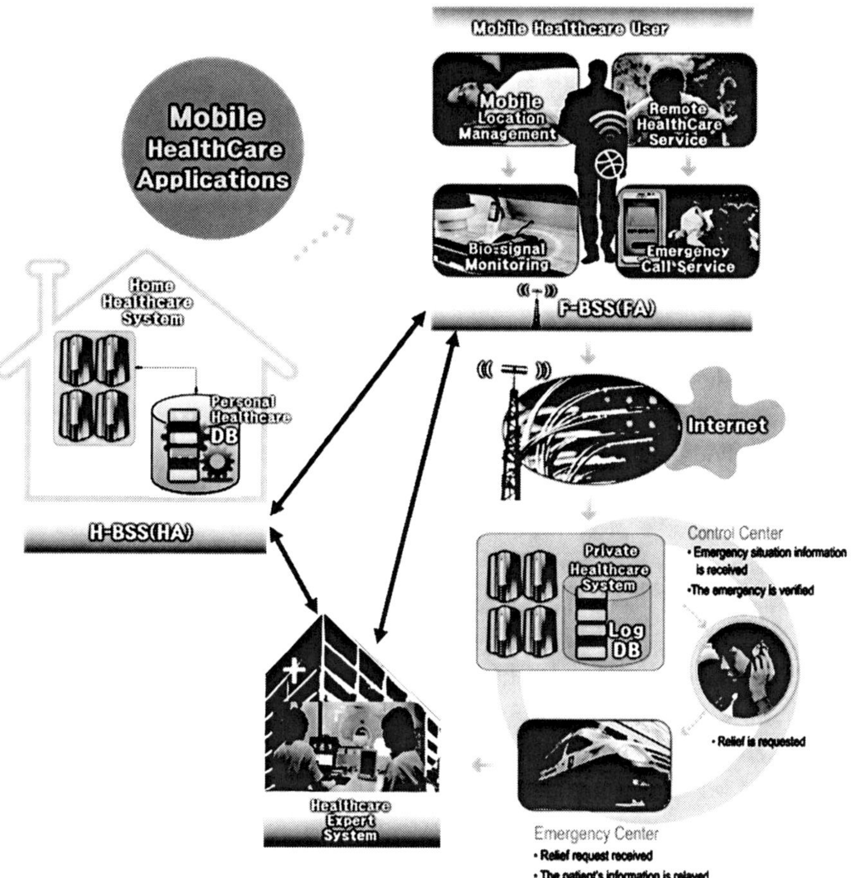

It provides the sensed information to a home medical station or doctor. It analyzes the details of the patient's healthcare information and it also delivers the doctor's instructions. It can provide selective medical knowledge using the healthcare expert system, which accumulates the know-how of physicians and healthcare professionals. It can deliver the healthcare information and treatment methods such as the type of workout for a patient.

The applications that take advantage of mobile healthcare services are as follows.

A *health-related sport information system* can provide the knowledge services using an intelligent database. Such a system can be applied to monitoring the health and conducting sports training. The health management system including diet is implemented. A health management cycle including amount of food, amount of exercise and resting time, etc is established in order to improve stamina and physical strength, etc. This system can be applied to health management of an ordinary person and record management of sports players.

The *cloud expert system* can provide medical knowledge services using an intelligent database. Such a system continuously constructs medical knowledge using intelligent logic and verified knowledge patterns. The cloud system expands the coverage of the medical knowledge system to a virtual and large database present in the space of the Internet. This space created for the virtual knowledge can integrate or interconnect with the distributed knowledge resources of medical experts via the Internet.

A *mobile healthcare information* system can be used in the field of health and medical forensics applications. Forensics applications require a forensics information guide and healthcare data logging as countermeasures against medical accidents. For example, forensics logging collects the data about the user context and constructs an indexing structure that can be used to search for specific data. The forensics data structure consists of a user id, a user location, a user health state (ECG, respiration, body-temperature, etc.), a dosage, etc. on the path of a mobile user. The forensics logic involves the use of event-based logging and the processing of checkpoints using registered events. The system operators can register the specific events into a dataset that can be stored in a health/medical forensics database.

Emergency relief services support applications that process events of interest to a user. It provides a health medical service whereby a user monitors and detects the status of one's own body. The service then informs by means of an emergency alarm, which alerts to an abnormal health state or other dangerous environmental information. An emergency call is placed to the doctor on call and to a home station. In response, critical analysis and the instructions of the doctor are passed onto the user. Normally, a user's health status and the response thereto are provided to the user in the form of the amount of exercise, an exercise class, etc.

As *military, police, and firefighting services, the biorhythm and survival status information, etc* of mobile user are identified in order to support the performance of public mission-critical applications of military, policy and fire fighting, etc. Therefore, the optimum mission performance information environment will be established. This guides various strategic activities including placement, role and method of mission performer.

THE ARCHITECTURE AND COMPONENTS OF MOBILE HEALTHCARE

The architecture and components of mobile healthcare are shown in Figure 3. It is based on three cloud systems, each of which interacts with the mobile healthcare client, the closed intranet background computing, and Internet open services, respectively.

The first mobile healthcare client layer in the top level imports the sensing event-data from a mobile user or an environmental sensor and exports the data for reporting using the mobile cloud with mobile healthcare agents. The human health-related data and the data about device internals are collected by the mobile embedded station (MES or attached mobile terminal) of each mobile user. The collected data is transferred into the next layer, which is a closed layer taking place in the background, by a base support station (BSS or namely Sync center), which is interconnected with the Intranet infrastructure (namely, an Infra-Network). The mobile networks support external wireless networking (namely Ex-Network) based on an infrastructure network (namely, Internet-working) which is ad-hoc networks that provide direct communication among mobile users. The Ex-Network can include such wireless local networks as BAN/PAN. It dynamically supports user's status sensing network environments based on the location, dangerous event, contact user, etc. of mobile users. The mobile healthcare users can dynamically form a mobile healthcare group over such wireless networks. Such a mobile healthcare client layer should take into account user mobility and sensing data; hence, the *mobility issue* applies to this phase.

Mobile cloud operates the mobile agents on MES terminal for information transfer of an individual mobile healthcare use. It can support user mobility, wireless transmission of bio-information sensing data, and seamless transmission.

Figure 3. Mobile cloud healthcare architecture

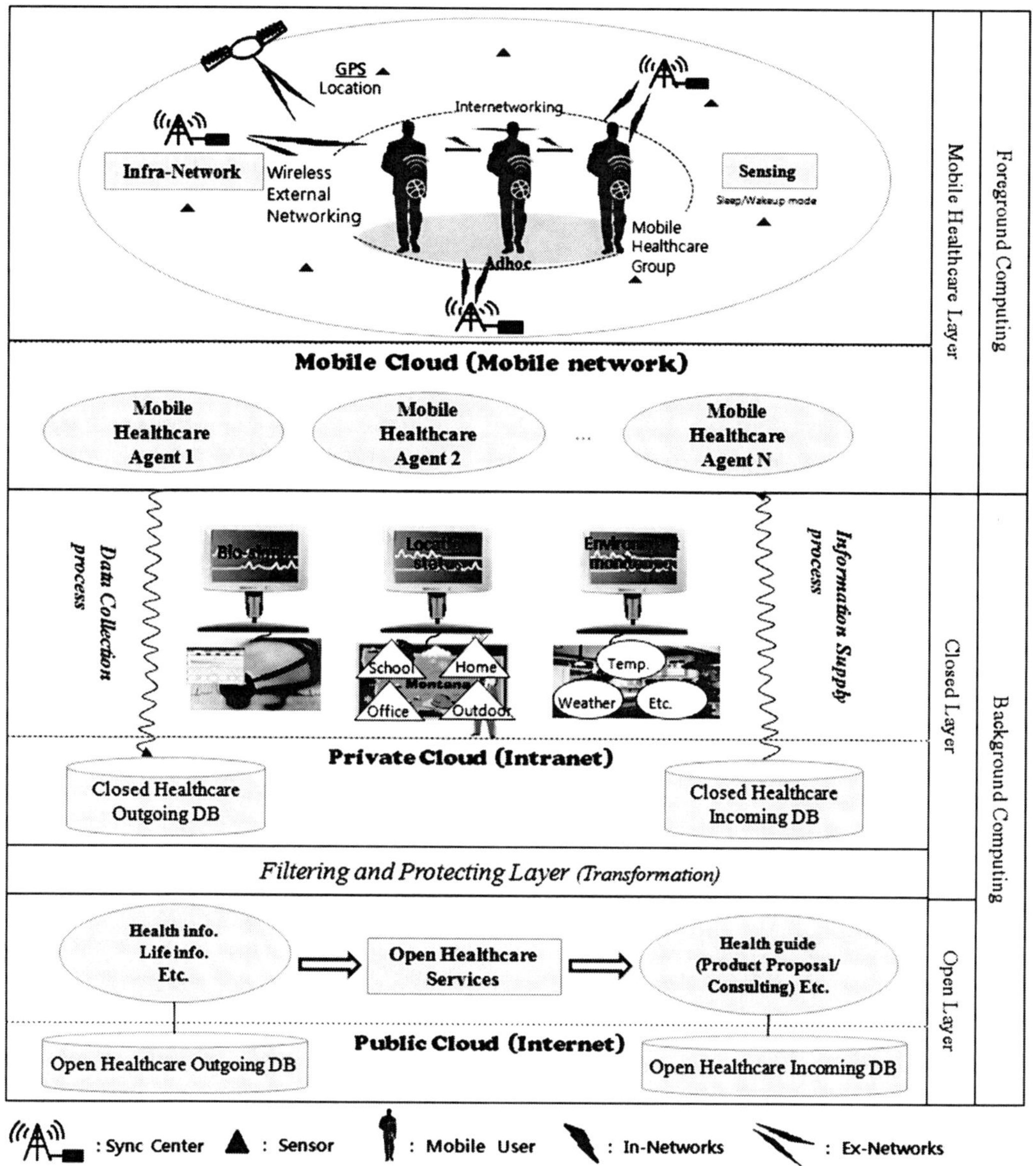

Secondly, a closed layer manages the closed healthcare database and the log data of mobile-healthcare-users by providing background-support infrastructure, which is provided by an operating company or hospital. This closed layer receives the healthcare data collected by mobile users from the upper mobile-healthcare-client layer, analyzes real-time event data or non-real-time planning data, and reports information to the mobile user.

Also, it provides filtering and transformation services between the mobile healthcare client layer and the Internet open service layer. This closed layer should offer support for personal information protection and security services in order to provide safe mobile healthcare client computing; this is the *security issue*. A private cloud running on the intranet executes user's device backup, data analysis, control and feedback, location management, etc as the server and center in the rear of the mobile healthcare users.

Finally, an Internet-open-service layer provides, based on the Internet, the available non-security data about human-life related healthcare information service. Also, this layer provides each mobile user's interesting healthcare information as feedback to a mobile healthcare client layer at the top level. This open layer should have high transfer speed and provide convenient user access so that information can be provided rapidly, so that the issue present in this layer is *performance*. Private cloud support a variety of valuable health information services such as health guide, health information sharing, health life-cycle management for supporting mobile healthcare on the Internet.

Overall, the raw data that originated with a mobile user in the first mobile healthcare client layer is collected after passing through the second closed layer into a third open layer in a downward data collection process which is shown in Figure 3. Figure 3 also shows how the collected data is analyzed, filtered, and stored in both the second and the third layers. The service information produced by the third service layer is delivered to the mobile user in the top layer, which is the mobile healthcare client layer, by an upward-oriented healthcare information support process. The download data collection process collects information about healthcare and living from a mobile user. The upload information support process provides a health guide and other guidance for a mobile user.

In order to maximize the portability and mobility of mobile healthcare user, implementing embedded client of healthcare device depends on the implementation of lightweight, thin, small, and flexible devices. Such mobile healthcare client devices are classified into input devices, output devices, computing devices, and network device. The individual devices develop implementation characteristics independently while two or more device modules can be integrated as single device module. An integrated single module configuration lowers the probability of being exposed to defects because of its concise structure and economical because the production cost is lowered. Also, the dual configuration of client device consolidates system stability as it consolidates the restoration ability followed by defect and failure.

User mobility supports user location recognition and location tracing. Such attribute supports various healthcare services based on user location. For example, it supports emergency call and rescue service of acute patients.

Data mobility supports connectivity and synchronization between healthcare client and data backup center. Data connectivity means supporting the path where the data gathered at the client gets sent to the server and the data at the backup server gets sent to the client. Data synchronization means the data store at the client and the same data stored at the server must be identical.

Service mobility supports disconnected operations and service migration using checkpoint and log in order to guarantee performance and stability of the healthcare and application service which is being executed. Disconnected operations means the fact that the performing service should be recovered and performed continuously when the client gets disconnected. Service migration is the process of moving the location of BSS (Background Support Station) depending on the movement of healthcare user by organizing the mobile agent that supports the client. The relationship between mobile health client and mobile agent is composed of 1:1 mapping structure. This structure can be extended as 1: n or n: 1 relation. For the recovery during client or service disconnection, checkpoint or log is stored periodically or non-periodically during the normal healthcare information service.

Background cloud computing components support real-time mobile healthcare. In mobile healthcare computing, it is an important issue to provide real-time cloud computing model using integrated wireless and wired network environments. The components of real-time healthcare are a *mobile embedding component* and a *background support component.*

The internal component can be virtualized in order to support the optimal real-time mobile communication and computing. From the sensing node to the embedded mobile station, the embedded components are unified by the virtualization of resources within a mobile embedded device, and they can be selectively used to provide optimal real-time computing.

The computing component can be virtualized to create a background computing system including the second closed layer and the third open layer that can support the real-time mobility of a mobile healthcare user. In the external system of mobile healthcare service, the virtualization of components requires not only that the wire-

less base stations, user location be virtualized, the Internet and network be virtualized, but also that the servers be virtualized, and that there be the virtualization of healthcare applications and interfaces. In particular, a system optimizing real-time mobility can be configured by identifying and selecting the factors influencing real-time processing. Also, virtualization can provide a virtual API and libraries so that versatile healthcare information services can be easily developed.

Figure 3 shows the cloud computing structure for mobile healthcare. The one showing network configuration of transmitting the healthcare information of mobile user and mobility model of mobile client is Figure 4. In Figure 4, the wearable healthcare user attaching MES device transmits body signal through Foreign BSS. At the Home BSS of home or hospital where the background

Figure 4. Wearable mobility model and computing components in mobile healthcare

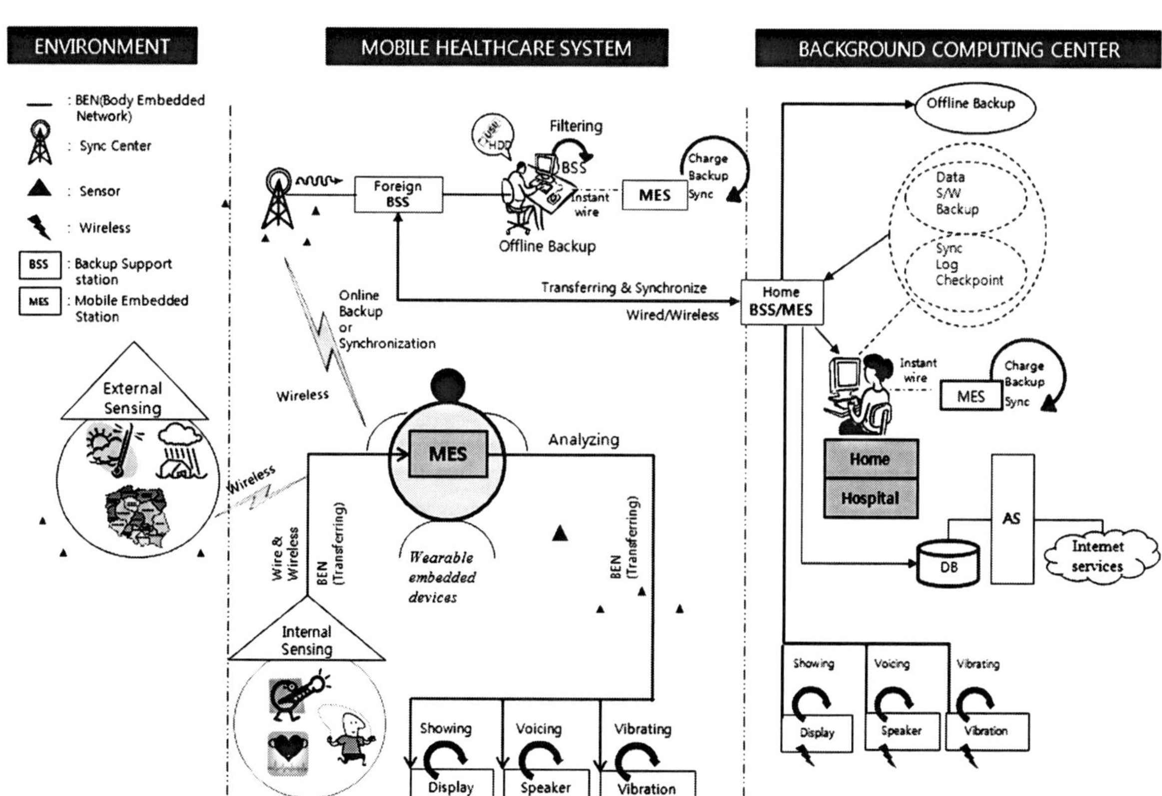

computing center of wearable user is located, the synchronization with offline backup of mobile healthcare client is supported.

The wearable computing system can be provided as a mobile healthcare platform as shown in Figure 4. Each device component is interconnected via a wired or wireless transmission network. In the instance depicted, the following components are present.

MES (Mobile Embedded Station): An MES is an embedded or connected to digital garment, which is interconnected with internal sensors by means of a wireless connection or wired conduction fibers. The MES is also connected with external sensors by a wireless local network. It supports applications that deal with events of interest to the user. The status of an MES can be assigned that of My MES, to invoke a user, or Friend MES, which is connected to a garment friend by P2P communications as shown in Figure 4.

Sensors: Sensors detect the origination of events that have occurred in the human body or the external environment in real time. The internal sensors can sense the body temperature, respiration, ECG, etc. whereas external sensors detect the temperature, weather, location, etc.

BSS (Background Support Station): A BSS is located on a wired link and supports data transfer and the processing of MES in the background. It provides background application services that enable background knowledge monitoring, knowledge information analysis, etc. It can support data exchange with other BSSs. A BSS provides the functions of power charging, data synchronization or backup with an MES (Mobile Support Station). It transfers data over wired/wireless global foreign networks to a home BSS or Monitoring and Syncing Center (MSC). It can also support a monitoring service using peer-to-peer communication over a wireless local network. BSSs may be classified into a Home BSS and a Foreign BSS as Figure 4. The Home BSS originates and registers an MES with itself. Here, a Home BSS is a computing system that creates and registers

a wearable host, and manages the home address of the host. It manages the mobile position and open Internet services of a wearable healthcare host using a background-computing center (Figure 4). Secondly, the Foreign BSS is a BSS that is visited by a foreign MES. A "Foreign BSS" is a computing system that registers a visiting wearable host, and manages the foreign address of the visiting wearable host.

DB (database): The DB stores the information about running applications and the resource information of a wearable healthcare user.

AS (application server): An application server is connected to a gateway system to provide Internet open services. The gateway system is located between the Internet and Internet provides information about security, data filtering, firewall operations, etc. An open user accesses various community services using an application server accessed over the Internet. The BSS interconnects with Internet by means of an application server (AS) as shown in Figure 4.

The issues and requirements related to mobile healthcare architecture and components are as follows. As the mobile cloud architecture of Figure 3 is interworked with three cloud systems, the healthcare data transmission interface must be supported. The transmission network must provide effective and high performance transmission ability in the infrastructure aspect. And the wire network healthcare information transmission path configuration must be changed depending on the mobile network environment of mobile healthcare client. For example, the transmission performance and transmission cost vary depending on the information transmission path of the instance where mobile user connects to wide area mobile network (3G/4G) and local wireless network (WLAN). The migration technique for location synchronization of mobile agent that effectively supports information transmission depending on the moving position of mobile client is required. To improve information protection between the 2rd closed layer and the 3rd open layer or efficiency of information access, the configuration of computing system supporting filtering logic and semantic information selection logic (for example, expert system) is required. To support information gathering and information interaction of the mobile healthcare users in Figure 3 and Figure 4, the integrated mobile cloud network configuration is required for supporting the virtualized access of ad-hoc and infrastructure wireless network. In order to provide warning and health guide services satisfactorily for the user by analyzing the body signal information gathered by mobile healthcare client MES of Figure 4, the output device to feedback information to the mobile client such as display, speaker and vibration is required.

MOBILE HEALTHCARE INFORMATION FLOWS

For the satisfactory information transmission of mobile healthcare, seamless data transfer must be supported. To construct the seamless data flow, the heterogeneous network integration, the disconnected operations, and the communication link redundancy are important issues.

To configure heterogeneous cloud system as single information transmission flow, a compatible interface for information security and information transmission of bio-signal must be supported. Also in order to configure by integrating the mobile healthcare cloud system, the components for minimum basic standard configuration and open interface specification must be proposed (*Heterogeneous network integration*).

The disconnected operation in mobile healthcare is a method for minimizing the side effect of disconnecting healthcare data transmission followed by cutoff of network resources or failure of transmission node. The methods of backing up the body signal at the transmission terminal of the part where transmission cutoff has occurred or evading by predicting transmission cutoff re required (*Disconnected operations*).

The transmission stability and transmission performance are maximized by overlapping two or more transmission links between nodes to guarantee transmission stability. Therefore, the method of configuration by overlapping the link of part with high transmission failure rate and low transmission performance as priority is required (*Link redundancy*).

Figure 5 shows the system process chain that analyzes the mobile healthcare information flow based on a linear model. The components chained together include a healthcare sensor (HS), a mobile embedded station (MES), a foreign agent (FA) or foreign background support station (F-BSS), a home agent (HA) or home background support station (H-BSS), and the Internet.

The system process chain provides information service flow. This process chain embodies the entire service platform of mobile healthcare computing system from the body sensor to the application server in the sequence shown in Figure 5. The computing and communication components of the mobile healthcare system chain are present in the following sequence.

HS transmits the gathered body signal based on the body embedded network (BEN) configured as wire link. When the information gathered at many HS's are gathered at the MES, the data must be synchronized depending on the time.

MES supports memory buffering in order to solve the transmission speed gap between HS and F-BSS. And MES supports disconnected operations in order to overcome the cutoff of vulnerable wireless link while transmitting data to F-BSS through wireless link.

For monitoring the internal and external interacting environments of the moving MESs, a short-distance network configuration is required as BAN/PAN. It can dynamically transmit the mobility status-sensing events related to the location, dangerous event, contact user, etc. of mobile users.

F-BSS transmits the data transmitted from many mobile clients as the base station of AP or 3G/4G of wireless LAN. Therefore, an independen-

Figure 5. The computing chain and components in mobile healthcare

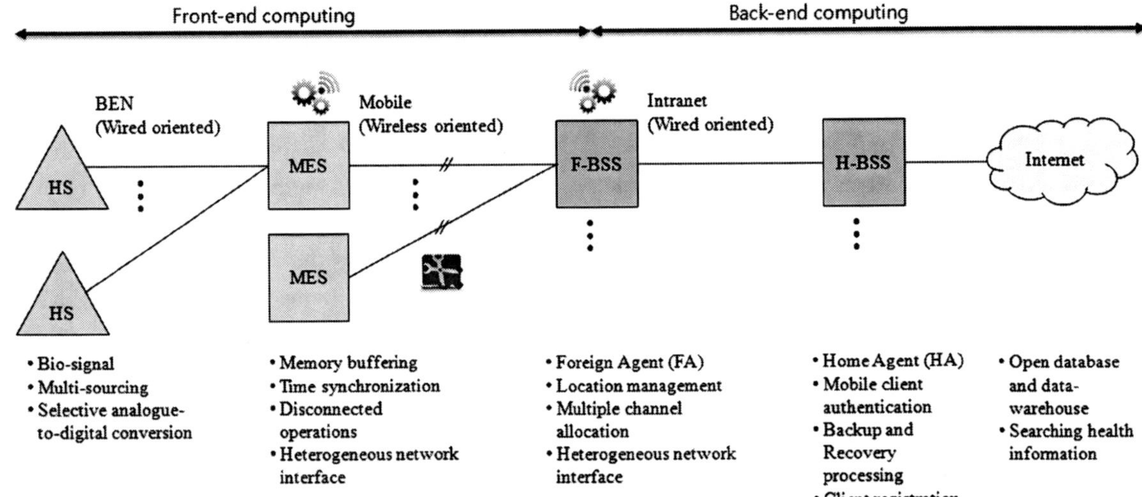

dent multiple channel allocation for each client. To support data transmission of mobile client, the foreign agent is supported. And management is required for the seamless data transmission of mobile client. F-BSS transmits the bio-signal gathered from each mobile client to the H-BSS where the corresponding mobile client is registered through private intranet.

H-BSS supports the authentication service to check whether the mobile client registered to one's own. H-BSS registers the newly created mobile healthcare client and operates home agent in order to support the transmission of mobile client. In order to minimize the data loss of mobile client registered to them, the backup and recovery process are supported. Then this gets redefined as shared database for the open service of health information of mobile healthcare client accumulated at many H-BSS. The internet based health information service users access after searching the information they desire by connecting to the database.

In Figure 5, the heterogeneous network interface is an important factor for MES and F-BSS. In H-BSS, data filtering and security of heterogeneous network are important factors. Especially,

link redundancy and disconnected operation are important in a wireless link connecting MES and F-BSS.

In order to maximize system flexibility and scalability in the mobile healthcare computing chain, the installation of cloud system is required. In the front-end computing part of Figure 5, mobile personal cloud system is the main foundation for supporting mobility and various terminal interface of mobile healthcare client. And the back-end computing part is classified as private cloud and public cloud as two sub-parts. F-BSS and H-BSS are configured as private cloud while Internet part is configured as public cloud.

However, such cloud system configuration is configured independently from the applied service and can be flexibly and selectively configured depending on installation cost, system scale and required performance, etc. Figure 6 shows the information flow in the mobile healthcare client aspect. These mobile client based data flows create their own bio-signal information and form the following cycles after wearing the wearable embedded devices. The healthcare information of mobile client is mainly classified into two types. They are forward direction information flow sending by gathering information collected from the user and the feedback information flow such as guide information, etc according to setup info or analysis result for data gathering of user. Process convert can internally switch each unit process of MES in Figure 6.

In the forward information flow, the embedded MES of mobile user gathers digital bio-signal data, user location and environment information, etc. next the gathered information is periodically or non-periodically transmitted to BSS. In the feedback information flow on the contrary, the command of BSS or healthcare guide information are transmitted to the MES of mobile user to change the settings of mobile user. Also, the necessary healthcare information is designated by setting up the interested health information of

mobile user to the MES. The following service process provides the logic sequences to mobile healthcare computing system.

First, the MES goes through three sub-processing steps as shown in Figure 6. In the first sub-process (1 of Figure 6), a mobile user selects an interesting keyword for each life sector. In the second sub-process (2 of Figure 6), mobile information including the user position, object event, etc. related to the data of interest to the user given in the previous step is often gathered into MES. In the third sub-process (3 of Figure 6), it performs real-time health monitoring services for the information of interest to the user and the mobile resources including clothing-attached sensors, MES, etc. For mobile healthcare applications, the messages including ECG, body temperature,

Figure 6. Mobile healthcare client and information flows

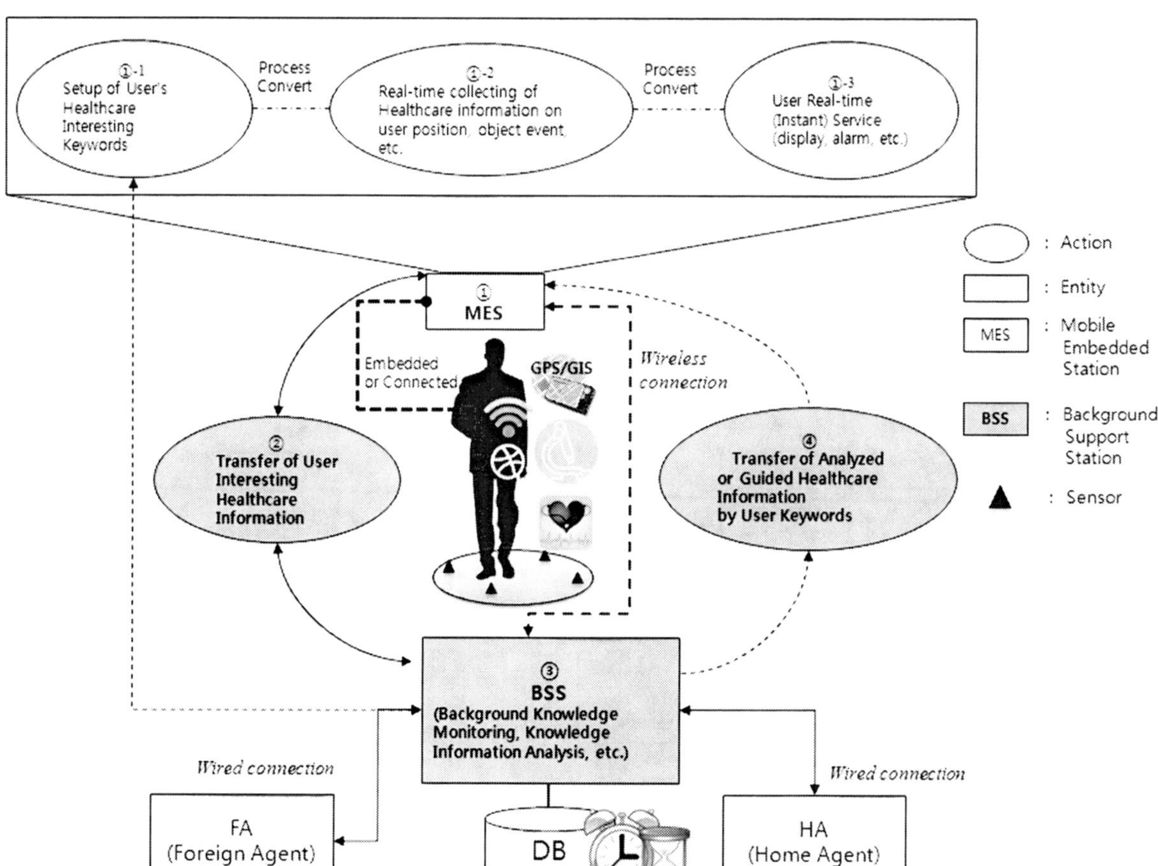

respiration, etc. containing health-related information are displayed or are presented in the form of an alarm.

Next, it transfers information analyzed or guided by the keywords of interest to the user between the MES and the BSS. The real-time event information collected by the MES is transferred to the BSS, or the application information analyzed by the BSS is fed back or provided to the MES.

Finally, the guided information is transmitted to the MES of a mobile user from the BSS. The information is analyzed or guided according to the keywords of interest to the user and the knowledge in the DB on the BSS.

The mobile healthcare client of Figure 6 can be applied as wearable client model. The wearable computing requires methods such as synchronization, high real-time and emergency network, etc. It requires step by step synchronization method to guarantee integrity of information transmitted as stepped from the wearable healthcare client to the server. And a high real-time support method is necessary in order to improve low real-time due to long transmission distance of data transmis-

sion path. Finally, a new emergency networking method is necessary in order to safely transmit the emergency information of wearable user.

The information flow processes for mobile healthcare users may be generally represented by the seven processes shown in Figure 7, which depicts the detailed flow of information for a mobile healthcare computing system from the body sensor to the application server using a forward sequence of events. The forward sequence can be applied in reverse to create a backward sequence, which would indicate the flow of data from the application server to the sensor.

First, the healthcare-data generation process detects its sensing information using a body textile or an environmental sensor. If necessary, the key-in process is performed by a mobile user. Environmental events or unexpected bio-signal events are randomly generated on the MES of a mobile healthcare user. The raw sensory data is transferred to the MES over a wired digital yarn or wireless medium on a user body. Data generation using the digital garment system is divided into data about the internal resources of the digital clothing and

Figure 7. The detailed information flow process for mobile healthcare

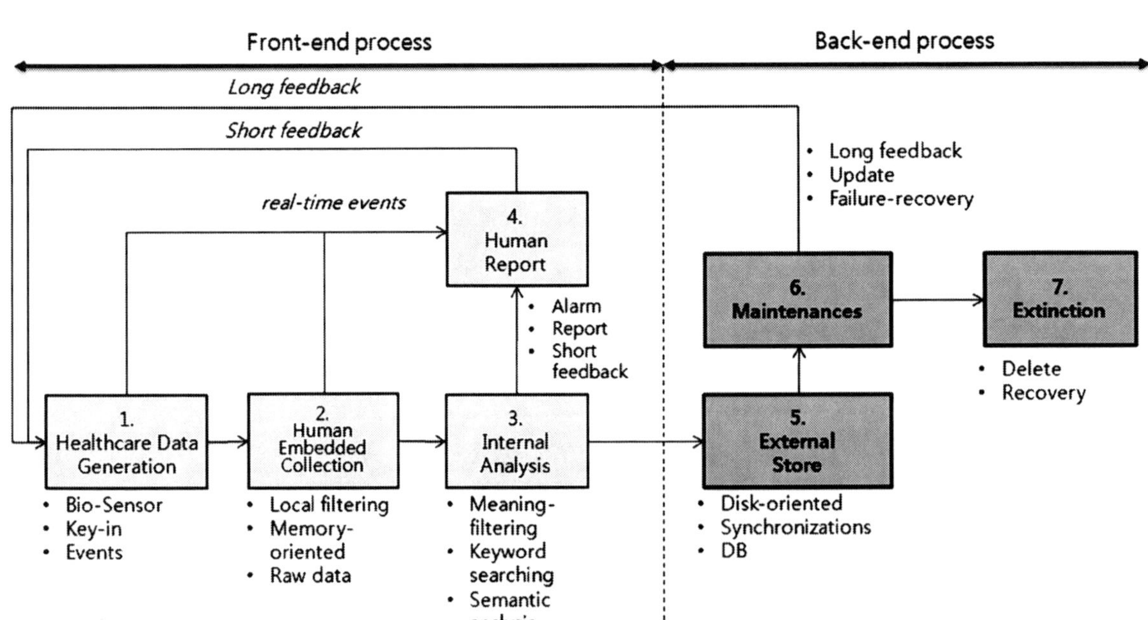

data about the external environmental resources. The internal resources as biosensors, key-in, etc. occurs the internal events. Biosensors detect the human health-related events in a body-embedded sensor network. Using key-in devices, the user will enter the user events. The external environmental resources occurs the external events as follows. Environmental sensors detect the environment around the mobile users using natural resources such as the temperature and weather. Event messages are occurred by an emergency caused by an artifact around the mobile users.

Second, the human embedded collection process collects the raw data or local filtered data and sends it to the memory of the MES. Data collection is performed by the MES embedded on a mobile client. The MES locally receives raw physical data over wired or wireless links from the internal or external resources of its mobile client. Data that has been buffered, filtered, and locally collected on the MES can be stored by performing a manual offline backup. The MES executes the following operations. Periodic or non-periodic filtering is supported (*Local filtering*). Memory buffering supports real-time transfers, which relay the filtered data from the MES to the BSS, or vice versa (*Memory buffering*). The received raw data is transformed into the formatted standard-format of thee BSS on the Intranet (*Raw-data formatting*).

Third, the collected data in the MES is quickly analyzed using the keywords of interest to the mobile user. Also, the data is filtered by using the semantic meanings. Local analysis is promptly performed by MESs such as smart phones. Keywords of interest to a user are searched, sorted, and evaluated. The keywords are found and sorted (*Searching keywords*). The event messages related to the keywords of user interest are accepted; otherwise, they are discarded (*Filtering meanings*). The meaning of the filtered event-message is compared with that of the user-interest keywords, and the analysis results are passed onto the subsequent report process (*Semantic analysis*).

Fourth, the human report process feeds the quickly analyzed information back to a mobile healthcare user over a digital yarn/wireless network, and the reporting data is then output via embedded media by such means as a local display, creating a voice using a local speaker, and creating vibrations using a local vibrator. This report process passes a real-time response message received from step 1 to step 3 above to the MES user. An MES user is informed by an emergency alarm (*Alarm*). Local-based report services can be supported by BSS (*Report*). The response messages corresponding to real-time events can be reported (*User short feedback*).

Fifth, the fast filtered data of the third process can be stored externally on disk storage. Local data can be transferred over wireless external networks to the BSS (Monitoring and Syncing Center) to be monitored and synchronized. The stored data requires synchronization to ensure the integrity of the bio-signal data. All MES data is accumulated onto a disk-based database (DB) and is statistically analyzed by a BSS such as a server computer. The operations of this process take place on the medium of storage (*Disk-oriented storage*). Data and status of each MES should be continuously synchronized with BSS storage (*Synchronizations*). The forecasting services are mainly provided by statistical analysis (*Long feedback*). Managing the DB has the privileges to perform creation, update, and deletion on a database (*DB management*).

Sixth, for the healthcare data maintenance, an update strategy and a failure-recovery process are activated for each MES. The transferring and synchronizing of global information takes place between friendly users over wired/wireless global home networks. Data to be filtered and globally collected on the BSS can be stored by performing a backup manually offline. The update process is keeps the data up to date with the program and device status of the MES (*Update*). The failure-recovery process supports a recovery process of the data and the program for a failed MES (*Failure-recovery*).

Seventh, in the registration and extinction process, all the resources of a mobile healthcare system can be removed or destroyed in this extinction process. Initial setup and registration of all global resources including the MES and BSS is performed (*Registration*). Final removal of all global resources including the MES and BSS is performed (*Delete*) Recovery processes of a device-failed MES and a failed BSS are supported (*Recovery*)

The processes of steps 1 to 4 occur on the MES and are called *front-end processes*. The cycle processes of steps 5 to 7 take place on the BSS and are referred to as *back-end processes*. All of these steps require real-time or non real-time feedback to their routines.

FUTURE RESEARCH DIRECTIONS

In this section, the issues that mobile healthcare will be faced with in the future are presented.

The current healthcare information system and service status show the following characteristics. First, the hospital or healthcare center oriented medical information system is consolidated. Second, the private medical information system within the wire and wireless intranet based limited range (security system oriented) must be consolidated. Third, the gathering (group and classification) oriented medical information system installation, in other words the symptom oriented medical information or treatment information system must be continuously developed. In order to develop the healthcare information system currently established based on hospital or healthcare support center, the following requirements must be improved.

First, the shift of medical information paradigm for the proposal of new preventive healthcare information system is required. It is necessary to build up healthcare information service of pre-venting disorders targeting healthy people from being patient treatment oriented medical service. This provides personal disease history prediction service as an implementation of healthcare expert system based on building up personal disease history DB, family disease history DB and group disease history DB.

Second, it must be expanded and built as a daily healthcare information production system producing healthcare information out of patient's or ordinary person's daily information from the medical information center oriented medical information production system.

Third, the buildup of individual oriented customized healthcare information system from being gathering (group) centered is required: Personal medical information device (personal health and medical information analysis indicator role is necessary), personal healthcare self-treatment information device, digital healthcare garment, personal healthcare sensing module and building up network are necessary.

Fourth, the alternative toward compatibility and convergence with the existing medical information system is required.

Fifth, the buildup of new personal or group medical information life cycle system is required. This would be building up the life cycle system of healthcare information production, storage, distribution and extinction, etc.

Sixth, preparing opportunity for popularization of existing high priced healthcare devices: The disease free health service of human race is implemented by extending healthcare service accessibility of general public through implementation of economic value according to lighter healthcare devices, implementation of mass production system and popularization of information healthcare technology followed by application of information technology.

There are many issues and problems to using mobile healthcare computing and these should be accordingly addressed. The following is a list that the author has compiled.

Embedded sensing networking: Conductive fibers are required to collect or deliver the sensory information in real-time and to deliver it safely. Also, a Personal Area Network (PAN) or a Body Embedded Network (BEN) is required in order for the installation of additional sensory devices to be rendered convenient

Dynamic binding and tuning of mobile healthcare device: This binding requires garment binding or user binding by means of changing a personal garment or the user of a garment, respectively. Also, creating this binding requires that the tuning of a real-time garment system be dependent on the status of every garment user.

Cost effectiveness: The procurement of new digital garments entails the increased expense of the new garments. The price of the new garments can be from several fold higher to dozens of times more expensive. Therefore, there is a need for the production of digital garments to use standardized production methods and standardized components in order to realize low cost when placed on the market.

Backup-support services: This is related to real-time user state analysis, database construction, and intelligent system construction. Real-time user state analysis provides instant and powerful analysis of a garment user. This real-time analysis is performed using a background system like BSS, which supports the real-time monitoring of user events. Secondly, database construction is associated with the continuous compilation of a database to perform statistical analysis of garment users and their environments. Finally, intelligent system construction is helpful because to make the response of a digital garment user successful, the interaction and guidance of application services for the garment user are required. Otherwise, the user instructions are updated or changed dependent on the intelligent logic and statistical data.

More enhanced personal security: The central location of the personal information is the closed layer consisting of the Intranet on which the BSS is located. Because the privacy of individuals becomes more concentrated on the BSS on the closed layer than on the existing desktop or a centralized server, the importance of security should receive more emphasis. Mobile cloud security supports the security cloud configuration, which is required for supporting dynamic security based on context-awareness.

Lightweight mobile device: Mobile healthcare devices still heavy. It needs continuously to make the mobile devices lightweight.

Side-effects: Some mobile devices can consist of a lot of wiring and can cause irritation in heat and headaches. Such side-effects should be avoided or prevented using the advanced technologies and methods.

Privacy and Security: Mobile healthcare devices can invade privacy because of being tracked wherever you go. And they can be used to gain an unfair advantage over others such as hacking.

Safety and QoS: For safe information transmission, it needs the fault-recovery processes that can immediately recover its connections *when a mobile* healthcare device is disconnected. Also, the differential performance quality should be supported for different healthcare applications.

Scalability and Portability: Scalability should ensure the continued scalability of the system resources, due to the increase in the number of users of mobile healthcare. Portability is to support the user's devices replacement, the program transplant, etc using the mobile agent technique. Mobility cloud should be supported to ensure a seamless user-mobility.

CONCLUSION

This chapter firstly described the mobile healthcare system architecture and components, which emphasized the lightweight mobile client and devices and the flexibility and scalability of background healthcare supporting components. Secondly, it presented the information data flows and cycles for supporting mobile healthcare computing. Finally, it described various applications and health-medical issues and characteristics. The following objectives will be presented in order to build up the mobile healthcare information system described in this chapter.

Firstly, a medical service that can be accessed at any time and place will be implemented by discovering various mobile healthcare services continuously and developing the mobile healthcare information lifecycle.

Secondly, a universal economic medical information system will be implemented by spreading low cost individual healthcare information devices in order to implement the personal healthcare service.

Thirdly, a healthcare information expert system will be built in order to switch the healthcare service from background healthcare service to prevention-oriented forefront healthcare service.

Lastly, the subject of healthcare service must be extended from patient-oriented to medical staff such as doctors or nurses. A convenient and safe healthcare information system should be established for monitoring and caring for the health status of medical staff which is not building up healthcare information devices and system as a tool for medical activity (such as treatment).

Through accomplishment of such goals, a harmonious and cooperative healthcare information system between the patient, the family, the doctor and the hospital can be achieved.

Also, the mobile cloud, the private cloud and the public cloud must configure the overall system by combining the following characteristics of their own in order to build up a mobile healthcare cloud system.

Firstly, a mobile healthcare cloud must satisfactorily support the synchronization between various mobile devices, as well as having easy interface design and user mobility.

Next, a private cloud must consolidate the performance of elements such as the cloud system, system safety and information security.

The public cloud must support system scalability in order to consolidate usability through the development of various applications, and consolidate economic efficiency by lowering service cost and support large-scale users.

REFERENCES

Akyildiz, I. F., Su, W., Sankarasubramaniam, Y., & Cayirci, E. (2002). A survey on sensor network. *IEEE Communications Magazine*, 102–114. doi:10.1109/MCOM.2002.1024422

Barbará, D. (1999). Mobile computing and databases-A survey. *IEEE Transactions on Knowledge and Data Engineering*, *11*(1). doi:10.1109/69.755619

Bertucci, G. (2007). Compendium of ICT applications on electronic government: Vol. 1. *Mobile applications on health and learning*. New York: Department of Economic and Social Affairs, United Nations.

Bujnoch, Z. (2013). Enabling collaborative workflows: Shaping the future of mobile healthcare. *Frost & Sullivan*. Retrieved from http://www.frost.com

Coyle, S. (2009). *BIOTEX–Bio-sensing textiles for healthcare*. Paper presented at Smart Textiles Salon. Ghent, Belgium.

Dash, S. K., Mohapatra, S., & Pattnaik, P. K. (2010). A survey on applications of wireless sensor network using cloud computing. *International Journal of Computer Science & Emerging Technologies*, *50*(1).

Dinh, H. T., Lee, C., Niyato, D., & Wang, P. (2011). A survey of mobile cloud computing: Architecture, applications, and approaches. In *Wireless Communications and Mobile Computing*. Hoboken, NJ: Wiley. Retrieved from http://onlinelibrary.wiley.com/doi/10.1002/wcm.1203/abstract

Estrin, D. (2001). Comm'n sense: Research challenges in embedded networked sensing. *UCLA Computer Science Department Research Review*. Retrieved from http://lecs.cs.ucla.edu

Geier, J. (2007). *Wireless network industry report*. Wireless-Nets, Ltd.

Germanakos, P., Mourlas, C., & Samaras, G. (2005). A mobile agent approach for ubiquitous and personalized ehealth information systems. In *Proceedings of the Workshop on 'Personalization for e-Health' of the 10th International Conference on User Modeling (UM'05)*, (pp. 67–70). eHealth.

Gough, C. (2009). *Industry brief: Healthcare cloud security*. Intel IT Center.

HL7. (2012). Retrieved from http://www.hl7.org/Special/committees/mobile/index.cfm

Harold, P. (2007). MyHeart - Fighting cardiovascular diseases through prevention and early diagnosis. *Philips Research Password, 29*, 12–15.

Huang, P. (2000). *Promoting wearable computing: A survey and future agenda*. Academic Press.

Hyek, P. (2013). mHealth: Mobile technology poised to enable a new era in health care. *Ernst & Young*. Retrieved from http://www.ey.com/Publication/

Kay, M., Santos, J., & Takane, M. (2011). mHealth new horizons for health through mobile technologies. In Global Observatory for eHealth. Geneva: WHO Press.

Logicworks. (2013). *Logicworks healthcare cloud*. Retrieved from http://www.logicworks.net

Malhotr, K., Gardner, S., & Rees, D. (2005). Evaluation of GPRS enabled secure remote patient monitoring system. [Riga, Latvia: ASMTA.]. *Proceedings of ASMTA, 2005*, 41–48.

mHealth. (2012). *Wikipedia*. Retrieved from http://en.wikipedia.org/wiki/MHealth#Definitions

Miller, F. (2004). Wearables–Clothing with a sixth sense. *Fraunhofer magazine*, 38-39.

Nguyen, V. (2000). *Mobile computing & disconnected operation: A survey of recent advances*. Retrieved from http://www.cis.ohio-state.edu/~jain/cis788-95/mobile_comp/index.html

Park, S., & Jayaraman, S. (2003). Enhancing the quality of life through wearable technology. *IEEE Engineering in Medicine and Biology Magazine*. PMID:12845818

Pfaltz, M. C., Grossman, P., Michael, T., Margraf, J., & Wilhelm, F. H. (2010). Physical activity and respiratory behavior in daily life of patients with panic disorder and healthy controls. *International Journal of Psychophysiology, 78*, 42–49. doi:10.1016/j.ijpsycho.2010.05.001 PMID:20472006

Rehman, A., Mustafa, M., Javaid, N., Qasim, U., & Khan, Z. A. (2012). Analytical survey of wearable sensors. In *Proceedings of BioSPAN with 7th IEEE International Conference on Broadband and Wireless Computing, Communication and Applications (BWCCA)*. Victoria, Canada: IEEE.

Rimal, B. P., Choi, E., & Lumb, I. (2009). A taxonomy and survey of cloud computing systems. In *Proceedings of Fifth International Joint Conference on INC, IMS and IDC*. IEEE.

Schadow, G., Mean, C. N., & Walker, D. M. (2006). The HL7 reference information model under scrutiny. *Master of Industrial Engineering, 124*, 151–156. PMID:17108519

Sloninsky, D., & Mechael, P. N. (2008). *Towards the development of a mhealth strategy: A literature review*. Geneva: World Health Organization.

Smith, B., & Ceusters, W. (2006). HL7 RIM: An incoherent standard. *Studies in Health Technology and Informatics*, *124*, 133–138. PMID:17108516

Tubaishat, M., & Madria, S. (2003). Sensor networks: An overview. *IEEE Potentials*, *22*(2), 20–23. doi:10.1109/MP.2003.1197877

Zawoad, S., & Hasan, R. (2013). *Cloud forensics: A meta-study of challenges, approaches, and open problems*. Retrieved from http://arxiv.org/abs/1302.6312

Chapter 41
Inclusive Technology for Rural Development:
Rural Call Centre in Orissa, India

Sanjay Mohapatra
Xavier Institute of Management, India

Neha Agarwal
Xavier Institute of Management, India

ABSTRACT

This is a research work on usage of information and communication technology to address the loopholes in the existing system in rural India and suggest an improved way of catering to basic utility services to common people for betterment of their life. The work links all utility related discrete businesses on a common platform and creates a win-win situation for all stakeholders. The model proposed is trying to use mobile phones as a universal communication tool while providing social services in a rural call centre. The work also addresses the relative ranking of services in rural areas based on baseline survey as rural people spend 80% of their expense on obtaining health, transport, and education related information by frequent visits to urban areas. If this model is implemented then it will save time, cost and transport expenses on frequent visit and customer will enjoy the information, tips, and emergency guide line.

INTRODUCTION

Glancing at some rural growth centres and some of the successes of the poverty alleviation schemes, one can easily conclude that the rural economy of India is opening up and developing. Yet, a closer look will show that the rural economy continues to be a stratified and fractured economy, with masses of livelihood seekers near and below the poverty line are being excluded from the benefits of the economic growth. There are many reasons for this and lack of proper education has been found to be a major stumbling block (Agarwal, 2006). Electronic learning or e-learning as it is better known as has come to revolutionize the way education is imparted. Over time there has been increased penetration of information and communication technology in the rural areas. It has opened ways of educating people of all ages and all abilities (Singh, 2005). Success stories like

DOI: 10.4018/978-1-4666-8756-1.ch041

e-choupal etc. have opened our eyes to the fact that there is a greater need for a wide range of business development services (BDS) to actually enable the rural consumers realise their true business acumen (Agarwal, 2006; Labelle, 2005; Hario, 2008; Mohapatra et al., 2008; Senteni, 2006). There has always been a great deal of information asymmetry among the rural consumers regarding market information, about various services like education, transportation, health, government schemes, loans etc. (Brownder et al., 2005; Shen, 2005; Upton et al., 2004). This study aims to find out the relevant information gaps existing in the areas of education, health, govt. schemes etc. and suggest a framework and approach of the use of information and communication technology platform in providing inclusive and sustainable development for the rural poor.

LITERATURE REVIEW

With advent of technological revolution, relationship between technology, information and knowledge have impacted business models of many organizations. Drucker (1965) stated that creation, organization and institutionalization of knowledge was the first technological revolution in history. However, this relationship has gone through a paradigm shift. Porter (1979) talked of five forces that are important for any organization to maintain its competitive edge. Technology had tremendous impact on the same forces (Porter, 2001) and for organizations, role of technology on these forces for development and maintenance of competitive edge has changed over time. Laszlo and Laszlo (2002) argue that there was greater focus on internal processes aiming at production and managerial efficiency during the first half of the twentieth century. Then technology led competition and economic expansions brought change in focus and it shifted to inclusive technologies, where bottom of pyramid stand to gain the most (Prahlad, 2004) as consumers. Prahlad

(2004) argued that using inclusive technology, not only bottom of pyramid can get benefits, but the organizations will also get profit for sustainability.

Computer and internet led technologies in villages are likely to create a material culture of its own. Farmers or villagers are likely to adopt this culture fast, if they receive enough attention and respect from marketers. It seems that marketers have realized or understood this and they seem to be capitalizing upon attention and respect element (Prahalad, C.K. 2004). However it has to be further explored up to what extent the dignity is created amongst farmers through e –initiatives in India. In the subsequent section, we explore literature work in this area. The next section is divided into following sections – what is inclusive technology, ICT for development (ICT4D), role of ICT in rural development, Call Centre, rural call centre and role of rural call centre in development process.

INTRODUCTION TO INCLUSIVE TECHNOLOGY

Social inclusion is defined as the extent to which an individual or community can fully participate in a society. The access to technology and the ability to use it also influences social inclusion to some extent. There exists a barrier in accessing technology by rural masses which can be categorised as follows:

1. Access to physical resources (hardware)
2. Access to digital information such as software and content
3. Skills that people need to access the devices

The addressal of these issues does not guarantee that the technology will be adopted by its intended users. According to the unified theory of acceptance and use of technology model a technology must be perceived as beneficial, easy to use, and socially endorsed with adequate infrastructure in place to support its use (Venkatesh et al., 2003). There exists disparity in opportunities available to people in rural and urban areas through information and communication technologies. There exists barrier to the use and acceptance of these technologies in rural areas. 'Inclusive technology' is defined as a technology which overcomes the barriers in using technology that are inherent within a community in order to increase the available opportunities (Pitula, 2007). The technology should be relevant to the needs of the community and must be affordable and sustainable. For example, mobile penetration has incredibly grown in India over the past years and at the beginning of 2009, there were more than 370 million subscribers, many of them coming from rural areas. However, even if the masses have an access to mobile connectivity, most of the handsets' potential is still untapped - as the content delivered is often not directly related to their livelihood and their environment. Rural communities certainly need local information concerning health, education, government services and other valuable information that can improve their livelihood and meet their daily needs (www. dcontent.in, 2010).

The Technology Achievement Index is a measure of how well a country is creating and diffusing technology and building a human skill base, reflecting capacity to participate in the technological innovations of the network age. It was introduced by UNDP and it helps policy makers to define technology strategies (www. wto.org, 2010).

TAI measures achievements in four areas:

- Technology creation as measured by the number of patents granted to residents and by receipts of royalties and license fees from abroad;
- Diffusion of recent innovations as measure by the number of Internet hosts per capita;
- Diffusion of old innovations (telephones/ capita, electricity consumption/capita); and

- Human skills as measured by mean years of schooling and the gross tertiary science enrolment ratio (Labelle, 2005).

Countries with the highest TAI have policies that are based on the belief that ICTs enable economic and social development (Table 1) (www. ibid.information.co.in, 2010).

INTRODUCTION TO RURAL CALL CENTRE

India has rapidly achieved the status of being the most preferred destination for business process outsourcing for companies located in the US and Europe, the reason being availability of low cost skilled manpower, English speaking population

Table 1. Countries with the highest TAI, Source: IBID

TAI Rank	TAI
Leaders	
Finland	0.744
United States	0.733
Sweden	0.703
Japan	0.698
Korea, Republic of	0.666
Netherlands	0.630
UK	0.606
Canada	0.589
Australia	0.587
Singapore	0.585
Germany	0.583
Norway	0.579
Ireland	0.566
Belgium	0.553
New Zealand	0.548
Austria	0.544
France	0.535
Israel	0.514

and appropriate infrastructure. With the BPO industry flourishing in India more and more companies began establishing operations in the metropolitan cities to capitalize on the available human resource talent and physical infrastructure. But the expansion caused intense competition. There was a high employee turnover and increased training and recruitment costs for many BPO companies. Keeping these factors in mind many BPO companies set up operations in smaller towns and villages. The benefits that were derived from the rural operations were low cost of operations and lower attrition levels (www.knowledge.wharton. edu, 2010). Non-urban BPOs or rural BPOs are on the rise, the reason being low cost. India's BPO industry is lagging behind due to rising expenses. There has been an increase in employee salary as well as training and recruitment costs. To curb people costs, many companies looked for recruitment in rural areas but found that fewer candidates would sign on due to high cost of living in towns. The same authors also argue that the existence of a BPO industry relies on cost effectiveness. By moving jobs to rural areas, companies and clients take advantage of significantly reduced operating costs. Most companies setting up BPO operations in rural India operate as third-party service providers to multiple clients. There is a tremendous opportunity for non-urban BPOs in domestic voice [i.e., call centers] and non-voice businesses, and international non-voice work. The rural call centre concept in India is catching up. Many organisations have implemented the rural BPOs. In July 2008 HDFC setup a BPO centre at Tirupati in Andhra Pradesh state through its subsidiary Atlas Documentary facilitators. It employs around 550 employees who are involved in non-core operations replacing 1000 employees in Mumbai and Chennai.

The Tata Group's rural BPO known as Uday (www.udayngo.org, 2010) is an initiative of the community service arm of group company Tata Chemicals where around 200 people are employed at the two BPO centres in Gujarat and UP.

Desicrew, a rural BPO concept incubated by IIT Chennai's Rural Technology Business Incubator. It used the network created by common service centre initiative which aims to set up one computer in each village across the country. Recent developments have also taken place (www.washingtonpost.com, 2010) in the area of providing health related information by a call centre to the rural masses. India's National Population Stabilization Fund has opened a call centre to provide reliable information to anonymous callers about reproductive health, family planning or contraception. The call centre fills a critical information gap that exists in Indian society about reproductive health issues. It caters to the population in rural areas who are underserved by health care and social workers.

'Soochna se Samadhaan' is an initiative of One World South Asia (www.solutionexchange-un. net.in, 2010). One world South Asia with support from British Telecom and CISCO systems are piloting the service in North India in partnership with other civil society organizations. It seeks to benefit the largest section of the population of India, the farmers, by providing them, at their door step, with need based information on basic agricultural practices in the local language which is also expected to help improve production, storage, marketing etc. It also aims to serve the grassroots communities with information and knowledge from other sectors like education, health, livelihoods, grievances, RTI etc.

GAP IDENTIFICATION FROM LITERATURE

Though there have been a lot of advances in the technological field for rural development but still there exists a barrier in accessing technology by rural masses. The need of the hour is to provide a beneficial and easy to use technology for the people. Again to derive benefits from ICT there needs to be a certain level of economic development in a country. It is a tool to empower communities and helps them become self-sufficient in meeting their basic needs and reach their full potential. To widen the range of employment opportunities offered by ICTs, networking and telecommunications facilities are being improved in order to generate more number of jobs in the non-software ICT service sectors, especially internet supported call centres and transcription work.

The concept of rural call centre is on the rise and is benefiting the rural masses by generating employment opportunities and empowering them. Apart from that a few initiatives have also been taken in providing the services to the rural customers for a social cause. 'Soochna se Samadhaan', an initiative of One World South Asia is one such initiative which seeks to benefit the farmers by providing them information on basic agricultural practices in local language. The existing rural BPOs mainly provide knowledge services in health and agriculture sectors. There exists a lot of scope and opportunity in providing other basic knowledge services through a rural call centre which are important from the development point of view of rural masses. The rural communities also need local information concerning education, government services and other valuable information that can improve their livelihood and meet their daily needs. Based on the gaps as identified, the objective has been set for the research work.

FIELD STUDY

This section contains research objective, scope of the study, methodology adopted for collecting data, data collection and findings. Based on the gaps found in literature review, we have formulated objectives in research objective section while scope of the research explain the rural area covered for research within stipulated time frame. Methodology section explains sample design, sources of data and analysis plan after collecting data. Under data collection and findings section, the manuscript explains characteristics of data such

as demographic profile such as age, sex, income, education and preferences to different services categorized by demographic profile.

OBJECTIVE

The study would focus on finding the most important services based on several parameters like age, income, gender and occupation. Lastly, the research would focus on developing a framework to analyse the feasibility analysis of such a model based on the metrics designed using the balance score card approach.

For this we would like to focus on the following aspects:

- Identifying the information gap across various categories of services
- Finding the relative importance of services required by the villagers and the particulars under each category.
- Analysis of changes at different levels viz. village level, entrepreneur level, Implementation partner level and the Area level at large (qualitative and quantitative aspects as would be defined in the questionnaire for the aforesaid purpose) using a balance score card approach.

SCOPE

Due to time constraint, the sample size for the survey was limited to 80 respondents, 40 each from the villages Balianta and Balakati, which were situated near to our institute. The findings of the report are based on data analysis, observations, interviews and documentation. Given the number of interviews possible within the stipulated period, the study does not aim at providing clear cut answers to the aforesaid objectives but certainly would provide a food for thought to carry on further research. The aim of the study is to analyse and find the service prioritization matrix for the services required by the villagers and provide suggestions for possible alternatives for access and management of information in rural areas.

METHODOLOGY

For data collection a pre-structured questionnaire was administered. For all the different stakeholders (community and individuals) associated with model personal interviews were conducted. A survey was conducted for the villages for problem identification and need assessment. The research topic was defined using quantifiable variables for carrying out suitable analysis and drawing necessary conclusions.

Sample design

Balianta and Balakati villages were selected for the study because these villages are nearer to the city and since the number of farmers is less in the villages, the information gap in non farming activities can be identified. The sample size was taken to be 40 in each village. The process of stratified random sampling was followed for selecting the sample. Thus, the total sample size was eighty households. The villagers were interviewed with a pre-structured interview schedule for assessing the impact of the internet and communication technology regarding social, economic, technological and environmental aspects. The villagers were also interviewed for the study of impact assessment.

Data and Its Sources

The study was based on primary data. The relevant data was collected on pre-structured interview schedules from the households through personal interview.

Analysis Framework

To study the impact of Internet and communication technology in villages, analysis was done with tools like Likert scale, STEEPLE analysis. Simple descriptive methods like percentages and averages were used for the study. Further, focus group discussions, personal interviews and survey using pre-structured questionnaire were conducted to know the relative importance of the services required by the villagers from the call centre and the lacunas in terms of information gaps that need to be addressed.

DATA COLLECTION

In total, there were eighty (80) data were collected from different villages. The sample had a good variety in terms of its characteristics and hence can be concluded that they represented the population. Table 2 shows distribution of total sample size in different sections.

FINDINGS

The responses obtained through questionnaire and qualitative study was analysed which led to the following observations (in terms of percentage of respondents) as shown in table 3. Detailed explanations are given under different section heads.

Distribution of People According To Occupation Who Have Given High Preference to Different Services

Health Service

35% of businessmen gave very high preference to health related information.

Table 2. Sample characteristics

	GENDER	AGE	INCOME	OCCUPATION
MALE	56			
FEMALE	24			
Less than 18		0		
18 to 25 yrs		32		
26 to 35 yrs		36		
More than 35		12		
Less than ` 1000			12	
`1000 to 5000			40	
` 5001 to 8000			16	
` 8001 to 10000			12	
More than ` 10000			0	
Business Man				36
Farmer				8
Driver				16
Student				12
House Wife				8

It was found from the survey that health related information is mostly required by the people who are into business activities. They are of the opinion that because of frequent travel and untimely food and drinking habits they usually fall sick and therefore emergency health care services relat-

Table 3. Percentage wise distribution of respondents for different services

	Health Services	Emergency Services	Education Services	Govt. Schemes	Agriculture	Insurance	Loan
Business Men	36	50	14	37	0	60	35
Driver	21	25	28	37	0	30	20
Farmer	14	6	14	13	100	10	45
House Wife	8	0	0	13	0	0	0
Student	21	19	44	0	0	0	0
Less than 1000	21	13	29	12	0	0	0
1001 to 5000	50	55	43	50	100	100	86
5001 to 8000	14	19	14	25	0	0	14
8001 to 10000	15	13	14	13	0	0	0
More than 10000	0	0	0	0	0	0	0
Less than 18 yrs	0	0	0	0	0	0	0
18 to 25 yrs	57	100	86	37	100	10	57
26 to 35 yrs	29	0	0	25	0	70	29
More than 35 yrs	14	0	14	38	0	20	14

ing to common cold, fever, dysentery is mostly required by them. The percentage values are depicted in table3.

Emergency Services

In this category it was seen that about 50% of the sample constituted by the business class feel that they require the emergency services. These services are those which should be provided as when required. Under this category services relating to health, disaster, security and any other emergency issue are included. The percentage values are depicted in the table3.

Education

42.85% of the sample constituted by students feels that education related information services should be provided in the call centre because there exist a lot of information asymmetry among the students relating to their career prospects issue. Information relating to vacancies in colleges, application dates, coaching facilities etc. is the need of the hour for the student community.

The relative importance of mandi prices, weather related information, durable related information is low in the community as none of the respondents from the various occupational classes rated them as very important. The reasons for the same could be the mercurial nature of the services, mandi prices and weather related information. Similarly with growing demand of the microfinance in the rural areas loan services were rated as most important by the business community (57.14%) as they require financial assistance to run their micro enterprises.

Government Related Schemes

These were rated important equally by the businessmen and driver because they always seek for employable opportunities in the government sector because they feel it's relatively stable.

Most of the people sampled belonged to the category of businessmen. Here its found out that the majority of the businessmen have giver their preference to the services govt. related schemes. So govt related schemes can be considered as one of the services (please refer table 3).

Since the businessmen constituted the majority of the sample the services for which businessmen have obtained the highest percentage value will be taken into consideration. So health related information needs to be considered in this case. Similarly the services education, loan, emergency services, insurance related service will be considered which will be later sorted using a matrix.

Distribution of People According To Income Who Have Given High Preference to Different Services

Table 4 shows distribution of the sample as per income level (monthly income). Based on their income level, we have numbered them as income category 1,2,3,4 and 5 etc. In our entire discussion in this section we would refer to this categorization of income.

Agriculture

From the table 3 it can be inferred that people in the monthly income range of 1000-5000 feel that agriculture related information is very important for them. Information relating to agriculture inputs like seed, fertiliser, pesticide etc. on a timely

Table 4. Income distribution of the sample

Income Category	
1	Less than Rs.1000
2	Rs.1000-Rs.5000
3	Rs.5001-8000
4	Rs. 8001-Rs.10000
5	>Rs.10000

basis will help them to increase their income, but because of the absence of the same they are unable to monitor and thereby fail to control the crop loss.

Health

It is seen that 21.42%people with income less than Rs.1000 per month feel that health related information is very much required. This is because the lower strata income people are unable to afford basic health facilities regarding hospital services, diagnostic centres etc.

Emergency

56.25% of the population with the income range of 1000-5000 income feel that they require them. This may be due to the reason that the people require readily available information on emergency services (table 3).

Education

People belonging to the income group Rs.1000-5000 per month feel that education related information is very much required. This mainly caters to the population which is not financially well off. So they are concerned about their child's education. That is the reason why they prefer availing education related information. Preferences for education service have been given in table 3.

Government Related Schemes

People belonging to the income group Rs.1000-5000 per month feel that government related information is very much required. This mainly caters to the population which is not financially well off. So they are concerned about the various government opportunities for job and other opportunities.

Insurance and Loan

People belonging to the income group Rs.1000-5000 per month feel that insurance related information is very much required. The income to which they belong is not so high so they to overcome any untoward incident they prefer to have information related to insurance related schemes. People belonging to the income group Rs.1000-5000 per month feel that loan related information is very much required. The income to which they belong is not so high so they usually have a need to avail loan facility (please refer table 3).

In the sample the majority is constituted majority of people belonging to the income group Rs.1000-5000. So government scheme related information needs to be considered in this case. Similarly it is considered that the services education, loan, emergency services, health, insurance related service which will be later sorted using a matrix.

Distribution of People According To Age Who Have Given High Preference to Various Services

Agriculture

Agriculture related service is mainly preferred by the respondent belonging to the age group 18-25 years. This is mainly because the people belonging to this age group have newly started doing agriculture and they think that to tackle agriculture related issues they need to avail information related to the same. Table 5 shows preference of different services with respect to age group.

Transport

Transport related service is mainly preferred by the respondent belonging to the age group 18-25 years. This is mainly because the people belonging

Table 5. Preferences of different age groups with respect to different services

Age group	Agriculture	Transport	Govt. schemes	Health	Education	Loan
<18	0	0	0	0	0	0
18-25	100	100	37.5	57.14286	85.71429	57.14286
26-35	0	0	25	28.57143	0	28.57143
>35	0	0	37.5	14.28571	14.28571	14.28571

to this age group need to commute for study and business purpose so they need to avail this facility.

Govt. Schemes

The govt schemes are mainly preferred by the people belonging to age group 18-25 and greater than 25. It was because this age group constitutes majority of people who are working and need more options to switch for or students who would be searching for new opportunities.

Health

Health services are mostly preferred by people belonging to the age group 18-25 years of age.

Education

The education related information is mostly needed by people belonging to the age group 18-25. This is because this age group mainly comprises of students who would like to go for higher studies and look for similar options.

Loan

Loan related information is mostly preferred by people belonging to the age group 18-25, this is because at this age the people mostly look out for new options like looking for a new job, starting business etc. or availing study loans for higher studies.

Emergency

Emergency related information is mainly preferred by people belonging to age group 18-25. Since the age group 18-25 years constituted the majority of the sample, the services for which this age group has obtained the highest percentage value will be taken into consideration. So health related information needs to be considered in this case. Similarly the services education, loan, emergency services, and insurance related services will be considered which will be later sorted using a matrix

Distribution of People According To Gender Who Have Given High Preference to Different Services

- **Agriculture:** Agri related services were mainly preferred by male. This is because in the village the farmer community mainly comprised of the male.
- **Govt schemes:** Govt. schemes are mostly preferred by male this was because the male members are mainly in search for employment opportunity as compared to females.
- **Education:** Education related service was mainly preferred by male Insurance: male
- **Loan:** Male
- **Emergency:** Male

Since the gender male constituted the majority of the sample, the services for which this gender has obtained the highest percentage value will be taken into consideration. So health related information needs to be considered in this case. Similarly the services education, loan, emergency services, insurance and health related services will be considered which will be later sorted using a matrix.

Service Priority Matrix

From the above observation across the various parameters the service priority matrix (table 6) is being constructed which will provide information about relative importance of various services that are to be provided in the call centre.

A 50% cut-off was assumed for benchmarking the importance of services. Based on the above matrix the relative importance of the services is as follows:

1. Loan
2. Emergency
3. Agri
4. Health
5. Govt. schemes
6. Education

Since the village is largely dominated by the business class people a direct co-relation between the services provided and the utility received can be seen.

From the service priority matrix after relative importance of services are defined it is very important to identify the particulars (essential information) under each category of service.

From the focus group discussion and personal interviews it was found that the following type of information is required under each of the top six categories of services which are as in table 7.

THE MODEL: RURAL CALL CENTRE

After analysing the services required under each category, the next step is to suggest a platform for the dissemination of information. To this end, a rural BPO will help us bridge the gap of information asymmetry by providing adequate services at affordable prices to the right customer at the right time. At a time when BPO units in urban centres have put on hold hiring plans, rural BPO centres seem to be sprouting at various locations, offering jobs to young people from tier II and tier III towns who would otherwise have been forced to migrate to the bigger cities for employment. Thus the rural BPO will not only be an information service provider but also generate income for the unemployed people, carving the way towards equitable sustainable development.

The model comprises of a rural call centre which is the information centre. The rural call centre will have all the relevant information related to the various services that has been short listed. The data collection team which comprises of the village level staff will be responsible for collection and updating of the information. The staff will be guided by the data screening specialist who will be responsible for the sorting of data

Table 6. Aggregating the services with respect to age, income and gender

Parameter / Services	Service1	Service2	Service3	Service 4	Service 5	Service 6
Occupation	Loan	Emergency				
Age	Agri	Transportation	Emergency	Health	Loan	
Income	Agri	Insurance	Loan	Emergency	Govt	Health
Gender	Agri	Insurance	Loan	Emergency	Govt	Education

Table 7. Summarizing the findings

Services	Type of information	Preferred by			
		Occupation	Monthly income	Age	Gender
LOAN	Name of the bank	Businessmen	Rs.1000-5000	18-25	Male
	Prevailing interest rate				
	Type of loans				
	Repayment schedule				
	Collateral/guarantee				
	Distance of the bank from the village				
	Contact person				
	Phone number				
EMERGENCY	Hospital	Businessmen	Rs.1000-5000	18-25	Male
	Technicians(Electrician/Plumber)				
	Police station				
	Fire Brigade				
	Post Office				
	Fair price shop				
	Petrol pump				
AGRICULTURE	Agri inputs	Farmers	Rs.1000-5000	18-25	Male
	Resource person				
	Government offices				
	Credit schemes				
	Storage facilities				
	Market information				
	Logistics provider				
HEALTH	Hospital	Drivers and businessmen	Rs.1000-5000	18-25	Male
	Specialist				
	OPD timings				
	Medicine store				
	Diagnostic centre				
	Rate chart for pathological tests				
	Appointment(specialised services)				
	Contact person				
	Distance				
GOVT SCHEMES	Ongoing govt. schemes	Drivers and businessmen	-	26-35	Male
EDUCATION	Admission dates	Students male and female equally	-	Under 18 and 18-25	Both male and female
	Eligibility criteria				
	Application form cost				
	Contact person				
	Location				
	Distance from village				
	Coaching/tuition facilities				

and make it available to the call centre in a usable form (information). The rural masses will be the customers who can make a call to the call centre and can avail the facility of obtaining information from the various sectors. The call centre will have a tie-up with the various clients who will act as a source of revenue for the call centre. For e.g. the various private institutions can have a tie up with the call centre. These institutions will provide relevant information with the call centre which can then share with the caller.

In case a customer query is not processed in a given amount of time the rural call centre takes some amount of buffer time in order to process the call (a day or two) and then revert back to the customer. In this way maintaining positive customer relationship will promote the customer spread positive word of mouth about the call centre.

The rural call centre architecture will have the following features:

- State of the art computerization with fully automated call desks.
- Uninterrupted and backup power supply.
- Fully redundant voice and data communications with security.
- Dedicated and high speed internet connectivity for 100% uptime and availability
- Scalable capacity.
- Duplicated system to ensure uninterrupted call reception and uninterrupted internet connectivity.
- Security by tight infrastructure access levels protected by multi layered physical and logical security.

ROAD MAP

Before setting up the call centre in the areas prospective villages would be identified based on mapping exercises. For identification of villages we would partner with the local NGOs and civil society organisations. Information regarding parameters like name of the village, block, district, location status, total no. of households, total population, major occupation of the villagers, distance of village from the NGO, electrification status, condition of supply, awareness about internet and communication technology would be collected.

After the collection of village data the location of the call centre would be finally decided by the management team based on the feasibility analysis which would be done on parameters like centralised location of the place from all the villages, availability of resources like manpower, electricity etc., and interest of the various stakeholders.

REVENUE MODEL

In the initial days of operation of the call centre the revenue will be generated from the company and service providers regarding which the information will be provided by the customer executives to the rural consumers. For e.g. the name of the bank providing the loan will always try to acquire new set of customers and therefore would like to use the platform for its advertisement and brand promotion. Similarly a coaching centre would like to increase the number of enrolment and thereby

Table 8. Roadmap

0-1 month	Baseline survey
2- 6month	Construction of BPO, hiring of manpower, Identification of village contact person and entrepreneur who owns the service station,
7-12 month	Training of staff in terms of data collection team, data screening specialist, data base manager, project officer, administrative staff etc.
13-18 month	Launch of the call centre operations, data base management and updation, promotion and advertisement
19-24 month	Expansion of services in different blocks and replication of the model
25-36	Full scale operation of call centre operations Franchising and finding new partners who can take the similar model in other districts of the state.

its popularity. Through our service he can get the market penetration in the untapped but potential areas. On a later stage after customers start realising the importance of the service the concept of a calling card will be introduced which the user has to buy for a limited validity period and a specified talk time for using our service. As per our estimate in a normal scenario the rural call centre will cater to the needs of one Gram Panchayat with population of around 8000-1000 initially.

CONCLUSION

Majority of people live in inaccessible areas, furthermore illiteracy, ignorance and lack of proper communication leads to lesser utilization of available resources. High cost of transportation facilities and lack of investment for creation of service in rural areas creates a deficit of services in these areas. This project aims to deliver required services to the unmet population at their door step through telecommunication in a cost-effective manner.

The project had been specifically planned according to the bottom of pyramid approach which addresses large and simple needs of the customers. The project mainly uses the existing relevant technologies which are affordable by the common man. The age limit of average Indians lies in the range of 25-35 years, and majority of the population are acquainted by the usage of the Information and communication technologies, and in the coming years when they will move to a higher age group these types of services will be beneficial for them in future. The project is having a competitive edge over other system because it is one of the simplest manners to get connected to a service provider, without hesitation.

The management structure will help in promotion of workers participation of all fronts bringing about a holistic development of the village by generating gainful employment opportunities. It would also help in addressing the gender issues in development and other social taboos. This village would serve as a role model for other villages to learn the importance of leadership and social entrepreneurship. Though many initiatives are being taken for rural development, much more needs to be done to integrate efforts and make socio-economic development more rurally inclusive. To this end, we hope that our research and submissions will generate pro-active strategies to effectively help the rural poor.

The proposed model has been discussed with practitioners and several non government organisations (NGO). Detailed discussions have been carried out with different stakeholders and we are in the pilot stage of implementation. The results so far have been encouraging and we hope the same model can be applied to other developing countries with similar demographic profile. It will be interesting to watch the results from this experimentation in other parts of the world.

REFERENCES

Agrawal, B. C. (2006). Communication technology and rural development in India: Promises and performances. *Indian Media Studies Journal*, *1*(1), 1–10.

Anand, S., Patra, B. P., & Kumar, I. (2007). Cognitive justice for consumers: Mediation through efficiency of information exchanges. Indian Institute of Management Kozhikode. In *Conference Proceeding, International Conference on Marketing and Society*.

Andres, R. & Kelly, J. (2009). Non-profit and for profit convergence: Are non-profits increasingly adopting private sector practices. *International Journal of Society Systems Science*, *1*(4), 307-324

Annamalai, K., & Rao, S. (2003). *Case study series. Michigan Business School*. Department of Corporate Strategy and International Business.

Barton, B. (2003). The internet's impact on agricultural input distribution channels. *Review of Agricultural Economics*, *25*(1), 14–21. doi:10.1111/1467-9353.00042

Biyani, K. (2006). *It happened in India*. New Delhi, India: Rupa & Co.

Bonabeau, E. (2009). Decisions 2.0: The power of collective intelligence. *MIT Sloan Management Review*, *50*(2), 45–52.

Bowonder, B., Gupta, V., & Singh, A. (2005). *Developing a rural market e-hub: The case study of e–Choupal experience of ITC*. Retrieved October 30, 2005, from http://planningcommission.nic.in/reports/sereport/ser/stdy_ict/4_e-choupal%20.pdf

Corney, J. R., Torres-Sánchez, C., Jagadeesan, A. P., Yan, X. T., Regli, W. C., & Medellin, H. (2010). Role of technology in rural call centre. *Advanced Engineering Informatics*, *24*(3), 243–250. doi:10.1016/j.aei.2010.05.011

Economic Times.com (2010). *Gender equality. Women lead the way in rural BPOs*. Retrieved from http://economictimes.indiatimes.com/Infotech/Gender_equality_Women_lead_the_way_in_rural_BPOs/articleshow/3072242.cms. 2010

Hart, S. L., & London, T. (2005). *Developing native capability what multinational corporations can learn from the base of the pyramid*. Stanford Social Innovation Review Summer.

ibid. (2010). Retrieved from http://www.ibid.informindia.co.in

Knowledge for Development. (2010). Retrieved from http://www.knowledgefordevelopment.com

Leimeister, J. M., Huber, M., Bretschneider, U., & Krcmar, H. (2009). Leveraging crowdsourcing: Activation-supporting components for IT-based ideas competition. *Journal of Management Information Systems*, *26*(1), 197–224. doi:10.2753/MIS0742-1222260108

Mario, O. G. (2008). The role of BPOs in rural transformation: The GramIT experience, *IDCA Conference*, New Delhi, India.

Marker, P., McNamara, K., & Wallace, L. (2002). The significance of information and communication technologies for reducing poverty. *Department for International Development, London*. Retrieved from http://www.dfid.gov.uk/

Mohapatra, S., & Raha, N. (2008). Role of IT for poverty alleviation for weavers in Orissa, India. In R. Dr Gera (Ed.), *Advances in Technology and Innovations in Marketing*. New Delhi: Macmillan.

Nasscom. (2009). *The Indian I.T. strategy*. New Delhi, India: NASSCOM. Retrieved from http://www.NASSCOM.org

Oecd. (2010). Retrieved from http://www.oecd.org

Pitula, K., & Radhakrishnan, T. (2007). A conceptual model of inclusive technology for information access by the rural sector. *Proceedings of the HCII Conference*. doi:10.1007/978-3-540-73279-2_28

Porter, M. E., & Millar, V. E. (2001). How Information gives you competitive advantage. *Harvard Business Review*, 149–174.

Prahalad, C. K. (2004). *The fortune at the bottom of the pyramid: Eradicating poverty through profits*. Wharton School Publishing.

Prahalad, C. K. (2004). *The fortune at the bottom of the pyramid: Eradicating poverty through profits*. Wharton School Publishing.

Prahalad, C. K., & Ramaswamy, V. (2004). *The future of competition: Co creating unique value with customers*. Harvard Business School Press.

Prahalad, C. K., & Ramaswamy, V. (2004). *The future of competition: Co creating unique value with customers*. Harvard Business School Press.

Senteni, A., & Johari, A. (2006). Information and communications technology integration and developmental intervention: Enabling knowledge creation and capacity building in developing countries' organizations. *Educational Technology Research and Development, 54*, 299–300.

Sharp, D. (2003). Knowledge management today: Challenges and opportunities. *Information Systems Management, 20*(2), 32–37.

Shen, R. (2005, May 16-19). Expansion of ITC's eChoupal initiative in ASEAN countries via FDI: An interactive case study. UNITAR/SHU Series on International Economics and Finance. Foreign Direct Investment for Development Financing. Organized jointly by UNITAR and the Stillman Schools of Business at Seton Hall University (SHU), Hiroshima, Japan.

Shiva, V. (1997). *Biopiracy: The plunder of nature and knowledge.* Cambridge, UK: South End Press.

Simon, H. A. (1968). The future of information processing technology. *Management Science, 14*(9), 619–624. doi:10.1287/mnsc.14.9.619

Singh, N. (2005). Information technology and India's economic development, in India's emerging economy: Performance and prospects in the 1990S and beyond (pp. 244-245). Oxford University Press.

Solution Exchange. (2010). Retrieved from http://www.solutionexchange-un.net.in

U Penn. (2010). Retrieved from http://knowledge.wharton.upenn.edu/india/article.cfm?articleid=4450

Udayngo. (2010). Retrieved from http://www.udayngo.org

Umit, T., Basoglu, N. A., & Tugrul, U. D. (2010). Rural call centre a reality with technology. International Journal of Information Systems in the Service Sector, 2(1), 71-93.

Unhchr. (2010). Retrieved from http://www.unhchr.ch/udhr/lang/eng.htm

Upton, D. M., & Fuller, V. A. (2004). *The ITC e-Choupal initiative.* Harvard Business School.

Van der Velden, M. (2005). Programming for cognitive justice towards an ethical framework for democratic code. *Interacting with Computers, 17*(1), 105–120. doi:10.1016/j.intcom.2004.10.004

Venkatesh, V., Morris, M. G., Davis, G., & Fred, D. (2003). User acceptance of information technology: Toward a unified view. *Management Information Systems Quarterly, 27*(3), 425–478.

Visvanathan, S. (1998). A celebration of difference: Science and democracy in India. *Science, 280*, 5360–5375.

Visvanathan, S. (2001). Knowledge and information in a network society. *Seminar.*

Visvanathan, S. (2002). *Transfer of technology. International Encyclopedia of Social and Behavioral Sciences.* Oxford, UK: Elsevier Science.

Von-Pischke, J. (1989). *Finance at the frontier: Debt capacity and the role of credit in developing the private economy. Economic Development Institute of the World Bank.* Washington, DC: The World Bank.

Washington Post. (2010). Retrieved form http://www.washingtonpost.com/wpdyn/content/article/2009/01/04/AR2009010401502.html

WTO.org (2010). Retrieved from http://www.wto.org/english/thewto_e/whatis_e/tif_e/agrm6_e.htm

This work was previously published in the International Journal of Information Systems in the Service Sector (IJISSS), 6(2); edited by John Wang, pages 1-17 copyright year 2014 by IGI Publishing (an imprint of IGI Global).

Chapter 42
Distributed Leadership and Its Applications in Health Care Settings:
Social Media Perspective

Vida Farzipour
University of London, UK

ABSTRACT

In this chapter, I go through distributed leadership which is one of the mainstreams of plural leadership from social media perspective. In addition, the attributes and variants of distributed leadership are covered in this chapter. The role of social media to help the distribution of power and increasing engagement to enhance the quality of care and patient safety is also addressed in the health care context. It is concluded that Understanding distributed leadership and its application in the health care setting is largely related to the appreciation of the political and social power that currently exists.

INTRODUCTION

With the advent of the 21st century, the discourse of leadership has changed and new vocabularies have entered into the language of leadership: shared, dispersed, distributive, collaborative, collective, co-operative, concurrent, co-ordinated, and co-leadership - all encouraging the concept that leadership needs to be plural. Thus, "Leadership in the plural" has been developed by leadership authors in response to the critiques of heroic models of leadership (Fletcher, 2004; Uhl-Bien, 2006). Fletcher (2004) emphasised that the focal point of

plural leadership is that less hierarchical leadership is needed in organisations where leadership responsibilities can be distributed throughout the organisation. Effectively, distributed leadership and shared leadership are the most commonly used terms to describe similar structures (James, 2011), however, more effort has been put into publishing on distributed leadership in the UK (Bolden, 2011).

"Distributed leadership has become a popular 'post heroic' (Badaracco 2001) representation of leadership which has encouraged a shift in focus from the attributes and behaviours of individual

DOI: 10.4018/978-1-4666-8756-1.ch042

'leaders' (as promoted within traditional trait, situational, style and transformational theories of leadership) to a more systematic perspective, whereby 'leadership' is conceived of as a collective social process emerging through the interactions of multiple actors (Uhl-Bien 2006)" (Cited in Bolden, 2011, p. 251). Distributed leadership has been developed widely by the work of researchers in education (Spillane, 2006; Gronn, 2002) and has become one of the mainstreams of plural leadership in which leadership responsibilities are shared among different people throughout the organisation and beyond its boundaries over time to achieve effective organisational outcomes (Denis et al., 2012).

Organizations are facing many unsolved problems, accompanied by the difficulty of meeting all followers' expectations (Currie & Lockett, 2011). There is no doubt that leadership is important throughout all organizations because many leadership issues cannot be solved by single leaders as they may not have adequate and appropriate information to make effective decisions (James, 2011; Pearce and Conger, 2003; Heifetz, 1994). Therefore, distributed leadership offers a potential answer to these problems by increasing employees' autonomy and empowering them to take on leadership roles and work collaboratively (Buchanan, Addicott, Fitzgerald, Ferlie, & Baeza, 2007). On the other hand, in modern organizations, communities need to be established where individuals "share the experience of serving as a leader, not sequentially, but concurrently and collectively" (Raelin, 2005, p. 18). It is good practice when leaders are acknowledged to be supported by a network of employees throughout an organization, engaging in leadership practice collaboratively and spontaneously but not necessarily known as leaders (James, 2011).Therefore, here we can see the value of distributed leadership. "Distributed leadership is viewed as desirable in public services because it is inclusive and aligns

with recent organizational restructuring towards the flatter organization. It may foster collaborative and ethical practice and avoid alienation associated with lack of power by those positioned as followers. And it is considered to be particularly appropriate for complex, contemporary organizations, where knowledge is distributed" (Currie & Lockett, 2011, p. 287).

The interest of applying distributed leadership within healthcare has started recently, which is now widely acknowledged to be the responsibility of everyone within the organization, and a distributed culture of leadership is encouraged throughout the organisation (James, 2011; No More Heroes, 2011; Rowling, 2012). The NHS in England is incredibly complex, consisting of various organisations such as hospital trusts, teaching hospitals and primary care trusts with their own unique characteristics. They are performing within a pluralistic environment that involves doctors, patients, nurses, professional staff, managers and politicians from diverse cultures, mentalities and clinical and political attitudes. The variety of groups working in the health care sector, the hierarchical structure and political influences all combine to make effective change hard to achieve in the NHS. In spite of these difficulties, the NHS has experienced dramatic changes in its history in terms of leadership. Hartley and Benington (2010) also argued that due to the financial crisis and decline in public expenditure, there has been more focus on the leadership and the role of leaders in the health and social care sectors. In spite of the constant drive towards the provision of an excellent service over the last few years, the health sector has experienced severe failures in terms of quality of care and patient safety (Watcher, 2010). These significant failures, especially those from Mid-Staffordshire NHS Trust, have highlighted the crucial role of leadership in finding a solution to improve the safety and quality of care (Francis, 2010). However, it is very important to decide on the leadership that would be effective and more appropriate for health care structure with a view to enhancing quality and safety. In recent years, the NHS has tended to distribute leadership to create a flatter structure among its units; this has been implemented to try to achieve its goals in improving the quality of health services (e.g. James, 2011; Rowling, 2012). In addition, health service users' expectations, as well as public expectations, put more pressure on health policy makers to improve the quality of care and patient safety by setting practical goals and standards in the NHS (Griffith's Report, 1983).

Nowadays the Internet plays an important role in our daily life which encourages the growing use of social networks among all ages. It provides an environment for collaborating and sharing information (Von Muhlen & Ohno-Machado, 2012) for all participants. Furthermore, an increase in the use of social media by clinical staff (Vance, Howe, & Dellavalle, 2009; Von Muhlen & Ohno-Machado, 2012) can facilitate the distribution of leadership in health care by promoting the collaboration and interaction between patients and health professionals. They can easily be engaged in leadership activities and decision making online through social media. Applying IT in health care can help health care to achieve its goals and objectives such as reducing costs, enhancing the quality of care, increase access to health care information and increase the effectiveness and efficiency of the services (Castro, 2009).

Towards these ends, the author in this research is looking at previous studies on distributed leadership, especially those which have been carried out in health care systems including NHS England. In this research, focus will be on distributed leadership and its association and impact on patient outcomes and patient engagement to respond to a gap in application of distributed leadership and its benefits in health care from social media perspective.

RESEARCH BACKGROUND

Application of Distributed Leadership in Health Care Settings

"England represents a 'fast mover' regarding implementation of transformational leadership and distributed leadership within public service organizations (PSOs). Policy-makers have acted in two ways to encourage more effective leadership of PSOs. Firstly, they have implemented structural reform away from markets and hierarchies (in rhetorical terms at least), towards network forms of service delivery. Secondly, they have implemented large-scale leadership education initiatives to orientate public service leaders towards distributed leadership" (Currie & Luckett, 2011, p 293). Because of the way that NHS practice is changing, the model of the 'romantic' or 'superhero' leader is ill-suited to current demands (James, 2011, p.18) and the post heroic model is needed in the NHS (No More Heroes, 2011) in which everybody can play a part by spreading responsibilities to achieve desired goals. So the NHS needs leadership, not only from "the board to the ward" but also across its boundaries into the wide variety of institutions with which it interacts, such as social care and local government. There now needs to be a move from heroic leadership to shared and distributed leadership in which everybody is involved to achieve excellent health care outcomes (Ham, 2008; Mountford & Webb, 2009; James, 2011; McKee, Charles, Dixon-Woods, Willars, & Martin, 2013). With this in mind, allied to government policy in health and social care, the coalition government has decided to apply Mr. Darzi's reform in his Next Stage Review report (Department of Health, 2008) which promotes distribution of leadership to clinicians. Therefore, the government is keen to engage general practitioners to take a lead in "planning and commissioning of health and social care in England" (Currie and Lockett, 2011, p.

292). Consequently, more effort has been made to distribute leadership to patients too (Department of Health, 2010). Thus, Sharing leadership is needed in health care and it cannot be led just by managers and left in the hands of the few; doctors, clinicians, nurses and other health professionals should be involved to achieve excellent health care outcomes (Ham, 2008; Mountford & Webb, 2009; McKee et al, 2013).

A healthcare setting is an appropriate context to be investigated for different reasons. Firstly, improving patient outcomes (quality of care and patient safety) is crucial to healthcare and it is valued politically and socially. Better patient outcomes have been in deficit for the last few years due to several failures and despite health-care attempts to improve the quality and safety of care delivered to patients (McKee et al, 2013). However, heroic models of leadership have failed to improve quality of care and patient safety as it cannot be achieved by individual managers alone. Staff and patients should be involved in leadership practice; leadership needs to be distributed across the organization (McKee et al., 2013). Secondly, the hieratical structure of the NHS (top-down) is working against those leaders who try to share leadership. In addition to this hierarchical and bureaucratic structure of the NHS (Mintzberg, 1979), traditional professional hierarchy (Martin, 2008), concentration of power (Fitzgerald & Ferlie, 2006) and the paternalistic and authoritarian stance (Bate, 2000) may constrain and restrict the distribution of leadership. Thus, this vertical structure needs to become flatter to provide a capacity for everybody to be engaged in leadership practice which is a crucial part of health policy. Thirdly, the relationship between managers and clinicians is very important in today's complex structure of health care; there are power bases across the organization and this may cause conflict between those groups (McKee et al., 2013). An important tool to minimise the conflict in health care is increasing clinical engagement in leadership roles (Ham & Dickinson, 2008; No More Heroes, 2011). Finally, health care provision in the UK is conducted in a complex organization and is regarded as a fast mover in policy reform and restructuring (Martin, Currie, & Finn, 2009). Therefore, this complex, pluralistic organization cannot be managed with low quality standards of management and leadership; there has been scrutiny of moves to implement an effective leadership style, recently recognized as distributed leadership (e.g. McKee, 2013; The King's Fund report, 2011, 2012).

There has been limited research into the significance of distributed leadership effect on organizational performance. In spite of this, Agle, Nagarajan, Sonnenfeld, and Srinivasan (2006), and De hoogh et al. (2004) note that distributed leadership has been widely used by policy-makers to improve organizational performance of public service organizations, including the NHS, by engaging stakeholders and service users to involve them in leadership tasks (Currie, Boyett, & Suhomlinova, 2005).

The Application of Social Media in Health Care

The accessibility of the internet has provided great opportunities for people to use social media to communicate online (Gruzd, Wellman, & Takhteyev, 2011). Having access to customer's information and reviews provided invaluable sources for other customers (Senecal & Nantel, 2004). "By using social media, consumers can create content and offer valuable advice to others (Füller et al. 2009, cited in Hajli, 2014). This new development has seen online communities and an electronic network of individuals emerge on social platforms where members share information globally and quickly" (Molly, McLure & Samer, 2005, cited in Hajli, 2014). The rise of using online communities and social media promoted customer involvement (Park, Lee & Han, 2007) and information sharing (Chen & Whinston, 2011a). Communities will form the next generation of online businesses which provide the opportunities for a better customer-manager relationship in organisations (Ridings & Gefen 2004).

The United Kingdom is one of the developed countries where the government invested in health IT as a single-payer health care system (Smee, 2007). The NHS is one of the largest employers in the world and its National programme for IT is one of the most expensive eHealth programmes in the world (Gerard, 2006). In health care online health portals provide web-based health services and information for people to manage their own health care needs (Castro, 2009). Applying IT in health care system can reduce medical errors and improve patient safety (Lucian et al, 2005).

These days more health care centers are providing health and medical information through social media (Van de Belt, 2012) and the use of social media by clinical staff has increased dramatically in recent years (Vance et al., 2009; Von Muhlen & Ohno-Machado, 2012). It gives the opportunity to health care providers to increase patients' awareness of their own disease and treatment options (Prasad, 2013). Multiple actors in the health care are needed to promote the use of IT and online communities. Strong leadership is also required to coordinate the stakeholders' actions and obtaining a common goal in the NHS which is improving quality of care and patient safety. Therefore, the distribution of leadership can facilitate achieving this goal (Castro, 2009). The use of social media is an important skill for leaders in health care. It can be achieved by applying distributed leadership in which staff and patients can be engaged in leadership activities and decision making. Social media facilitate this engagement and make the interaction between patient and health professional more effective (Iverson, Howard & Penney, 2008; Chretien, Azar, & Kind, 2011) and enables patients to manage their illnesses. In addition, reliable medical information needs to be provided online to make sure that patients have access to authentic and standard information: this is an important responsibility of clinicians (Prasad, 2013). Ef-

fectively, patient can trust more on online medical information. Thus, "The concept of the "e-patient" represents a fundamental change in the role that a number of patients wish to play in managing their health care, reflecting more proactively with less hierarchical health care delivery, signaling more collaboration" (Prasad, 2013, p.493).

According to Prasad (2013, p.492) "Social media can be used to increase compliance with medications, patient support, and education, and links with patient support groups; encourage institutional loyalty; and enhance the overall physician-patient interaction, which itself can often be time restricted". Main purposes of using social media in health care are: firstly, patients who have same disease sharing their experience and support each other emotionally (Hardiker & Grant, 2011) and obtain information on disease and treatment (Van de Belt, 2012; Eysenbach, 2008). Secondly, social media can improve the communication and interaction between health care staff and patient (Bosslet, Torke, Hickman, Terry & Helft 2011; Cline & Haynes, 2001). Thirdly, using social media is cost-efficient (Van de Belt, 2012): this is a crucial point for the NHS that trying to reduce costs as well as improving quality of care. An important application of IT in health care is that it enables and empowers people to manage their own health care effectively by communicating with health care providers (Castro, 2009). It matches with the recent NHS effort to be patient-centric and try to engage patients in decision making of their own care by distribution of leadership and facilitate it by using Internet and online communities. Social media can be a complementary of the application of distributed leadership and facilitate engaging employees and patients in leadership activities and decision making.

What Is Leadership?

The theories of leadership started with trait and behavioural style by focusing on personal characteristics, traits and behaviour of leaders and went through contingency theory before moving towards transformational, transactional and heroic models of leadership then ending with post-heroic models of leadership. Therefore, post-heroic approaches such as distributed leadership, collaborative leadership and shared leadership have been more influential styles of leadership in recent years. However, distributed leadership seems to be a much more universal idea which creates a concrete base for other new leadership models.

It was traditionally believed that leadership cannot spread to the lower levels of an organization; this was a fundamental assumption until recently. It was assumed that a leadership model can be conceived as a tripod of leaders, followers and organizational goals (Bennis, 2007). So, the focus of leadership development traditionally was on improving leaders' traits, influencing followers and achieving organizational goals. Contrary to this popular view, Drath et al. (2008) believed that this construction (leaders, followers and common goals) is limited. While Drath et al. (2008) were not against using the idea of the leadership tripod, they suggested adding another approach. They believed that the essence of leadership is constructed of three leadership outcomes -direction, alignment and commitment. Direction is a collective agreement on goals, aims and responsibility. Alignment is a collective coordination of knowledge and tasks that are effective. Commitment is the enthusiasm of people to merge their personal interests into the collective interests of the organization. The focus of this approach is on how members can collectively generate these outcomes rather than focusing on leaders, followers and shared goals.

"Leadership is relational (Uhl-Bien, 2006) and contextual (Osborn, Hunt, & Jauch, 2002); it is insufficiently explained by the notion of leaders and followers" (James, 2011, p. 5). Moreover, Clegg, Kornberger, and Pitis (2008, p. 662) define leadership as "the process of directing, controlling, motivating and inspiring staff towards the realization of stated organizational goals". Leadership has been seen as a process in Clegg's et al. (2008)

definition which simply means it can be carried out by a group as a shared distributed responsibility, not necessarily by an individual. Therefore, leadership is considered to be "the outcome of dynamic, collective activity through the building of relationships and networks of influence. It is therefore as much bottom up as top down, with more egalitarian interactions where the person labelled 'leader' behaves in a less hierarchical way than leaders traditionally have done. Roles may even change, with someone labelled 'leader' in one situation but 'follower' with the same people in others. Leadership creates an environment where new knowledge – collective learning – can be co-created and implemented rather than just the implementation of a top leader plan" (James, 2011, p. 6). Broadening the perception of new models of leadership and its patterns are needed for leadership development; otherwise the organization will end up with a system of trial and error without developing appropriate leadership behaviour.

Theoretical Roots of Distributed Leadership

According to Oduro (2004), the story of distributed leadership goes back to 1250 BC, noting that "one of the most ancient leadership notions recommended for fulfilling organizational goals through people" (p. 4). However, Harris (2009) believed that the idea of distributed leadership can be attributed to the mid 20th century. Gronn (2000) is also in agreement with Harris that the idea of distributed leadership was first mentioned by the Australian leadership theorist Gibb in 1954. In his handbook of social psychology he explicitly states that "leadership is probably best conceived as a group quality, as a set of functions which must be carried out by the group" (Gibb, 1954, cited in Gronn 2000, p. 324; Bolden, 2011, p. 252). Gronn (1999) alluded to Gibb's idea that leadership is normally distributed and dispersed rather than being under the control of one person. He also argued that we should look at leadership in a distributed form in the current century (Gronn, 2000). He stated that " The reality, in fact, is that the leadership of organizations is normally distributed, dispersed and diffused rather than concentrated in one or a few hands"(Gronn, 1999, p. 3). Moreover, Currie et al. (2011) also state that it was Gibb who first used a distributed pattern of leadership in 1954, but this remained inactive until its revival by Brown and Hosking in 1986. Similarly, Yasini, Arasteh, Ebrahim, and Zeinabadi (2012) argued that distributed leadership has been used from the 1950s, and has been re-reviewed by Elmore (2000), Spillane (2001) and Gronn (2002) to build a theoretical framework for it at the beginning of the 21st century. Since then, it has been considered by a number of different authors in different contexts. Thus, the twenty first century model places emphasis on delegated responsibility among various organizational groups while moving towards sharing values, culture and traditions (Elmore, 2000).

What Is Distributed Leadership?

There is no agreed definition of distributed leadership as there are some ambiguities about what should be distributed and by whom. Different authors have defined distributed leadership in various ways (Peck & Dickinson, 2008); Raelin (2005, p. 18) defined distributed leadership as a process in which activities are concerned with establishing communities in which "everyone shares the experience of serving as a leader, not sequentially, but concurrently and collectively". Moreover, Spillane (2005, p.149) stated that "distributed leadership is often cast as some sort of monopolistic construct when, in fact, it is merely an emerging set of ideas that frequently diverge from one another". In addition, Fitzgerald and Buchanan (2013) have given an empirical description of distributed leadership with three elements; senior leaders, credible leaders and people who are willing to be involved in change attempts.

According to Elmore (2000, p. 13), "Leadership is the guidance and direction of instructional improvement". He focused on distributed leadership in schools in which leadership responsibilities were distributed among people across the school so as to achieve shared values and a shared culture (Elmore, 2000).

In distributed leadership "appointed leaders are seen as one voice among many in a larger coordinated social process" (Uhl-Bien, 2006, p. 662), but the 'leaders' themselves may change over a period of time. In addition, Huffington et al. (2004) stated that implementing distributed leadership needs an appreciation of the psychological and emotional challenges that leaders are facing; also needed a change in attitudes towards the concept of leadership and also a perception of leadership tasks at different levels. This does not mean that leaders do not require developing their own personal skills and capabilities. These are needed in learning how to cope with new situations and tasks (James, 2011; James & Ladkin, 2008). Buchanan et al. (2007) also opined that "Leadership needs to be numerous, brief, transient, fluid, migratory, ambiguous and distributed, with many leadership actors engaging and disengaging over time" (cited in Currie and Lockett, 2011, p. 291). According to Spillane (2001), distributed perspective makes leadership more than a set of traits or behaviours; it becomes a series of tasks, and leadership will move from an individual to a web of leaders, followers and situation.

Merha, Smith, Dixon, and Robertson (2006) focused the effect of distributed leadership on performance by using a social networks analysis. They found that certain kinds of centralized leadership structures are related to better team performance. They also suggested that a distributed leadership structure can be different according to structural characteristics; this can have important implications for team performance. On the other hand, Bolden (2011) concluded that usage of distributed leadership depends on different contexts, region and countries. This was done by reviewing conceptual and empirical literature on the concept of distributed leadership to find its origins, and its similarities and differences with shared, collective, collaborative, emergent, democratic and co-leadership. Moreover, Fitzsimons et al., (2011) identified four different patterns of shared and distributed leadership; "relational-entity, relational-structural, relational-processual, and relational-systemic". In the literature they raised fundamental points about how we think about development and the practice of leadership.

Gronn (2002) looked at distributed leadership as a unit of analysis and more specifically as a numerical action and as a concertive action. He believes that during the past two decades we were preoccupied by individual heroic models of leadership and now the time for distributed leadership has come (Gronn, 2000). He also pointed out that distributed leadership can potentially be a solution to the current conception of leadership (Gronn, 2000). He supports the distributed leadership pattern that Gibb had in mind in his study. This generated further work in various studies in the area of distributed leadership (Gronn, 2002).

Patterns of Distributed Leadership

In this section, the author will discuss different patterns of distributed leadership as explored by Gronn (2002) which have also been taken into consideration by other authors (e.g. Currie and Luckett, 2011; James, 2011):

1. **Numerical Action Perspective:** Gronn (2002, p. 429) points out "If focused leadership means that only one individual is attributed with the status of leader, an additive or numerical view of distributed leadership means the aggregated leadership of an organization is dispersed among some, many, or maybe all of the members". The numerical aspect of Gronn's definition of distributed leadership does not ignore individuals who may do more work than their colleagues.

However, it aims to provide more opportunities for all members of the organization to experience leadership to some extent (Wenger, 2000).

2. **Concertive Action Perspective:** Gronn's (2002) holistic sense of distributed leadership is known as 'concertive action' rather than aggregated individual acts in the numerical sense. "Gronn (2002) uses the term 'concertive' action to explain distributed leadership as spontaneous collaboration, intuitive working relations and institutionalized practice, which together represent an increasing degree of institutionalization – from unplanned, short-term collaborations to formalised organizational structures. A brief explanation of each element can be seen as following:

a. **Spontaneous Collaboration:** Spontaneous collaboration occurs in the work place, where more than two individuals with different skills and expertise from different organizational levels unify to pool their skills and regularize conduct to do a task and provide opportunities for synergy, the trigger for continuous collaboration (Gronn, 2002).

b. **Intuitive Working Relations:** Intuitive working relations involve a shared role that appears when two or more people develop a close working relationship within an implicit framework of understanding each other (Gronn, 2002). In this regard, Gabarro (1978, p. 294) found that the mutual influence that people can have on one another in such a relationship was ''very much dependent on how much that person was trusted by the other''.

c. **Institutionalized Practices:** Working together can be viewed as evolving into a concertive structure which may be grafted onto an existing formal framework of governance (Gronn, 2002). This form of distributed leadership institutionalizes formal structures or mechanisms either by design or adaption (Gronn, 2002).

3. **Conjoint Agency:** Conjoint agency is a co-ordination of each unit member's individual acts with the overall plans which are merged from their own and their peers' plans (Gronn, 2002). Currie and Lockett (2011, p. 289) define conjoint agency as "the direction of leadership influence". Conjoint agency involves two patterns: Firstly, the experience of synergy is seen as purely internal to the concertive unit, while the second is reciprocal influence which is both internal and external (Gronn, 2000). Discussing the experience of synergy, Follett (1973, p. 162) says that each unit member "calls out something from the other, releases something, frees something, opens the way for the expression of latent capacities and possibilities" (cited in Gronn, 2002). In reciprocity, "two or more parties influence one another; this occurs in a manner akin to 'a zigzagging spiral' or a 'virtuous cycle', with each person in these arrangements bearing the accumulated effects of successive phases of influence as they begin to influence one another again" (Gronn, 2002, cited in Currie & Lockett, p. 289). In doing so, in their relations with their colleagues, they are open themselves to the influence of their peers and may influence them in return (Gronn, 2002).

Distributed Leadership Variants

To some authors (e.g. Pearce & Conger, 2003; Katzenbach & Smith, 1993; Sims & Lorenzi, 1992), distributed leadership does not mean avoiding leadership hierarchy, but instead identifies the application of distributed leadership in a top-down fashion such as super leadership (leaders develop the leadership qualities of others), team leadership (leadership qualities are promoted in team players by a leader's mentoring role), collective leadership (leadership is shared within a strategic group) and shared leadership; these are more conjoint and less concertive. On the other hand, another group of researchers regard distributed leadership as a bottom-up activity such as collaborative leadership or a structure with nobody in charge (e.g. Buchanan et al., 2007); these are more concertive and less conjoint (Currie & Lockett, 2011). Currie and Lockett (2011) merged literatures that have already been published in the area of distributed leadership and developed a spectrum of distributed leadership variants. Distributed leadership seems to be a much more global notion and can be pictured as a broad spectrum which represents these smaller entities of leadership. Following, is a brief explanation of distributed leadership variants.

Concertive Model: Different people with various backgrounds collaborate autonomously, pool their expertise, share their roles and establish close relationships (Gronn, 2002).

Conjoint Model: Is the direction of leadership effect which relates to the adjustment and simultaneity of leadership activity within different people, resulting in interpersonal synergy and reciprocal influence (Gronn, 2002).

Currie and Lockett (2011) made it clear that concertive action and conjoint agency are complementary parts of distributed leadership and the absence of one cannot lead to pure distributed leadership. More clearly, the absence of conjoint agency will lead to diffusion in the direction of leadership and there will be no synergy and mutual influence. On the other hand, the absence of concertive action will lead to a direction of a number of leadership activities without any synergy and reciprocal influence (Currie & Lockett, 2011).

Nobody in Charge Model: In the model that Buchanan et al., (2007) developed "nobody is in charge and everybody is in charge", meaning that there is no formal manager or leader but that every individual has a leadership role. This causes inter-relationships to be developed. This model is in contrast to individualistic heroic models of leadership.

Collaborative Model: The purpose of a collaborative model is to create a reciprocal inter-relationship between individuals' actions (Currie & Lockett, 2011). However, the collaboration structures are usually controlled by external agencies (Huxham & Vangen, 2000).

Collective Model: This model emphasizes the effect of external organizations, such as government policy, on the enactment of distributed leadership in health care organizations (Denis, Lamothe, & Langley, 2001). In their investigation, Denis et al. (2001) focused on how context can develop the interactions between leadership actors; this is aligned with the distributed leadership structure demonstrated by Spillane (Spillane et al, 2004; Spillane, 2005; Spillane & Diamond, 2007). In addition, this model concludes that a variety of expertise, skills and influence is essential (Denis et al., 2001). The model of collective leadership seems to be more formal than collaborative leadership and 'nobody in charge' approaches (Currie & Lockett, 2011).

Shared Leadership re-envisions the 'who' (leadership representing a set of practices that can and should be enacted by actors at all levels, rather than a set of personal characteristics and attributes located in a senior level manager), the 'what' (leadership is a group phenomenon, with followers playing a role in influencing and creating leadership) and the 'how' (focus on skills and abilities required to create conditions in which collective learning can occur) of leadership (Currie & Lockett, 2011, p. 290).

Super Leadership places emphasis on empowering people to be able to lead themselves (Sims & Lorenzi 1992). This model helps people to be independent from others, especially formal leaders, and will help to increase their motivation and develop their capacity (Currie & Lockett, 2011).

Team Leadership: Katzenbach and Smith (1993) asserted that team leadership is a process in which leaders act as coaches who facilitate leadership development among others, remove barriers and create opportunities for them to be active team players and enhance their confidence and commitment.

Transformational Leadership: "Transformational leaders are those who stimulate interest among their followers to view their work from new perspectives, who generate awareness of the vision of the organization, who develop in their followers' higher levels of ability and potential and who motivate their colleagues and followers to look beyond their own interests towards those that will benefit the group. Their key behaviours include empowerment, role modelling, creating a vision, acting as change agents and making the norms and values of the group clear to all" (McLaurin & Al Amri, 2008, p. 333; Brown & Mitchell, 2010). To achieve superior results, they behave in different ways by using factors known as the Four I's (McLaurin & Al Amri, 2008). These elements are idealised influence, inspirational motivation, intellectual stimulation and individualised consideration (Bass, 1985; Bryman, 1992). "Idealised influence displays leaders as the most respectful, trustworthy and admirable people, highlighting characteristics such as setting a vision and articulating it so that it will be accomplished; it describes how leaders share risks with their followers in line with ethical principles. Inspirational motivation describes how leaders encourage their employees to achieve a vision by creating both an individual and team spirit. Intellectual stimulation explains how leaders promote their employees' innovative and creative skills through problem solving, questioning assumptions and approaching old problems in entirely new ways, without criticising employees for their mistakes. Finally, individual consideration emphasizes a leader's mentoring role and the development of learning opportunities" (Bass, Avolio, Jung & Berson, 2003, p. 208). Most scholars in management suggest that managers and supervisors owe their employees an ethical approach that reflects a transformational leadership model (Caldwell, 2011).

The Rationales behind Distributed Leadership

The heroic model of leadership could not appropriately display the real nature of leadership (Fletcher & Kaeufer, 2003; Seers, Keller & Wilkerson, 2003; Gronn, 2003). Due to the limitations of individualistic and heroic models of leadership, attention has moved towards the promotion of distributed leadership (Currie at al., 2009a, b & c). Following the emphasis on leadership in the' Modernising Government' white paper (Cabinet Office, 1999, p. 57), policy-makers in England focused on developing and promoting leadership in public services such as the Home Office, the police services, education and the NHS (Currie & Lockett, 2011). Effectively, distributed leadership seen as the more favourite models of leadership for policy makers. According to Fletcher (2004, p. 650) "post heroic leadership re-envisions the 'who' and 'where' of leadership by focusing on the need to distribute the tasks and responsibilities of leadership up, down, and across the hierarchy. It re-envisions the 'what' of leadership by articulating leadership as a social process that occurs in and through human interactions, and it articulates the 'how' of leadership by focusing on the more mutual, less hierarchical leadership practices and skills needed to engage collaborative, collective learning. It is generally recognized that this shift – from individual to collective, from control to learning, from 'self' to 'self-in-relation', and from power over to power with – is a paradigm shift in what it means to be a positional leader. Moreover, Berg (1998) believes that distributed leadership creates a learning organizational environment in which people who have less power do not feel isolated from a group or an activity, so that everybody is involved in leadership practice. By doing this, the dependent status of followership will be removed and leader-centrism will be prevented. In a distributed leadership approach, individuals do not receive any direction, but are given narrative and resources enable them to make collective achievements; this encourages creativity and initiative. For these reasons, and also due to the failure of individualistic and heroic models of leadership, distributed leadership has gained its credible status among other approaches of leadership (Currie & Lockett, 2011; Heifetz, 1994).

Distributed Leadership and Service Improvement in the NHS

The NHS needs a high quality and effective leadership but the complexities of this massive organization have not been fully considered (Rowling, 2012). For this reason, the future of leadership and management in the NHS has been investigated by a commission which has been established by the King's Fund (2011). In this report (No More Heroes, 2011) all the evidence from different sources has been collected to explore which model of leadership is most appropriate for the NHS. In addition, the crucial role of managers in supporting clinical staff has been emphasized to ensure improved patient care as well as the running of the NHS more effectively. In this report, it has been argued that the NHS must turn away from heroic models of leadership and move towards a 'shared and distributed' model not only from the board to the ward but also across the whole organization. Thus, leaders need to work with others to achieve their goals, engage followers and work throughout the organization to deliver high quality patient care.

In addition, Fitzgerald et al. (2013) studied distributed leadership in English healthcare settings. In their study, the patterns of distributed leadership have been analyzed to see whether they have the ability to effect service improvements. Their findings can be categorised as: a pattern of widely distributed leadership and greater service improvement are associated; the presence of effective hybrid roles and better outcomes are associated; distributed leadership was reinforced by the pre-existing relationships between management and professional groups. In addition, the superior role of hybrid leaders in the NHS was recognized, resulting in better health outcomes and service improvement (Fitzgerald et al., 2013). In this regard, Currie and Lockett (2011) recognized distributed leadership as a 'panacea' for policy makers to effect improvement in the performance of health and social care organizations based on the work of Hennessey (1998) and Kakabadse et al. (2003).

Distributed Leadership and Engagement in the NHS

McKee et al. (2013) showed an explicit role of distributed leadership in the NHS in his research, pointing out that engagement of all staff in leading on patients' safety resulted in positive outcomes. It is crucial to engage nurses and allied health professionals to encourage them to take on leadership roles, thus creating a climate in which individuals can improve services and care (James, 2011). Having engaged and motivated employees results in having less mistakes and delivering a high quality health service (Rowling, 2012; Prins et al., 2010), having lesser turnover rates and absenteeism with a high profile of commitment and ethics (Rowling, 2012), having more secure patient care (Laschinger & Leiter, 2006), enhancing performance (Salanova, Agut & Peiro, 2005), improving patient experience and decreasing mortality rates (West & Dawson, 2012)

Patient engagement is also seen to be very important. Empowering patients in order to engage them in their own care, decision making and working closely with their doctors helps to meet their needs. Patient experience is greatly associated with staff involvement (Rowling, 2012). Engaging patients is a crucial part of health policy. The Department of Health (2000) emphasized that services should be shaped based on the taste and preferences of patients as well as their needs. In 2007, World Class Commissioning tried to merge patient and public involvement (PPI) by embedding them into the instructions of services. In 2008, it was stated that patients must be empowered in terms of better choice, more information and more influence (Department of Health, 2008). In 2009, the NHS Constitution stated that patients have the right to influence the level of care and services they receive (Department of Health, 2009b). In 2010, Liberating the NHS emphasized shared decision making between patients and clinicians by stressing that the objectives of health care can only be achieved if patients are fully involved in their own care (Department of Health, 2010).

The Use of Web 2.0 in Health Care

"Web 2.0 is a new advancement, which has transferred the internet to a social environment by introducing social media, where individuals can interact and generate content online" (Lai & Turban, 2008, cited in Hajli, 2014). Web 2.0 was proposed in 2004 in order to facilitate communication and enhance collaboration among people through social media (Antheunis, Tates, & Nieboer, 2013). O'Reilly (2006, p. 4) stated that "Web 2.0 is a set of economic, social, and technology trends that collectively form the basis for the next generation of the Internet–a more mature, distinctive medium characterized by user participation, openness, and network effects". In addition, Hansen (2008, p. 2) defined "Web 2.0 is a term which refers to improved communication and collaboration between people via social networking".

The use of Web.2 in healthcare is identified as Health 2.0, Medicine 2.0 or ehealth (Eysenbach, 2008; Van de Belt et al., 2012). Several authors noted that applying ehealth (Health 2.0, Medicine 2.0) is changing the way patients and health staff communicate or interact (Chou, Hunt, Beckjord, Moser & Hesse, 2009, Eysenbach, 2008; Van de Belt et al., 2012; Chretien et al., 2011). An important notion of Health 2.0 is patient empowerment 2.0 that has been defined by Bos et al. (2008) as "the active participation of the citizen in his or her health and care pathway with the use of information and communication technologies".

Therefore, Health 2.0 enhances the collaboration between health professionals and patients. It also provides an opportunity for patients to engage in their own care (Van de Belt et al., 2012), facilitates patient access to health-related information and empowers them to make better choices.

The Use of Online Communities in Health Care

"An online community is a *virtual community* whose members interact with each other primarily via the Internet. An online community can also act as an *information system* where members can post, comment on discussions, give advice or collaborate. The members of online communities use Internet to interact socially (Preece, 2000). There is no need to use complex technology; email-based online community can be set up to be used by users (Johnson & Ambrose, 2006). Online communities give this opportunity to patients to share their feelings and support each other emotionally: this will make them to feel less loneliness and improve their compliance with treatment. There will be also less psychological issues such as anxiety and depression (Battles & Wiener, 2002). In addition, the use of online communities helps patients to understand their treatment better by sharing the information with people who are in the same condition and help each other to take the necessary actions towards this. Moreover, health care applications delivered via telecommunications, or "telehealth," have great potential to facilitate the provision and receipt of high quality health care by reducing geographic barriers to care" (Castro, 2009, p.7).

"The development of patient-centric, online portals is in line with a broader trend in health care to use IT to create a more patient-centric approach to health care. Online health portals range from basic portals that provide patients with basic medical information on illnesses and drugs, to more advanced portals that provide online access to health care services, to even more advanced portals that provide access to personalized medical information" (Castro, 2009, p.7). The eHealth portal in the NHS is called NHS direct that guide people for the most relevant and appropriate treatment (nhsdirect, 2014). Moreover, it provides the variety of health service information and advice for people such as responding people's online questions in securely or providing telephone advice and information.

Limitations of the Study

Like other research, this study has a number of limitations. Firstly, there is limited access to health care units to carry out a comparative study in a big scale. Secondly, the study aim to use secondary data which not publically available and there may be a mismatch between the time of conducting the interviews and the time for collection of data by the hospital (secondary data); this needs to be carefully considered.

FUTURE RESEARCH DIRECTION

This critical literature review has provided good insight for future research. The author suggests:

- Due to the dramatic change that the NHS is experiencing in terms of leadership at the moment, longitudinal research with the application of different methods should be conducted. This will gain a deep understanding of this phenomenon (distributed leadership) and its impacts, especially from employees' perspective and patients' perspective.
- The hybrid role of health professionals (doctors, nurses, physiotherapist and so on) is crucial to improving the quality of care and service in health care. Therefore, more attention should be paid to this phenomenon with a recommendation made for future research in this area.

- Further research is also needed to study the application of distributed leadership in different contexts internationally (cross-cultural) as well as in private sectors. More data will enable better generalization of the findings.

Implication of the Study

The theoretical implication of this research is to provide a foundation for the application of distributed in healthcare by using online communities and social media. The study also shows that social media can improve quality of care and patient safety by increasing social interactions between patients and health providers.

CONCLUSION

A critical literature review has been conducted to investigate the concept of distributed leadership and its association and impact on patient outcome and patient engagement in a health care setting through social media perspective. As it has been seen in the literature there was no agreed definition of distributed leadership, but it is often identified as a process in which everyone should take part in leadership activities concurrently and collectively. Despite the fact that the debate on distributed leadership started in the 1950s, but recently the NHS has put more emphasis on the use of distributed leadership. In addition, recent medical leadership development programmes (2013 & 2014) have been based on the characteristics of a distributed model of leadership.

England health care (NHS) is a massive, complex and hierarchical organization with a variety of professionals with different backgrounds, values and cultures. In addition, the NHS has experienced severe failures in terms of quality of care and patient safety, making the role of leadership even more important. The NHS cannot be managed with low quality standards of leadership. Therefore, distributed leadership has been proposed as a model of effective leadership in health care with a view to improve the quality of care, patient safety and health services by engaging staff from different levels of the organization as well as engaging patients and others. The rationale behind the application of distributed leadership in health care can be summed up as firstly, leading such a complex organization cannot be the sole responsibility of an individual, so clinicians, nurses and other staff should be engaged in leadership practice to improve the quality of health care services. Secondly, the hybrid role of staff is also crucial. Thirdly, the success in adapting to the dramatic changes which the NHS is experiencing at the moment is very much dependent on the application of new concepts in leadership (distributed leadership).

Moreover, Health care providers can improve the quality of care by using the social media and knowing how patients use them. Online communities help patients to share their knowledge about disease and its treatment and also support and be supported emotionally. It also has great social and economic influences on health care. Social media enhances the communication between doctors and patients. However, clinicians must be very cautious of the security of the social network they are using to communicate with patients so as to maintain patients' privacy and confidentiality. Therefore, implementing distributed leadership, employees' engagement and patients' engagement can be facilitated by using social media.

In summary, we should go beyond the description of distributed leadership and pay more attention to how leadership can be distributed (Currie & Lockett, 2011) and by whom. Understanding distributed leadership and its application in the health care setting is largely related to the appreciation of the political and social power that currently exists (Gosling et al, 2009). Strong leadership is needed to remove the barriers on eHealth and health IT adoption in health care system.

REFERENCES

Agle, B. R., Nagarajan, N. J., Sonnenfeld, J. A., & Srinivasan, D. (2006). Does CEO charisma matter? An empirical analysis of the relationships among organizational performance, environmental uncertainty, and top management team perceptions of CEO charisma. *Academy of Management Journal*, *49*(1), 161–174. doi:10.5465/AMJ.2006.20785800

Antheunis, M. L., Tates, K., & Nieboer, T. E. (2013). Patients' and health professionals' use of social media in health care: Motives, barriers and expectations. *Patient Education and Counseling*, *92*(3), 426–431. doi:10.1016/j.pec.2013.06.020 PMID:23899831

Bass, B. M. (1985). *Leadership and performance beyond expectations*. Academic Press.

Bass, B. M., Avolio, B. J., Jung, D. I., & Berson, Y. (2003). Predicting unit performance by assessing transformational and transactional leadership. *The Journal of Applied Psychology*, *88*(2), 207–218. doi:10.1037/0021-9010.88.2.207 PMID:12731705

Bate, P. (2000). Changing the Culture of a Hospital: From Hierarchy to NetworkedCommunity. *Public Administration*, *78*(3), 485–512. doi:10.1111/1467-9299.00215

Battles, H. B., & Wiener, L. S. (2002). Starbright World: Effects of an electronic network on the social environment of children with life-threatening illnesses. *Children's Health Care*, *31*(1), 47–68. doi:10.1207/S15326888CHC3101_4

Bennis, W. (2007). The challenges of leadership in the modern world: Introduction to the special issue. *The American Psychologist*, *62*(1), 2–5. doi:10.1037/0003-066X.62.1.2 PMID:17209674

Berg, D. N. (1998). Resurrecting the muse: Followership in organizations. *The psychodynamics of leadership*, 27-52.

Bolden, R. (2011). Distributed leadership in organizations: A review of theory and research. *International Journal of Management Reviews*, *13*(3), 251–269. doi:10.1111/j.1468-2370.2011.00306.x

Bos, L., Marsh, A., Carroll, D., Gupta, S., & Rees, M. (2008, July). Patient 2.0 Empowerment. In SWWS, 164-168.

Bosslet, G. T., Torke, A. M., Hickman, S. E., Terry, C. L., & Helft, P. R. (2011). The patient–doctor relationship and online social networks: Results of a national survey. *Journal of General Internal Medicine*, *26*(10), 1168–1174. doi:10.1007/s11606-011-1761-2 PMID:21706268

Brown, M. E., & Mitchell, M. S. (2010). Ethical and unethical leadership. *Business Ethics Quarterly*, *20*(4), 583–616. doi:10.5840/beq201020439

Bryman, A. (1992). *Charisma and Leadership in Organizations*. Newbury Park, CA: Sage.

Buchanan, D. A., Addicott, R., Fitzgerald, L., Ferlie, E., & Baeza, J. I. (2007). Nobody in charge: Distributed change agency in healthcare. *Human Relations*, *60*(7), 1065–1090. doi:10.1177/0018726707081158

Caldwell, C. (2011). Duties Owed to Organizational Citizens –Ethical Insights for Today's Leader. *Journal of Business Ethics*, *102*(3), 343–356. doi:10.1007/s10551-011-0819-8

Castro, D. (2009). *Explaining international IT application leadership: Health IT*. Available at SSRN 1477486.

Change Foundation. (2011). *Using social media to improve healthcare quality*. Retrieved from https://www.changefoundation.ca/docs/social-mediatoolkit.pdf

Chen, J., Xu, H., & Whinston, A. B. (2011). Moderated online communities and quality of user-generated content. *Journal of Management Information Systems*, *28*(2), 237–268. doi:10.2753/MIS0742-1222280209

Chou, W. Y. S., Hunt, Y. M., Beckjord, E. B., Moser, R. P., & Hesse, B. W. (2009). Social media use in the United States: Implications for health communication. *Journal of Medical Internet Research, 11*(4), e48. doi:10.2196/jmir.1249 PMID:19945947

Chretien, K. C., Azar, J., & Kind, T. (2011). Physicians on twitter. *Journal of the American Medical Association, 305*(6), 566–568. doi:10.1001/jama.2011.68 PMID:21304081

Clegg, S., Kornberger, M., & Pitis, T. (2008). *Managing and organizations: an introduction to theory and practice* (2nd ed.). Los Angeles, CA: Sage Publications Inc.

Cline, R. J., & Haynes, K. M. (2001). Consumer health information seeking on the Internet: The state of the art. *Health Education Research, 16*(6), 671–692. doi:10.1093/her/16.6.671 PMID:11780707

Currie, G., Boyett, I., & Suhomlinova, O. (2005). Transformational leadership within secondary schools in England. A panacea for organizational ills? *Public Administration, 83*(2), 265–296. doi:10.1111/j.0033-3298.2005.00450.x

Currie, G., Koteyko, N., & Nerlich, B. (2009a). The dynamics of professions and development of new roles in public services organizations: The case of modern matrons in the English NHS. *Public Administration, 87*(2), 295–311. doi:10.1111/j.1467-9299.2009.01755.x

Currie, G., & Lockett, A. (2011). Distributing leadership in health and social care: Concertive, conjoint or collective? *International Journal of Management Reviews, 13*(3), 286–300. doi:10.1111/j.1468-2370.2011.00308.x

Currie, G., Lockett, A., & Suhomlinova, O. (2009). The institutionalization of distributed leadership: A 'Catch-22' in English public services. *Human Relations, 62*(11), 1735–1761. doi:10.1177/0018726709346378

Currie, G., Lockett, A., & Suhomlinova, O. (2009b). Leadership and institutional change in the public sector: The case of secondary schools in England. *The Leadership Quarterly, 20*(5), 664–679. doi:10.1016/j.leaqua.2009.06.001

De Hoogh, A., den Hartog, D., Koopman, P., Thierry, H., van den Berg, P., van der Weide, J., & Wilderom, C. (2004). Charismatic leadership, environmental dynamism, and performance. *European Journal of Work and Organizational Psychology, 13*(4), 447–471. doi:10.1080/13594320444000164

Denis, J. L., Lamothe, L., & Langley, A. (2001). The dynamics of collective leadership and strategic change in pluralistic organizations. *Academy of Management Journal, 44*(4), 809–837. doi:10.2307/3069417

Department of Health. (2000). *The NHS Plan: A plan for investment, a plan for reform. Cm 4818-I.* London: Department of Health. Available at: www.dh.gov.uk/en/Publicationsandstatistics/Publications/PublicationsPolicyAndGuidance/DH_4002960

Department of Health. (2008). *Next Stage Review: High Quality Care for All.* London: DH.

Department of Health. (2009b). *The NHS Constitution for England* (2009 edition). London: Department of Health. Available at: www.dh.gov.uk/en/ Publicationsandstatistics/Publications/PublicationsPolicyAndGuidance/DH_093419

Department of Health. (2010). *Equity and Excellence: Liberating the NHS.* London: DH.

Drath, W. H., McCauley, C. D., Palus, C. J., Van Velsor, E., O'Connor, P. M., & McGuire, J. B. (2008). Direction, alignment, commitment: Toward a more integrative ontology of leadership. *The Leadership Quarterly, 19*(6), 635–653. doi:10.1016/j.leaqua.2008.09.003

Elmore, R. F. (2000). *Building a new structure for school leadership*. Washington, DC: The Albert Shanker Institute.

Eysenbach, G. (2008). Medicine 2.0: Social networking, collaboration, participation, apomediation, and openness. *Journal of Medical Internet Research, 10*(3), e22. doi:10.2196/jmir.1030 PMID:18725354

Fitzgerald, L., & Ferlie, E. (2000). Professionals: Back to the future? *Human Relations, 53*(5), 713–739. doi:10.1177/0018726700535005

Fitzgerald, L., Ferlie, E., McGivern, G., & Buchanan, D. (2013). Distributed leadership patterns and service improvement: Evidence and argument from English healthcare. *The Leadership Quarterly, 24*(1), 227–239. doi:10.1016/j.leaqua.2012.10.012

Fitzsimons, D., James, K., & Denyer, D. (2011). Alternative Approaches for Studying Shared and Distributed Leadership. *International Journal of Management Reviews, 12*(3), 313–328. doi:10.1111/j.1468-2370.2011.00312.x

Fletcher, J., & Kaufer, K. (2003). *Shared leadership. Shared Leadership: Reframing the how's and whys of leadership*. London: Sage. doi:10.4135/9781452229539.n2

Fletcher, J. K. (2004). The paradox of postheroic leadership: An essay on gender, power, and transformational change. *The Leadership Quarterly, 15*(5), 647–661. doi:10.1016/j.leaqua.2004.07.004

Follett, M. P., Urwick, L. F., & Metcalf, H. C. (1973). *Dynamic administration: the collected papers of Mary Parker Follett*. Harper & Brothers Publ.

Francis, R. (2010). *Independent Inquiry into care provided by Mid Staffordshire NHS Foundation Trust January 2005-March 2009*. The Stationery Office.

Fund, K. (2011). *The Future of Leadership and Management in the NHS. No More Heroes*. London: The Kings Fund.

Gabarro, J. J. (1978). The development of trust, influence, and expectations. *Interpersonal behaviour: Communication and understanding in relationships, 290*, 303.

Gibb, C. A. (1954). Leadership. In G. Lindzey (Ed.), Handbook of social psychology (Vol. 2). Academic Press.

Gosling, J., Bolden, R., & Petrov, G. (2009). Distributed leadership in higher education: What does it accomplish? *Leadership, 5*(3), 299–310. doi:10.1177/1742715009337762

Gronn, P. (1999). *A realist view of leadership*. Paper presented at the ELOAusAsia on-line conference "Educational leadership for the new millennium–leaders with soul," Parramatta, Australia.

Gronn, P. (2000). Distributed properties: A new architecture for leadership. *Educational Management and Administration, 28*(3), 317–338. doi:10.1177/0263211X000283006

Gronn, P. (2002). Distributed leadership as a unit of analysis. *The Leadership Quarterly, 13*(4), 423–451. doi:10.1016/S1048-9843(02)00120-0

Gruzd, A., Wellman, B., & Takhteyev, Y. (2011). Imagining Twitter as an imagined community. *The American Behavioral Scientist, 55*(10), 1294–1318. doi:10.1177/0002764211409378

Hajli, M. N. (2014). A study of the impact of social media on consumers. *International Journal of Market Research, 56*(3), 388–404. doi:10.2501/IJMR-2014-025

Ham, C. (2008). Doctors in leadership: Learning from international experience. *The International Journal of Clinical Leadership, 16*(1), 11–16.

Ham C, Dickinson H (2008). *Engaging Doctors in Leadership: What we can learn from international experience and research evidence?* NHS Institute for Innovation and Improvement.

Hansen, M. M. (2008). Versatile, immersive, creative and dynamic virtual 3-D healthcare learning environments: A review of the literature. *Journal of Medical Internet Research, 10*(3), e26. doi:10.2196/jmir.1051 PMID:18762473

Hardiker, N. R., & Grant, M. J. (2011). Factors that influence public engagement with eHealth: A literature review. *International Journal of Medical Informatics, 80*(1), 1–12. doi:10.1016/j.ijmedinf.2010.10.017 PMID:21112244

Harris, A. (2009). *Distributed leadership: What we know*. Springer Netherlands. doi:10.1007/978-1-4020-9737-9

Hartley, J., & Benington, J. (2010). *Leadership for Healthcare*. Bristol: Policy Press. doi:10.1332/policypress/9781847424877.001.0001

Heifetz, R. A. (1994). *Leadership without Easy Answers*. Cambridge, MA: The Belknap Press of Harvard University Press.

Hosmer, L. T. (2007). *The Ethics of Management* (6th ed.). New York: McGraw-Hill.

Huffington, C., James, K., & Armstrong, D. (2004). *What is the emotional cost of distributed leadership. Working Below the Surface: The Emotional Life of Contemporary Organizations*. London: Karnac.

Huxham, C., & Vangen, S. (2000). Leadership in the shaping and implementation of collaboration agendas: How things happen in a (not quite) joined-up world. *Academy of Management Journal, 43*(6), 1159–1175. doi:10.2307/1556343

Iverson, S. A., Howard, K. B., & Penney, B. K. (2008). Impact of internet use on health-related behaviours and the patient-physician relationship: A survey-based study and review. JAOA. *The Journal of the American Osteopathic Association, 108*(12), 699–711. PMID:19075034

James, K., & Ladkin, D. (2008). Meeting the challenge of leading in the 21st century: Beyond the 'deficit model' of leadership development. *Leadership learning: Knowledge into action*, 13-34.

James, K. T. (2011). *Leadership in context lessons from new leadership theory and current leadership development practice. Commission on Leadership and Management in the NHS*. The King's Fund.

Johnson, G. J., & Ambrose, P. J. (2006). Neo-tribes: The power and potential of online communities in health care. *Communications of the ACM, 49*(1), 107–113. doi:10.1145/1107458.1107463

Katzenbach, J. R., & Smith, D. K. (1993). *The Wisdom of Teams: Creating the High Performance Organization*. Boston, MA: Harvard Business School.

Laschinger, H. K. S., & Leiter, M. P. (2006). The impact of nursing work environments on patient safety outcomes: The mediating role of burnout engagement. *The Journal of Nursing Administration, 36*(5), 259–267. doi:10.1097/00005110-200605000-00019 PMID:16705307

Martin, G. P. (2008). 'Ordinary people only': Knowledge, representativeness, and the publics of public participation in healthcare. *Sociology of Health & Illness, 30*(1), 35–54. doi:10.1111/j.1467-9566.2007.01027.x PMID:18254832

Martin, G. P., Currie, G., & Finn, R. (2009). Leadership, service reform, and public-service networks: The case of cancer-genetics pilots in the English NHS. *Journal of Public Administration: Research and Theory, 19*(4), 769–794. doi:10.1093/jopart/mun016

McKee, L., Charles, K., Dixon-Woods, M., Willars, J., & Martin, G. (2013). 'New'and distributed leadership in quality and safety in health care, or 'old'and hierarchical? An interview study with strategic stakeholders. *Journal of Health Services Research & Policy*, *18*(2suppl), 11–19. doi:10.1177/1355819613484460 PMID:24121833

McLaurin, J. R., & Al Amri, B. (2008). Developing an understanding of charismatic and transformational leadership, Proceedings of the Academy of Organizational Culture, Communications and Conflict, 13(2), 15-19.

Mehra, A., Smith, B. R., Dixon, A. L., & Robertson, B. (2006). Distributed leadership in teams: The network of leadership perceptions and team performance. *The Leadership Quarterly*, *17*(3), 232–245. doi:10.1016/j.leaqua.2006.02.003

Mintzberg, H. (1979). *The Structuring of Organizations*. Englewood Cliffs, NJ: Prentice Hall.

Mountford, J., & Webb, C. (2009). When clinicians lead. *The McKinsey Quarterly*.

Oduro, G. K. (2004, September). Distributed leadership in schools: What English headteachers say about the" pull" and" push" factors. In *British Educational Research Association Annual Conference* (pp. 16-18).

Osborn, R. N., Hunt, J. G., & Jauch, L. R. (2002). Toward a contextual theory of leadership. *The Leadership Quarterly*, *13*(6), 797–837. doi:10.1016/S1048-9843(02)00154-6

Park, D. H., Lee, J., & Han, I. (2007). The effect of on-line consumer reviews on consumer purchasing intention: The moderating role of involvement. *International Journal of Electronic Commerce*, *11*(4), 125–148. doi:10.2753/JEC1086-4415110405

Pearce, C. L., & Conger, J. A. (2003). *Shared Leadership: Reframing the How's and Whys of Leadership*. Thousand Oaks, CA: Sage.

Peck, E., & Dickinson, H. (2008). *Managing and leading in inter-agency settings*. Policy Pr.

Prasad, B. (2013). Social media, health care, and social networking. *Gastrointestinal Endoscopy*, *77*(3), 492–495. doi:10.1016/j.gie.2012.10.026 PMID:23410701

Preece, J. (2000). *Online communities: Designing usability and supporting socialbilty*. John Wiley & Sons, Inc.

Prins, J. T., Hoekstra-Weebers, J. E., Gazendam-Donofrio, S. M., Dillingh, G. S., Bakker, A. B., Huisman, M., & Van Der Heijden, F. M. et al. (2010). Burnout and engagement among resident doctors in the Netherlands: A national study. *Medical Education*, *44*(3), 236–247. doi:10.1111/j.1365-2923.2009.03590.x PMID:20444054

Raelin, J. A. (2005). We the leaders: In order to form a leaderful organization. *Journal of Leadership & Organizational Studies*, *12*(2), 18–30. doi:10.1177/107179190501200202

Ridings, C. M., & Gefen, D. (2004). Virtual community attraction: Why people hang out online. *Journal of Computer-Mediated Communication*, *10*(1), 1–10.

Robinson, P., Tyndale-Biscoe, J. (2011, November). What makes a top hospital. *CHKS*.

Rowling, E. (2012). *Leadership and Engagement for Improvement in the NHS: Together we can*. Report from The King's Fund Leadership Review.

Salanova, M., Agut, S., & Peiro, J. M. (2005). Linking organizational resources and work engagement to employee performance and customer loyalty: The mediation of service climate. *The Journal of Applied Psychology*, *90*(6), 1217–1227. doi:10.1037/0021-9010.90.6.1217 PMID:16316275

Seers, A., Keller, T., & Wilkerson, J. (2003). Can team members share leadership. *Shared leadership: Reframing the hows and whys of leadership*, 77-102.

Senecal, S., & Nantel, J. (2004). The influence of online product recommendations on consumers' online choices. *Journal of Retailing*, *80*(2), 159–169. doi:10.1016/j.jretai.2004.04.001

Sims, H. P. Jr, & Lorenzi, P. (1992). *The new leadership paradigm: Social learning and cognition in organizations*. Sage Publications, Inc.

Smee, C. (2000). United Kingdom. *Journal of Health Politics, Policy and Law*, *25*(5), 945–951. doi:10.1215/03616878-25-5-945 PMID:11068739

Spillane, J. P. (2005). *Distributed leadership*. San Francisco, CA: Jossey Bass.

Spillane, J. P. (2005, June). Distributed leadership. *The Educational Forum*, *69*(2), 143–150. doi:10.1080/00131720508984678

Spillane, J. P., & Diamond, J. B. (Eds.). (2007). *Distributed leadership in practice*. New York: Teachers College, Columbia University.

Spillane, J. P., Halverson, R., & Diamond, J. B. (2001). Investigating school leadership practice: A distributed perspective. *Educational Researcher*, *30*(3), 22–28. doi:10.3102/0013189X030003023

Spillane, J. P., Halverson, R., & Diamond, J. B. (2004). Towards a theory of leadership practice: A distributed perspective. *Journal of Curriculum Studies*, *36*(1), 3–34. doi:10.1080/0022027032000106726

Uhl-Bien, M. (2006). Relational leadership theory: Exploring the social processes of leadership and organizing. *The Leadership Quarterly*, *17*(6), 654–676. doi:10.1016/j.leaqua.2006.10.007

Van de Belt, T. H., Berben, S. A., Samsom, M., Engelen, L. J., & Schoonhoven, L. (2012). Use of social media by Western European hospitals: Longitudinal study. *Journal of Medical Internet Research*, *14*(3), e61. doi:10.2196/jmir.1992 PMID:22549016

Vance, K., Howe, W., & Dellavalle, R. P. (2009). Social internet sites as a source of public health information. *Dermatologic Clinics*, *27*(2), 133–136. doi:10.1016/j.det.2008.11.010 PMID:19254656

Von Muhlen, M., & Ohno-Machado, L. (2012). Reviewing social media use by clinicians. *Journal of the American Medical Informatics Association*, *19*(5), 777–781. doi:10.1136/amiajnl-2012-000990 PMID:22759618

Wachter, R. M. (2010). Patient safety at ten: Unmistakable progress, troubling gaps. *Health Affairs*, *29*(1), 165–173. doi:10.1377/hlthaff.2009.0785 PMID:19952010

Wenger, E. (2000). Communities of practice and social learning systems. *Organization*, *7*(2), 225–246. doi:10.1177/135050840072002

West, M., & Dawson, J. (2012). *Employee Engagement and NHS Performance*. The King's Fund. Retrieved from www.kingsfund.org.uk/leadershipreview

What is NHS Direct. (n.d.). Retrieved from www.nhsdirect.nhs.uk/article.aspx?name=WhatIsNHSDirect> (accessed 10 September 2014).

Yasini, A., Arasteh, H., Ebrahim, A., Zeinabadi, H. (2012). Distributed leadership. *Science Journal of Public Management, 12*, 129-148.

KEY TERMS AND DEFINITIONS

Distributed Leadership: A process in which everyone can take part in leadership activities concurrently and collectively.

eHealth: The electronic transition of health care resources and information.

Engagement: The act of being involved or take part in an activity.

Leadership: Is the process of guiding, stimulating and inspiring people towards organisational purposes.

Patient Safety: The avoidance of mistake and negative impact on patients related to health care.

Quality of Care: The degree to which care is clinically effective and safe and provides a positive experience for patients.

Social Media: Internet based applications and tools that enable people to create, share ideas and information in virtual networks.

This work was previously published in the Handbook of Research on Integrating Social Media into Strategic Marketing edited by Nick Hajli, pages 303-323 copyright year 2015 by Business Science Reference (an imprint of IGI Global).

Chapter 43
The Benefits of Big Data Analytics in the Healthcare Sector:
What Are They and Who Benefits?

Andrea Darrel
University of Southern Queensland, Australia

Timothy Hardie
Lakehead University, Canada

Margee Hume
University of Southern Queensland, Australia

Jeffery Soar
University of Southern Queensland, Australia

ABSTRACT

The benefits of big data analytics in the healthcare sector are assumed to be substantial, and early proponents have been very enthusiastic (Chen, Chiang, & Storey, 2012), but little research has been carried out to confirm just what those benefits are, and to whom they accrue (Bollier, 2010). This chapter presents an overview of existing literature that demonstrates quantifiable, measurable benefits of big data analytics, confirmed by researchers across a variety of healthcare disciplines. The chapter examines aspects of clinical operations in healthcare including Cost Effectiveness Research (CER), Clinical Decision Support Systems (CDS), Remote Patient Monitoring (RPM), Personalized Medicine (PM), as well as several public health initiatives. This examination is in the context of searching for the benefits described resulting from the deployment of big data analytics. Results indicate the principle benefits are delivered in terms of improved outcomes for patients and lower costs for healthcare providers.

INTRODUCTION

Biomedical informatics is the science of information applied to medicine and is "distinct from related fields like computer science, statistics and biomedicine, which have different objects of study"(Bernstam, Smith, & Johnson, 2010). Biomedical informatics incorporates a "core set of methodologies for managing data, information and knowledge" (Sarkar, 2010) with the goal of "improving the quality and safety of healthcare while reducing the costs" (Hersh, 2009).

DOI: 10.4018/978-1-4666-8756-1.ch043

Advances in biomedical informatics have been proceeding at an astonishing pace, with some notable successes and some equally notable setbacks. The following chapter offers a comprehensive review of what benefits, and what drawbacks, current research into the application of big data analytics to healthcare and biomedical engineering have revealed, in an effort to guide further research and to understand more clearly what benefits arise where big data intersects with healthcare, and to whom those benefits accrue.

According to a McKinsey report (2011) on the potential financial savings to be harvested from big data analytics, healthcare is particularly rich in opportunity. Clinical operations, payment and pricing, R&D, public health and new business models all have the potential to benefit from the analysis of large sets of data. Preliminary investigation reveals that there have been many documented, quantified gains that accumulate to improve physician performance, provide better guidance for treatment, dramatically improve patient outcomes and significantly lower costs for hospitals, insurers and co-payees.

The looming demographic shift in the United States and other developed nations portends health care costs that will consume a significant portion of national budgets in the years to come, and delivering better health care to more people for less cost will be a critical policy issue (Ahern, Smith, Topol, Mack, & Fitzgerald, 2013; Bloom, Börsch-Supan, McGee, & Seike, 2012; Morton & Weng, 2013; Vogeli et al., 2007).

BACKGROUND

What Is Big Data?

In general, we can define big data as pools of information so large that conventional analytical techniques cannot make sense of them (Bertot, Jaeger, & Grimes, 2010). In a very real sense, the definition is a moving target. As our capacity to store information increases and techniques to analyze that data continue to develop and improve, the amounts of data that constitute big are similarly changing.

1 bit = binary digit
8 bits = 1 byte
1024 bytes = 1 kilobyte
1024 kilobytes = 1 megabyte
1024 megabytes = 1 gigabyte
1024 gigabytes = 1 terabyte
1024 terabytes = 1 petabyte
1024 petabytes = 1 exabyte
1024 exabytes = 1 zettabyte
1024 zettabytes = 1 yottabyte
1024 yottabytes = 1 brontobyte
1024 brontobytes = 1 geobyte

Since launching the National Archives and Records Administration in 2005 (Sproull & Eisenberg, 2005), the amount of information in the form of archival records the US government is managing has grown from 17 terabytes (TB) to 142 TB as of 2012, representing over 7 billion electronic artifacts, a number that is projected to continue to grow (Reed, Murray, & Jacobson, 2013).

Two important characteristics distinguish big data from ordinary data:

1. The efficacy of standard analytical techniques
2. The dynamic nature of the analysis.

Big data is any dataset that "exceeds the processing capabilities of conventional database systems" (Gupta, Gupta, & Mohania, 2012), and big data is analyzed and processed in real time, allowing human decision makers to use the data to guide their behaviour as the analysis is unfolding.

To illustrate the analytical complexity of "big data", consider the following: credit card companies routinely collect transaction information on millions of customers, amounting to very large datasets (Steffes, Murthi & Rao, 2011). That data can be mined using traditional analytical techniques to detect spending patterns and predict future transactions, information that is packaged and sold to direct marketing firms, who target products and services based on those spending patterns (Bult & Wansbeek, 1995). While the dataset being used is very large, the analytical techniques use straightforward estimation and inference calculations on a static dataset that is not being updated as the analysis proceeds. The dataset in this instance is simply "data".

If the exact same dataset consists of information that is changing at the time of analysis and the analytical techniques consist of advanced algorithms that mine the data without human supervision or prompting after initial installation, it becomes "big data". The dataset of spending patterns can now allow banks to detect fraudulent use of credit cards as it happens, through the use of algorithms that use associative learning rules to classify transactions into different risk categories. Field applications have demonstrated that these real time programs allow banks to detect 95% of fraudulent card use as it occurs (Ogwueleka, 2011; Rani, Kumar, Mohan, & Shankar, 2011).

Neural network and artificial intelligence algorithms running behind standard bank software can potentially detect the use of a credit card and then combine that information with other data sources such geolocation information and social media to offer services or discounts tailored to specific customers. Banks have not been eager to embrace the use of social media in their marketing efforts, but the capability to do so exists, and is continuing to grow (Mitic, 2012).

That may seem far-fetched, but when Hurricane Sandy struck the Atlantic coast of the United States in 2012, the Federal Emergency Management Agency (FEMA) created an innovative partnership with private companies and other federal agencies that used Twitter hashtags, Instagram photos, geo-tagged photos from the Civil Air Patrol (CAP) and sensor data from the National Oceanic and Atmospheric Administration (NOAA) to target

areas in need of supplies, and kept a pulse on how the community was responding to disaster relief efforts, all assisted by the advanced algorithms of big data analytics (Mapcite, 2013).

When it comes to healthcare, the opportunity for big data to deliver tangible benefits is very real, and healthcare in particular is embracing the potential of big data analytics.

Exploring the existing literature, Jourdan (2008) found five areas of research that were of interest to investigators:

1. **Artificial Intelligence:** Algorithms and applications that address classification, prediction, web mining, and machine learning.
2. **Benefits:** How businesses have used data warehousing, data mining, and/or enterprise wide BI systems to achieve some measurable financial benefit.
3. **Decision:** Using data modeling, decision-making and decision modeling to improve overall decision making.
4. **Implementation:** Using data warehousing, data mining, customer relationship management (CRM), enterprise resource planning (ERP), knowledge management systems (KMS), and eBusiness projects to address project management issues.
5. **Strategy:** How to apply BI tools and technologies.

After analyzing 167 papers in the BI literature area, Jourdan (2008) comes to the conclusion that Strategy is the most discussed topic (59 papers), followed by Artificial Intelligence (37 papers) and discussions surrounding Implementation (35 papers). Using BI to improve Decision-Making is of less interest (26 papers) and the accrued Benefits of BI is the least studied area (10 papers). Jourdan (2008) theorizes that one of the difficulties faced by researchers trying to identify the specific benefits is quantifying exactly how the use of big data results in an advantage to the firm.

At the end of this chapter, readers should have a clear understanding of what big data is and why it is important, why healthcare practitioners and various other stakeholders pursue big data analytics, what benefits have been shown to arise from those initiatives, how those benefits are defined, and what the future could look like as more and more data becomes available for analysis.

MAIN FOCUS OF THE CHAPTER

Issues, Controversies, Problems

When businesses use big data to enhance their competitiveness, both the process and the product are often referred to as "business intelligence". The process concerns the methods that businesses use to collect and analyze information that is of value to them. The product is the information that allows businesses to predict how "competitors, suppliers, customers, technologies, acquisitions, markets, products and services, and the general business environment" are likely to respond to various stimuli (Vedder, 1999).

For both private and public organizations, a benefit can be defined as anything that enhances the organization's ability to carry out its mission, or in other words, to enhance competitive advantage. A competitive advantage is achieved when outcomes (whether in terms of profits or attaining goals) consistently exceed the average within a defined industry (Porter, 2008). Porter defines two basic types of benefits that can enhance an organization's competitive advantage: cost advantage and differentiation advantage.

A *cost advantage* arises when an organization can deliver the same products or services as competitors at a lower cost, and a *differentiation advantage* arises when an organization can deliver products or services with benefits that exceed those of the competition. For the purposes of this chapter, in recognition of the fact that healthcare organizations and firms can be motivated by a profit incentive, but are not necessarily, benefits are defined in Table 1.

For many nationalized health care systems, market forces are not material in determining costs, but this does not reduce the pressures on these systems to deliver maximum value for taxpayer money. A looming demographic crisis and a rapidly aging population has exerted tremendous pressure on many national health systems to address the costs of delivering services (Meijer, Wouterse, Polder, & Koopmanschap, 2013). A primary driver for developing and deploying advanced analytics is to reduce the costs of delivering healthcare products and services, and many big data applications are successful in achieving significant savings.

Improved productivity in the field of healthcare includes delivering products and services more efficiently, which may or may not result in a cost advantage. A major aspect of productivity is reduced morbidity and negative health outcomes for patients, which is a social good in and of itself, with the added advantage of cost savings when complications leading to death are prevented from occurring in the first place, saving both the patient's life and the expense of treating the complication.

Table 1. Cost advantages of big data applied to healthcare

Cost Advantages	Applied to Healthcare Using Big Data
Lower Costs	Activities that allow healthcare organizations to provide the same products or services at a lower cost than previously achieved
Improved Productivity	Activities that allow healthcare organizations to deliver their products or services in a more efficient or effective way than previously achieved
Increased Market Share	Activities that allow healthcare organizations to capture a greater share of the market or to identify new markets
Price Premium	Activities that allow healthcare organizations to charge more for products or services
Limiting Liability	Activities that allow healthcare organizations to limit their exposure to liability claims

Increasing market share through capturing market share from competitors or by identifying new markets takes two distinct forms in the healthcare sector. The healthcare organizations primarily interested in capturing increased market share are pharmaceutical companies and medical device and equipment manufacturers (Costa, 2013), although private hospitals have also used big data analytics to draw more insured patients to highly rated hospitals and surgeons (Marjoua, Butler, & Bozic, 2012). When healthcare providers identify and reach underserved populations of patients, particularly vulnerable patients, they are in effect discovering new markets for products and services.

The ability to charge a price premium comes into effect in the healthcare sector as physician payment models shift from fee-for-service plans, which reward volume, to performance-based pricing plans, which reward outcomes. Physicians achieve a price premium for their services when they are able to produce the best patient outcomes or achieve cost controls. Physicians working with terminal patients in particular are rewarded when they are able to achieve costs controls while still affording maximal care to patients, and a failure to replace fee-for-service payment plans reduces physician's willingness to use best-practices and standard protocols identified through big data analytics (Neumann, Palmer, Nadler, Fang, & Ubel, 2010; Timbie, Fox, Van Busum, & Schneider, 2012).

Performance based pricing plans allow physicians to test the cost efficacy of new treatment regimens, supported by big data analytics. Value-based pricing (VBP) models in Sweden identified Acomplia as a potentially effective treatment for obesity related diabetes, and a set reimbursement plan was put into place, contingent upon outcomes, allowing physicians to either switch treatment or continue at substantially reduced costs, in effect delivering a price premium (Persson, Willis, & Odegaard, 2010).

Limiting liability is a concern for many healthcare practitioners, and the use of big data specifically generates significant benefits in the pharmaceutical silo of the healthcare sector. The use of big data in designing clinical trials, analyzing and aggregating trial results and monitoring the efficacy of approved treatments is greatly assisted by the advanced analytics of big data.

Estimates about the cost of bringing new drugs to market vary widely, with some pharmaceutical companies estimating their costs in the low range of $90 million and others reporting an upper limit of $880 million, an almost tenfold difference in estimated costs. Systematic reviews of cost reporting reveal that there are no gold standards of reporting in this area, and all drug development cost claims should be subject to reasonable audit and disclosure criteria (Morgan, Grootendorst, Lexchin, Cunningham, & Greyson, 2011). What is more well-known is the cost of getting it wrong. When drug companies introduce products that are subsequently shown to be harmful, they are held to liability claims that are significantly in excess of even the highest estimates of development costs. In 2012, GlaxoSmithKline (GSK) was ordered to pay a $3 billion dollar settlement for promoting two products for off-label use that were later shown to have harmful side effects. Since 2009, the US government has collected more than $11 billion dollars in liability claims against pharmaceutical companies (Outterson, 2012). Pharmaceutical and insurance companies are thus highly motivated to reduce their liability and big data plays a big role in their ability to do that.

Unsurprisingly, the majority of benefits arising from the use of big data analytics in the health care sector relate to reducing costs and improving productivity.

Big data is demonstrably effective at achieving some of those savings across a number of fields. In the following section, we will examine the use of big data to lower costs and improve productivity, as it applies to:

- Cost Effectiveness Research (CER)
- Clinical Decision Support Systems (CDS)
- Transparency
- Remote Patient Monitoring (RPM)
- Public Health Administration (PHA)
- Personalized Medicine (PM).

Methodology

Potentially relevant articles were identified using keyword searches and then divided into two categories: those that appeared relevant based on abstract and title, and those that appeared relevant but required careful review as the abstract and title provided insufficient information. Full text retrievals were carried out for articles with titles and abstracts that appeared relevant, which were then evaluated for the following criteria:

- Use of large datasets
- Use of advanced analytics
- Use of dynamic data.

Articles that did not meet the criteria were excluded from analysis. The same procedure was deployed for articles that appeared relevant but contained insufficient information in the title and abstract alone. After the first section on comparative effectiveness research was conducted, the parameters for publication dates were tightened, as evidence demonstrated that virtually no use of big data analytics could be detected prior to 2009. A second reviewer confirmed article relevance and verified the application of exclusion/inclusion criteria (see Figure 1).

CLINICAL OPERATIONS

Clinical operations in healthcare are all the actions that relate to the patient bedside, including diagnosing and monitoring the course of disease or trauma or other injury, and all observations and treatments administered, many of which are now collected in the form of digital records. Electronic Health Records (EHR) have the potential "for establishing new patient-stratification principles and for revealing unknown disease correlations" (Jensen, Jensen, & Brunak, 2012). Advances in medical genomics brings the possibility of personalized medicine based on a specific patient's gene sequence closer to fruition, and while there are challenges in integrating genomic data into EHR, advanced data analytics present a "promising means of disseminating genetic testing into diverse care settings (Kho et al., 2013).

Clinical operations represent a fertile ground for the use of big data to lower the costs of delivering medical services and products and to improve outcomes for patients. Specific clinical operations that have successfully deployed big data to achieve measurable, quantifiable benefits:

1. Cost Effectiveness Research (CER)
2. Clinical Decision Support (CDS) software systems
3. Transparency
4. Remote Patient Monitoring (RPM)
5. Personalized Medicine (PM).

Cost Effectiveness Research (CER)

Cost Effectiveness Research (CER) is based on the idea that healthcare resource allocation decisions can be guided by considering the costs of a particular treatment in relation to the expected benefits. The basic principles of CER are as follows:

- The ratio of net health-care costs to net health benefits provides an index by which priorities may be set.
- Quality-of-life concerns, including both adverse and beneficial effects of therapy, may be incorporated in the calculation of health benefits as adjustments to life expectancy.

Figure 1. Flow chart of results from the literature

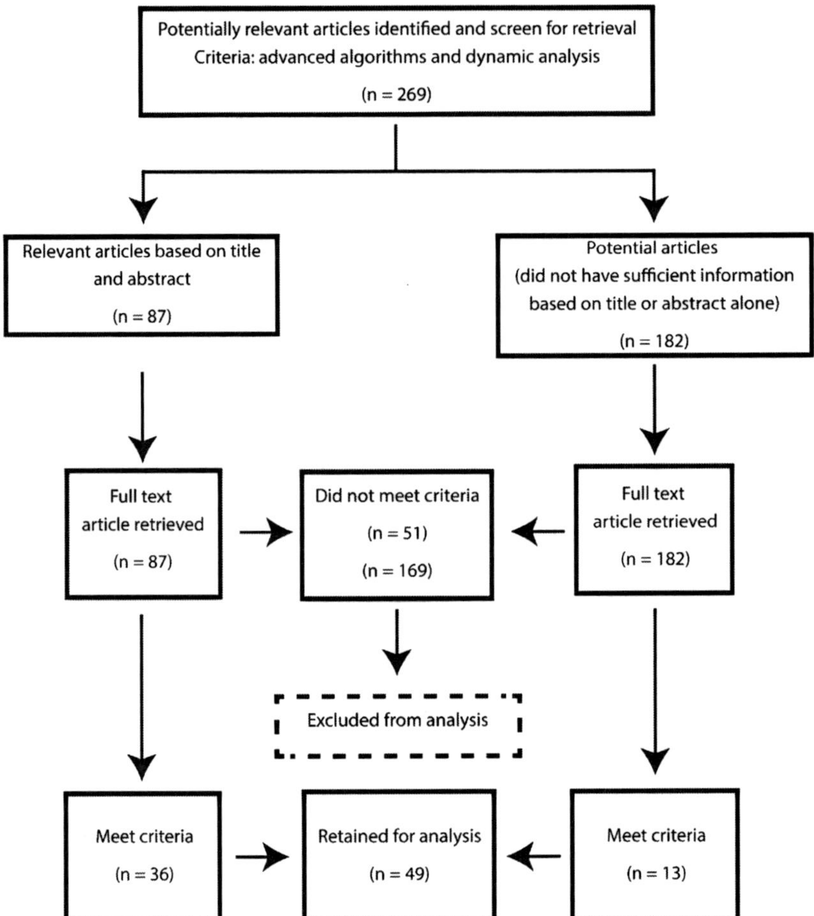

- The timing of future benefits and costs may be accounted for by the appropriate use of discounting.
- Current decisions must inevitably be based on imperfect information, but sensitivity analysis can increase the level of confidence.
- Analyses should be adaptable to the needs of various health-care decision makers, including planners, administrators and providers (Weinstein & Stason, 1977).

CER considers not just financial costs, but also a broader societal perspective that accounts for "benefits, harms and costs to all parties", including patients, care providers, insurers and auxiliary product and service providers (Russell, Gold, Siegel, Daniels, & Weinstein, 1996). CER is not intended to limit or restrict access to treatments or medicines, but rather "to provide healthcare decision makers, and patients and their personal physicians with more and potentially better information to help choose the best intervention, and thereby facilitate the best possible patient outcomes" (Siegel et al., 2012).

When the analytical tools of big data are applied to CER, the emphasis is on "the generation and synthesis of evidence that compares the benefits and harms of alternative methods to prevent, diagnose, treat and monitor a clinical condition or to improve the delivery of care" (Gandjour, 2011). Early advocates for CER and big data analytics predicted that "better information will result in better health outcomes and more effective use of resources" (Sox & Greenfield, 2009). CER has been promoted as an essential aspect of health care reform, given its potential to "prevent blunt incentives from inadvertently harming patients and to foster intelligent changes that can improve both the efficiency and the quality of care" (Mushlin & Ghomrawi, 2010).

The vast majority of published work in the realm of CER either uses static data and traditional analytic techniques, disqualifying it from consideration as an example of big data, or theorizes only probable outcomes (Avorn & Fischer, 2010; Chalkidou et al., 2009; Fischer & Avorn, 2004). For example, a standard decision tree-analysis on the cost effectiveness of a particular vaccination strategy was conducted on 180 000 infants in the Netherlands (Rozenbaum et al., 2010), which is undeniably a very large sample size, but the analytical techniques were of a standard variety and the data was static during analysis.

Existing evidence shows a promising confirmation of the predicted benefits of CER. The following table summarizes literature that confirms at least one benefit of big data analytics in the area of CER per publication (see Table 2).

While the macro justification for CRE is aimed at lowering costs of delivering medical services (Orszag & Emanuel, 2010), at the practitioner level, the emphasis remains on patient health and improving outcomes with cost savings only a secondary benefit, an initiative described as "goal-oriented patient care" (Reuben & Tinetti, 2012) across a wide variety of medical specialities. The following table illustrates the journals that published at least one article on CER, demonstrating how widespread the adoption of CER is across medical disciplines.

Clinical Decision Support Systems (CDS)

Clinical Decision Support Systems (CDS) are software programs that anticipate probable outcomes of particular treatment strategies by comparing the proposed treatment to previous patient outcomes. The software mines digital patient records and offers therapeutic suggestions and recommendations for the current patient based on what tended to work for previous patients presenting the same symptoms (Berner, 2007). These suggestions are offered at the time a decision about a particular therapy or regimen occurs, thereby meeting the two criteria for big data: large datasets are considered and the analysis happens in real time as the decisions are made.

CDS systems are primarily designed to address quality issues by providing practitioners with guidelines that have been proven to work in the past (Romano & Stafford, 2011). They are not intended to replace the judgement of individual practitioners faced with unique patients, but rather meant to act in a support capacity by revealing probable outcomes based on previous applications (Trowbridge & Weingarten, 2001). For maximum efficacy, CDS systems need to:

1. Provide decision support automatically as part of clinician workflow.
2. Deliver decision support at the time and location of decision making.
3. Provide actionable recommendations.
4. Use a computer to generate the decision support, without requiring clinician initiative (Kawamoto, Houlihan, Balas, & Lobach, 2005).

CDS system efficiency has a built in requirement for big data analytics, since the maximum productivity and efficacy of these systems are effected when the analysis takes place in real time, at the time and location of the decision making (Wright et al., 2009). The use of CDS systems is by far the most explored topic in big data analytics and clinical operations, likely due to the fact that many of these systems operate in conjunction with computerized Physician Order Entry (POE) systems, which have been in place since the late

Table 2. Demonstrated benefits of CER

Citation	Benefit	Summary of Findings
(Kremers et al., 2011)	Lower costs, improved productivity through better patient outcomes	Medical records generated by different healthcare providers over many years to specific individuals are linked in a single database that enables long term, population based planning for rheumatic disease treatment in a constantly changing population
(Abernethy et al., 2010)	Lower costs, improved productivity through better patient outcomes	An insurance provider serving more than 8 million patients maintains a database of patient records and 300 standard treatment protocols for cancer and analyzes best treatment options in real time, providing patients and doctors with best option suggestions at the time of treatment
(F Akram, J H Kim, & K N Choi, 2013)	Improved productivity through better detection of malignancies	Digital mammograms are pre-processed using advanced algorithms, removing digital obstacles such as labels, scanning and taping artifacts and physical obstacles such as pectoral muscles for use in CAD programs that alert radiologists to problems as files are examined
(S Ayyachamy & M Vasuki, 2013)	Lower costs through appropriate treatment regimens and improved productivity through better patient outcomes	Content Based Medical Image Retrieval (CBMIR) extracts stored images from a database using a variety of transforms (Fourier, discrete cosine, etc) and analyzes their visual content to assist both physicians and CAD programs in recognition, diagnosis, and treatment of lesions under consideration
(Du, 2010)	Improved productivity through elimination of unnecessary imaging analysis	The use of unsupervised data mining algorithms to detect microscopic cell abnormalities in digital images containing large numbers of cells, to help guide medical imaging choices.
(Prasad, Zimmermann, Prabhu, & Pai, 2010)	Lower costs through reduction of false positive identifications for breast cancer	Automatic classification of breast cancer tissue stains into positive or negative through the use of image analysis algorithms that draw on a large set of images collected in a university database
(Z. Chen et al., 2013)	Lower costs through elimination of unnecessary treatment and improved productivity through better patient outcomes	Replacing binary models of toxicity in cancer trials with an algorithm that detects and analyzes toxicity continuously calculating next dose levels from existing data
(Lacson et al., 2012)	Improved productivity through enhanced patient safety by alerting all caregivers of critical diagnostic results	Automated retrieval of radiology reports that cite critical imaging findings to enhance communication of critical results between caregivers
(Su, Wang, Jiao, & Guo, 2011)	Improved productivity through better and faster detection of breast cancer	Automatic detection and classification of breast tumors in ultrasonic imaging without any manual intervention using a self-organizing neural network that detects areas of interest by analyzing pixel textures and other digital morphologies
(Skounakis et al., 2010)	Lower costs and improved productivity through accurate and early detection of cancer	An open access interactive platform for 3D tomographic datasets that combines manual and semi-automatic segmentation techniques with integrated correction tools to identify tumors, and that can be adapted by different caregivers to plan treatments accordingly

1990s (Bates, 1998; Bates et al., 1999). Most of these early POE systems were aimed at preventing medication errors which are both costly and lead to negative patient outcomes. The dataset consists of pharmaceutical compound characteristics and counter-indications, potential over-dosages and under-dosages based on unique patient records that generate alerts for the prescribing physician at the time the order is entered.

The central benefit described in the literature relates to improved productivity through better patient outcomes, but by eliminating inadequate treatments which can lead to complications, and superfluous treatments which can lead to unnecessary costs, they also provide a lower costs benefit. When a busy emergency room used a CDS system that assessed patients and then alerted nursing staff to prompt patients to consider seasonal influenza vaccinations, they were able to capture market share from private physicians and realize a profit from the additional vaccinations (Venkat et al., 2010). Even so, the principle motivator was to increase the uptake in vaccinations rates, and the financial benefit was of secondary consideration.

Unlike CER, which is very often prompted by a desire to reduce the costs of delivering high quality healthcare, CDS systems are almost uniformly designed to achieve higher productivity through better outcomes for patients (Moxey et al., 2010). Bright et al. (2012) compared 148 different CDS randomized trials and found that while patient outcomes were improved, there was little evidence to support a claim for consistent economic savings.

While a significant percentage of the articles returned after a keyword search for CDS do describe benefits, many of them do not meet the criteria for inclusion in the study, because the datasets they describe are historical and the analysis is static (Eppenga et al., 2012; Krasowski & Penrod, 2012; Scharnweber et al., 2013).

The papers in Table 3 describe CDS systems using big data analytics to improve productivity and reduce costs.

Transparency

The issues of transparency and the application of big data analytics fall into four broad categories:

1. Sharing of clinical trials data
2. Sharing of patient information between healthcare providers
3. Sharing of information between patients and healthcare providers
4. Evaluating healthcare organizations and providers for effectiveness.

Pharmaceutical companies and other healthcare service providers and researchers within the private sector have tended to see clinical trials data as commercially proprietary information and have resisted the call to register and reveal the results of clinical trials, despite evidence that some firms have engaged in data suppression, misrepresentation and manipulation (Bian & Wu, 2010). In a particularly egregious example of data suppression, GlaxoSmithKline (GSK) was sued for suppressing reports of suicidal thinking, leading to physician over-prescription, especially amongst children, for a popular antidepressant (Sibbald, 2004), prompting New York State Attorney to demand that GSK develop and maintain an online clinical trials registry that includes information about safety, efficacy, side effects, methodologies and early terminations, but this requirement was not extended to all other drug companies.

By 2008, the World Medical Association revised the Declaration of Helsinki to include the requirement that "every clinical trial must be registered in a publicly accessible database before the recruitment of the first subject" (WorldMedicalAssociation, 2013). The main purpose of trial registration is to reduce or eliminate publication and reporting bias, whereby only positive and commercially valuable results are released, to provide reliable evidence for decision making, protecting public health and reducing liability for healthcare providers (Krleža-Jerić & Lemmens, 2009). The creation of these large, publicly available databases immediately opens the possibility for big data analytics to mine the data for relationships and correlations that may not be easily detected by any other means.

The benefits of transparency in clinical trials data relate primarily to improved productivity through improved outcomes for patients and reduced costs through the elimination of collecting new data when sufficient data already exists, and by increasing the probability that the trial will reach conclusion.

Gotzsche (2011) identifies four specific benefits of mandatory data sharing:

Table 3. Demonstrated benefits of CDS

Citation	Benefit	Summary of Findings
(Bates et al., 1999)	Improved productivity through appropriate dosing and avoidance of errors, and lower costs through avoidance of complications and over-prescription of potentially costly treatments	An 86% decrease in medication errors following the implementation of computerized physician order entry (POE). Upon entering the order, the computer generated appropriate does and frequencies, displayed relevant laboratory data, screening orders for allergy and drug interactions, assisting physicians in making the best orders for individual patients
(Robbins et al., 2012)	Improved productivity through better patient outcomes	Automatically generated computer alerts to inform both patients and care-givers of virologic failure and 11 over other abnormal lab results for patients with HIV, facilitating appointment rescheduling and repeated lab testing
(Kozel, 2012)	Improved productivity through better patient outcomes and lower costs through avoidance of serious complications	Automated protocols for newborns added to electronic records to automatically detect risk factors for hypoglycemia, reducing nursing errors in detecting those factors from 21% to 5%.
(Seidling et al., 2010)	Lower costs through avoidance of over-prescribing costly medications and improved productivity through better patient outcomes by avoiding toxic drug doses	An algorithm extracting relevant patient information and comparing that information with upper dose limits for various compounds instantly alerts physicians at the time a drug order is entered that upper limits may be compromised specific to individual patients
(Venkat et al., 2010)	Capturing market share by offering seasonal influenza vaccines in ER departments	Patients presenting at emergency rooms are entered into a EHR system, which evaluates their suitability for seasonal flu vaccinations and then prompts nursing staff to offer it, resulting in greater uptake of flu shots at a profit for the ER
(Haut, Lau, Kraenzlin, & et al., 2012)	Improved productivity through better patient outcomes	An evidence based algorithm identifies patient risk stratification levels and recommends appropriate treatment regimens for venous thromboembolism in trauma patients
(Bressan, James, & McGregor, 2012)	Improved productivity through better neonatal patient outcomes	The Artemis System for monitoring neonatal patients for signs of infection is optimized to include data streams from infusion pumps, EEG monitors and cerebral oxygenation monitors assisting care providers with decision making during critical prematurity
(Verberne et al., 2012)	Improved productivity through better colorectal cancer patient outcomes	An intelligent algorithm monitors lab results for colorectal cancer patients automatically issuing letters to patients to attend follow up appointments, scheduling appointments urgently when lab results indicate
(Raja et al., 2012)	Lower costs through the elimination of unnecessary imaging	Historical patient records were mined to create a CDS system that assists physicians in determining if current emergency room patients require computed tomographic (CT) pulmonary angiography for the diagnosis of pulmonary embolism
(McLachlan, Wells, Furness, Jackson, & Kerr, 2010)	Improved productivity through better patient outcomes, particularly for ethnic and low-income patients	CDS deployed to address care disparities arising from patient's ethnic or socioeconomic status in cardiovascular risk management post myocardial infarction. The use of EHR and automatic detection of risk factors enhanced care for patients who might otherwise have received inadequate care
(Ongenae, Dhaene, De Turck, Benoit, & Decruyenaere, 2010)	Improved productivity through better patient outcomes by early detection of sepsis in an ICU unit	Machine Learning Techniques augment the medical time series collected for a specific patient in the ICU and then calculates the probability the patient is septic
(Mariotti, Gentilini, & Dapor, 2013)	Improved productivity through the efficient use of specialists.	Patients waiting to see orthopaedic and ENT specialists were grouped according to explicit clinical indicators and on clinical priorities and appointments were automatically generated, resulting in enhanced agreement between primary and specialist providers.

continued on following page

Table 3. Continued

Citation	Benefit	Summary of Findings
(Cho, Park, Kim, Lee, & Bates, 2013)	Improved productivity through the prevention of pressure ulcers in critically ill patients.	A predictive decision model embedded within an EHR prompted staff in an ICU to take preventative measures to present pressure ulcers in vulnerable patients, reducing the prevalence of pressure ulcers by tenfold.
(Smith, Murphy, et al., 2013)	Improved productivity through improved follow-up for patients returning abnormal cancer related test results	Automated, system wide tracking of cancer-related abnormal test results lacking follow-up documentation generated context specific prompts to care providers
(Graven, Allen, Smith, & MacDonald, 2013)	Improved productivity through reduced mortality rates	The entire country of Belize experienced reduced mortality rates in eight disease management algorithm domains that used automated alerts to coordinate care
(Ip et al., 2012)	Improved productivity through improved screening of PAP tests for patients at the Mayo Clinic.	50 000 PAP results were examined to develop a CDS to identify abnormal test results, which was then combined with screening and management guidelines, generating alerts for care providers.
(Suganthi & Madheswaran, 2012)	Improved productivity through improved detection of malignant breast tumors	Neural networks and a multi-objective genetic algorithm are deployed to detect malignant tumors using texture and shape features extracted from mammograms, automatically advising clinicians of potential breast cancers.

1. Better results through harm reduction,
2. Reduced incentive to cheat when results can be confirmed independently,
3. Improved efficiency by eliminating the need to collect data where sufficient data exists,
4. Meta-analyses based on published summary data would be much more reliable.

Gotzsche notes a potential harm that can arise from data sharing – that anyone with an agenda "could selectively interpret the data in a way that furthers this agenda (p.6), but suggests that making data widely available would allow those agendas to be challenged as easily as they can be asserted.

Much of the current literature on the benefits of transparency in the sharing of clinical trial data remains speculative, but almost all literature specifically identifies the potential for big data analytics to deliver both lower costs and improved productivity (Mello et al., 2013). Mello identifies nine specific benefits of sharing clinical trial data and the principal beneficiaries which are analyzed in Table 4.

The following papers confirm at least one of the benefits identified by Mello and Gotzsche, delivered through the use of advanced algorithms

analyzing dynamic data in real time. While much literature exists describing the benefits of open clinical trials, only those specifically describing the use of big data analytics are included in the analysis. Large sample sizes are insufficient for inclusion if the data is not analyzed using advanced algorithms that offer correctives or other information at the time of the trial. For example a study of over 5000 patients randomly prescribed medication to treat diabetes was not included because the analysis used traditional proportional hazards regressions to evaluate historical data that was not changing at the time of analysis (Ginsberg et al., 2010). In contrast, a study of over 20 000 clinical trials conducted at Pfizer was used to create a database of historical controls in the area of pain management, allowing future pain control trials to partially reduce their need to subject some trial participants to a placebo arm by automatically displaying the results from previous studies when new trials are initiated (Desai, Bowen, Danielson, Allam, & Cantor, 2013). While double-blind, randomized trials remain the preferred methodology for clinical trial research (Avins, Cherkin, Sherman, Goldberg, & Pressman, 2012), the reality is that

Table 4. Potential benefits of sharing clinical trial data

Primary Beneficiaries Benefit	Public or Patients	Research Participants	Scientific Community	Regulators	Trial Sponsors
Encourage accurate characterization of the benefits and risks of drugs in research reports, improving public confidence in clinical research and pharmaceuticals	x		x	x	x
Improving surveillance of drug safety and effectiveness	x		x	x	
Facilitate secondary analysis of clinical trial data to explore new scientific questions	x		x		x
Speed innovation	x		x		x
Enable patients and advocacy groups to learn more about their specific medical problems	x				
Ensure that research participants are not exposed to unnecessary risks		x	x		
Ensure that research subjects' participation advances science		x	x		
Achieve operational efficiencies in conducting clinical trials			x		x
Inform strategic decisions about potential avenues of research and development			x		x

participants do not like being part of the placebo group and will often drop out of a study if they feel that is the case, seriously compromising the research (Llewellyn-Thomas, McGreal, Thiel, Fine, & Erlichman, 1991). The creation of an historical controls database, containing the data from placebo groups allows researchers to reduce the number of patients receiving placebos while maintaining the integrity of the trial.

The scarcity of literature in the area is likely the result of the fact that despite strenuous calls to do so, most trial results are simply not reported. Huser & Cimino (2013) found that of 8907 trials registered at ClinicalTrials.gov, only 9.2% reported results by both registry and publication. For the cited examples, the principle benefit realized was improved productivity through appropriately selecting trial participants based on combined results from previous trials and other data sources (see Table 5).

Remote Patient Monitoring (RPM)

Remote Patient Monitoring (RPM) is an aspect of telemedicine that requires the use of big data analytics almost by definition. Defined broadly, telemedicine "is the use of electronic information and communications technologies to provide and support health care when distance separates the participants" (Field & Grigsby, 2002). Historically, telemedicine used video and land based communications to deliver health services to remote populations (see Table 6).

A very early project involving NASA, the Tohono O'odham Indian Nation, the Lockheed Missile and Space Company, the Indian Health Service and the Department of Health, Education and Welfare demonstrated "the feasibility of a consortium of public and private partners working together to provide medical care to remote

Table 5. Demonstrated benefits applied to transparency

Citation	Benefit	Summary of Findings
(Fenstermacher, Wenham, Rollison, & Dalton, 2011)	Improved productivity through better outcomes for cancer patients and lower costs by identifying clinical trial participants	Over 100 000 patients records are continuously updated and monitored for participation in appropriate cancer clinical trials
(Li et al., 2013)	Improved productivity by increasing clinical trial participants leading to better drug development	Automating clinical trial eligibility by recognizing medication attributes using natural language processing
(Desai et al., 2013)	Improved productivity through better outcomes for patients in pain therapeutic area and lower costs by increasing the likelihood that clinical trial participants will continue trial by reducing randomization factor	20 000 Pfizer trials were mined to examine effects on placebo subjects and used to create a historical placebo group database to supplement distribution calculations for future placebo groups
(Fraccaro, Dentone, Fenoglio, & Giacomini, 2013)	Improved productivity through the creation of patient cohorts for enrollment in clinical trials in the areas of HIV and eye diseases	A web-based Clinical Data Management System captures patient information from EHRs and allows simultaneous sharing of the information for multicenter research, automatically generating patient cohorts specific to each center
(Ginn, Alexander, Edelstein, Abedi, & Wixon, 2013)	Improved productivity through sharing of results from gene therapy trials across the internet	A searchable database records the results from all gene therapy trials around the world, accessible on the internet to all future researchers

Table 6. Telehealth definitions

	Definition
Telehealthcare	The use of any information technology to provide healthcare at a distance
Telemedicine	The use of electronic information and telecommunication technologies to support long distance health care, patient and professional health care, patient and professional health related education, public health and health administration
Telemonitoring	Monitoring patients who are not at the same location as the health care provider
Remote Patient Monitoring	The use of technology to enable monitoring of patients outside of conventional clinical settings

populations via telecommunication" as early as the 1970s (Freiburger, Holcomb, & Piper, 2007). These early telemedicine initiatives did not require the use of advanced data analytics, but rapid advances in both communications and medical technology have made RPM considerably more complex than simple videoconferencing.

RPM involves continuous monitoring of the "physiological status of patients using heterogeneous sensors such as blood pressure, weight, blood glucose, and/or physical activity sensors in order to shift medical services from hospital and clinical settings to an in-home monitoring scenario" (Lan et al., 2012). The principal ratio-nale behind early RPM systems is to improve the delivery of health care services for better patient outcomes, especially when those patients were underserved (Shea et al., 2006). Using a variety of sensors and wireless technology to monitor "multiple biological and environmental signals simultaneously, the RPM system can also provide alarms/alerts for the patient or the caregiver in real time so that the patient gets assistance in a timely manner when an acute event occurs" (Joshi, Moradshahi, & Goubran, 2013).

While improved outcomes for patients are still an important feature of RPM, the benefits of big data analytics in this area related primarily to reduced costs (Baker, Johnson, Macaulay, & Birnbaum, 2011; Cryer, Shannon, Van Amsterdam, & Leff, 2012; Klersy et al., 2011). When the data generated by RPM is processed using an analytics engine that provides "intelligent back-end processing and machine learning algorithms", the rate of false negatives falls dramatically as opposed to conventional RPM (Lee et al., 2013). This means that rates of readmission for any particular condition declines, as the advanced algorithms of big data analytics are far better at detecting which patients require readmission than human interpreters, who tend to be risk adverse and recommend readmission if there is any doubt in their minds (Radhakrishnan, Jacelon, & Roche, 2012). Despite the quantifiable benefits both in terms of reduced patient morbidity and lower costs, less than half of eligible patients are enrolled in RPM programs for implantable cardioverter-defibrillators, indicating that the area of RPM is likely to continue to experience significant growth (Akar et al., 2013).

While most of the articles describe the benefits of remote and automated monitoring of implantable devices, which are more effective in detecting adverse cardiac events than clinical evaluations (Guédon-Moreau, Mabo, & Kacet, 2013), another interesting application involves the use of Interactive Voice-Response Systems (IVR) for the management of chronic diseases (Piette, 2000). Patients suffering from mental health issues (Baer et al., 1995; González, Costello, La Tourette, Joyce, & Valenzuela, 1997; Kobak et al., 1997), diabetes (Mahoney, Tennstedt, Friedman, & Heeren, 1999; Piette & Mah, 1997; Piette, McPhee, Weinberger, Mah, & Kraemer, 1999), heart failure (Patel & Babbs, 1992), drug and alcohol addictions (Alemi et al., 1994; Perrine, Mundt, Searles, & Lester, 1995), lower back pain (Millard & Carver, 1999) and patients undergoing outpatient chemotherapy (Christ & Siegel, 1990) were all monitored using IVR which was consistently more effective, or at least *as* effective as a traditional clinical assessment at identifying patients requiring clinical follow-ups. The use of software and automated telephone inquiry systems result in dramatically lower costs as routine follow-ups with human caregivers are targeted at those patients who require additional attention. IVR technology that includes big data analytics results in health care providers receiving alerts as the software analyzes the responses to questions, allowing the "clinical team to intervene sooner when a patient's symptoms worsen" (Rich, Howe, Larson, & Chuang, 2013). The potential to deliver IVR and provide caregivers with real time analytics is a topic of considerable interest, but the true potential of combining IVR data with other data sources to alert patients and/or providers has

Table 7. Future applications

Technology	Potential Medical Applications
High frequency electromagnetic wave sensors (microwaves)	• Detect changes in heart and respiratory rates by measuring vibrations on the body surface • Detect changes in sympathovagal balance as a measurement of stress • Low power Doppler radar to detect respiratory rates in newborns, alerting caregivers when no movement is detected
Frequency modulated continuous wave radar	• Detection of physical orientation of bodies • Monitoring nighttime movements of patients with dementia, which is associated with increased rates of injury • Monitoring vital signs through evaluation of signal echoes
Infrared thermography	Rapid detection of infectious disease in airports and other areas when large numbers of people congregate
Global positioning systems	Enable rapid response to cardiac events through the use of wearable ECG monitors that continuously convey data via smartphones

(Jose & Jingle, 2013; Suzuki & Matsui, 2012)

yet to be realized (Willig et al., 2013). See Table 7 for potential future applications.

Table 8 describes several different areas in which RPM and the use of big data analytics resulted in lower costs by avoiding costly readmissions. Articles that described RPM through the use of telephone or video communications were not included, and only those articles that referenced RPM through the use of big data analytics and real time alerts/alarms were considered, which is not to say that RPM through more traditional, static communications is not of value. Medicare patients with heart failure who were monitored via video and land based telephone lines experienced fewer hospitalization events and subsequently lower costs accrued to the hospitals (Pekmezaris et al., 2012).

A meta-analysis of all RPM strategies for patients with heart failure demonstrates that either continuous device monitoring with a Human-to-Machine (HM) interface or structured telephone support with Human-to-Human (HH) interaction reduces mortality rates, but RPM with HM interaction is more cost effective (Pandor et al., 2013).

Personalized Medicine (PM)

Personalized Medicine (PM) uses "modern imaging and exploratory technologies to disclose genomic, proteomic and epigenetic information peculiar to each patient, in the effort to individualize prognosis and therapeutic care" (Nicolaidis, 2013). Big data in biomedicine is "driven by

Table 8. Demonstrated benefits of RPM

Citation	Benefit	Summary of Findings
(Varma & Michalski, 2013)	Lower costs by preventing readmission following heart implants	Patients monitored remotely were automatically alerted to follow-up appointments at regular intervals post-implant, resulting in better adherence to follow-up protocols and better detection of adverse events
(Abraham, 2013)	Lower costs by preventing readmission following heart implants	Patients monitored remotely were alerted to adverse events using a pulmonary artery pressure measurement system which automatically detects the onset of heart failure permitting intervention before more serious events that require hospitalization occur
(Mabo et al., 2012)	Lower costs by preventing readmission following implantation of a pacemaker	Data collected from pacemakers automatically transmits to a data service center for analysis and alerts are sent to health care providers when adverse advents are detected, permitting interventions to take place before more serious complications arise
(Varma, Pavri, Stambler, & Michalski, 2013)	Lower costs through same day detection of implantable cardioverter –defibrillator malfunction	ICD devices continuously monitored for malfunction and alerts automatically generated when malfunctions were detected, allowing repairs to be made before adverse events occurred undetected
(Zanaboni et al., 2013)	Lower costs through reduced hospital admissions	Patients with implantable cardiac devices monitored remotely had lower hospital admission rates in all studies examined
(Kosse, Brands, Bauer, Hortobagyi, & Lamoth, 2013)	Lower costs through the detection of preventable falls among elderly patients	Intelligent alarms monitor physical parameters and alert caregivers to changes that indicate a potential fall, reducing falls by 77% with minimal false alarms
(Pecchia, Melillo, & Bracale, 2011)	Lower costs through the early detection of problematic heart arrhythmias	Historical ECG records were mined to create classification rules for arrhythmias and patients with implantable heart devices were monitored for adverse signals which triggered automatic alerts to health care providers
(Amir, Wolf, Rappaport, & Abraham, 2012)	Lower costs through early detection of pulmonary congestion leading to heart failure	Remote detection of pulmonary congestion using dielectric senor technology
(Arasaratnam et al., 2012)	Lower costs through appropriate dosage	Automated, remote site dose monitoring for patients undergoing cardiac catheterization provides consistent optimal dosage instructions automatically to remote clinics

the single premise of one day having personalized medicine programs that will…establish the causal genetic factors that could help manage the golden triangle of treatment: the right target, the right chemistry, the right patient" (see Figure 2) (Costa, 2013).

Ten years after the completion of the Human Genome Project, progress towards the goal of PM has stalled, largely because the science is harder than expected and because economic incentives are not aligned to invest in diagnostics (Lester, 2009; Towse, Ossa, Veenstra, Carlson, & Garrison, 2013).

While PM makes use of large sets of data stored digitally, not all PM is based on analytics that qualify as "big data". Some of the obstacles to reaching the full potential inherent in big data and PM include:

- Lack of an appropriate computational infrastructure and architecture to generate, maintain, transfer and analyze large data sets,
- Integrating that data with *omics* data and other data sets, such as imaging and patient clinical records,
- Managing the costs associated with generating, storing and analyzing data,
- Difficulties in transferring data from one location to another (usually done by mailing external hard drives),
- Maintaining the security and privacy of the data (Costa, 2013).

Personalized medicine represents the clinical area that originally showed the most promise in terms of deploying big data analytics, but has proven to be the most difficult to implement. Specific barriers to implementation:

- **Scientific Challenges:** Including identifying clinically significant genetic markers, limiting off-target effects of gene therapy, and conducting clinical trials to identify

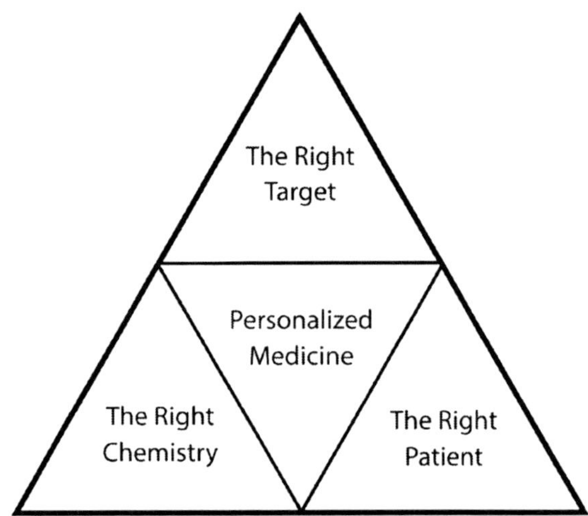

Figure 2. The golden triangle

genetic variants associated with a particular drug response.

- **Regulatory Challenges:** Including defined regulatory pathways for coordinated approval of co-developed diagnostics and therapies, the development of risk-based reviews to assess validity and utility, and ensuring data transparency.
- **Commercialization Challenges:** Including creating downstream market opportunities and enticing private sector participants to explore how new understandings of genes, proteins and pathways can lead to new and better drug targets, accelerating and sharing the costs of preclinical development phases, and formalizing partnerships between private and public sector organizations.
- **Data Challenges:** Including the development of tissue banks containing specimens along with information linking them to clinical outcomes, sufficient processing power to retain and analyze massive sets of information, and enhanced ability to share and move data between sites.
- **Translational Challenges:** Including the development of a standard ontology and evaluation tools, such as biomarkers and

assays, the inclusion of pharmacogenomics information in drug labelling, standardizing the accuracy of diagnostic tests and clarifying the processes manufacturers must follow regarding claims about how treatments, and diagnostics work (Hamburg & Collins, 2010).

Despite these limitations, researchers and technology developers continue to explore opportunities to realize the promise of big data and personalized medicine. The New York Genome Center (NYGC) and IBM announced an initiative to use IBM's Watson cognitive system to deliver personalized treatment options for aggressive genetic cancers like glioblastoma, a type of brain cancer that kills 13 000 people each year in the United States. Waston is a "new class of software, services and apps that think, improve by learning, and discover answers and insights to complex questions from massive amounts of Big Data" (NYGC, 2014). Dr. R. Kravitz (2014) notes that personalized medicine in terms of phenotypes and patient preferences offers ample opportunities to deliver patient specific treatment options without necessarily relying on genomic data.

Public Health Administration (PHA)

According to the World Health Organization (WHO), public health refers to all organized measures (whether public or private) to prevent disease, promote health, and prolong life among the population as a whole. Its activities aim to provide conditions in which people can be healthy and focus on entire populations, not on individual patients or diseases. Thus, public health is concerned with the total system and not only the eradication of a particular disease. The three main public health functions are:

1. The assessment and monitoring of the health of communities and populations at risk to identify health problems and priorities.

2. The formulation of public policies designed to solve identified local and national health problems and priorities.
3. To assure that all populations have access to appropriate and cost-effective care, including health promotion and disease prevention services.

Public health initiatives include:

- Vaccination and control of infectious diseases,
- Motor vehicle safety,
- Safer workplaces,
- Safer and healthier foods,
- Safe drinking water,
- Healthier mothers, babies and families,
- Decline in deaths from preventable illnesses such as heart disease, diabetes and cancer (Bonita, Beaglehole, & Kjellstrom, 2006).

Public health providers have been using very large, novel sources of data since 1999, making this section of healthcare one of the earliest adopters of huge datasets to prompt actions in very close to real time. These early initiatives do not meet both criteria for big data analytics, however, as the methods used to analyze the data were not automated, did not use advanced mining algorithms or any kind of machine learning and analyzed static data that was not changing at the time of analysis.

Epidemiology, a subset of public health is defined as the "study of all health and disease" (Morris, 1975), although in more colloquial uses it refers to the study of infectious disease outbreaks, specifically. Digital epidemiology, e-epidemiology and Tele-epidemiology all refer to the use of novel data sources to track infectious disease.

Traditionally, epidemiology has been based on data collected by public health agencies through health personnel in hospitals, doctors offices and out in the field (Salathe, Freifeld, Mekaru,

Tomasulo, & Brownstein, 2013). The use of data generated by weather, satellite and ocean technologies created advanced opportunities to detect and respond to infectious disease outbreaks, but digital epidemiology in this form still used standard analytics on static data.

The French National Space Agency (CNES) has carried out several Tele-epidemiology projects that have allowed public health officials to detect infectious disease outbreaks almost as soon they happen.

Some early successes in Tele-epidemiology include:

- **S2E Guyana:** Dengue fever in Guyana.
- **EMERCASE:** Rift Valley fever in Senegal and Southern Mauritania.
- **S2E Argos:** Tropical diseases in Niger and Burkina Faso.
- **S2E Migrating:** Avian flu in the Camargue area of France, a joint project with the National Institute for Health and Medical Research (INSERM).
- **MATE:** Dengue fever in Argentina, a joint project with the Argentinean Spatial Agency (CONAE).
- **BIBO:** Avian flu, a joint project with the Chinese Space Agency (CRESDA).
- **VIBRIO:** Cholera in the Mediterranean. (Marechal, Ribeiro, Lafaye, & Güell, 2008).

The prime driver for these initiatives is to create or amplify the effects of Early Warning Systems (EWS) to prevent the spread of disease (Thomson & Connor, 2001), which delivers two key benefits:

1. Improved productivity through a dramatic reduction in mortality and morbidity rates.
2. Lower costs through avoidance of economic impact of wide-spread infectious disease.

Public health care providers tend to be driven by the need to improve productivity and reduce the suffering and mortality associated with infectious disease outbreaks. "At its core, public health is concerned with promoting and protecting the health of populations" (Childress et al., 2002). Policy makers, in comparison, tend to be concerned with the economic impact of large scale disease outbreaks, and the impact can be significant. The aggregate annual economic cost of a dengue fever outbreak in Puerto Rico was estimated to be $46 million, and the weighted average cost of treatment per case is $3 078, representing 19% of the per capita GDP ($16 300 in 2010). Who pays these costs?

- 36% paid by government
- 40% incurred by households
- 18% incurred by insurance
- 6% incurred by employers. (Halasa, Shepard, & Zeng, 2012)

Both benefits tend to accrue together in the case of public health administration, and which benefit is stressed depends on whether the perspective of policy or provider is emphasized. In almost every case, both reduced morbidity and mortality and avoidance of costs occurs in tandem.

There are four specific ways that digital data can be used to study infectious disease dynamics:

1. Early detection of outbreaks
2. Continuous monitoring of disease levels
3. Assessment of health related behaviours relevant to disease control
4. Additional method for analyzing the period before an outbreak. (Salathe et al., 2013)

The opportunity for big data in public health administration is to capture data from novel sources such as social media, mobile telecommunications and the Internet to automatically detect opportunities to enhance public health and create alerts that notify relevant personnel at the moment the opportunity is detected.

Google Flu is an excellent example of how a machine algorithm can detect an outbreak of influenza long before health care personnel, by compiling a list of flu-related search words and tracking their entry into the search engine by geographic location (Olson, Konty, Paladini, Viboud, & Simonsen, 2013). Google Flu is not without flaws, and can often miss outbreaks (Olson, 2013), but as the search engine grows increasingly experienced, its abilities will improve. Combining the search engine with results from retail pharmacies, tracking both over the counter and prescription medicine orders for flu-related symptoms (Patwardhan & Bilkovski, 2012) or emergency room visits for flu-like symptoms (Dugas et al., 2012) increases the predictive efficacy of Google Flu. When the search engine data is further refined through the use of control engineering mathematical models that measure probabilistic dependence between latent state variables, and observed measurements generated by the search engine, the predictive power of the

enterprise to detect influenza outbreaks increases (Dukic, Lopes, & Polson, 2012).

The majority of the scholarly literature is concerned with developing the architecture to effectively initiate digital epidemiology that can generate alerts in real time, but little of this has been tested in the field to date. In a review of influenza syndromic surveillance in emergency rooms, none of the 58 studies reviewed made use of big data analytics (Hiller, Stoneking, Min, & Rhodes, 2013), although several stressed the potential big data might offer (Kass-Hout et al., 2012; Painter, Eaton, & Lober, 2013)

Researchers at Johns Hopkins have demonstrated that by mining over 2 billion tweets, Twitter can effectively be used to extract public health information regarding a variety of ailments and conditions, but that demonstration has not yet led to implementation of a Twitter based symptom surveillance program (Paul & Dredze, 2012). See Table 9 for a summary of public health and social media potential.

In a similar vein, researchers were able to illustrate and model individual behaviors using social media data that are capable of predicting

Table 9. Public health and social media potential

How to Use Twitter to Track Conditions Using Most Likely Words							
	Allergies	**Insomnia**	**Obesity**	**Injuries**	**Respiratory**	**Dental**	**Aches/Pains**
General	allergies nose eyes allergy allergic	sleep asleep fell awake hours	blood weight eat healthy fat	knee leg right ankle shoulder	throat stop better voice hurts	"ow" teeth tooth wisdom dentist	body needs neck hurts head
Symptoms	sneezing coughing cold nose runny	insomnia fall burning pain falling	pressure weight loss blood high	pain sore arthritis limping neck	cough coughing cold sneeze sneezing	pain toothache sore infection tooth	aches pain sore muscle aching
Treatments	medicine benadryl Claritin zyrtec drops	sleeping pills caffeine Tylenol pill	diet exercise dieting insulin exercising	surgery brace crutches physical therapy	medicine antibiotics codeine vitamin Tylenol	braces pain relief muscle surgery	massage exercise massages bath hot

(Paul & Dredze, 2012)

depression *before* onset by exploring language, emotion, style, egonetworks and user engagement to predict depressive episodes. The research found that depressive individuals demonstrated the following characteristics:

- Lowered social activity
- Greater negative emotions
- High self-attentional focus
- Increased relational and medicinal concerns
- Heightened expression of religious thoughts
- Usually belonged to highly clustered, close-knit networks
- Highly embedded with their audiences. (De Choudhury, Gamon, Counts, & Horvitz, 2013)

In theory, the observation of the above characteristics could trigger an alert to both the individual and a mental health care provider, but at the moment, the opportunity exists only in theory.

An interesting drawback to the use of internet or social media based data sources has to do with signal amplification. In 2011, a team of researchers discovered a link between the use of pravastatin in combination with paroxetine and hyperglycemia, which they confirmed by mining search engines for those specific keywords and related terms. Subsequent media attention to the relationship resulted in many more people searching for those terms, amplifying the signal power and suggesting, incorrectly, that more people were experiencing problems than was actually the case. "Search data are very sensitive to media, marketing and viral social influence … if there are murmurs there is a dangerous drug, people on the drug will look it up. They may not have the problem, they are just worried" (Kuehn, 2013). It's an on-going issue that architects and designers are attempting to address (Diaz-Aviles, Stewart, Velasco, Denecke, & Nejdl, 2012).

In the area of traffic management, much of the deployment of big data analytics is concerned with military surveying and mapping (Tang & Yuwen, 2013) or military logistics management (tracking personnel and equipment) (Becker et al., 2013). Additionally, most of the literature is concerned with developing the algorithms and architecture necessary to realize the potential benefits, but there have also been some notable successes at using data to improve public safety on the transportation network, both on the ground and in the air (see Table 10) which shows papers describing the actual deployment of big data analytics in the area of public health administration, and the benefits accrued.

FUTURE RESEARCH DIRECTIONS

This chapter organized the relevant literature into six distinct sections: Cost Effectiveness Research (CER), Clinical Decision Support Systems (CDS), Transparency, Remote Patient Monitoring (RPM), Personalized Medicine (PM), and Public Health Administration (PHA). Of the six areas investigated, CDS shows the most use of big data analytics, likely a result of the ability of algorithms to build on the vast data sources about drug regimes captured by automated physician order entry systems. CER has also has some notable successes, again building on the cached data sources maintained by pharmaceutical companies and insurance providers. Public health, with ample data sources to draw on has been successful in implementing some innovative big data strategies. RPM is just beginning to realize the potential in having advanced, learning algorithms monitor patients with both implantable and wearable devices, which both alert caregivers to potential problems (including device malfunction) and dramatically reduce rehospitalization rates by detecting problems at the earliest stages.

Table 10. Demonstrated benefits in the area of public health

Citation	Benefits Described	Summary of Findings
(Takeshi, Makoto, & Yutaka, 2010)	Improved productivity through quick notification and lower costs by alerting citizens to an earthquake in progress	Earthquakes greater than 3 on the seismic scale are detected through the continuous monitoring of Twitter and users in the area of the earthquake are notified that a quake is in progress allowing them to take protective actions
(Schmidt, 2012)	Improved productivity through quick notification and lower costs by alerting citizens to an outbreak in progress	Development of a iPhone application (HealthMap) that mines news websites, government alerts, eyewitness accounts and other data sources for reports of disease outbreaks and then delivers maps directly to users via mobile phones to alert them at the time an outbreak is detected
(Diaz-Aviles et al., 2012)	Improved productivity through quick notification and effective tracking of transmissions and lower costs by alerting citizens to an outbreak in progress	Twitter carefully monitored during an outbreak of *Enterohemorrhagic Escherichia coli* in Germany triggering alarms well before more established systems detected a problem, and effectively tracking transmission patterns
(Chunara, Andrews, & Brownstein, 2012)	Improved productivity through quick notification and effective use of resources and lower costs by alerting citizens to safe water sources and treatment centers before the cholera became serious	Creation of maps (using Health Map) that transmit real time data via mobile phones showing confirmed cases, location of hospitals, treatment centers, safe water installations and water points to combat the cholera epidemic after the 2010 earthquake in Haiti
(Larson et al., 2013)	Improved productivity through instant awareness of vaccine concerns in a specific location and lower costs through avoidance of preventable disease outbreaks	Real time monitoring of negative public opinions about vaccines over social media using Health Maps to allow immunization programs to tailor programs for greater uptake
(Gerz, Tafferner, Park, & Keis, 2012)	Lower costs through better prediction of weather conditions and improved productivity through enhanced safety	Algorithms combine radar, satellite and surface station data to detect snow fall and icing conditions at airports, and report weather conditions in real time, automatically alerting ground crews to changing or dangerous conditions
(Ovide, 2012)	Improved productivity through faster detection of traffic flow problems	Millions of cellphone and GPS signals are combined with car speed information, weather data and sports schedules to detect interruptions in traffic in Woodbridge, N.J., alerting traffic control personnel of problems

The biggest setbacks have occurred in the area of PM, where the sequencing of the human genome originally held such promise. The actual practice of genomic medicine has turned out to be vastly technically complex, and requires huge tissue and bio-banks to mine for information. As the technical and infrastructure problems are addressed, the potential for big data will become increasingly easier to harness.

CONCLUSION

In the healthcare sector of the economy, the application of big data analytics is motivated by the dual incentives to reduce the costs of delivering health-care services and products while improving the ability of healthcare providers to enhance patient outcomes. While costs pressures are significant, there is little evidence that cost alone motivates practitioners to embrace the opportunities and benefits of advanced analytics (Mueller & Szczesny, 2013; Smith, Saunders, Stuckhardt, & McGinnis, 2013; Tuckson, Newcomer, & De Sa, 2013). The benefits of big data accrue primarily to patients in terms of reduced morbidity and mortality rates, more effective and targeted treatments and better monitoring of chronic conditions, and to health services providers who are able to deliver more effective treatments and services while using healthcare resources more efficiently.

The two principle benefits tend to occur in tandem. In the case of RPM, reducing the costs of monitoring patients was a primary driver, but outcomes for patients were almost always improved as well.

Pharmaceutical companies and medical equipment providers are motivated to realize the benefits of capturing additional market share (Gagnon, 2013) and limiting liability (Jones, 2013), but the adoption of particular pharmaceutical regimes or specific equipment in the field is motivated by the initial two benefits of lowering costs while improving patient outcomes.

Table 11 summarizes the findings in each section analyzed.

Most of applications of big data analytics are in nascent stages of adoption. This is particularly true for personalized medicine, but efforts to create the large datasets and tissue banks necessary to realize the full potential of big data are underway, including efforts to communicate the vital importance of these datasets to both patients and practitioners alike. "The critical value of tissue bank samples, bioinformatics, and EMR in the early stages of the biomarker discovery process for personalized medicine is often overlooked", according to Suh et. al. (2013) but that is slowly

changing as the benefits of big data analytics accrue and become clear to all stakeholders.

The way forward will require that certain challenges, some very specific to healthcare, be tackled:

- Continual technical advances to store and efficiently access the rapidly expanding amount of data
- Ensuring patient privacy and security
- Collecting good data that is accurate and relatively complete
- Aligning economic incentives to encourage the development of diagnostics. (Adler-Milstein et al., 2013)

Big data is poised to reshape the way we live, work, and think. A worldview built on the importance of causation is being challenged by a preponderance of correlations. The possession of knowledge, which once meant an understanding of the past, is coming to mean an ability to predict the future. The challenges posed by big data will not be easy to resolve. Rather, they are simply the next step in the timeless debate over how to best understand the world. (Cukier & Mayer-Schoenberger, 2013).

Table 11. Summary of findings

Area of Inquiry	Benefit Observed	Primary Beneficiary
Cost Effectiveness Research	Lower costs Improved productivity	Healthcare providers Patients
Clinical Decision Support	Improved productivity Lower costs Increased market share	Patients Healthcare providers Health care providers
Transparency	Improved productivity	Patients
Remote Patient Monitoring	Lower costs	Healthcare providers
Public Health	Improved productivity Lower costs	Patients and the general public Transportation providers
Personalized Medicine	Improved productivity	Patients

REFERENCES

Adler-Milstein, J., Jha, A. K., Caballero, A. E., Davidson, J., Elmi, A., & Gavin, J. et al. (2013). Healthcare's "Big Data" Challenge. *The American Journal of Managed Care*, *19*(7), 537–538. PMID:23919417

Ahern, D. K., Smith, J. M., Topol, E. J., Mack, J. F., & Fitzgerald, M. (2013). Addressing the cost crisis in Health Care. *American Journal of Preventive Medicine*, *44*(1).

Akar, J. G., Bao, H., Jones, P., Wang, Y., Chaudhry, S. I., & Varosy, P. et al. (2013). Use of Remote Monitoring of Newly Implanted Cardioverter-Defibrillators: Insights From the Patient Related Determinants of ICD Remote Monitoring (PREDICT RM) Study. *Circulation*, *128*(22), 2372–2383. doi:10.1161/CIRCULATIONAHA.113.002481 PMID:24043302

Alemi, F., Stephens, R., Parran, T., Llorens, S., Bhatt, P., Ghadiri, A., & Eisenstein, E. (1994). Automated Monitoring of Outcomes Application to Treatment of Drug Abuse. *Medical Decision Making*, *14*(2), 180–187. doi:10.1177/0272989X9401400211 PMID:8028471

Avins, A. L., Cherkin, D. C., Sherman, K. J., Goldberg, H., & Pressman, A. (2012). Should we reconsider the routine use of placebo controls in clinical research? *Trials*, *13*(1), 44. doi:10.1186/1745-6215-13-44 PMID:22540350

Avorn, J., & Fischer, M. (2010). 'Bench to behavior': Translating comparative effectiveness research into improved clinical practice. *Health Affairs*, *29*(10), 1891–1900. doi:10.1377/hlthaff.2010.0696 PMID:20921491

Baer, L., Jacobs, D. G., Cukor, P., O'Laughlen, J., Coyle, J. T., & Magruder, K. M. (1995). Automated telephone screening survey for depression. *Journal of the American Medical Association*, *273*(24), 1943–1944. doi:10.1001/jama.1995.03520480063041 PMID:7783305

Baker, L. C., Johnson, S. J., Macaulay, D., & Birnbaum, H. (2011). Integrated telehealth and care management program for Medicare beneficiaries with chronic disease linked to savings. *Health Affairs*, *30*(9), 1689–1697. doi:10.1377/hlthaff.2011.0216 PMID:21900660

Bates, D. W. (1998). Effect of Computerized Physician Order Entry and a Team Intervention on Prevention of Serious Medication Errors. *Journal of the American Medical Association*, *280*(15), 1311. doi:10.1001/jama.280.15.1311 PMID:9794308

Bates, D. W., Teich, J. M., Lee, J., Seger, D., Kuperman, G. J., & Ma'Luf, N. et al. (1999). The impact of computerized physician order entry on medication error prevention. *Journal of the American Medical Informatics Association*, *6*(4), 313–321. doi:10.1136/jamia.1999.00660313 PMID:10428004

Becker, D., King, T. D., McMullen, B., Lalis, L. D., Bloom, D., Obaidi, A., & Fickitt, D. (2013). Big Data Quality Case Study Preliminary Findings. Bedford, MA: National Security Engineering Center.

Berner, E. S. (2007). *Clinical Decision Support Systems*. Springer Science+Business Media, LLC.

Bernstam, E. V., Smith, J. W., & Johnson, T. R. (2010). What is biomedical informatics? *Journal of Biomedical Informatics*, *43*(1), 104–110. doi:10.1016/j.jbi.2009.08.006 PMID:19683067

Bertot, J. C., Jaeger, P. T., & Grimes, J. M. (2010). Using ICTs to create a culture of transparency: E-government and social media as openness and anti-corruption tools for societies. *Government Information Quarterly*, *27*(3), 264–271. doi:10.1016/j.giq.2010.03.001

Bian, Z.-X., & Wu, T.-X. (2010). Commentary Legislation for trial registration and data transparency. *Trials*, *11*(64).

Bloom, D. E., Börsch-Supan, A., McGee, P., & Seike, A. (2012). Population Ageing: Macro Challenges and Policy Responses. *Global Population Ageing: Peril or Promise?*, 35.

Bollier, D. (2010). *The Promise and Peril of Big Data*. Paper presented at the Eighteenth Annual Aspen Institute Roundtable on Information Technology. Washington, DC. Retrieved from http://creativecommons.org/licenses/by-nc/3.0/us/

Bonita, R., Beaglehole, R., & Kjellstrom, T. (2006). *Basic Epidemiology*. Geneva, Switzerland: World Health Organization.

Bright, T. J., Wong, A., Dhurjati, R., Bristow, E., Bastian, L., & Coeytaux, R. R. et al. (2012). Effect of clinical decision-support systems: A systematic review. *Annals of Internal Medicine*, *157*(1), 29–43. doi:10.7326/0003-4819-157-1-201207030-00450 PMID:22751758

Bult, J. R., & Wansbeek, T. (1995). Optimal Selection for Direct Mail. *Marketing Science*, *14*(4), 378–394. doi:10.1287/mksc.14.4.378

Chalkidou, K., Tunis, S., Lopert, R., Rochaix, L., Sawicki, P. T., Nasser, M., & Xerri, B. (2009). Comparative effectiveness research and evidence-based health policy: Experience from four countries. *The Milbank Quarterly*, *87*(2), 339–367. doi:10.1111/j.1468-0009.2009.00560.x PMID:19523121

Chen, H., Chiang, R. H. L., & Storey, V. C. (2012). Business Intelligence and Analytics: From Big Data to Big Impact. *Management Information Systems Quarterly*, *36*(4), 1165–1188.

Childress, J. F., Faden, R. R., Gaare, R. D., Gostin, L. O., Kahn, J., & Bonnie, R. J. et al. (2002). Public Health Ethics: Mapping the Terrain. *Law. Medical Ethics (Burlington, Mass.)*, *30*(2), 170–178. doi:10.1111/j.1748-720X.2002.tb00384.x PMID:12066595

Christ, G., & Siegel, K. (1990). Monitoring quality-of-life needs of cancer patients. *Cancer*, *65*(S3), 760–765. doi:10.1002/1097-0142(19900201)65:3+<760::AID-CNCR2820651321>3.0.CO;2-F PMID:2302653

Costa, F. F. (2013). Big data in biomedicine. *Drug Discovery Today*. doi:10.1016/j.drudis.2013.10.012

Cryer, L., Shannon, S. B., Van Amsterdam, M., & Leff, B. (2012). Costs for 'hospital at home' patients were 19 percent lower, with equal or better outcomes compared to similar inpatients. *Health Affairs*, *31*(6), 1237–1243. doi:10.1377/hlthaff.2011.1132 PMID:22665835

Cukier, K., & Mayer-Schoenberger, V. (2013). The Rise of Big Data. *Foreign Affairs*, *92*(3), 27–40.

De Choudhury, M., Gamon, M., Counts, S., & Horvitz, E. (2013). *Predicting Depression via Social Media*. Redmond, WA: Microsoft.

Desai, J. R., Bowen, E. A., Danielson, M. M., Allam, R. R., & Cantor, M. N. (2013). Creation and implementation of a historical controls database from randomized clinical trials. *Journal of the American Medical Informatics Association*, *20*(e1), e162–e168. doi:10.1136/amiajnl-2012-001257 PMID:23449762

Diaz-Aviles, E., Stewart, A., Velasco, E., Denecke, K., & Nejdl, W. (2012). *Epidemic Intelligence for the Crowd, by the Crowd*. Paper presented at the ICWSM. New York, NY.

Dugas, A. F., Hsieh, Y. H., Levin, S. R., Pines, J. M., Mareiniss, D. P., & Mohareb, A. et al. (2012). Google Flu Trends: Correlation with emergency department influenza rates and crowding metrics. *Clinical Infectious Diseases*, *54*(4), 463–469. doi:10.1093/cid/cir883 PMID:22230244

Dukic, V., Lopes, H. F., & Polson, N. G. (2012). Tracking epidemics with google flu trends data and a state-space SEIR model. *Journal of the American Statistical Association*, *107*(500), 1410–1426. doi:10.1080/01621459.2012.713876

Eppenga, W. L., Derijks, H. J., Conemans, J. M., Hermens, W. A., Wensing, M., & De Smet, P. A. (2012). Comparison of a basic and an advanced pharmacotherapy-related clinical decision support system in a hospital care setting in the Netherlands. *Journal of the American Medical Association*, *19*(1), 66–71. doi:10.1136/amiajnl-2011-000360 PMID:21890873

Field, M. J., & Grigsby, J. (2002). Telemedicine and remote patient monitoring. *Journal of the American Medical Association*, *288*(4), 423–425. doi:10.1001/jama.288.4.423 PMID:12132953

Fischer, M. A., & Avorn, J. (2004). Economic implications of evidence-based prescribing for hypertension: Can better care cost less? *Journal of the American Medical Association*, *291*(15), 1850–1856. doi:10.1001/jama.291.15.1850 PMID:15100203

Freiburger, G., Holcomb, M., & Piper, D. (2007). The STARPAHC collection: Part of an archive of the history of telemedicine. *Journal of Telemedicine and Telecare*, *13*(5), 221–223. doi:10.1258/135763307781458949 PMID:17697507

Gagnon, J. P. (2013). The research manufacturing pharmaceutical industry. In M. I. Smith, A. I. Vertheimer, & J. E. Fincham (Eds.), *Pharmacy and the US Healthcare System* (p. 215). London: Pharmaceutical Press.

Gandjour, A. (2011). Prioritizing Comparative Effectiveness Research. *PharmacoEconomics*, *29*(7), 555–561. PMID:21534639

Ginsberg, H. N., Elam, M. B., Lovato, L. C., Crouse, J. R. III, Leiter, L. A., & Linz, P. et al. (2010). Effects of combination lipid therapy in type 2 diabetes mellitus. *The New England Journal of Medicine*, *362*(17), 1563–1574. doi:10.1056/NEJMoa1001282 PMID:20228404

González, G. M., Costello, C. R., La Tourette, T. R., Joyce, L. K., & Valenzuela, M. (1997). Bilingual telephone-assisted computerized speech-recognition assessment: Is a voice-activated computer program a culturally and linguistically appropriate tool for screening depression in English and Spanish? *Cultural Diversity and Mental Health*, *3*(2), 93–111. doi:10.1037/1099-9809.3.2.93 PMID:9231537

Gøtzsche, P. C. (2011). Why we need easy access to all data from all clinical trials and how to accomplish it. *Trials*, *12*(1), 249. doi:10.1186/1745-6215-12-249 PMID:22112900

Guédon-Moreau, L., Mabo, P., & Kacet, S. (2013). Current clinical evidence for remote patient management. *Europace*, *15*(suppl 1), i6–i10. doi:10.1093/europace/eut119 PMID:23737234

Gupta, R., Gupta, H., & Mohania, M. (2012). Cloud Computing and Big Data Analytics: What Is New from Databases Perspective? In S. Srinivasa & V. Bhatnagar (Eds.), *Big Data Analytics* (Vol. 7678, pp. 42–61). Springer. doi:10.1007/978-3-642-35542-4_5

Halasa, Y. A., Shepard, D. S., & Zeng, W. (2012). Economic cost of dengue in Puerto Rico. *The American Journal of Tropical Medicine and Hygiene*, *86*(5), 745–752. doi:10.4269/ajtmh.2012.11-0784 PMID:22556069

Hamburg, M. A., & Collins, F. S. (2010). The path to personalized medicine. *The New England Journal of Medicine*, *363*(4), 301–304. doi:10.1056/NEJMp1006304 PMID:20551152

Hersh, W. (2009). A stimulus to define informatics and health information technology. *BMC Medical Informatics and Decision Making*, 9(1), 24. doi:10.1186/1472-6947-9-24 PMID:19445665

Hiller, K. M., Stoneking, L., Min, A., & Rhodes, S. M. (2013). Syndromic Surveillance for Influenza in the Emergency Department–A Systematic Review. *PLoS ONE*, 8(9), e73832. doi:10.1371/journal.pone.0073832 PMID:24058494

Huser, V., & Cimino, J. J. (2013). Linking ClinicalTrials. gov and PubMed to Track Results of Interventional Human Clinical Trials. *PLoS ONE*, 8(7), e68409. doi:10.1371/journal.pone.0068409 PMID:23874614

Jensen, P. B., Jensen, L. J., & Brunak, S. (2012). Mining electronic health records: Towards better research applications and clinical care. *Nature Reviews. Genetics*, 13(6), 395–405. doi:10.1038/nrg3208 PMID:22549152

Jones, R. M. (2013). *A New World Order: The Expansion of Executive Corporate Liability in the Life Sciences Industry*. Student Scholarship, Paper 250.

Jose, J., & Jingle, I. B. J. (2013). Remote Heart Monitoring and Diagnosis Service Platform via Wearable ECG Monitor. *International Journal of Science, Engineering and Technology Research*, 2(5), 1095–1099.

Joshi, V., Moradshahi, P., & Goubran, R. (2013). *Operating system performance measurements for remote patient monitoring applications*. Paper presented at the Medical Measurements and Applications Proceedings (MeMeA). New York, NY.

Jourdan, Z., Rainer, R. K., & Marshall, T. E. (2008). Business Intelligence: An Analysis of the Literature. *Information Systems Management*, 25(2), 121–131. doi:10.1080/10580530801941512

Kass-Hout, T. A., Xu, Z., McMurray, P., Park, S., Buckeridge, D. L., & Brownstein, J. S. et al. (2012). Application of change point analysis to daily influenza-like illness emergency department visits. *Journal of the American Medical Informatics Association*, 19(6), 1075–1081. doi:10.1136/amiajnl-2011-000793 PMID:22759619

Kawamoto, K., Houlihan, C. A., Balas, E. A., & Lobach, D. F. (2005). Improving clinical practice using clinical decision support systems: A systematic review of trials to identify features critical to success. *British Medical Journal*, 330(7494), 765. doi:10.1136/bmj.38398.500764.8F PMID:15767266

Kho, A. N., Rasmussen, L. V., Connolly, J. J., Peissig, P. L., Starren, J., Hakonarson, H., & Hayes, M. G. (2013). Practical challenges in integrating genomic data into the electronic health record. *Genetics in Medicine*, 15(10), 772–778. doi:10.1038/gim.2013.131 PMID:24071798

Klersy, C., De Silvestri, A., Gabutti, G., Raisaro, A., Curti, M., Regoli, F., & Auricchio, A. (2011). Economic impact of remote patient monitoring: An integrated economic model derived from a meta-analysis of randomized controlled trials in heart failure. *European Journal of Heart Failure*, 13(4), 450–459. doi:10.1093/eurjhf/hfq232 PMID:21193439

Kobak, K. A., Dottl, S. L., Greist, J. H., Jefferson, J. W., Burroughs, D., & Mantle, J. M. et al. (1997). A computer-administered telephone interview to identify mental disorders. *Journal of the American Medical Association*, 278(11), 905–910. doi:10.1001/jama.1997.03550110043034 PMID:9302242

Krasowski, M. D., & Penrod, L. E. (2012). Clinical decision support of therapeutic drug monitoring of phenytoin: Measured versus adjusted phenytoin plasma concentrations. *BMC Medical Informatics and Decision Making*, 12(1), 7. doi:10.1186/1472-6947-12-7 PMID:22333264

Kravitz, R. L. (2014). Personalized Medicine Without the "Omics". *Journal of General Internal Medicine*, 29(4), 551–551. doi:10.1007/s11606-014-2789-x PMID:24504920

Krleža-Jerić, K., & Lemmens, T. (2009). 7th revision of the Declaration of Helsinki: Good news for the transparency of clinical trials. *Croatian Medical Journal*, 50(2), 105–110. doi:10.3325/cmj.2009.50.105 PMID:19399942

Kuehn, B. M. (2013). Scientists mine web search data to identify epidemics and adverse events. *Journal of the American Medical Association*, 309(18), 1883–1884. doi:10.1001/jama.2013.4015 PMID:23652502

Lan, M., Samy, L., Alshurafa, N., Suh, M.-K., Ghasemzadeh, H., Macabasco-O'Connell, A., & Sarrafzadeh, M. (2012). *WANDA: an end-to-end remote health monitoring and analytics system for heart failure patients*. Paper presented at the Conference on Wireless Health. New York, NY. doi:10.1145/2448096.2448105

Lee, S. I., Ghasemzadeh, H., Mortazavi, B., Lan, M., Alshurafa, N., Ong, M., & Sarrafzadeh, M. (2013). *Remote Patient Monitoring: What Impact Can Data Analytics Have on Cost?* Paper presented at the Wireless Health '13. Baltimore, MD. doi:10.1145/2534088.2534108

Lester, D. S. (2009). Will personalized medicine help in 'transforming' the business of healthcare? *Personalized Medicine*, 6(5), 555–565. doi:10.2217/pme.09.31

Llewellyn-Thomas, H. A., McGreal, M. J., Thiel, E. C., Fine, S., & Erlichman, C. (1991). Patients' willingness to enter clinical trials: Measuring the association with perceived benefit and preference for decision participation. *Social Science & Medicine*, 32(1), 35–42. doi:10.1016/0277-9536(91)90124-U PMID:2008619

Mahoney, D., Tennstedt, S., Friedman, R., & Heeren, T. (1999). An automated telephone system for monitoring the functional status of community-residing elders. *The Gerontologist*, 39(2), 229–234. doi:10.1093/geront/39.2.229 PMID:10224719

Manyika, J. Chui, M., Brown, B., Bughin J., Dobbs, R. Roxburgh, C. and Byers, A.H. (2011). *Big Data: The Next Frontier for Innovation, Competition and Productivity*. San Fransisco: McKinsey Global Institute.

Mapcite. (2013). *How Emergency Managers Can Benefit from Big Data*. Retrieved 23/10/13, 2013, from http://www.mapcite.com/posts/2013/july/how-emergency-managers-can-benefit-from-big-data.aspx

Marechal, F., Ribeiro, N., Lafaye, M., & Güell, A. (2008). Satellite imaging and vector-borne diseases: The approach of the French National Space Agency (CNES). *Geospatial Health*, 3(1), 1–5. PMID:19021103

Marjoua, Y., Butler, C. A., & Bozic, K. J. (2012). Public Reporting of Cost and Quality Information in Orthopaedics. *Clinical Orthopaedics and Related Research*, 470(4), 1017–1026. doi:10.1007/s11999-011-2077-6 PMID:21952744

Meijer, C., Wouterse, B., Polder, J., & Koopmanschap, M. (2013). The effect of population aging on health expenditure growth: A critical review. *European Journal of Ageing*, 1–9. doi:10.1007/s10433-013-0280-x

Mello, M. M., Francer, J. K., Wilenzick, M., Teden, P., Bierer, B. E., & Barnes, M. (2013). Preparing for responsible sharing of clinical trial data. *The New England Journal of Medicine*. PMID:24144394

Millard, R. W., & Carver, J. R. (1999). Cross-sectional comparison of live and interactive voice recognition administration of the SF-12 health status survey. *The American Journal of Managed Care*, 5(2), 153. PMID:10346511

Mitic, M., & Kapoulas, A. (2012). Understanding the role of social media in bank marketing. *Marketing Intelligence & Planning, 30*(7), 668–686. doi:10.1108/02634501211273797

Morgan, S., Grootendorst, P., Lexchin, J., Cunningham, C., & Greyson, D. (2011). The cost of drug development: A systematic review. *Health Policy(Amsterdam), 100*(1), 4–17. doi:10.1016/j.healthpol.2010.12.002 PMID:21256615

Morris, J. N. (1975). *Uses of Epidemiology*. Edinburgh, UK: Churchill Livingstone.

Morton, L. W., & Weng, C.-Y. (2013). Health and Healthcare Among the Rural Aging. In N. Glasgow & E. H. Berry (Eds.), Rural Aging in 21st Century America (Vol. 7, pp. 179-194). Springer Netherlands. doi:10.1007/978-94-007-5567-3_10

Moxey, A., Robertson, J., Newby, D., Hains, I., Williamson, M., & Pearson, S.-A. (2010). Computerized clinical decision support for prescribing: Provision does not guarantee uptake. *Journal of the American Medical Informatics Association, 17*(1), 25–33. doi:10.1197/jamia.M3170 PMID:20064798

Mueller, S., & Szczesny, A. (2013). *Cost Pressure, Rationalization, Specialization and the Quality of Health Care*. Social Sciences Research Network.

Mushlin, A. I., & Ghomrawi, H. (2010). Health Care Reform and the Need for Comparative-Effectiveness Research. *The New England Journal of Medicine, 362*(3), e6. doi:10.1056/NEJMp0912651 PMID:20054035

Neumann, P. J., Palmer, J. A., Nadler, E., Fang, C.-H., & Ubel, P. (2010). Cancer Therapy Costs Influence Treatment: A National Survey Of Oncologists. *Health Affairs, 29*(1), 196–202. doi:10.1377/hlthaff.2009.0077 PMID:20048377

Nicolaidis, S. (2013). Personalized medicine in neurosurgery. *Metabolism, 62*, S45–S48. doi:10.1016/j.metabol.2012.08.022

NYGC. (2014). *The New York Genome Center and IBM Watson Group Announce Collaboration to Advance Genomic Medicine*. Retrieved April 17, 2014, 2014, from http://www.nygenome.org/news/new-york-genome-center-ibm-watson-group-announce-collaboration-advance-genomic-medicine/

Ogwueleka, F. N. (2011). Data Mining Application in Credit Card Fraud Detection System. *Journal of Engineering Science and Technology, 6*(3), 311–322.

Olson, D. R. (2013). *How Accurate Is Google Flu Trends? A Comparative Study of Internet Search Data and Public Health Syndromic Surveillance for Monitoring Seasonal and Pandemic Influenza, 2003-2013*. Paper presented at the 2013 CSTE Annual Conference. New York, NY.

Olson, D. R., Konty, K. J., Paladini, M., Viboud, C., & Simonsen, L. (2013). Reassessing Google Flu Trends Data for Detection of Seasonal and Pandemic Influenza: A Comparative Epidemiological Study at Three Geographic Scales. *PLoS Computational Biology, 9*(10), e1003256. doi:10.1371/journal.pcbi.1003256 PMID:24146603

Orszag, P. R., & Emanuel, E. J. (2010). Health care reform and cost control. *The New England Journal of Medicine, 363*(7), 601–603. doi:10.1056/NEJMp1006571 PMID:20554975

Outterson, K. (2012). Punishing Health Care Fraud–Is the GSK Settlement Sufficient? *The New England Journal of Medicine, 367*(12), 1082–1085. doi:10.1056/NEJMp1209249 PMID:22970920

Painter, I., Eaton, J., & Lober, B. (2013). Using Change Point Detection for Monitoring the Quality of Aggregate Data. *Online Journal of Public Health Informatics, 5*(1). doi:10.5210/ojphi.v5i1.4597

Pandor, A., Gomersall, T., Stevens, J. W., Wang, J., Al-Mohammad, A., & Bakhai, A. et al. (2013). Remote monitoring after recent hospital discharge in patients with heart failure: A systematic review and network meta-analysis. *Heart (British Cardiac Society)*, *99*(23), 1717–1726. doi:10.1136/heartjnl-2013-303811 PMID:23680885

Patel, U. H., & Babbs, C. F. (1992). A computer-based, automated, telephonic system to monitor patient progress in the home setting. *Journal of Medical Systems*, *16*(2-3), 101–112. doi:10.1007/BF00996591 PMID:1402436

Patwardhan, A., & Bilkovski, R. (2012). Comparison: Flu Prescription Sales Data from a Retail Pharmacy in the US with Google Flu Trends and US ILINet (CDC) Data as Flu Activity Indicator. *PLoS ONE*, *7*(8), e43611. doi:10.1371/journal.pone.0043611 PMID:22952719

Paul, M. J., & Dredze, M. (2012). A model for mining public health topics from Twitter. *Health*, *11*, 16–16.

Pekmezaris, R., Mitzner, I., Pecinka, K. R., Nouryan, C. N., Lesser, M. L., & Siegel, M. et al. (2012). The impact of remote patient monitoring (telehealth) upon Medicare beneficiaries with heart failure. *Telemedicine Journal and e-Health*, *18*(2), 101–108. doi:10.1089/tmj.2011.0095 PMID:22283360

Perrine, M. W., Mundt, J. C., Searles, J. S., & Lester, L. S. (1995). Validation of daily self-reported alcohol consumption using interactive voice response (IVR) technology. *Journal of Studies on Alcohol and Drugs*, *56*(5), 487. PMID:7475027

Persson, U., Willis, M., & Odegaard, K. (2010). A case study of ex ante, value-based price and reimbursement decision-making: TLV and rimonabant in Sweden. *The European Journal of Health Economics*, *11*(2), 195–203. doi:10.1007/s10198-009-0166-1 PMID:19639352

Piette, J. D. (2000). Interactive voice response systems in the diagnosis and management of chronic disease. *The American Journal of Managed Care*, *6*(7), 817–827. PMID:11067378

Piette, J. D., & Mah, C. A. (1997). The feasibility of automated voice messaging as an adjunct to diabetes outpatient care. *Diabetes Care*, *20*(1), 15–21. doi:10.2337/diacare.20.1.15 PMID:9028687

Piette, J. D., McPhee, S. J., Weinberger, M., Mah, C. A., & Kraemer, F. B. (1999). Use of automated telephone disease management calls in an ethnically diverse sample of low-income patients with diabetes. *Diabetes Care*, *22*(8), 1302–1309. doi:10.2337/diacare.22.8.1302 PMID:10480775

Porter, M. E. (2008). *Competitive advantage: Creating and sustaining superior performance.* Simon and Schuster.

Radhakrishnan, K., Jacelon, C., & Roche, J. (2012). Perceptions on the Use of Telehealth by Homecare Nurses and Patients With Heart Failure: A Mixed Method Study. *Home Health Care Management & Practice*, *24*(4), 175–181. doi:10.1177/1084822311428335

Rani, J. K., Kumar, S. P., Mohan, U. R., & Shankar, C. U. (2011). Credit Card Fraud Detection Analysis. *International Journal of Computer Trends and Technology*, *2*(1), 24–27.

Reed, J., Murray, K., & Jacobson, M. (2013). Digitization Standards at the National Archives and Records Administration. *Archiving Conference*, 2013(1), 211-215.

Reuben, D. B., & Tinetti, M. E. (2012). Goal-oriented patient care--an alternative health outcomes paradigm. *The New England Journal of Medicine*, *366*(9), 777–779. doi:10.1056/NEJMp1113631 PMID:22375966

Rich, J., Howe, J., Larson, L., & Chuang, C. (2013). Implementing Interactive Voice Recognition Technology to Activate Vulnerable Patients. *Journal of the International Society for Telemedicine and eHealth, 1*(1), 3-11.

Romano, M. J., & Stafford, R. S. (2011). Electronic health records and clinical decision support systems: Impact on national ambulatory care quality. *Archives of Internal Medicine, 171*(10), 897–903. doi:10.1001/archinternmed.2010.527 PMID:21263077

Rozenbaum, M. H., Sanders, E. A. M., van Hoek, A. J., Jansen, A. G. S. C., van der Ende, A., & van den Dobbelsteen, G. et al. (2010). Cost effectiveness of pneumococcal vaccination among Dutch infants: Economic analysis of the seven valent pneumococcal conjugated vaccine and forecast for the 10 valent and 13 valent vaccines. *BMJ (Clinical Research Ed.), 340*(1), c2509. doi:10.1136/bmj.c2509 PMID:20519267

Russell, L. B., Gold, M. R., Siegel, J. E., Daniels, N., & Weinstein, M. C. (1996). THe role of cost-effectiveness analysis in health and medicine. *Journal of the American Medical Association, 276*(14), 1172–1177. doi:10.1001/jama.1996.03540140060028 PMID:8827972

Salathe, M., Freifeld, C. C., Mekaru, S. R., Tomasulo, A. F., & Brownstein, J. S. (2013). Influenza A (H7N9) and the importance of digital epidemiology. *The New England Journal of Medicine, 369*(5), 401–404. doi:10.1056/NEJMp1307752 PMID:23822655

Sarkar, I. N. (2010). Biomedical informatics and translational medicine. *Journal of Translational Medicine, 8*(22), 12. PMID:20187952

Scharnweber, C., Lau, B. D., Mollenkopf, N., Thiemann, D. R., Veltri, M. A., & Lehmann, C. U. (2013). Evaluation of medication dose alerts in pediatric inpatients. *International Journal of Medical Informatics, 82*(8), 676–683. doi:10.1016/j.ijmedinf.2013.04.002 PMID:23643148

Shea, S., Weinstock, R. S., Starren, J., Teresi, J., Palmas, W., & Field, L. et al. (2006). A randomized trial comparing telemedicine case management with usual care in older, ethnically diverse, medically underserved patients with diabetes mellitus. *Journal of the American Medical Informatics Association, 13*(1), 40–51. doi:10.1197/jamia.M1917 PMID:16221935

Sibbald, B. (2004). Legal action against GSK over SSRI data. *Canadian Medical Association Journal, 171*(1), 23-23a.

Siegel, J. P., Rosenthal, N., Buto, K., Lilienfeld, S., Thomas, A., & Odenthal, S. (2012). Comparative Effectiveness Research in the Regulatory Setting. *Pharmaceutical Medicine, 26*(1), 5–11. doi:10.1007/BF03256887

Smith, M., Saunders, R., Stuckhardt, L., & McGinnis, J. M. (2013). *Best care at lower cost: the path to continuously learning health care in America.* National Academies Press.

Sox, H. C., & Greenfield, S. (2009). Comparative Effectiveness Research: A Report From the Institute of Medicine. *Annals of Internal Medicine, 151*(3), 203–205. doi:10.7326/0003-4819-151-3-200908040-00125 PMID:19567618

Sproull, R. F., & Eisenberg, J. (2005). Building an electronic records archive at the National Archives and Records Administration recommendations for a long-term strategy (p. xii). Retrieved from http://ezproxy.usq.edu.au/login?url=http://site.ebrary.com/lib/unisouthernqld/Doc?id=10082366

Suh, K. S., Sarojini, S., Youssif, M., Nalley, K., Milinovikj, N., & Elloumi, F. et al. (2013). Tissue banking, bioinformatics, and electronic medical records: The front-end requirements for personalized medicine. *Journal of Oncology*, *368751*. doi:10.1155/2013/368751 PMID:23818899

Suzuki, S., & Matsui, T. (2012). *Remote sensing for medical and health care applications*. Remote Sensing-Applications. doi:10.5772/36924

Tang, L., & Yuwen, J. (2013). *The Study on Digital Traffic Service System and Key Technologies of Location Based Service*. Paper presented at the 2013 the International Conference on Remote Sensing, Environment and Transportation Engineering (RSETE 2013). New York, NY. doi:10.2991/rsete.2013.148

Thomson, M. C., & Connor, S. J. (2001). The development of Malaria Early Warning Systems for Africa. *Trends in Parasitology*, *17*(9), 438–445. doi:10.1016/S1471-4922(01)02077-3 PMID:11530356

Timbie, J. W., Fox, D. S., Van Busum, K., & Schneider, E. C. (2012). Five Reasons That Many Comparative Effectiveness Studies Fail To Change Patient Care And Clinical Practice. *Health Affairs*, *31*(10), 2168–2175. doi:10.1377/hlthaff.2012.0150 PMID:23048092

Towse, A., Ossa, D., Veenstra, D., Carlson, J., & Garrison, L. (2013). Understanding the Economic Value of Molecular Diagnostic Tests: Case Studies and Lessons Learned. *Journal of Personalized Medicine*, *3*(4), 288–305. doi:10.3390/jpm3040288

Trowbridge, R., & Weingarten, S. (2001). Clinical decision support systems. *Making health care safer: A critical analysis of patient safety practices. Evidence Report/technology Assessment*, 43.

Tuckson, R. V., Newcomer, L., & De Sa, J. M. (2013). Accessing genomic medicine: Affordability, diffusion, and disparities. *Journal of the American Medical Association*, *309*(14), 1469–1470. doi:10.1001/jama.2013.1468 PMID:23571584

Vedder, R. G., Vanecek, M. T., Guynes, C. S., & Cappel, J. J. (1999). CEO and CIO perspectives on competitive intelligence. *Communications of the ACM*, *42*(8), 108–116. doi:10.1145/310930.310982

Venkat, A., Chan-Tompkins, N. H., Hegde, G. G., Chuirazzi, D. M., Hunter, R., & Szczesiul, J. M. (2010). Feasibility of integrating a clinical decision support tool into an existing computerized physician order entry system to increase seasonal influenza vaccination in the emergency department. *Vaccine*, *28*(37), 6058–6064. doi:10.1016/j.vaccine.2010.06.090 PMID:20620167

Vogeli, C., Shields, A. E., Lee, T. A., Gibson, T. B., Marder, W. D., Weiss, K. B., & Blumenthal, D. (2007). Multiple Chronic Conditions: Prevalence, Health Consequences, and Implications for Quality, Care Management, and Costs. *Journal of General Internal Medicine*, *22*(3), 391–395. doi:10.1007/s11606-007-0322-1 PMID:18026807

Weinstein, M. C., & Stason, W. B. (1977). Foundations of cost-effectiveness analysis for health and medical practices. *The New England Journal of Medicine*, *296*(13), 716–721. doi:10.1056/NEJM197703312961304 PMID:402576

Willig, J. H., Krawitz, M., Panjamapirom, A., Ray, M. N., Nevin, C. R., & English, T. M. et al. (2013). Closing the Feedback Loop: An Interactive Voice Response System to Provide Follow-up and Feedback in Primary Care Settings. *Journal of Medical Systems*, *37*(2), 1–9. doi:10.1007/s10916-012-9905-4 PMID:23340825

WorldMedicalAssociation. (2013). World Medical Association declaration of Helsinki: Ethical principles for medical research involving human subjects. *Journal of the American Medical Association.*

Wright, A., Sittig, D. F., Ash, J. S., Sharma, S., Pang, J. E., & Middleton, B. (2009). Clinical Decision Support Capabilities of Commercially-available Clinical Information Systems. *Journal of the American Medical Informatics Association, 16*(5), 637–644. doi:10.1197/jamia.M3111 PMID:19567796

KEY TERMS AND DEFINITIONS

Artificial Intelligence: Algorithms and applications that address classification, prediction, web mining and machine learning.

Big Data: Pools of information so large that conventional analytical techniques cannot make sense of them. Requires use of dynamic data that is changing at the time of analysis, advanced algorithms and very large datasets.

Biomedical Informatics: The science of information applied to medicine.

Business Intelligence: The use of data to enhance competitiveness.

Clinical Decision Support Systems: Software programs that anticipate probable outcomes of particular treatment strategies by comparing the proposed treatment to previous patient outcomes.

Clinical Operations: All the actions that relate to the patient bedside, including diagnosing and monitoring the course of disease or trauma or other injury, and all observations and treatments administered.

Competitive Advantage: Anything that enhances an organization's ability to carry out its mission.

Cost Advantage: Arises when an organization can deliver the same products or services as competitors at a lower cost.

Cost Effectiveness Research: Healthcare resource allocation guided by considering the costs of a particular treatment in relation to the expected benefits.

Differentiation Advantage: Arises when an organization can deliver products or services with benefits that exceed those of the competition.

Electronic Health Record: A digital copy of a patient's health record.

Epigenetics: The study of heritable changes in gene activity which are not caused by changes in the DNA sequence.

Genomics: A discipline in genetics that applies recombinant DNA, DNA sequencing methods and bioinformatics to sequence, assemble, and analyze the structure and function of genomes (the complete set of DNA within a single organism).

Improved Productivity: Delivering products and services more efficiently, which may or may not result in a cost advantage.

Metabolomics: The study of the unique chemical fingerprints that specific cellular processes leave behind.

Personalized Medicine: The use of modern imaging and exploratory technologies to disclose genomic, proteomic and epigenetic information peculiar to each patient, in the effort to individualize prognosis and therapeutic care.

Price Premium: The ability to charge a higher price for a product or service that has greater perceived value than competing products or services.

Proteomics: The study of the function and structure of the complete set of proteins produced or modified by an organism or system.

Public Health Administration: All organized measures (whether public or private) to prevent disease, promote health, and prolong life among the population as a whole.

Remote Patient Monitoring: Continuous monitoring of the physiological status of patients using heterogeneous sensors such as blood pressure, weight, blood glucose, and/or physical activity sensors in order to shift medical services from hospital and clinical settings to an in-home monitoring scenario.

Transparency: Sharing of information between healthcare providers, patients and other health care organizations.

Tele-Epidemiology: The study of human and animal epidemics, the spread of which is closely tied to environmental factors. By combining data from various earth-orbiting satellites, hydrology data and clinical data from humans and animals, outbreaks of infectious disease can be predicted with accuracy.

This work was previously published in Big Data Analytics in Bioinformatics and Healthcare edited by Baoying Wang, Ruowang Li, and William Perrizo, pages 406-439 copyright year 2015 by Medical Information Science Reference (an imprint of IGI Global).

Chapter 44
Communication between Power Blackout and Mobile Network Overload

Christian Reuter
University of Siegen, Germany

ABSTRACT

In cases of power outages the communication of organizations responsible for recovery work (emergency services, public administration, energy network operators) to the public poses several challenges, primarily the breakdowns of many communication infrastructures and therefore the limitations of the use of classical communication media. This paper surveys technical concepts to support crisis communication during blackouts. Therefore it first investigates the perception and information demands of citizens and communication infrastructures in different scenarios. Furthermore, it analyzes communication infrastructures and their availability in different scenarios. Finally it proposes 'BlaCom', an ICT-based concept for blackout communication, which addresses the time span between the occurrence of the energy blackout and the possible overload of the mobile phone network. It combines general information with location-specific and setting-specific information, was implemented as a prototype smartphone application and evaluated with 12 potential end users.

1. INTRODUCTION

The 2012 blackout in India (670 million affected), the 2009 blackout in Brazil and Paraguay (87 million), the 2006 European blackout (10 million) and the 2003 Northeast blackout in the United States and Canada (55 million) show that big power outages still occur all over the world. The constant electricity supply became increasingly important over the recent decades because large

parts of our infrastructure only function with electricity. Therefore the occurrence of power outages is a growing problem (Birkmann et al., 2010). This does not only concern the economy or private households, but all basic (critical) infrastructures like water and food or information and communication technology in general (Lorenz, 2010). The dependency on a functioning electricity supply is very high, so that a long outage is highly problematic (Deutscher Bundestag, 2011;

DOI: 10.4018/978-1-4666-8756-1.ch044

Holenstein & Küng, 2008). Even though the probability for power outages is relatively low and the average duration of such blackouts e.g. in Western Europe only amounts to few minutes, the general preparation for potential crisis situations is rather poor (Birkmann et al., 2010). If a power outage takes place, communication tools, and almost all further infrastructures, will fail after a certain time, which can entail serious consequences especially in the case of long outages (Deutscher Bundestag, 2011; Hiete et al., 2010). Such long blackouts do not only mean a physical, but also a psychological burden for the affected people (Volgger et al., 2006). Uncertainty and feelings of anxiety, as well as the need for information emerge.

In terms of the communication matrix for social software in crisis management (Reuter et al., 2012), four different cases for information and communication in such a situation can be distinguished (Figure 1) depending on a distinction of (a) organizations and the (b) public as the (i) sender and the (ii) receiver of information. On the inter-organizational level organizations of crisis response communicate with each other often using radio communication, which is less affected by working electricity due to emergency power units (bottom left). On the public level,

citizens and volunteers communicate with each other in the real or via social media such as Twitter or Facebook (top right). This citizen-generated content is also being analyzed by crisis response organizations (bottom left). Besides the communication among the citizen, it is also very important that organizations responsible for recovery work inform the public (top left)

This work focuses on crisis communication between authorities/organizations and the people affected by a power outage (citizens), as marked in Figure 1. It focuses on which and how crisis-related information should be provided to the public.

Based on a previous short paper (Reuter, 2013) this paper outlines the perception of the population, their demands for information as well as relevant communication media and their availability during power outages. Furthermore it presents an ICT-based prototypically implemented concept for crisis communication and the results of its evaluation. This paper reports from a project focusing on coping and recovery work during big to medium power outages (Wiedenhoefer et al., 2011). Therefore organizations responsible for recovery work and crisis communication, such as emergency services like the police and fire department and infrastructure suppliers, such as

Figure 1. Focus of the study using the "crisis communication matrix" (Modified) (Reuter et al., 2012)

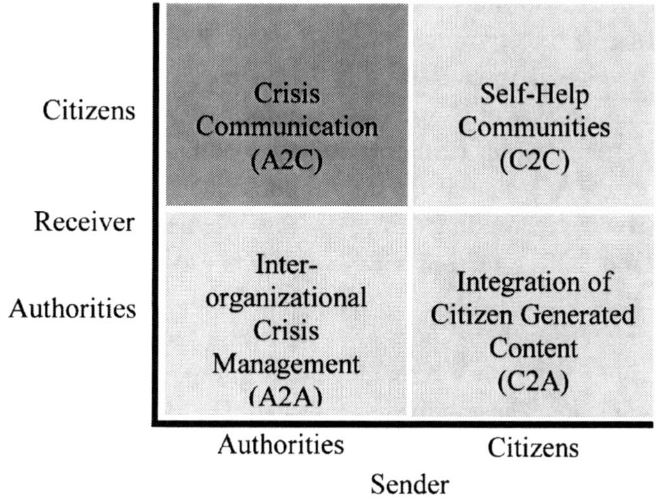

energy network operators, are part of the collaborative project aiming to improve both information sharing (Ley et al., 2014) as well as mobile collaboration (Reuter et al., 2014). However, the aim of this work is also to research how to provide the citizens with information about emergencies during power breakdowns, focusing on the time span between the occurrence of the power blackout and the breakdown of communication infrastructures due to mobile network overload.

2. INFORMATION NEEDS IN POWER OUTAGES BY CITIZEN

Because electricity has become indispensable in everyday life, there is a strong dependency on an intact supply infrastructure (Birkmann et al., 2010). Typically, citizens only notice the underlying infrastructure when the electricity supply fails and only then become aware of their dependency on electricity in their daily lives (Lorenz, 2010). Power outages are seen as annoying, but not as threatening. Furthermore, a functioning electricity supply is taken for granted – the possibility of a long power outage is not considered (Holenstein & Küng, 2008, 14). By putting an emphasize on a functioning electricity supply and by not taking possible consequences into consideration, the potential threat is underestimated (Birkmann et al., 2010, 82). Reflecting on such situations is seen as less important than dealing with daily problems (Quarantelli, 1999, 27). Moreover, the population's self-help capacity decreases because of its growing dependence on the electricity supply (Lorenz, 2010, 40). According to the German Federal Administration Office (Bundesverwaltungsamt, 2001) it can be assumed that self-protection will stagnate at the current low level.

From the citizen's perspective, the responsibility for civil protection lies with other actors, especially with the federal state. Those citizens who had to repeatedly deal with crisis situations are the only exception for practiced self-protection

(Bundesverwaltungsamt, 2001). As a consequence, existing concepts for risk communication are widely unknown within the population (Helsloot & Beerens, 2009, 31; Lorenz, 2010, 38; Menski & Gardemann, 2008, 65). Memories of events, in which people were affected only slightly or for a short period of time, are often forgotten, so that no arrangements for better self-protection in the future are made (Holenstein & Küng, 2008, 22; Menski & Gardemann, 2008, 5). Additionally, power outages are seen as unique incidents with the result that a repetition of such an incident is mentally out ruled by those affected (Lorenz, 2010, 31). The availability of groceries and drinking water in private households has decreased noticeably because of the permanent availability of these goods in stores. Keeping large quantities of food has become rare, especially in cities (Menski & Gardemann, 2008, 39). This can in part be explained by the absence of shortages in supply over recent decades. To sum up, it can be said that power outages seldom happen in Western Europe, so that the population is not aware of the risk of a long power outage and is not well prepared for such an incident.

Information is of great importance in such uncertain situations. Before and during power outages there are different information demands on behalf of the population. Before a crisis, information is necessary for sensitizing and crisis preparation. The awareness of a threat is essential for implementing prevention measures (Genen, 2009, 64). At first, citizens have to be informed about existing hazard potentials and their probabilities, and – if foreseeable – possible consequences. This makes a better preparation possible because citizens then have a rough idea of what to do when a crisis occurs (Volgger et al., 2006, 8). Especially recommendations regarding the preparation and assessment of the emerging threat are useful (Volgger et al., 2006, 16). The distribution of such information can take place in many different ways. Basic plans and instructions, including best practices, are a simple solution for emergencies. For this kind of information, Coombs (2009, 105) uses the term "instructing information". This is information that shows the people affected how to protect themselves. It is imperative that warnings are issued before a crisis occurs (Geenen, 2009, 64; Volgger et al., 2006, 16). For predictable crises, detailed warnings have to be announced on every channel available as early as possible. Thus, the citizens are given a time frame large enough for individual preparations.

During the crisis a demand for orientation information generally exists, so that those affected can comprehend the crisis situation. According to a network operator (Nilges et al., 2009) and an empirical study (Klauser et al., 2008, 3) a consistent and transparent provision of information to the population is necessary. The duration of the power outage is undoubtedly the most urgently needed piece of information. If this information is not available, at least an estimation of the time frame will be required in order to be able to better adjust to the new situation. If no information is passed on, the feeling of uncertainty – of being left alone – will intensify, especially in longer outages. If communication is generally possible but fails because of problem with the information transmission (e.g. hotline overload so that callers are redirected to unspecific recorded messages), those affected will quickly feel as if they are not being taken seriously (Klauser et al., 2008, 4). This is also the case when confronting affected citizens with standardized, unspecific information (Holenstein & Küng, 2008, 5). Because of failures in the pre-crisis communication, those affected will additionally also need all the information which should have been communicated in the context of risk communication. Thus, "instructing information" is required, which is adapted to the current crisis situation (Klauser et al., 2008, 5). According to Lorenz (2010, 29), the need of information should optimally correspond to the specific demand, as well as

the existing fears and hardships of the population and also be as precise and detailed as possible. In case of longer power outages, there also exists an information demand for how to deal with scarce resources and how and where mutual help is necessary and possible. This information exchange requires dialogic forms of communication. However, this seems to be hardly realizable – especially for widespread and long power outages. Moreover, Coombs (2009, 106) mentions "adjusting information", which helps those affected to deal with the crisis situation psychologically. He also mentions the "golden hour", the response time of 60 minutes or less for first adjusting information. Klafft (2014) highlights current issues in crisis communication and alerting, such as strategies for the implementation of individualization in the alerting system as well as adaptive multi-channel alerting.

To sum it up, the most information demands exist: (1) Warnings: Once a crisis is predictable for the crisis management, the affected population must be informed of possible damages and threats. (2) Crisis-related information: information about the duration, the area affected (i.e. the dimension of the crisis), as well as the cause (only conditional) in order to adjust to the crisis at best. (3) Communication channels: information about which communication channels can be used. Particularly in longer crises it is important to minimize the information deficit. Additionally, the citizens are told where precise information can be found (Geenen, 2009, 86).

3. COMMUNICATION INFRASTRUCTURES AND THEIR AVAILABILITY DURING POWER OUTAGES

The use of communication infrastructures is necessary to cover the citizens' information demands. The German Federal Parliament (Deutscher Bundestag, 2011, 4-6) analyzed the risks for modern societies in a widespread and long power outage, with the result that the consequences can be summed up to damages of severe quality because of the almost total dissemination of the living and working environment by electric driven devices. The consequences for information technology and telecommunication are expected to be dramatic. Regarding communication technology, a power outage can be divided into different scenarios broken down by duration (Deutscher Bundestag, 2011; Hiete et al., 2010). Here, a transceiver needs to be available.

Table 1 shows that major parts of the communication system are currently not suitable for long and widespread power outages. For short power outages, communication can be ensured with the aid of analog telephony as well as battery-driven devices as long as the communication infrastructure is not damaged or overloaded. For locally restricted power outages, under certain circumstances, mobile telephony and mobile Internet connections can be maintained by surrounding base stations that are not affected by the outage. In every other scenario it can be assumed that technical dialogic communication is not possible (Deutscher Bundestag, 2011, 104).

In the area of *fixed-line telephony,* the digital devices will immediately stop working. The same is true for the base stations of *mobile networks,* whereas the mobile devices may still work for a few days, if they are fully charged. Neverthe-

less, a mobile network overload will most likely occur because of the increased traffic volume. Cell broadcast, a mobile technology allowing messages to be broadcasted to all mobile devices within the cell, is used by Wireless Emergency Alerts (WEA), a "public safety system that allows customers who own certain wireless phone models and other enabled mobile devices to receive geographically-targeted, text-like messages alerting them of imminent threats to safety in their area" (Federal Communications Commission, 2013). It is an initiative of the Federal Communications Commission (FCC), along with the Federal Emergency Management Agency (FEMA) and the wireless industry. However, in Germany cell broadcast is currently not provided by telecommunication companies caused by the lack of appropriate business models[1].

Mass media are available due to emergency power capacities (e.g. newspaper publishers); particularly radio, because it can also be received by battery-driven devices. According to Andersen and Spitzberg (2009, p.221), communication has to be redundant, both in the selection of the transmission media, as well as regarding the sources of information. Therefore, as many information channels as possible should be covered. Communication should also not only be run as a one-way communication. The *Radio Data System* (RDS), a data stream, which offers the standard functions of automatic program search and alternate frequencies through Traffic Message Channel (TMC), is

Table 1. Availability of media in different scenarios (Deutscher Bundestag, 2011)

#	Medium	Scenario A (<8h)	Scenario 2 (8-24h)	Scenario 3 (>24h)
1	Telephony	Yes, but maybe overloaded	No	No
2	Cell phone	Yes, but maybe overloaded	No	No
3	Internet (via cell phone)	Yes, but maybe overloaded	No	No
1-3	(if telephone switch central office / base station is not affected)	Yes, but maybe overloaded	Yes	Yes
4	Television	No	No	No
5	Radio (battery-powered receiver unit provided)	Yes	Yes	Yes

used by navigation devices for traffic messages and is also broadcasted via radio. In the USA, such concepts already exist when using RDS for weather alerts and other potential emergencies. RDS can be extended by further services – the radio text can be transmitted, which consists of up to 64 characters, and can also be used for rudimental information. Over the years, however, the distribution of battery-operable devices (transistor radios or corded telephones) has decreased; a fact which is often only realized during a power outage (Holenstein & Küng, 2008).

Further capabilities to warn the population were decreased throughout the 1990s (Geenen, 2009, 98; Menski & Gardemann, 2008, 28). *Sirens* were taken out of service or were handed over to the communities and not all siren warning systems are equipped with an emergency power supply. Only about one third can be used for warning the population (Menski & Gardemann, 2008, 28). Additionally, Helsloot and Beerens (2009) present non-technical communication concepts, which could be utilized during power outages: vans equipped with speakers, flyers, information points and meetings. This is all necessary in order to be able to reach a high percentage of people.

Due to the *Internet* and its mobile use, a variety of different ways of communication are now available. Classic services, such as websites and e-mail exist and more recent social services available in a mobile version, are chats, microblogging services and social networking services, all of which are used in a crisis (Palen & Liu, 2007). Social media services are being implemented by individuals in a self-organizing activity (Reuter et al., 2013); however crisis management organizations can "take advantage […] for their crisis response as long as they take precautions to maintain their proprietary data" (Jennex, 2010). Latonero & Shklovski (2011) present an example, where the Los Angeles Fire Department using Twitter for emergency management. By doing this, one way communication (broadcasting) as well as dialogic

communication (e.g. answering questions) is realized. A journey with about 500 students researched the availability of social media during the 2011 San Diego/Southwest Blackout: "Contrary to expectations, the cell phone system did not have the expected availability, and as a result, users had a difficult time using social media to status/contact family and friends" (Jennex, 2012). Another study discusses the utilities' efforts to ensure communication in case of blackout during Y2K (Jennex, 2004): Concerning the preparations for ensuring communications a conclusion is to utilize multiple communication methods including wired and wireless networks as well as the suggestion to do not solely reliability of the Internet. In order to make such communication also available during *power outages*, Hossmann et al. (2011) present a disaster mode of Twitter, which may allow communicate to continue in case of network outages by using short radio technologies. Al-Akkad et al. (2013) "examine challenges people face in situations of disrupted network infrastructures" and found that people "often make creative use of the remains of the technological landscape". They propose architectural qualities fostering resilient technology among self-exposure (wireless hotspots), short-lived interactions, graceful degradation, self-management and viral deployment. Semaan and Mark (2011) describe resilience through technology adaptation, e.g. unintended uses, in Iraq. Panitzek et al. (2012) propose an emergency switch for privately owned wireless routers, which allows wireless routers to transition to an emergency mode creating a supportive wireless mesh network. However, none of the concepts enables the comprehensive provision of information during power outages.

The number of crisis-specific *mobile applications* for iOS (MissionMode, 2012a) as well as Android (MissionMode, 2012b) is increasing (see Table 2). Besides general crisis applications, which enable an interactive display of catastrophes on a map ('Disaster Alert', 'Disaster Radar'), sharing information ('Real Time Warning'), collecting eyewitness reports ('EarShot'), or live broadcasts of emergency services and infrastructure providers ('EmergencyRadio'), there are applications, which send push-notifications when entering a current danger area ('Katwarn'). There are also many applications for special crisis situations, such as earthquakes (e.g. 'Earthquake Alert'), storms (e.g. 'Hurricane Tracker'), floods ('Flood Watch'), wild fires ('Wildfires'), or epidemics (e.g. 'HealthMap'). Furthermore applications with 'instructing information', such as a pocket reference for first responders including crisis-checklists ('NIMS ICS Guide'), as well as for the purpose of prevention ('FEMA') exist. Google Now and Maps forward automatic notifications for locally relevant warnings – independently from crisis-specific apps installed – for Android smartphones since the second quarter 2013. Applications, which explicitly consider the individual needs for information as well as the specifics of blackout situations, are currently not available.

Table 2. Overview of mobile crisis applications for iOS and Android

Name	iOS	Andr.	Focus	Description/Speciality
Centers for Disease Control		x	Epidemic	News, updates, extracts from social media
Disaster Alert	x	x	Catastrophe	List and interactive map for displaying catastrophes
Disaster Radar	x		Catastrophe	Interactive map for displaying catastrophes globally
EarShot	x		Eye witness	Collecting eyewitness reports including pictures
Earthquake Alert		x	Earthquakes	Real-time information
Earthquake!		x	Earthquakes	Information provided over the last 24 hours; display on a map
Emergency Radio	x		Radio	Live broadcast of emergency services and infrastructure providers in the USA
FEMA	x		Instruction	Information for prevention and crisis-checklists in crises
Flood Watch	x		Floods	Displaying floods with changing trends
HealthMap		x	Epidemic	Overview on epidemics, location-specific warnings
Hurricane Express	x		Hurricane	Data on storms in America, weather forecasts
Hurricane Hound		x	Hurricane	Marking potential development regions
Hurricane Tracker	x		Hurricane	Live videos, localized information, warnings
KATWARN		x	Danger	Notification when entering a current danger area
Latest Quakes		x	Earthquakes	Information on earthquakes including filtering option
NIMS ICS Guide	x	x	Instruction	Pocket reference for first responders, crisis-checklist
OnGuard Weather Alerts		x	Weather	Location-specific weather alerts
Outbreak Near Me	x		Epidemic	Real-time capturing of spread, submitting information
RadarScope	x		Weather	Overview on storms from 155 different radar information sites
Real time Warning		x	Warning	Crises worldwide including the option to share information
Shelter View	x		Instruction	Display of shelters (gymnasiums etc.)
Storm Shield		x	Weather	Weather information for storms
StormEye		x	Weather	Displaying storms in the surroundings
Tsunami Alert		x	Tsunami	Real-time alerts for tsunamis
Wildfires		x	Wildfires	Message option: „I'm OK"

4. 'BLACOM': CONCEPT FOR INTERNET-BASED BLACKOUT COMMUNICATION

Although radio is undoubtedly the most reliable medium for information transmission, it currently cannot be used to meet target-group-specific information demands (Deutscher Bundestag, 2011, 116). In addition the distribution of transistor radios independent from electricity is progressively decreasing (Holenstein & Küng, 2008). As depicted in the previous section, many communication media fail when power breaks down. Mobile communications are rudimentarily maintained through emergency power, whereas, however, rather unimportant base stations, which normally serve to optimize network coverage, are shut down, by which the network becomes overloaded more quickly for a large number of phone calls. Figure 2 clarifies this sequence by reference to a timeline. Because of the time span available between emergency power supply and the overload of mobile communications (punctured in Figure 2) the target-group-specific transmission of preferably small amounts of data compared to manual calls of the affected customers at power

suppliers and emergency services is comprehensible and reasonable. Cell broadcast would be an additional way to inform all people, but it does not allow sending tailored information and is not available in Germany.

The aim of the concept is to cover the timespan between the occurrence of the power outage and the mobile network overload.

In order to address these points we have decided to conceptualize and implement an application for mobile-independent, battery-powered, internet-enabled smartphones and tablets. They are usually usable also after the actual communication channels fail and, at the same time, enable detailed and individual interaction. We aimed to proactively meet the information needs of the affected based on experiences of previous crises or trainings (Reuter et al., 2009) in order to reduce the amount of manual requests, which can become a quantitative problem for the respective emergency services (Ley et al., 2012). As a consequence the overload of the mobile communication network should be prolonged as long as possible by the decreased number of phone calls.

At this, the following core functionalities have to be considered:

Figure 2. Blackout and its consequences for mobile communication to illustrate the time frame (own illustration)

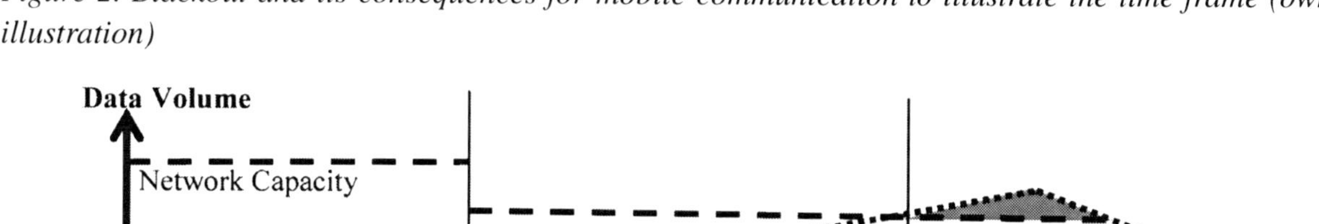

4.1. Feature A: Location-Specific Information

Depending on the location a user needs different information. Providing him all information at any place might lead to information overload instead valuable information. As a first step, the concept intends to automatically locate the user. Of course the user has to allow the application to use the location based on sensors – if no location sensor is available it is possible to enter the location manually. Based on the location of the user location-specific crisis-related information (e.g. the duration of the outage or specific warnings, contact points in the surroundings, emergency accommodations, positions of hospitals nearby, help request) are given. The content of the messages might be based on standardized libraries (Niebla et al., 2012). Energy network operators are willing to provide this information instead of having thousands of calls, which cannot be answered in that amount during power outages. With such information also the amount of information that needs to be transferred can be reduced. Furthermore energy network operators are not always willing to provide all citizens an overview about the supply rate of the whole area, but their specific situation.

4.2. Feature B: Setting-Specific Information

Information needs are not only based on the position but vary according to specific, individual requirements of each citizen. Such requirements result from, for instance, disease specifics (e.g. dialysis patient), family specifics (e.g. parents of young children) or demographic specifics (e.g. age) and implicate the necessity for targeted information supply. The concept contains an option to configure one's own profile in order to, for example, determine language, age and further parameters as well as to activate or deactivate special information types.

4.3. Feature C: General Information

Besides the characterization of location- and setting-specific information (Figure 3), which enables individual information supply, the category of general information is necessary as well. For instance, it consists of 'best practices', manuals or infrastructure information, which are permanently available in a further category.

Figure 3. Information depended on the (1) locations and (2) settings of the recipient (own figure)

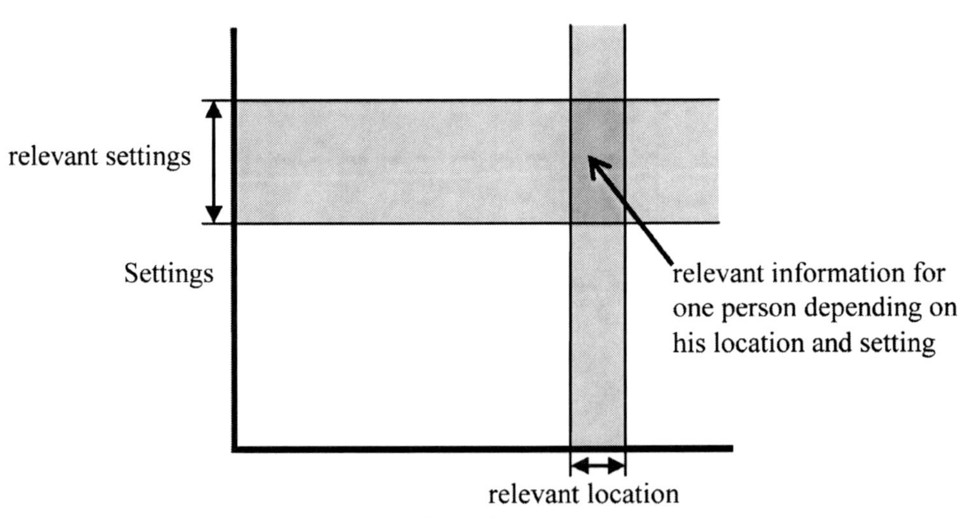

4.4. Feature D: Handling Network Breakdowns

In order to be better prepared for blackouts the characteristics of such scenarios have to be considered. In case of energy breakdowns it is very likely that the mobile networks will also break down, at least after a certain time they are often not continuously available. A native smartphone application or an installed program has an advantage compared to a web site where information is always available once it is downloaded, even if the network breaks down. To assess the actuality, the time of the latest update (relevant for temporary power outages) should be displayed as well as the availability of new information. When the networks are available again new information should be downloaded directly and automatically prioritized.

4.5. Feature E: Integration of Emergency Services and Energy Network Operators

To enable up-to-date information, a close connection to existing systems is necessary. Energy network operators might be motivated to provide information in order to relieve emergency services and overloaded hotlines from relatively uncritical problems.

5. DEVELOPMENT AND EVALUATION OF THE 'BLACOM'-PROTOTYPE

In order to test the acceptance of the concept we have implemented a clickable prototype, which represents all functionalities but, however, in the first phase, does not have access to real-time information and contains pre-defined demo data (Figure 4).

The concept, implemented as a prototype, was evaluated in a qualitative summative evaluation that included 12 participants (Table 3) (duration: Ø 35 minutes; bandwidth: 20-40 minutes). The participants were chosen based on previous knowledge regarding power outages and risk preparation, as well as technical understanding in order to be able to assess the operability and the benefit more profoundly, and availability. In the beginning, the possible problem scenario was explained to the users. Especially those problems that are often underestimated and forgotten and mainly occur during longer blackouts (e.g. the failures of inventory control systems or water supply) were mentioned. Afterwards, the main idea of the concept – information transmission as early as possible – and its functionality were presented. The participants were then told to use the prototype by themselves using the "thinking

Figure 4. Screenshot of the prototypical application concept "Blacom" for blackout communication

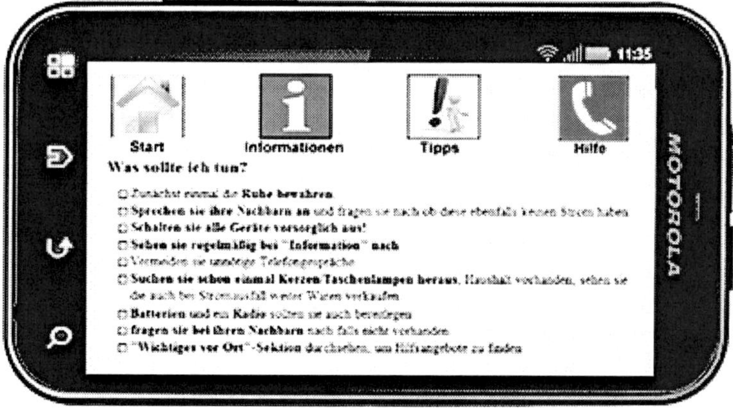

Table 3. Overview about the participants of the qualitative summative evaluation

Participant	Gender	Age	Profession
E1	male	56	Master craftsman
E2	female	54	Translator
E3	male	21	Student of Business Administration
E4	male	24	Student of Economics
E5	male	23	Student of Civil Engineering
E6	male	24	Student of Political Science
E7	male	20	Apprentice of cook
E8	male	23	Student of Information Systems
E9	male	23	Student of Computer Science
E10	female	25	Student of Sociology
E11	male	54	Electrician
E12	male	49	Teacher

aloud" method (Nielsen, 1993). The evaluation was recorded and the statements were then classified and analyzed.

The evaluation consisted of three parts (Table 4): First, an introduction with the description of a blackout scenario and possible reasons, second, the presentation of the concept and a walkthrough of the prototype and third, questions related to the usability, usefulness of the categories, if the information is complete, the motivation of using it and perceived problems and suggested extensions.

5.1. Results of the Evaluation

5.1.1. Why and How Long

Throughout the evaluation, the information perceived as the most relevant, was that on the current crisis situation, especially about the duration and the scale:

Of course I want to know: why and how long? (E11, 35:15).

The transparent presentation of this information at any time during the use was of great importance for the participants: *"What is definitely good here is that the* [name of the] *incident is transparent here every time"* (E4, 22:00). It was emphasized that, particularly in the area of the behavior tips and the current information, the conciseness of the statement is vital: *"At a first glance, I want to see what it is about"* (E1). The information should be as short as possible, that is to say with little text, only highlighting the central information in the area of the behavior tips was considered good and necessary (E1, E2).

5.1.2. Local Help and Volunteer Services

Another participant introduced the aspect of self-help / volunteerism (E6, 22:45). With this, a further category for local help services driven by citizens could be added. Examples for such a service could be childcare or shelter offered by private persons. At the same time, however, it was suggested that such help services should be managed centrally: citizens could offer their help via central information points and would then be added to the system. Moreover, it should be considered if, besides the information category, the other categories could also be updated during an incident (E4, 26:00). Then it would be foreseeable if emergency shelters were occupied or if further telephone numbers were added.

Table 4. Concept of the evaluation

Phase	Description
1. Introduction	- Description of a blackout scenario - Description of possible problems within that scenario
2. Concept	- Presentation of the Concept - Walkthrough
3. Questions	- Usability - Usefulness of categories - Complete information - Motivation of using it - Problems / extensions

5.1.3. No Motivation of Using the System before Crisis

Only a few participants were interested in using the program and in already receive information before a crisis:

Electricity comes from the socket. It has always come from there. In order to create a motivation one would have to deliberately turn off the electricity every now and again. Illusionistic indeed, but probably the only way (E11, 29:15).

Statements from several participants mirrored the tendencies mentioned in the literature, to not, or only seldom deal with a crisis before it happens:

I then have this tool, so that in case of an emergency: when I click there I know how to behave optimally (E12).

In the opinion of the respondents, it does not seem possible to motivate people to deal with risk preparation. Certain incentives also need to be created to deal with such a program. The idea was expressed (E3, E9) that social networks offer an appropriate way for spreading the application because they are used by those affected by a crisis. The publication of that information on Facebook or Twitter with a link to the app download would be appropriate. At the same time, concerns regarding their reliability and trustworthiness, and the users trust in them, were expressed (E12). Two participants (E4, 29:00, E6, 30:01) had the idea that such a tool could be pre-installed on all new devices, similar to emergency numbers. A further suggestion was to combine text messages linking to the application (E3).

5.1.4. Sources of Information

There is a clear result that information about the broker of a piece of information is of great importance to the participants:

You want to know from whom the information is (E12).

In order to promote the use of the program, it was also suggested to eventually extend the problem areas so that it could be used in everyday life and the users could already get used to the program (E7, 13:30). The uncertainty regarding the availability of an Internet connection was also addressed. A respondent noted that laptops were less important than smartphones, because the use of smartphones is more widespread and they are better integrated into everyday life (E7, 14:30). Finally, the distribution of smartphones and laptops was seen negatively (E10, 37:30). Clearly, not every person affected has such a device at hand and that is why the concept can at best be a supplement to existing ways of communication.

5.1.5. Summary: When, How Long and Who

All in all, the evaluation revealed that the concept was considered useful by all participants. The design was said to be optimizable in parts, however, it was adequate and appropriate for the objective. All participants stated that either one or maybe even all information categories would be useful. Almost all participants could imagine using the suggested concept, if it was implemented adequately. But at the same time they mentioned at the beginning not to deal with such information before a power outage. Especially displaying the relevant information for those affected (when, how long), the information sources (for rating) and helping to spread the information was of high importance.

6. CONCLUSION

The aim of this paper is to discuss the use of information technology for power outage communication to the public. Based on previous work, the perception of power outages by the population, their information needs and the availability of communication infrastructures are summarized. Based on these requirements for citizen communication, the paper presents a concept of a crisis application providing relevant information, which was realized as a prototype in order to evaluate its acceptance.

The probability for power outages in Western Europe is very low. However, if a power outage occurs, a need for information on behalf of the population will emerge. At the same time, several types of communication media will not be available, so that others will then be overloaded (Birkmann et al., 2010; Deutscher Bundestag, 2011) due to increased use. In order to eliminate this dilemma, it seems to be reasonable to automatically provide relevant information for the citizens in addition to dialogic communication. This would aim to cover the information demands of the population, as well as reduce the overload of other communication media. For instance it could dramatically decrease the number of phone calls made to emergency hotlines. Mobile smartphone applications used on battery-powered devices are one possibility in order to support information management during power outages. Derived from the requirements we identified, a concept and its manifestation in a mobile application for providing relevant information has been presented and, later on, has been evaluated with potential users.

The ICT-based concept for blackout communication 'BlaCom', presented in this work, for mobile devices (laptop, smartphone, tablet computer) includes (1) general information (e.g. recommendations for action during power outages), (2) location-specific information (e.g. the duration of the outage or specific warnings, surrounding contact points, emergency accommodations, help request) and (3) setting-specific information (people with specific needs, like dialysis patients, people with little children or older people) about the current crisis situation, in order to provide relevant information and to reduce the amount of data that needs to be transferred. The evaluation revealed that especially the reason and the expected duration of the power outage are of great interest. It also became clear that the motivation to proactively inform the population is not existent. One possibility to deal with this problem is to integrate the functions into an emergency services app that also allows people to be located in case of emergencies and therefore might provide a motivation. Another possibility is to integrate the app into smart metering applications, provided by energy network operators. But organizations responsible for infrastructures should, at any rate, make their critical information available for smartphones. Identifying the sources to establish trust in the future was seen as important. Furthermore, the availability of the Internet was mentioned as a potential problem. As a consequence it must be stated that the concept can only be used as a supplement to other communication channels.

This work has limitations: First, it focused on the situation in Western Europe. In other parts of the world the status of energy networks and the information needs of the public may be different. Second, the concept was tested with a rather small group of citizen (n=12), just in order to get some feedback about the general conceptual decisions. In future work the concept might be refined by an energy network operator and tested with a higher amount of people. Third, smartphones do not (yet) cover the entire public, so that, at present, the population can only be reached partially. As a consequence our concept cannot be seen as a comprehensive solution but as an additional form of communication, which, in a simple way, enables to make use of the time span between normal operation and overload of mobile communications in order to meet special information needs of the population and to reduce the number of phone calls at hotlines as well as their work load. To efficiently make use of the limited infrastructure capacity for a longer time the reservation of bandwidth from mobile networks by power suppliers would be conceivable. Fourth, people are also communicating with family and friends, which has not been covered by this concept. This contribution just focuses on alert messages to the population. Despite the restrictions such a concept, in our opinion, is reasonable because, if mobile communication is possible, concepts are needed for using the network more efficiently.

Before establishing the concept for power suppliers and emergency services as well as in everyday life of the population further research is necessary, especially regarding the question on how the population can be motivated for prevention measures and to proactively use such an application. The pre-installation of warning applications (e.g. in Google Maps), the integration of the functionalities in a dedicated emergency services application, which additionally enables the localization of citizens in crisis situations, or the integration into smart-metering-applications, which are provided by power suppliers, could be possible. By integrating such concepts into applications already established in the population the obstacle for the intrinsically motivated use could be overcome more easily.

ACKNOWLEDGMENT

We like to thank the participants of our study for their fruitful comments. This paper is an enhanced and improved version of a paper presented at the 2013 International ISCRAM Conference (Reuter, 2013) as well as at the 2013 GI Conference (Reuter & Ludwig, 2013). This research has been financed by the projects 'InfoStrom', funded by a grant of the German Federal Ministry for Education and Research (No. 13N10712), as well as the project 'EmerGent', funded by a grant of the European Union (FP7 No. 608352).

REFERENCES

Al-Akkad, A., Ramirez, L., Denef, S., Boden, A., Wood, L., Büscher, M., & Zimmermann, A. (2013). "Reconstructing Normality": The Use of Infrastructure Leftovers in Crisis Situations As Inspiration for the Design of Resilient Technology. In *Proceedings of the Australian Computer-Human Interaction Conference* (pp. 457–466).

Andersen, P. A., & Spitzberg, B. H. (2009). Myth and Maxims of Risk and Crisis Communication. In R. L. Heath & D. O'Hair (Eds.), *Handbook of Crisis Communication* (pp. 206–226). New York: Routledge.

Birkmann, J., Bach, C., Guhl, S., Witting, M., Welle, T., & Schmude, M. (2010). *State of the Art der Forschung zur Verwundbarkeit Kritischer Infrastrukturen am Beispiel Strom / Stromausfall. Risk Management.* Berlin, Germany. Retrieved from http://www.sicherheit-forschung.de/schriftenreihe

Bundesverwaltungsamt. (2001). *Zweiter Gefahrenbericht der Schutzkomission beim Bundesminister des Inneren - Bericht über mögliche Gefahren für die Bevölkerung bei Großkatastrophen und im Verteidigungsfall* (Zivilschut.). Bundesverwaltungsamt.

Coombs, W. T. (2009). Conceptualizing Crisis Communication. In R. L. Heath & D. O'Hair (Eds.), *Handbook of Risk and Crisis Communication* (pp. 99–118). New York: Routledge.

Deutscher Bundestag. (2011). *Gefährdung und Verletzbarkeit moderner Gesellschaften – am Beispiel eines großräumigen und langandauernden Ausfalls der Stromversorgung* (T. Petermann, H. Bradke, A. Lüllmann, M. Poetzsch, & U. Riehm, Eds.).

Federal Communications Commission. (2013). Consumer Guide: Wireless Emergency Alerts (WEA). Retrieved from http://transition.fcc.gov/cgb/consumerfacts/wea.pdf

Geenen, E. M. (2009). Warnung der Beölkerung. In Schutzkommission beim Bundesminister des Inneren (Ed.), Gefahren und Warnung (pp. 61–102). Bonn.

Helsloot, I., & Beerens, R. (2009). Citizens' response to a large electrical power out-age in the Netherlands in 2007. *Journal of Contingencies and Crisis Management, 17*(1), 64–68. doi:10.1111/j.1468-5973.2009.00561.x

Hiete, M., Merz, M., Trinks, C., Grambs, W., & Thiede, T. (2010). Krisenmanagement Stromausfall (Langfassung) - Krisenmanagement bei einer großflächigen Unterbrechung der Stromversorgung am Beispiel Baden-Württemberg. (Innenministerium Baden-Württemberg & Bundesamt für Bevölkerungsschutz und Katastrophenhilfe, Eds.). Stuttgart.

Holenstein, M., & Küng, L. (2008). Stromausfall - was denkt die Bevölkerung. *Sicherheit, 2008*(3), 61.

Hossmann, T., Legendre, F., Carta, P., Gunningberg, P., & Rohner, C. (2011). Twitter in Disaster Mode : Opportunistic Communication and Distribution of Sensor Data in Emergencies. In *Proceedings of ExtremeCom* (pp. 1–6). Manaus, Brazil: ACM Press. doi:10.1145/2414393.2414394

Jennex, M. E. (2004). Emergency Response Systems: The Utility Y2K Experience. [JITTA]. *Journal of Information Technology Theory and Application, 6*(3), 85–102.

Jennex, M. E. (2010). Implementing Social Media in Crisis Response Using Knowledge Management. [IJISCRAM]. *International Journal of Information Systems for Crisis Response and Management, 2*(4), 20–32. doi:10.4018/jiscrm.2010100102

Jennex, M. E. (2012). Social Media – Viable for Crisis Response? Experience from the Great San Diego/Southwest Blackout. [IJISCRAM]. *International Journal of Information Systems for Crisis Response and Management, 4*(2), 54–68. doi:10.4018/jiscrm.2012040104

Klafft, M. (Ed.). (2014). *Current Issues in Crisis Communication and Alerting*. Fraunhofer Verlag.

Klauser, R., Pipek, V., & Rusch, G. (2008). *Störfall-Kommunikation*. Siegen: Interner Bericht des Instituts für Medienforschung der Universität Siegen.

Latonero, M., & Shklovski, I. (2011). Emergency Management, Twitter, and Social Media Evangelism. [IJISCRAM]. *International Journal of Information Systems for Crisis Response and Management, 3*(4), 1–16. doi:10.4018/jiscrm.2011100101

Ley, B., Ludwig, T., Pipek, V., Randall, D., Reuter, C., & Wiedenhoefer, T. (2014). Information and Expertise Sharing in Inter-Organizational Crisis Management. [JCSCW]. *Computer Supported Cooperative Work: The Journal of Collaborative Computing, 23*(4-6), 347–387. doi:10.1007/s10606-014-9205-2

Ley, B., Pipek, V., Reuter, C., & Wiedenhoefer, T. (2012). Supporting Improvisation Work in Inter-Organizational Crisis Management. In *Proceedings of the Conference on Human Factors in Computing Systems (CHI)* (pp. 1529–1538). Austin, USA: ACM Press. doi:10.1145/2207676.2208617

Lorenz, D. F. (2010). *Kritische Infrastrukturen aus Sicht der Bevölkerung*. Forschungsforum Öffentliche Sicherheit der FU Berlin. Retrieved from http://www.sicherheit-forschung.de/schriftenreihe/

Menski, U., & Gardemann, J. (2008). *Auswirkungen des Ausfalls Kritischer Infrastrukturen auf den Ernährungssektor am Beispiel des Stromausfalls im Münsterland im Herbst 2005*. Münster: Fachhochschule Münster. Retrieved from http://www.hb.fh-muenster.de/opus/fhms/volltexte/2011/677/pdf/Stromausfall_Muensterland.pdf

MissionMode. (2012a). 15 Disaster and Crisis Apps for iPhone and iPad. Retrieved from http://blog.missionmode.com/blog/15-disaster-and-crisis-apps-for-iphone-and-ipad.html

MissionMode. (2012b). 15 Disaster and Crisis Apps for Android. Retrieved from http://blog.missionmode.com/blog/15-disaster-and-crisis-apps-for-android.html

Niebla, C. P., Chaves, J. M., Ramirez, J., Mendes, M., & Ferrer, M. (2012). The Benefits of Alerting System Based on Standardised Libraries. In *Proceedings of the International Disaster and Risk Conference* (pp. 557–560).

Nielsen, J. (1993). *Usability Engineering*. San Francisco, USA: Morgan Kaufmann.

Nilges, J., Balduin, N., & Dierich, B. (2009). Information and Communication Platform for Crisis Management (IKK). In *Proceedings of the International Conference and Exhibition on Electricity Distribution (CIRED)*. Prague, Czech Republic. Retrieved from http://ieeexplore.ieee.org/xpl/articleDetails.jsp?tp=&arnumber=5255837&contentType=Conference+Publications&sortType=asc_p_Sequence&filter=AND(p_IS_Number:5255237)&pageNumber=24

Palen, L., & Liu, S. B. (2007). Citizen communications in crisis: anticipating a future of ICT-supported public participation. In *Proceedings of the Conference on Human Factors in Computing Systems (CHI)* (pp. 727–736). San Jose, USA: ACM Press. doi:10.1145/1240624.1240736

Panitzek, K., Schweizer, I., Schulz, A., Bönning, T., Seipel, G., & Mühlhäuser, M. (2012). Can We Use Your Router, Please? Benefits and Implications of an Emergency Switch for Wireless Routers. *International Journal of Information Systems for Crisis Response and Management, 4*(4), 59–70. doi:10.4018/jiscrm.2012100104

Quarantelli, E. L. (1999). *Summary of 50 years of research findings disaster related social behavior*. Disaster Research Centre University of Delaware.

Reuter, C. (2013). Power Outage Communications: Survey of Needs, Infrastructures and Concepts. In T. Comes, F. Fiedrich, S. Fortier, J. Geldermann, & T. Müller (Eds.), *Proceedings of the Information Systems for Crisis Response and Management (IS-CRAM)* (pp. 884–889). Baden-Baden, Germany.

Reuter, C., Heger, O., & Pipek, V. (2013). Combining Real and Virtual Volunteers through Social Media. In T. Comes, F. Fiedrich, S. Fortier, J. Geldermann, & T. Müller (Eds.), *Proceedings of the Information Systems for Crisis Response and Management (ISCRAM)* (pp. 780–790). Baden-Baden, Germany.

Reuter, C., & Ludwig, T. (2013). Anforderungen und technische Konzepte der Krisenkommunikation bei Stromausfall. In M. Hornbach (Ed.), Informatik 2013 - Informatik angepasst an Mensch, Organisation und Umwelt (pp. 1604–1618). Koblenz, Germany: GI-Edition-Lecture Notes in Informatics (LNI).

Reuter, C., Ludwig, T., & Pipek, V. (2014). Ad Hoc Participation in Situation Assessment: Supporting Mobile Collaboration in Emergencies. [TOCHI]. *ACM Transactions on Computer-Human Interaction, 21*(5), 1–26. doi:10.1145/2651365

Reuter, C., Marx, A., & Pipek, V. (2012). Crisis Management 2.0: Towards a Systematization of Social Software Use in Crisis Situations. [IJIS-CRAM]. *International Journal of Information Systems for Crisis Response and Management, 4*(1), 1–16. doi:10.4018/jiscrm.2012010101

Reuter, C., Pipek, V., & Mueller, C. (2009). Avoiding crisis in communication: A computer-supported training approach for emergency management. [IJEM]. *International Journal of Emergency Management, 6*(3-4), 356–368. http://www.inderscience.com/search/index.php?action=record&rec_id=31571 doi:10.1504/IJEM.2009.031571

Semaan, B., & Mark, G. (2011). Technology-mediated social arrangements to resolve breakdowns in infrastructure during ongoing disruption. [TOCHI]. *ACM Transactions on Computer-Human Interaction, 18*(4), 1–21. doi:10.1145/2063231.2063235

Volgger, S., Walch, S., Kumnig, M., & Penz, B. (2006). *Kommunikation vor, während und nach der Krise - Leitfaden für Kommunikationsmanagement anhand der Erfahrungen des Hochwasserereignisses Tirol 2005*. Innsbruck: Amt der Tiroler Landesregierung, Abteilung Öffentlichkeitsarbeit in Zusammenarbeit mit SVWP Kommunikationsmanagement und dem Management Center Innsbruck (MCI). Retrieved from http://www.tirol.gv.at/fileadmin/www.tirol.gv.at/themen/tirol-und-europa/downloads/Publikation_Krisen-_und_Risikokommunikation.pdf

Wiedenhoefer, T., Reuter, C., Ley, B., & Pipek, V. (2011). Inter-organizational crisis management infrastructures for electrical power breakdowns. In *Proceedings of the Information Systems for Crisis Response and Management (ISCRAM)*. Lisbon, Portugal.

ENDNOTES

[1]   http://www.teltarif.de/i/cellbroadcast.html

This work was previously published in the International Journal of Information Systems for Crisis Response and Management (IJISCRAM), 6(2); edited by Murray E. Jennex and Bartel Van de Walle, pages 38-53 copyright year 2014 by IGI Publishing (an imprint of IGI Global).

Chapter 45
E–Government for Health Facilities in Africa

Paul Macharia
National AIDS and STIs Control Programme, Kenya

Davies Kimanga
Health Information Systems, Kenya

Onesimus Kamau
e-Health Unit, Kenya

ABSTRACT

Low and Middle Income Countries (LMICs) face healthcare worker shortages, skill mix imbalances, and maldistributions; there is concern in their quality and productivity. Africa's infrastructural developments also are way behind the rest of the world, and this gap is widening. Scalable, cost-effective, and long-term strategies in healthcare services are greatly needed. This chapter explores how Information and Communication Technologies (ICTs) could play an important role in improving healthcare. Components of e-health, an emerging field in medicine, clinical care, and public health are discussed. The role of m-health is explored, identifying the benefits of integrating mobile phone technologies in healthcare. To meet the health financing deficiencies, the chapter also explores how Bring-Your-Own-Device (BYOD) could drive healthcare professionals' productivity through increased workplace flexibility.

INTRODUCTION

Access to healthcare services and the existence of a functioning health system are taken for granted in the developed world. However in sub-Saharan Africa, due to limitations in funding, staffing, training and other manifestations of essential infrastructure the quality of healthcare is below expectations. A higher prevalence of infectious diseases also greatly impacts life expectancy and mortality rate among productive segments of the population (Stilwell et al, 2005).

Initiatives aimed at facilitating the widespread deployment of Information and Communication Technologies (ICTs) to support the operations of health delivery systems could address health needs of Sub-Saharan Africa. Use of ICTs in healthcare as a tool for collecting community information;

DOI: 10.4018/978-1-4666-8756-1.ch045

linking health care professionals and enhancing health administration, remote diagnostics and distribution of medical supplies would positively impact health outcomes (Hongoro et al, 2004).

BACKGROUND

e-Government can be defined as a Country's use of innovative Information and Communication Technologies (ICTs) to provide its citizens with convenient access to information and services (Fang, 2002). Although e-Government is a global phenomenon, additional effort is needed to make it work in developing Countries (Schuppan, 2009). Scalable, cost-effective and long term strategies in preventive and curative care services are greatly needed. Information and Communication Technologies (ICTs) can play an important role in improving health systems (Lucas, 2008). e-health is an emerging field in medicine, clinical care and public health where health services and information is delivered or enhanced through Information and Communication Technologies (Eysenbach, 2001).

ISSUES

Sub-saharan Africa faces a shortage of health workers hampering the capacity to improve health outcomes (WHO, 2008), ICTs can bridge this gap by bringing great benefit to health care systems in the areas of medical information, clinical data exchange and treatment (Ojo, 2006). e-health can provide an opportunity to extend healthcare ability to meet patient needs in a manner that supplements traditional delivery of health care (Juma et al, 2012). An increase in cheaper, efficient and reliable mobile phones avails technological opportunities to offer m-health solutions for preventive and curative care services in low and middle income countries (Tamrat & Kachnowski, 2012).

Mobile phones can revolutionize health care services offering immediate and secure access to critical clinical information when needed to provide patient care (Phillips et al, 2010). Health care facilities have demonstrated that quality of care can greatly improve to meet patient needs if use of ICTs is increased in ways that improve service delivery by health care providers to their patients (Bates, 2002).

CHALLENGES

Human resources to provide healthcare in low and middle income countries are in very short supply, WHO estimates a deficit equivalent to about 2.4 million doctors, nurses and mid-wives worldwide with sub-Saharan Africa accounting for over two thirds of this deficit (Anyangwe & Mtonga, 2007). There are also very serious concerns about the quality and productivity of this workforce (Hongoro et al, 2004). Most African Countries are faced by worker shortage, skill mix imbalance, maldistribution, negative work environment, and weak knowledge base (Chen et al, 2004). This health workforce is also under assault by HIV/AIDS, out-migration, and inadequate investment affecting the capacity to delivery healthcare in an equitable way (Stilwell et al, 2004).

Africa's infrastructural developments are way behind the rest of the world and this gap is widening. Infrastructure in Africa is very expensive with very high tariffs compared to any other parts of the world. (Foster & Briceño-Garmendia, 2010). Power shortage in Africa has been on the increase in recent years affecting economic growth and productivity. Generation capacity is inadequate, electrification is limited, the services are unreliable and very costly (Rosnes et al, 2011).

Africa accounts for 25 percent of the global disease burden; however Africa has less than 1 percent of global health spending and with only 2 percent of the global health workforce. Low levels of per capita income, mixed or limited growth prospects, and low domestic revenue mobilization potential in many countries make health financing very challenging (Union & HIV, 2007).

OPPORTUNITIES

As an innovative way to face the challenges in health systems in low- and middle-income countries, m-Health offers an opportunity to bridge the gap to barriers including lack of infrastructure, access to information and enough health care providers to deliver affordable high quality healthcare (Bastawrous et al, 2012).

The m-Health Alliance defines mobile health as;

The use of mobile-based or mobile-enhanced solutions to deliver healthcare. The ubiquity of mobile devices in the developed or developing world presents the opportunity to improve health outcomes through the delivery of innovative medical and health services with information and communication technologies to the farthest reaches of the globe.

The use of mobile technologies to support healthcare objectives has the potential to transform health care delivery. Mobile technologies are experiencing rapid advancements creating new opportunities for the integration of mobile health into existing e-health services and catalyzing the use of m-health in provision of health care (Kay et al, 2012, Evans 2013). There are over 5 billion wireless subscribers worldwide with over 70% of these residing in low- and middle income countries. This access to mobile phone technology can be a very ideal platform in the provision of quality health care (Bastawrous et al, 2012).

To achieve Millennium Development Goals (MDGs) low and middle-income countries are using m-Health as a complementary strategy for strengthening health systems. m-Health is already being applied in maternal and child health, and programmes, including HIV/AIDS, malaria, and tuberculosis (TB) (Kay et al, 2012).

To meet the health financing deficiencies, Bring your own device (BYOD) described as "the trend by employees to use their own devices on the job "disrupting" the traditional model in which IT had full control over corporate productivity tools but also driving greater employee productivity through increased workplace flexibility" (Dell. com) can improve access to affordable healthcare by clinical staff using their own mobile devices to provide services (Bastawrous et al, 2012). To maximize on the potential benefits of BYOD, set of rules governing a corporate IT department's level of support for employee-owned PCs, smartphones and tablets should be enforced (Steele, 2011).

Formulation of policy to regulate the use of Electronic Medical Records (EMRs) systems supported by portable mobile devices to safeguard patient information should be of paramount importance. Interoperability of EMRs systems supporting mobile devices will increase data sharing leading to better health outcomes. Stringent network controls should be enforced to ensure proper monitoring and control of mobile devices (wordpress.com).

Most healthcare providers work in multiple facilities. Due to the nature of their work these providers need to access patient details instantly to provide healthcare support. EMRs should be enabler to the health provider's professional obligations. The BYOD concept can address and facilitate health providers ever growing needs of secure remote access to patient confidential data.

To secure EMRs supporting BYOD concept, device provisioning to access the system is paramount. The mobile devices should be well documented and managed by the system's administrators. Policies on data security and privacy should be enforced to keep patient data uncompromised. To ensure optimum working of EMRs, the mobile devices should be within network bandwidth (Meru Networks, 2013).

FUTURE RESEARCH DIRECTIONS

BYOD as an emerging trend offers opportunities in setting and scaling up access to technology at the work place. Future research could address integration of Electronic Medical Records (EMRs) Systems with mobile technologies and how health providers' devices could securely be integrated to the EMRs in an effort to provide quality healthcare services.

CONCLUSION

E-health presents an opportunity to improve healthcare in sub-Saharan Africa. Technology could address the shortage of qualified health professionals; facilitate access to care from remote locations and scale-up healthcare services with lean staff. However deliberate efforts to build infrastructural capacity in power generation, access to mobile phone technologies should be fast tracked and made available in affordable and cost effective ways. Health professionals' skill mismatch, maldistribution and weak knowledge base must also be effectively addressed.

REFERENCES

Anyangwe, S., & Mtonga, C. (2007). Inequities in the Global Health Workforce: The Greatest Impediment to Health in Sub-Saharan Africa. *International Journal of Environmental Research and Public Health*, 4(2), 93–100. doi:10.3390/ijerph2007040002 PMID:17617671

Bastawrous, A., Hennig, B., & Livingstone, I. (2013). mHealth Possibilities in a Changing World. Distribution of Global Cell Phone Subscriptions. *Journal of Mobile Technology in Medicine*, 2(11S), 22–25. doi:10.7309/jmtm.2.1.4

Bates, D. W. (2002). The quality case for information technology in healthcare. *BMC Medical Informatics and Decision Making*, 2(1), 7. doi:10.1186/1472-6947-2-7 PMID:12396233

Chen, L., Evans, T., Anand, S., Boufford, J. I., Brown, H., & Chowdhury, M. et al. (2004). Human resources for health: Overcoming the crisis. *Lancet*, 364(9449), 1984–1990. doi:10.1016/S0140-6736(04)17482-5 PMID:15567015

Dell.com. (n.d.). *What is BYOD?*. Retrieved February 24, 2014, from http://www.dell.com/learn/us/en/555/solutions/byod

Evans, J. (2013). *Unlocking the potential in mobile phones for Cancer Care*. Retrieved February 24, 2014, from http://medicmobile.org/2013/05/03/unlocking-the-potential-in-mobile-phones-for-cancer-care/

Eysenbach, G. (2001). What is e-health? *Journal of Medical Internet Research*, 3(2), e20. doi:10.2196/jmir.3.2.e20 PMID:11720962

Fang, Z. (2002). E-government in digital era: concept, practice, and development. *International Journal of the Computer, the Internet and Management*, 10(2), 1-22.

Foster, V., & Briceño-Garmendia, C. (Eds.). (2010). *Africa's infrastructure: A time for transformation*. World Bank Publications.

Haines, A., Sanders, D., Lehmann, U., Rowe, A. K., Lawn, J. E., & Jan, S. et al. (2007). Achieving child survival goals: Potential contribution of community health workers. *Lancet*, 369(9579), 2121–2131. doi:10.1016/S0140-6736(07)60325-0 PMID:17586307

Hongoro, C., & McPake, B. (2004). How to bridge the gap in human resources for health. *Lancet*, 364(9443), 1451–1456. doi:10.1016/S0140-6736(04)17229-2 PMID:15488222

Juma, K., Nahason, M., Apollo, W., Gregory, W., & Patrick, O. (2012). *Current Status of E-Health in Kenya and Emerging Global Research Trends 1*.

Kay, M., Santos, J., & Takane, M. (2011). mHealth: New horizons for health through mobile technologies. World Health Organization.

Lucas, H. (2008). Information and communications technology for future health systems in developing countries. *Social Science & Medicine*, *66*(10), 2122–2132. doi:10.1016/j.socscimed.2008.01.033 PMID:18343005

Meru Networks. (2013). *BYOD in Healthcare Improving Clinician Productivity and Patient Satisfaction*. Retrieved February 24, 2014, from http://www.merunetworks.com/collateral/white-papers/byod-in-healthcare-whitepaper.pdf

Ojo, T. (2006). Communication networking: ICTs and health information in Africa. *Information Development*, *22*(2), 94–101. doi:10.1177/0266666906065549

Phillips, G., Felix, L., Galli, L., Patel, V., & Edwards, P. (2010). The effectiveness of M-health technologies for improving health and health services: A systematic review protocol. *BMC Research Notes*, *3*(1), 250. doi:10.1186/1756-0500-3-250 PMID:20925916

Rosnes, O., & Shkaratan, M. (2011). *Africa's power infrastructure: investment, integration, efficiency*. World Bank Publications.

Schuppan, T. (2009). E-Government in developing countries: Experiences from sub-Saharan Africa. *Government Information Quarterly*, *26*(1), 118–127. doi:10.1016/j.giq.2008.01.006

Snow, R. W., Guerra, C. A., Noor, A. M., Myint, H. Y., & Hay, S. I. (2005). The global distribution of clinical episodes of Plasmodium falciparum malaria. *Nature*, *434*(7030), 214–217. doi:10.1038/nature03342 PMID:15759000

Steele, C. (2011). *BYOD policy*. Retrieved February 24, 2014, from http://searchconsumerization.techtarget.com/definition/BYOD-policy

Stilwell, B., Diallo, K., Zurn, P., Vujicic, M., Adams, O., & Dal Poz, M. (2004). Migration of health-care workers from developing countries: Strategic approaches to its management. *Bulletin of the World Health Organization*, *82*(8), 595–600. PMID:15375449

Tamrat, T., & Kachnowski, S. (2012). Special delivery: An analysis of mHealth in maternal and newborn health programs and their outcomes around the world. *Maternal and Child Health Journal*, *16*(5), 1092–1101. doi:10.1007/s10995-011-0836-3 PMID:21688111

Union, A. (2007). *HIV, O*. Health Financing in Africa.

Wordpress.com BYOD Issues and Solutions for Healthcare Safekeeping. (n.d.). Retrieved February 24, 2014, from: http://curemd.wordpress.com/2013/06/04/byod-issues-and-solutions-for-healthcare-safekeeping/

World Health Organization. (2008). *Global Atlas of the Health Workforce Geneva*. Retrieved February 24, 2014, from http://www.who.int/healthinfo/systems/WHO_MBHSS_2010_section2_web.pdf

ADDITIONAL READING

Buchan, J., & Sochalski, J. (2004). The migration of nurses: Trends and policies. *Bulletin of the World Health Organization*, *82*(8), 587–594. PMID:15375448

Chandrasekhar, C. P., & Ghosh, J. (2001). Information and communication technologies and health in low income countries: The potential and the constraints. *Bulletin of the World Health Organization*, *79*(9), 850–855. PMID:11584733

Chen, C., Haddad, D., Selsky, J., Hoffman, J. E., Kravitz, R. L., Estrin, D. E., & Sim, I. (2012). Making sense of mobile health data: An open architecture to improve individual-and population-level health. *Journal of Medical Internet Research, 14*(4), e112. doi:10.2196/jmir.2152 PMID:22875563

Eberhard, A., Foster, V., Briceño-Garmendia, C., Ouedraogo, F., Camos, D., & Shkaratan, M. (2008). Underpowered: the state of the power sector in Sub-Saharan Africa.

Fraser, H. S., & St John, D. M. (2000). Information technology and telemedicine in sub-Saharan Africa: Economical solutions are available to support health care in remote areas. *BMJ: British Medical Journal, 321*(7259), 465–466. doi:10.1136/bmj.321.7259.465

Free, C., Phillips, G., Galli, L., Watson, L., Felix, L., & Edwards, P. et al. (2013). The effectiveness of mobile-health technology-based health behaviour change or disease management interventions for health care consumers: A systematic review. *PLoS Medicine, 10*(1), e1001362. doi:10.1371/journal.pmed.1001362 PMID:23349621

Free, C., Phillips, G., Watson, L., Galli, L., Felix, L., & Edwards, P. et al. (2013). The effectiveness of mobile-health technologies to improve health care service delivery processes: A systematic review and meta-analysis. *PLoS Medicine, 10*(1), e1001363. doi:10.1371/journal.pmed.1001363 PMID:23458994

Gerber, T., Olazabal, V., Brown, K., & Pablos-Mendez, A. (2010). An agenda for action on global e-health. *Health Affairs, 29*(2), 233–236. doi:10.1377/hlthaff.2009.0934 PMID:20348066

Hongoro, C., & McPake, B. (2004). How to bridge the gap in human resources for health. *Lancet, 364*(9443), 1451–1456. doi:10.1016/S0140-6736(04)17229-2 PMID:15488222

Källander, K., Tibenderana, J. K., Akpogheneta, O. J., Strachan, D. L., Hill, Z., & ten Asbroek, A. H. et al. (2013). Mobile health (mHealth) approaches and lessons for increased performance and retention of community health workers in low-and middle-income countries: A review. *Journal of Medical Internet Research, 15*(1), e17. doi:10.2196/jmir.2130 PMID:23353680

Kaplan, W. A. (2006). Can the ubiquitous power of mobile phones be used to improve health outcomes in developing countries. *Globalization and Health, 2*(9), 399–404. PMID:16719925

Lehmann, U., Van Damme, W., Barten, F., & Sanders, D. (2009). Task shifting: The answer to the human resources crisis in Africa? *Human Resources for Health, 7*(1), 49. doi:10.1186/1478-4491-7-49 PMID:19545398

Mbarika, V. W., Okoli, C., Byrd, T. A., & Datta, P. (2005). The Neglected Continent of IS Research: A Research Agenda for Sub-Saharan Africa. *Journal of the Association for Information Systems, 6*(5).

Mosse, E. L., & Sahay, S. (2003). Counter Networks, Communication and Health Information Systems. In organizational information systems in the context of globalization (pp. 35-51). Springer US.

Mutula, S. M. (2008). Comparison of sub-Saharan Africa's e-government status with developed and transitional nations. *Information Management & Computer Security, 16*(3), 235–250. doi:10.1108/09685220810893199

Narasimhan, V., Brown, H., Pablos-Mendez, A., Adams, O., Dussault, G., & Elzinga, G. et al. (2004). Responding to the global human resources crisis. *Lancet, 363*(9419), 1469–1472. doi:10.1016/S0140-6736(04)16108-4 PMID:15121412

Ndou, V. (2004). E-government for developing countries: opportunities and challenges. *The Electronic Journal of Information Systems in Developing Countries, 18.*

Øvretveit, J., Scott, T., Rundall, T. G., Shortell, S. M., & Brommels, M. (2007). Improving quality through effective implementation of information technology in healthcare. *International Journal for Quality in Health Care*, *19*(5), 259–266. doi:10.1093/intqhc/mzm031 PMID:17717038

Shaw, R. P., & Griffin, C. C. (1995).Financing health care in Sub-Saharan Africa through user fees and insurance.

Unwin, T., & Unwin, P. T. H. (Eds.). (2009). *ICT4D: Information and communication technology for development.* Cambridge University Press.

Walsham, G., & Sahay, S. (2006). Research on information systems in developing countries: Current landscape and future prospects. *Information Technology for Development*, *12*(1), 7–24. doi:10.1002/itdj.20020

Wilson, E. V. (2009). Patient-centered E-health. *Ann L. Fruhling. Pages, 157*, 167.

Yepes, T., Pierce, J., & Foster, V. (2009).Making Sense of Africa's Infrastructure Endowment: A Benchmarking Approach.

KEY TERMS AND DEFINITIONS

Bring-Your-Own-Device: Is a new concept in the use of user-owned computing hardware to access workplace resources.

Curative Care: These are services provided to patients suffering from health problems.

E-Health: Is the use of information and communication technologies to improve healthcare service delivery.

Healthcare Providers: They are frontline personnel providing clinical care to patients.

Interoperability: Is the ability of different information systems to access and share data.

Mm-Health: Is the use of mobile phone technologies to deliver health care services.

Quality of Care: Implies a service meeting minimum standards.

Chapter 46

Using Virtual Environments to Achieve Learner Outcomes in Interprofessional Healthcare Education

Michelle Aebersold
University of Michigan, USA

Dana Tschannen
University of Michigan, USA

ABSTRACT

The use of simulation in the training of healthcare professionals has become an essential part of the educational experience. Students and practitioners need to learn a variety of technical, interpersonal, and clinical judgment skills to be effective healthcare practitioners. Virtual simulation can provide an effective training method to facilitate learning and can be targeted to develop specific skills in the area of Interprofessional Education (IPE). This chapter reviews the literature around simulation techniques and outlines a development process that can be used to develop virtual simulations to meet a variety of learning objectives including IPE. Specific issues and solutions are also presented to ensure a successful educational experience.

INTRODUCTION

Quality and safety are ongoing concerns in the healthcare environment. A recent article in the Journal of Patient Safety found 210,000 patients die each year from preventable medical errors (James, 2013). The Joint Commission (2013) attributes over 70% of these errors to failures in communication, with the majority of failures oc-

curring between various disciplines. This has led to an increase focus in the area of interdisciplinary or interprofessional education (IPE). The World Health Organization (WHO) defines interprofessional education as "When students from two or more professions learn about, from and with each other to enable effective collaboration and improve health outcomes" (WHO, 2010, p.7) In May 2011, the Interprofessional Education Col-

DOI: 10.4018/978-1-4666-8756-1.ch046

laborative published a set of core competencies for interprofessional education, which included competencies related to values/ethics, roles/responsibilities, interprofessional communications and teams/teamwork (Interprofessional Education Collaborative Expert Panel, 2011). Many academic and practice institutions have struggled with the implementation of these competencies due to a variety of challenges in both space and cost barriers. One promising methodology that may assist in attainment of these core competencies includes simulation. This chapter will provide an example of the use of one type of simulation method; virtual simulation to address the growing need for IPE to improve competencies in the area of communication.

BACKGROUND

Patient safety is currently one of the most urgent issues facing our health care systems. Beginning with the Institute of Medicine's (IOM) (Kohn, Corrigan, & Donaldson, 2000) report on patient safety in which it was reported up to 98,000 people die each year because of medical errors, patient safety has become an urgent concern for both health care administrators and those educating the future generation of health care providers. The IOM (2003) has made recommendations on health care education focused around their vision, "All health professionals should be educated to deliver patient-centered care as members of an interdisciplinary team, emphasizing evidence-based practice, quality improvement approaches and informatics" (http://www.nap.edu/catalog/10681.html, p. 3). In particular their recommendations around teamwork include the need to develop skills around communication and collaboration. Evidence has shown that effective team performance requires team members effectively communicate with each other and have a shared goal; such as improving patient care (AHRQ, 2003). Additionally communication failures are at the

root cause of many sentinel events analyzed by The Joint Commission (a regulatory agency that accredits hospitals) (http://www.jointcommission.org/sentinel_event.aspx). Many factors including how different professions train their students to communicate create the challenges in communication that currently exist between physicians and nurses in particular (Leonard, Graham, & Bonacum, 2004).

As a result of this focus on fostering IPE many health science schools have focused efforts on utilizing simulation as a means to achieve competencies in this area. Several studies have been published in this area utilizes different approaches. In a study by Liaw and colleagues (2014) nursing and medical students engaged together in simulations using standardized patients and high-fidelity computerized mannequin simulators. The students played their respective roles in caring for a patient who was going in to septic shock and becoming quite ill. Students were able to practice skills such as roles, communication, teamwork and handoffs; meeting several IPE competencies. Pre/Post evaluation showed a significant improvement in self-confidence with no significant differences between groups and the participants were highly satisfied with their learning. In another study by Dillion, Noble and Kaplan (2009) nursing and medical students engaging in a mock cardiac arrest code blue simulation to determine their perception of the value of simulation as an IPE learning experience. The results showed the experience to be a positive one and an increase in understanding of both their own roles and the other person's roles were found. In other areas IPE is met through a combination of curricular activities and simulation activities.

Simulations as proposed in this chapter could be defined as educational simulations. Aldrich (2009) considers educational simulations as a subset of immersive learning simulations. He also classifies serious games as subset of immersive learning simulations as well as games. This is part of his overall taxonomy in which sims are the broad category that includes computer games for entertainment and immersive learning simulations for formal learning programs. Educational simulations are different from computer games because they do not have a goal of being necessarily fun but do focus on engagement. They are focused on specific learning goals and strive to increase the participant's skill level in the real world whereas serious games increase awareness of real-world topics and can be used for both entertainment and learning (Aldrige, 2009).

VIRTUAL REALITY SIMULATION IN HEALTH CARE

Creating a virtual reality simulation program to support IPE in health care requires the consideration of many factors to ensure a successful outcome. These factors include a thorough understanding of the skills needed by those in the health care profession, an understanding of educational pedagogies, the ability to develop virtual environments and simulations scenarios, and most importantly how to evaluate their effectiveness.

Required Skills

Health care practitioners need a variety of clinical skills, cognitive skills, and interpersonal skills to be effective in their roles. Clinical or technical skills generally involve learning how to do procedures and often simple repetitive practice can enable a high degree of proficiency. This practice can usually be set up in a skills lab area or in the patient care area where they can practice skills such as inserting a urine catheter or administering intravenous medications. Cognitive and interpersonal skills may require more complex training due to their complex nature and need to vary depending on the situation. Cognitive skills such as clinical reasoning is the process of collecting cues, processing information, coming to a an understanding of the patient problem or

situation, planning and implementing interventions, evaluating outcomes and finally reflecting upon and learning from the process (Hoffman, O'Donnell, & Kim, 2007; Levett-Joneseta, et al., 2010; Tanner, Padrick, Westfall, & Putzier, 1987). It allows the nurse or healthcare practitioner to build upon previously acquired knowledge and past experiences in order to deal with new or unfamiliar situations (Lapkin, Levett-Jones, Bellchambers, & Fernandez, 2010). Educating professionals to acquire the necessary skill set requires not only technical knowledge but artistry. Artistry is a kind of knowing that is different from professional knowledge. Some would say artistry is based on intuition or even pattern recognition and is found in nurses practicing at an expert level. There is recognition that both the art and science of health care is needed by practitioners to perform effectively (Schon, 1983). The greatest challenge for educators is often in teaching the artistry. Educators are also challenged with bridging the gap between the classroom and the clinical area. Health care practitioners need to make the connections between the didactic material they hear in lecture or other training venues with the actual patient care setting in which they care for patients. Health care can be chaotic and doesn't always conform to typical textbook clinical signs and symptoms. Initially students and beginning health care practitioners often engage in very deliberate problem solving efforts focusing on one issue at a time. Situational awareness or sense of salience allows health care practitioners to problem solve in novel situations using their professional knowledge base. The ability to focus on important aspects of a patient situation, ignore those that don't apply and be able to use their professional knowledge in addressing the situation is called salience (Benner et al. 2009) or situational awareness (Aldridge, 2009). Salience or situational awareness is usually a hallmark of an expert practitioner and develops over time given the right circumstances to support this learning. For example, a patient who has a serious blood stream infection will exhibit a constellation of signs and symptoms that include a low blood pressure, a high heart rate, a fever and a low urine output. That same patient may also have lung congestion that is not part of the signs and symptoms of the blood stream infection itself. A beginner will assess all the signs and symptoms and recognize they are abnormal but may not be able to separate out which ones go together to support the diagnosis of blood stream infection. An expert will be able to look at the entire constellation of signs and symptoms and recognize the patient has sepsis (a blood stream infection) that might be secondary to pneumonia (as noted by the lung congestion). They must develop these key skills to become an effective practitioner and in addition they must also learn to become an effective member of the health care team.

Health care practitioners also need key interpersonal and communication skills because they do not practice alone but are part of a team. Although they can learn about effective communication skills through a lecture or other didactic approach, only after 'practicing' these skills in a simulated environment can they gain the proficiency necessary for effective use in the high stakes, complex clinical environment. Several programs have been developed to educate practitioners around effective communication strategies. Crew Resource Management (CRM) (originally developed in the airline industry) has become a popular training methodology for nurses and physicians. Various communication techniques are taught in CRM including how to 'go up the chain of command' and get someone to address a critical patient situation. TEAMSTEPPS is another training program developed by the Agency for Healthcare Research and Quality (AHRQ). The focus of this training is on teamwork skills with effective communication being one of those skills. The training identifies key communication strategies that have been found effective in health care and uses demonstrations, role play and debriefing to teach these strategies. Teamwork itself is another critical interpersonal skill. Nurses and other health care practicitoners

need to know how to be team leaders as well as good followers. They often need to move between roles depending on the situation and can do that several times a day, often in very challenging and intense situations. All of these skills will enhance patient outcomes and patient safety and poor skills in these areas will potentially lead to poor patient outcomes (Mazzocco et al., 2009). Acquisition of these skills is often challenging as students and healthcare practitioners are not always exposed to the 'right' patient care experiences which will foster the development of these skills.

Conceptual Framework

The development of these skills requires an integrative learning environment where students and health care practitioners can learn didactic information and then use that information in the practice environment to attain proficiency of these crucial skills. In the field of healthcare nurses and other health care practitioners are expected to become, at the minimum competent in their work. New nurses are considered beginners trying to achieve a level of competency and the ability to provide safe care to their patients with some support from nurses at a higher level of expertise. Nurses need to quickly progress to a competent level. Although one could remain at the competent level, nurses need to continue on to become experts in their field to support the highest level of patient care outcomes possible. To do this requires more than just experience. Although experience alone will initially improve the nurse's skills, it is not sufficient to continue the growth and over time skills may decay. It is the opportunity to 'practice' their skills in a meaningful way that will contribute to the progression towards mastery. This is in line with the educational pedagogy developed by Ericsson, which supports that acquisition of skills requires practice.

Ericsson's (2004) expertise framework is based on the assumption that to acquire expert performance one must engage in deliberate practice activities that are focused on improving some aspect of performance. This expert performance will include clinical or technical skills, cognitive skills and interpersonal skills and a sense of salience or situational awareness. This experiential learning (learning by doing) framework is helpful in guiding educators in facilitating focused experiential learning opportunities. Health care professionals improve their skills with experience, however, Ericsson's theory posits that experts are those individuals who continue to improve beyond the level needed to perform adequately and become recognized as experts in their domain. This level of expertise is gained through deliberate efforts focused on improving selected skills or tasks. Schon's (1983) work highlights the need for professionals to reflect upon experiences in order to gain knowledge. Ericsson states this occurs when individuals are instructed to improve certain aspects of their performance for a well defined task and then given immediate detailed feedback on their performance which they can reflect upon and continue to practice during subsequent training sessions. This is based on the ability of educators and trainers to determine the types of representative tasks (knowledge and skills) that define the domain of practice. Individuals who do not engage in deliberate practice activities experience the decay or their skills over time or their skills can be outdated as new knowledge about practice is discovered. This framework of deliberate practice to educate and train professionals can be achieved through the use of educational simulations and serious games.

Simulation

Simulation is a technique currently being used by many educators in a variety of fields. Simulation has long been used in the military, aviation and nuclear power industries as part of their overall training and readiness programs. Health care facilities, medical and nursing schools have recently incorporated simulation in an effort to enhance learning related to procedural training, team training and individual learner training. Simulation in health care increases patient safety, improves clinical judgment and can be used to teach/evaluate specific clinical skills (Bearnson & Wiker, 2005).

In the world of medical simulations there are three classifications of simulations used: low-fidelity (non-computerized trainers that teach a specific task such as intravenous catheter insertion), mid-fidelity (standardized patients, computer programs, video games), and high-fidelity (computerized human patient simulator mannequins that respond to treatments) (Harder, 2010). Simulation is a practical and successful model which can be used to teach a variety of skills; psychomotor (technical), cognitive (clinical reasoning, decision making), and interpersonal (communication, teamwork). A key benefit to using simulation is its ability to mimic real life situations without putting patients at risk (Nehring & Lashley, 2004; Morgan, Cleave-Hogg, McIlroy, & Devitt, 2002). The benefits of simulation are well established in the literature (Buckley &Gordon, 2010; Harder, 2010; Lapkin, Levette-Jones, Bellchambers, & Fernandez, 2010; McGaphie, Issenberg, Petrusa, & Scalese, 2010; Orledge, Phillips, Murray &Lerant, 2012; Shearer, 2013; Cumin, Boyd, Webster & Weller, 2013).

In addition simulation can help health care professionals learn how to apply previously learned knowledge in novel situations. Research has shown that participation in simulations is effective in helping students manage scenarios they had not previously encountered when compared to other forms of education (Owen, Mugford, Follows, & Plummer, 2006). This also occurs in the area of skill transfer from a simulation environment to the actual practice environment. In a study on advanced life support training it was found that physicians who participated in simulations designed to teach them how to be an effective leader in a situation where a patient was experiencing a cardiac arrest, performed better during actual cardiac arrests

(Wayne et al., 2008). Simulation also provides opportunities for students and nurses to engage in deliberate practice using evidence-based or best practice guidelines (Aebersold, 2010). In addition, simulation has shown to improve student's level of confidence or self-efficacy (Scherer, Bruce, & Runkawatt, 2007; Morgan & Cleave-Hogg, 2002).

Virtual Simulation

Although much is known about simulation using high-fidelity mannequins, research is just starting to emerge around the use of virtual reality environments for simulation in health care. Educators are using a variety of platforms to build virtual reality environments to support simulations. Much of the work done has been in Second Life (SL), which to date, is the most popular and mature multi-user virtual environment used in education (Warburton, 2009). SL provides an accessible environment for learners to participate in simulation scenarios with other learners through the use of avatars (a virtual on-line persona) in a realistic setting that fosters learning. Using SL is not without its challenges (which will be discussed later), but it can support certain types of simulations without significant start up costs providing educators have access to an 'island' or space within SL to set up their learning environment. Through the use of avatars, learners can gain a feeling of being 'physically present' in the environment, yet it is still a safe, controlled setting where students can practice their skills and make mistakes without harming patients (Burgess, Slate, Rojas-LeBouef, & LaPrairie, 2010). The virtual environment has an advantage over traditional role play in a classroom because we can mimic the setting in which the learner will practice (i.e. hospital unit, emergency room, operating room, clinic). Conradi and colleagues (2009) found that paramedic students using SL for problem based learning, indicated the environment was more authentic and collaborative than paper-based problem solving scenarios. Our own work in SL has shown that

learners are more likely to take risks in using new skills or problem solving novel situations because it is their avatar doing the work and they have a degree of anonymity. Early research is showing that simulations conducted in virtual reality can be just as effective for learning as those done with traditional high-fidelity simulation using human patient simulators (Youngblood, Harter, Srivastava, Moffett, Heinrichs, & Dev, 2008).

Virtual simulations have a role to play in overall education of health care practitioners. They can be used effectively for creating deliberate practice scenarios for skill development such as cognitive and interpersonal skills. In particular they are useful for communication and teamwork skill development. The next section will describe how we developed our virtual environment using SL and how simulations are developed using a standardized process supported by Ericsson's (2004) deliberate practice framework.

Virtual Environment Development

Land in Second Life–owned by the University of Michigan Medical School–was used to create a space for training students in cognitive and interpersonal skills. An eight-bed virtual hospital unit occupies one floor of the six-story hospital building. To create a sense of realism, patient rooms are equipped with wall-mounted blood pressure gauges, bedside cardiac monitors, medical supply cabinets, a sink, a computer desk, and chairs. Additional equipment on the unit includes central desk and computer workspace, crash cart, medication dispensing unit, x-ray view boxes and wheelchairs. Although the hospital unit was initially set up for nursing students to use for virtual simulations, the environment is well suited for inter-professional education. Specifically, the space supports several avatars in each patient room at one time (8-10 avatars), with additional observation space on the exterior deck of the building (translucent wall so that observers can see into the unit).

Several SL features provide opportunities for information sharing and interaction among the interprofessional learners. For example, objects can be created for learners to interact with in order to gain clinical information about their patients, such as health history, current vital signs and assessment parameters. Notecards–developed prior to the educational session–can be shared with learners to give them information or cues to aid them during the simulation. The voice chat function also allows for synchronous communication among the interprofessional learners. In summary, the overall environment provides a realistic, dynamic space for active learning. The environment can quickly be adapted to support educational objectives for a variety of simulations, while still maintaining fidelity and a sense of realism.

Second Life Scenario Development Process

A standardized process for simulation development is needed to maximize fidelity of the simulation process. The five step process includes

1. Key concept identification,
2. Competency and standard mapping,
3. Scenario building,
4. Debriefing development, and
5. Beta testing and refinement (as needed) of the scenario (Tschannen & Aebersold, 2010).

This process has been successfully used for the development of simulations for diverse settings, including ambulatory care, acute care, community prevention and professional educational settings (Tschannen, Aebersold, Sauter & Funnel, 2013). For the purpose of this chapter, a detailed description of each phase in the process will be given. In addition, an exemplar will be developed using the phases in the process. The exemplar will focus on the use of effective communication strategies among the interprofessional healthcare team. Although the setting is within the healthcare environment, it can be applied to many other business-related industries where transfer of communication is critical.

Phase 1: Key Concept Identification

In Phase 1, key concepts or behaviors that are needed for success in a particular industry must be identified. This step requires the review of current industry standards of practice and key competencies. For healthcare, this includes the Institute of Medicine Reports, the Quality and Safety in Education (Cronenwett, et al., 2007) standard, the *Essentials of Baccalaureate Education for Professional Nursing* (2009), the Accreditation Council for Graduate Medical Education (ACGME) competencies (http://www.acgme.org/acgmeweb/Portals/0/PFAssets/ProgramRequirements/CPRs2013.pdf), and the Interprofessional Education Collaborative (Interprofessional Education Collaborative Expert Panel, 2011). As noted in these publications, interprofessional communication is a core competency for both physicians and nurses.

Exemplar: One of the most critical aspects in healthcare delivery is communication among the healthcare team. According to The Joint Commission, miscommunication is one of the primary root causes for sentinel events (The Joint Commission, 2013). When communication is effective among nurses and physicians, patient and professional outcomes improve, such as improved quality of care (Hamric & Blackball, 2007; Kramer & Schmalenberg, 2003) increased patient and professional satisfaction (Hamric & Blackball, 2007; Boyle & Kochinda, 2004) and greater intent to stay (Boyle & Kochinda, 2004; Krairiksh & Anthony, 2001). Breakdowns in communication between nurses and physicians can often result in errors, many of which are preventable (Solet, Norvell, Rutan, & Frankel, 2005). For this reason, every opportunity to 'practice' communication among members of the healthcare team is important.

Phase 2: Competency and Standard Mapping

The key concepts are mapped in phase 2 to clinical standards and competencies to ensure that the simulation focus is in alignment with current requirements. This phase is critical to ensuring the approach taken within the simulation scenario will assist in the development of the preferred competency.

Exemplar: The concept of communication is in alignment with many professional standards and core competencies. The Interprofessional Education Collaborative identified interprofessional communication as one of three competency domains. Specifically, members of the healthcare team must "Communicate with patients, families, communities, and other health professionals in a responsive and responsible manner that supports a team approach to the maintenance of health and the treatment of disease (pg 23)." Similarly, the *Essentials of Baccalaureate Education for Professional Nursing* (2009), which addresses stakeholders' recommendations for required core knowledge of all health care providers, identified communication as a critical component of education. Within the document, nine essentials are included covering a range of topics, including Essential (VI) which describes incorporation of "effective communication techniques, including negotiation and conflict resolution to produce positive professional working relationships (American Association of Colleges of Nursing, 2009, pg 22)." In the medical profession, residents must 'demonstrate interpersonal

and communication skills that result in the effective exchange of information and collaboration with patients, their families, and health professionals (pg 9)."

Understanding the types of communication techniques required for competent practice for the interprofessional team (e.g. collaboration, conflict management, and negotiation) helps in determining the type of scenario that needs to be presented. In this case, it is clear that the ability to communicate pertinent patient information in a succinct and efficient manner is necessary for safe and effective patient care. For this reason, the scenario should require a succinct patient communication between a nurse and physician.

Phase 3: Scenario Building

Scenario building (Phase 3) includes brainstorming clinical scenarios that will stimulate the desired response/behavior. To ensure successful development of a scenario, it is important to have experts in the field (related to the scenario topic) assisting with the scenario building. In an interprofessional education session, this requires engagement of all stakeholders (e.g. nurses and physician faculty). This helps with ensuring the fidelity or 'degree of realism' of the developed scenario through each stakeholder lense. An important next step is to decide the background needed for the scenario (in this case where in SL should the scenario be run?) and which roles are played by learners and which are played by facilitators or 'actors'. A storyboard outlining the key aspects of the scenario is needed to build the scenario. Elements of the storyboard should include the following: Key concepts, pre-requisites, timeframe, setting, participants, scenario design and timeline, and debriefing questions.

Once the simulation has been developed, the process in which students or learners will be evaluated on their performance must be considered. Educators can use standardized scales such as the Emergency Medicine Crisis Resource Management (EMCRM) tool, developed by Youngblood et al. (2008) or the Capacity to Rescue Instrument (CRI) developed by Aebersold (2008). The EMCRM was developed to evaluate the participant's crisis management skills and assesses their team leadership skills, including knowledge of the environment, utilization of information and resources, and overall ability to communicate and facilitate task completion. The CRI identifies key assessments and interventions that need to be performed in the simulation scenario to ensure a good patient outcome. Educators can also develop their own set of behaviors based on 'best practice' standards or current evidence-based practice guidelines. Performance, which can be measured individually or as a team, can then be reviewed during the debriefing session after the completion of the simulation scenario.

Exemplar: Prior to the simulation, medical and nursing students should be provided some pre-learnings related to the education content, which in this case, is communication among the interprofessional team. There are a variety of training programs available that focus on communication, including Medical Team Training, Crew Resource Management, and Team Strategies and Tools to Enhance Performance and Patient Safety (TEAMSTEPPS). CRM, for example, was developed by the National Center for Patient Safety at the VA (Sculi, 2010). Part of this training program provides an overview of key behaviors and strategies that are used by leaders and subordinates to ensure that effective teamwork and communication takes place, especially when safety is in question. The training also provides an overview of the effective followership algorithm shown in Figure 1. Effective Followership

Figure 1. Effective followership algorithm
© 2011, Fortis Business Media, LLC and Gary L. Sculli. Used with permission.

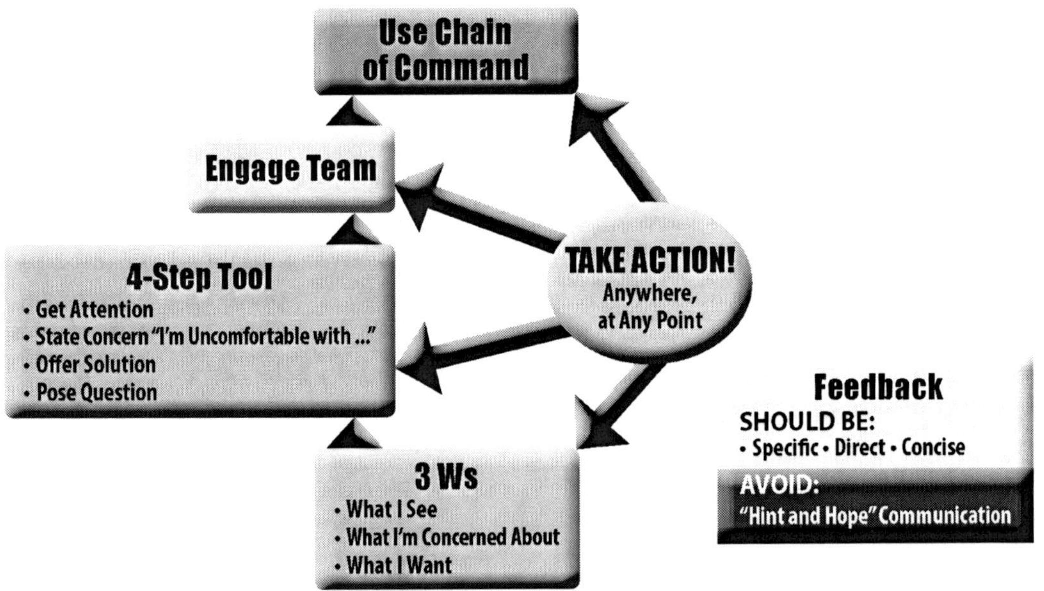

Algorithm, which includes specific communication strategies. Upon completion of the pre-learning, students can 'practice' the communication strategies identified in the training session while incorporating the specific experiences needed for the student to become competent (as deemed by industry standards).

A storyboard of the scenario should be developed. For the purpose of this exemplar, a storyboard, overviewing each element of the scenario was developed (Appendix). Once the storyboard has been developed, review of the scenario by experts in the field (e.g. communication and patient safety) should be conducted. Such feedback will aid in ensuring realism and fidelity in the scenario, as well as to ensure the most relevant evidence related to the themes are being highlighted in the scenario.

For the purpose of this scenario, a specific evaluation tool was not developed. The faculty should consider the student performance in relationship to the evidence based communication strategies learned in the CRM (i.e. effective followership algorithm). For example, did the nurse use the 3W's? The 4-step communication process? Was hinting and hoping avoided? Additionally, performance should be discussed during the debriefing session, which would occur at the conclusion of the simulation scenario.

Phase 4: Debriefing Development

This phase of the development is critical for success. Debriefing sessions provide an opportunity for participants to reflect on their performance (as well as the performance of other team members) and gain useful insights into behaviors and errors that contribute to the initiation and evolution of a crisis. Debriefing allows the learner to reexamine or reflect upon the simulation experience and supports the development of clinical reasoning skills (Dreifuerst, 2009). It is also important

to establish a trusting relationship between the facilitator and the learners (Wickers, 2010). The most effective debriefing strategy is debriefing with good judgment. In this strategy learners are required to reflect back on their experiences to make sense of what occurred. The facilitator also provides feedback to the learner on how they performed in the scenario (Rudolf, Simon, Dufresne, Raemer, 2006). According to a study conducted by Day and colleagues (2009), feedback provided during simulation has been shown to significantly improve performance over feedback given in the actual clinical site. Debriefing can also include feedback to participants based on their individual or group performance in the scenario as compared to a standardized measurement scale or a list of expected behaviors.

Exemplar: At the completion of the simulation, all participants would need to participate in the debriefing, which usually occurs in a classroom or conference room (e.g. unit conference room on SL unit). For this scenario, a focus would be on understanding how the interaction transpired. The debriefing should begin with a focus on the aspects of the simulation that went well (e.g. 'what do you feel went well during this scenario?'). Once positive aspects of the simulation are discussed, the facilitator should ask questions focused on the key concept of the simulation ('How would you describe the interaction between Nancy, the staff nurse, and Tracey, the physician?' What might the nurse have done differently? Was the 3W's approach used effectively and if not, how so?'). In addition, the debriefing session should highlight the critical points associated with effective communication, and clarification of the two strategies (e.g. 3 W's and Four step assertive communication strategy) should be given if needed. The staff nurses are given the opportunity to speak first and to reflect on their performance in the scenario. The physician and charge nurse should then be able to provide further feedback as to their reflection of the simulation. Observers may also provide some feedback as to how they might have done things differently.

Phase 5: Beta Testing and Further Refinement

The simulation should be beta tested with a group of individuals familiar with the topic of interest prior to implementation. In interprofessional simulations, it is important to ensure the diverse professions are accounted for in the beta test group. A diverse group will provide feedback to the fidelity of the scenario from all stakeholder perspectives. The beta test is an opportunity to 'test' the simulation and should be conducted in a manner similar to how one expects to implement the simulation to the targeted population. For example, if the scenario developed requires certain pre-work or supplies, all of this should be provided to the participants in the beta test. This helps to determine the effectiveness of the anticipated implementation process, as well as the overall fidelity of the scenario. This step in the process requires participants to provide feedback on all aspects of the simulation (i.e. scenario, implementation process, fidelity, etc). This feedback is then used to revise the scenario and the implementation process as needed.

Exemplar: For the purpose of the exemplar, the scenario should be beta tested with both nurse and medical faculty who also have completed the Crew Resource Management training. The purpose of the beta testing would be to test the process of setting up and running the scenarios and to pilot test the actual scenario with the interprofessional group. Faculty participating in the beta test would be brought to the simulation setting, provided the notecards (e.g. instructions) for the different roles, and provided the same

instructions as noted in the scenario (Appendix A). The simulation should run over approximately 15 minutes, with an additional 15 minutes allotted for the debriefing session. Faculty should be asked to share their input as to the fidelity and effectiveness of the implementation of the simulation used in the beta test. Specifically, questions related to the 'realness' and flow should be discussed (e.g. 'What (if any) changes would you make in the scenario of the implementation of the scenario when we implement this with our students?'). Feedback obtained from the beta test of the exemplar may include changes in wording and flow of the simulation

Scenario Implementation

Once the scenarios have been developed and adjustments made after the beta testing, they are ready to be used by learners. The virtual simulations are scheduled and 'run' by a trained facilitator who can oversee the simulation and effectively manage the debriefing directly after the simulation. Content experts may also be present to add to the experience during debriefing. The effectiveness of simulations can be evaluated by using standardized scoring templates during the scenario, having learners take a knowledge test or following the learners in the actual clinical site and observe their performance. Virtual simulations, as with all simulations are evaluated carefully during their execution for areas that might need further improvement.

ISSUES, CONTROVERSIES, PROBLEMS

Challenges occur in any new type of learning particularly when it includes technologies outside of the educator's control. There are advantages to using SL for educational purposes; it is free to users, can be downloaded on most computers without difficulty and basic navigation skills are easy for most people to learn. When using it for virtual simulations the learners usually only need basic navigation skills and do not require more advanced skills such as building objects or writing scripts. The educators, however, need to have access to space they can use which usually means having an island available and some type of building or structure to implement the virtual simulation. Many universities and even several health systems have invested in purchasing space (islands) in SL for training and education (both formal and informal). Challenges around using the space at a university or heath system are usually related to technology infrastructure and firewall issues. Computer labs on campus or training rooms often have closed systems that do not allow for the installation of programs such as SL without permission and support from the information technology (IT) departments. For example, prior to one of the virtual simulation days, a new version of SL was required prior to use of the software. We were unable to download the new version, thus the simulations were postponed (adding to student frustration). On the health system side, privacy issues exist as health care systems need to ensure protection of private health information and therefore several IT security measures and firewalls are in place, limiting the ability to incorporate a new software program such as SL.

Additional issues include skill set of the faculty or educator who is interested in using SL. As with many new technologies on campus that may be used by innovators or early adopters there is usually no internal IT support available. Often IT staff are not even familiar with the product. It then becomes the faculty/educator's responsibility to set up the space and manage the technology, including assisting students or learners with issues in downloading and using the program. Faculty/educators need to have skills to build their environments within SL and basic scripting skills are a minimal requirement for many virtual simulations. While it is possible to purchase many items that are needed, a working knowledge

of Prims (basic building blocks in SL) and scripting (to program object interactions) are usually necessary to understand how objects work. Faculty and educators find themselves functioning in several roles; developing the SL environment, developing and running the virtual simulations, and providing IT support to learners. One particular technology challenge for our work has been in getting learners to use the voice chat function. We found it necessary to use headsets to reduce the amount of background noise found with using laptop microphones. Learners often had difficulty getting their headsets to work and sometimes lost functionality part way through the simulations. Again some of this was due to using university/health system computers that faculty/educators did not have administrative access to so troubleshooting problems was difficult. It is also necessary for them to develop some skills with their avatars ahead of time to make full use of the training time.

Other concerns include privacy for participants during the virtual simulations and during the debriefing. In simulation, learners are encouraged to take risks and try new behaviors and skills that they have not mastered. During debriefing, learners are given critical feedback on their performance and it is sometimes very emotional, particularly if they did not do well and their 'virtual patient' did not have a positive outcome. When running simulation in a simulation lab using human patient simulators there are usually only the learners and faculty present. Even simulations that take place in situ (in the actual health care environment-hospital unit, emergency room) there is still a limited number of people around to observe. In SL if you are running the virtual simulation on an open island, any avatar can 'drop in' and watch. Even on a closed island, avatars that have permission to be on that island can observe or 'hear' or see what is happening. There are ways to mitigate this by placing up signs/barriers that tell other avatars there is a simulation in progress and it would be preferable not to have others observing.

SOLUTIONS AND RECOMMENDATIONS

Despite the challenges in using SL there are ways to minimize them and take full advantage of the benefits of SL for virtual simulations. One recommendation is getting the IT department involved in the beginning. You can add an IT member on your development team and encourage them to learn the program so they can be supportive. It is important that they understand this is a learning tool, not a game–such is the case with other forms of technology (i.e. clickers, video conferencing). Early research on the benefits of virtual simulation to learner development can be helpful in convincing others this is educational and not just 'fun'. Getting small grants from internal sources that support new types of learning or new uses for technology can also be helpful to educators/faculty in getting started. This money can be used to purchase items in SL or hiring a 'builder' or 'designer' to help with setting up the environment and even scripting objects.

In addition, thought must be given to the process of orienting students or learners to SL. We developed podcasts and an on-line orientation manual to use to assist learners in getting started. Learners would get instructions at the beginning of class or a few weeks ahead of training on downloading the program and setting up their avatars. This allows the learners time to practice navigation skills and getting to their destination for training so when they are scheduled for their virtual simulations time is not wasted on getting avatars ready to participate.

Finally the issue of privacy during virtual simulations and debriefing need to be addressed. Using SL exposes student to the potential of other avatars overhearing the conversations that occur. This can be mitigated by putting up a notification that simulations are in progress and please do not disturb. Local chat can be used and voice chat should be limited to the area needed by the participants.

FUTURE RESEARCH DIRECTIONS

Simulation is becoming integral to many areas of health professional education including IPE both in the classroom setting and in the work environment. The research is beginning to show the tremendous benefits of human patient simulation in helping learners develop both clinical/technical skills, cognitive skills (clinical reasoning) and interpersonal skills. Research in the area of virtual simulation is still very new. It is important as educators use technology like this to evaluate its effectiveness as a learning pedagogy in addition to evaluating technical aspects. Institutions will be more likely to fund and support virtual reality programs like SL if the benefits can be shown from a solid research and cost/benefit perspective. Future research is needed to identify the impact of virtual simulations on actual performance in the clinical setting. Our work has shown improvement in interpersonal skills using virtual simulation, but we are currently considering a methodology for following these students into the clinical setting to assess performance.

CONCLUSION

Simulations have been demonstrated to be a safe way to train health care practitioners and are used in a variety of settings. Virtual simulations, in particular, can provide an effective teaching methodology for use in health care practitioner education. The technology required can be easily obtained but requires planning and IT support to ensure it runs smoothly and learners are not frustrated by the technology challenges. The scenario development process outlined here can be used to develop simulations for a variety of settings including health care and IPE and can help faculty and educators design and conduct effective simulations.

REFERENCES

Aebersold, M. (2008). *Capacity to rescue: Nurse behaviors that rescue patients*. Retrieved from http://hdl.handle.net/2027.42/60718

Aebersold, M. (2010). Using simulation to improve the use of evidence-based practice guidelines. *Western Journal of Nursing Research*. doi:10.1177/0193945910379791 PMID:20876552

Aldridge, C. (2009). *The complete guide to simulations and serious games: How the most valuable content will be created in the age beyond Gutenberg to Google*. San Francisco, CA: Pfeiffer.

American Association of Colleges of Nursing. (2009). *The essentials of baccalaureate education for professional nursing practice faculty toolkit*. Author.

Bearnson, C. S., & Wiker, K. M. (2005). Human patient simulators: A new face in baccalaureate nursing education at Brigham Young University. *The Journal of Nursing Education, 44*, 421–425. PMID:16220650

Benner, P., Sutphen, M., Leonard, V., & Day, L. (2009). *Educating nurses: A call for radical transformation*. Carnegie Foundation.

Boyle, D. K., & Kochinda, C. (2004). Enhancing collaborative communication of nurse and physician leadership: Two intensive care units. *JONA, 34*(2), 60–70. doi:10.1097/00005110-200402000-00003 PMID:14770064

Buckley, T., & Gordon, C. (2011). The effectiveness of high fidelity simulation on medical–surgical registered nurses' ability to recognise and respond to clinical emergencies. *Nurse Education Today, 31*(7), 716–721. doi:10.1016/j.nedt.2010.04.004 PMID:20573428

Burgess, M. L., Slate, J. R., Rojas-LeBouef, A., & LaPraire, K. (2010). Teaching and learning in second life: Using the community of inquiry (CoI) model to support online instruction with graduate students in instructional technology. *The Internet and Higher Education, 13*(1-2), 84–88. doi:10.1016/j.iheduc.2009.12.003

Conradi, E., Kavia, S., Burden, D., Rice, A., Woodham, L., Beaumont, C., & Poulton, T. et al. (2009). Virtual patients in a virtual world: Training paramedic students for practice. *Medical Teacher, 31*(8), 713–720. doi:10.1080/01421590903134160 PMID:19811207

Council for Graduate Medical Education. (n.d.). Retrieved from http://www.acgme.org/acgmeweb/Portals/0/PFAssets/ProgramRequirements/CPRs2013.pdf

Cronenwett, L., Sherwood, G., Barnsteiner, J., Disch, J., Johnson, J., Mitchell, P., & Warren, J. et al. (2007). Quality and safety education for nurses. *Nursing Outlook, 55*(3), 122–131. doi:10.1016/j.outlook.2007.02.006 PMID:17524799

Cumin, D., Boyd, M. J., Webster, C. S., & Weller, J. M. (2013). A systematic review of simulation for multidisciplinary team training in operating rooms. *Simulation in Healthcare: Journal of the Society for Simulation in Healthcare*. doi: 10.1097/SIH.0b013e31827e2f4c

Day, T., Iles, N., & Griffiths, P. (2009). Effect of performance feedback on tracheal suctioning knowledge and skills: Randomized controlled trial. *Journal of Advanced Nursing, 65*(7), 14–23. doi:10.1111/j.1365-2648.2009.04997.x PMID:19457007

Dillon, P., & Noble, K. (2009). Simulation as a means to foster collaborative interdisciplinary education. *Nursing Education Perspectives, 30*(2), 87–90. PMID:19476071

Dreifuerst, K. T. (2009). The essentials of debriefing in simulation learning: A concept analysis. *Nursing Education Perspectives, 30*(2), 109–114. PMID:19476076

Ericsson, K. A. (2004). Deliberate practice and the acquisition and maintenance of expert performance in medicine and related domains. *Academic Medicine: Journal of the Association of American Medical Colleges, 79*(10Suppl), S70–S81. doi:10.1097/00001888-200410001-00022 PMID:15383395

Hamric, A. B., & Blackhall, L. J. (2007). Nursing-physician perspectives on the care of dying patients in intensive care units: Collaborations, moral distress, and ethical climate. *Critical Care Medicine, 35*(2), 422–429. doi:10.1097/01.CCM.0000254722.50608.2D PMID:17205001

Harder, N. B. (2010). Use of simulation in teaching and learning in health sciences: A systematic review. *The Journal of Nursing Education, 49*(1), 23–28. doi:10.3928/01484834-20090828-08 PMID:19731886

Hoffman, R., O'Donnell, J., & Kim, Y. (2007). The effects of human patient simulatiors on basic knowledge in critical care nursing with undergraduate senior baccalaureate nursing students. *Simulation in Healthcare, 2,* 110–114. doi:10.1097/SIH.0b013e318033abb5 PMID:19088615

Interprofessional Educational Collaborative Expert Panel. (2011). *Core competencies for interprofessional collaborative practice: Report of an expert panel*. Washington, DC: Interprofessional Education Collaborative.

IOM Health Professions Education. (n.d.). *A bridge to quality (free executive summary)*. Retrieved from http://www.nap.edu/catalog/10681.html

Joint Commission. (n.d.). Retrieved from http://www.jointcommission.org/sentinel_event.aspx

Kohn, L. T., Corrigan, J., & Donaldson, M. S. (Eds.). (2000). *To err is human: Building a safer health system*. Washington, DC: National Academy Press.

Krainkish, M., & Anthony, M. K. (2001). Benefits and outcomes of staff nurses' participant in decision making. *JONA, 31*(1), 16–33. doi:10.1097/00005110-200101000-00005

Kramer, M., & Schmalenberg, C. (2003). Securing good nurse/physician relationships. *Nursing Management, 34*(7), 34–38. doi:10.1097/00006247-200307000-00013 PMID:12843717

Lapkin, S., Levett-Jones, T., Bellchambers, H., & Fernandez, R. (2010). Effectiveness of patient simulation mannequins in teaching clinical reasoning skills to undergraduate nursing students: A systematic review. *Clinical Simulation in Nursing, 6*(6), e207–e222. doi:10.1016/j.ecns.2010.05.005

Leonard, M., Graham, S., & Bonacum, D. (2004). The human factor: The critical importance of teamwork and communication in providing safe patient care. *Quality & Safety in Health Care, 13*(suppl 1), i85–i90. doi:10.1136/qshc.2004.010033 PMID:15465961

Levitt-Jones, T., Hoffman, K., Dempsey, Y., Jeong, S., Noble, D., & Norton, C. et al.. (2010). The "five rights" of clinical reasoning: An educational model to enhance nursing students' ability to identify and manage clinically "at risk" patients. *Nurse Education Today, 30*(6), 515–520. doi:10.1016/j.nedt.2009.10.020

Liaw, S., Zhou, W., Lau, T., Siau, C., & Chan, S. (2014). An interprofessional communication training using simulation to enhance safe care for a deteriorating patient. *Nurse Education Today, 34*(2), 259–264. doi:10.1016/j.nedt.2013.02.019 PMID:23518067

Mazzocco, , Petitti, D. B., Fong, K. T., Bonacum, D., Brookey, J., Graham, S., & Thomas, E. J. et al. (2009). Surgical team behaviors and patient outcomes. *American Journal of Surgery*, *197*(5), 878–685. doi:10.1016/j.amjsurg.2008.03.002 PMID:18789425

McGaghie, W. C., Issenberg, S. B., Petrusa, E. R., & Scalese, R. J. (2010). A critical review of simulation-based medical education research: 2003-2009. *Medical Education*, *44*(1), 50–63. doi:10.1111/j.1365-2923.2009.03547.x PMID:20078756

Medical Teamwork and Patient Safety: The Evidence-Based Relationship. (2003). Agency for Healthcare Research and Quality.

Morgan, P. J., & Cleave-Hogg, D. (2002). Comparison between medical students' experience, confidence and competence. *Medical Education*, *36*(6), 534–539. doi:10.1046/j.1365-2923.2002.01228.x PMID:12047667

Morgan, P. J., Cleave-Hogg, D., McIlroy, J., & Devitt, J. H. (2002). Simulation technology: A comparison of experiential and visual learning for undergraduate medical students. *Anesthesiology*, *96*(1), 10–16. doi:10.1097/00000542-200201000-00008 PMID:11752995

Nehring, W. M., & Lashley, W. R. (2004). Current uses and opinions regarding human patient simulators in nursing education: An international survey. *Nursing Education Perspectives*, *25*(5), 244–248. PMID:15508564

Orledge, J., Phillips, W. J., Murray, W. B., & Lerant, A. (2012). The use of simulation in healthcare: From systems issues, to team building, to task training, to education and high stakes examinations. *Current Opinion in Critical Care*, *18*(4), 326–332. doi:10.1097/MCC.0b013e328353fb49 PMID:22614323

Owen, H., Mugford, B., Follows, V., & Plummer, J. L. (2006). Comparison of three simulation-based training methods for management of medical emergencies. *Resuscitation*, *71*(2), 204–211. doi:10.1016/j.resuscitation.2006.04.007 PMID:16987587

Rudolf, J. W., Simon, R., Dufresne, M. S., & Raemer, D. B. (2006). There is no such thing as non-judgmental debriefing: A theory and method for debriefing with good judgment. *Simulation in Healthcare*, *1*(1), 49–55. doi:10.1097/01266021-200600110-00006 PMID:19088574

Scherer, Y. K., Bruce, S. A., & Runkawatt, V. (2007). A comparison of clinical simulation and case study presentation on nurse practitioner students' knowledge and confidence in managing cardiac event. *International Journal of Nursing Education Scholarship*, *4*(1), 22. doi:10.2202/1548-923X.1502 PMID:18052920

Schon, D. A. (1983). *The reflective practitioner: How professionals think in action*. San Francisco, CA: Jossey Bass.

Sculi, G. L. (2010). *Nursing crew resource management*. VA National Center for Patient Safety.

Shearer, J. E. (2013). High-fidelity simulation and safety: An integrative review. *The Journal of Nursing Education, 52*(1), 39-45. doi:10.3928/01484834-20121121-01

Solet, D. J., Norvell, J. M., Rutan, G. H., & Frankel, R. M. (2005). Lost in translation: Challenges and opportunities in physician-to-physician communication during patient handoffs. *Academic Medicine*, *80*(12), 1094–1099. doi:10.1097/00001888-200512000-00005 PMID:16306279

Tanner, D. A., Padrick, K. P., Westfall, U. E., & Putzier, D. J. (1987). Diagnostic reasoning strategies of nurses and nursing students. *Nursing Research*, *36*(6), 358–365. doi:10.1097/00006199-198711000-00010 PMID:3671123

Tschannen, D., & Aebersold, M. (2010). *Second Life: Innovative simulation development-making it REAL!* Meaningful Play.

Tschannen, D., Aebersold, M., Sauter, C., & Funnell, M. M. (2013). Improving nurses' perceptions of competency in diabetes self-management education through the use of simulation and problem-based learning. *Journal of Continuing Education in Nursing, 44*(6), 257–263. doi:10.3928/00220124-20130402-16 PMID:23565600

Van Sickle, K. R., McClusky, D. A., Gallagher, A. G., & Smith, C. D. (2005). Construct validation of the ProMIS simulator using a novel laparoscopic suturing task. *Surgical Endoscopy and Other Interventional Techniques, 19*(9), 1227–1231. doi:10.1007/s00464-004-8274-6 PMID:16025195

Wayne, D. B., Didwania, A., Feinglass, J., Fudala, M. J., Barsuk, J. H., & McGaghie, W. C. (2008). Simulation-based education improves quality of care during cardiac arrest team responses at an academic teaching hospital: A case-control study. *Chest, 133*(1), 56–61. doi:10.1378/chest.07-0131 PMID:17573509

Wharburton, S. (2009). Second Life in higher education: Assessing the potential for and the barriers to deploying virtual worlds in learning and teaching. *British Journal of Educational Technology, 40*(3), 414–426. doi:10.1111/j.1467-8535.2009.00952.x

Wickers, M. P. (2010). Establishing the climate for a successful debriefing. *Clinical Simulation in Nursing, 6*(3), e83–e86. doi:10.1016/j.ecns.2009.06.003

World Health Organization (WHO). (2010). *Framework for action on interprofessional education & collaborative practice.* Geneva: World Health Organization. Retrieved August 30, 2014 from http://www.who.int/hrh/resources/framework_action/en/

Youngblood, P., Harter, P. M., Srivastava, S., Moffett, S., Heinrichs, W. L., & Dev, P. (2008). Design, development, and evaluation of an on-line virtual emergency department for training trauma teams. *Simulation in Healthcare, 3*(3), 146–153. doi:10.1097/SIH.0b013e31817bedf7 PMID:19088658

ADDITIONAL READING

Anderson, P., & Stephens, M. (2008). Wolverine Island. *EDUCAUSE Review, 43*(5). http://www.educause.edu/EDUCAUSE+Review/EDUCAUSEReviewMagazineVolume43/WolverineIsland/163175 Retrieved November 19, 2009

Boulos, M. N. K., Hetherington, L., & Wheeler, S. (2007). Second Life: An overview of the potential of 3-D virtual worlds in medical and health education. *Health Information and Libraries Journal, 24*(4), 233–245. doi:10.1111/j.1471-1842.2007.00733.x PMID:18005298

Cheal, C. (2009). Second life: Hype or learning? *On the Horizon, 15*(4), 204–210. doi:10.1108/10748120710836228

Clark, C.C. (1976) Simulation gaming: a new teaching strategy in nursing education. *Nurse Educ.*, Nov-Dec;1(4):4-9.

Fanning, R. M., & Gaba, D. M. (2007). The role of debriefing in simulation based learning. *Simulation in Healthcare, 2*(2), 115–125. doi:10.1097/SIH.0b013e3180315539 PMID:19088616

Gaba, D. M. (2004). A brief history of mannequin-based simulation and application. In W. F. Dunn (Ed.), *Simulators in critical care and beyond* (p. 130). Des Plaines, IL: Society of Critical Care Medicine.

Gaba, D. M., Howard, S. K., Fish, K. J., Smith, B. E., & Sowb, Y. A. (2001). Simulation-based training in anesthesia crisis resource management (ACRM): A decade of experience. *Simulation & Gaming*, 32(2), 175–193. doi:10.1177/104687810103200206

Garrison, D. R., Cleveland-Innes, M., & Fung, T. S. (2010). Exploring causal relationships among teaching, cognitive andsocial presence: Student perceptions of the community of inquiry framework. *The Internet and Higher Education*, 13(1-2), 31–36. doi:10.1016/j.iheduc.2009.10.002

Issenberg, S. B., McGaghie, W. C., Petrusa, E. R., Lee, G. D., & Scalese, R. (2005). Features and uses of high-fidelity medical simulations that lead to effective learning: A BEME systematic review. *Medical Teacher*, 27(1), 10–28. doi:10.1080/01421590500046924 PMID:16147767

Jeffries, P. R. (2005). A framework for designing, implementing, and evaluating simulations used as teaching strategies in nursing. *Nursing Education Perspectives*, 26(2), 96–103. PMID:15921126

Kamel-Boulos, M., Hetherington, L., & Wheeler, S. (2007). Second Life: An overview of the potential of 3-D virtual worlds in medical and health education. *Health Information and Libraries Journal*, 24(4), 233–245. doi:10.1111/j.1471-1842.2007.00733.x PMID:18005298

Kapp, K. M., & O'Driscoll, T. (2010) *Learning in 3D: Adding a New Dimension to Enterprise Learning and Collaboration*. NY: Wiley. Retrieved from: http://books.google.com/books?id=d6lSyf3HNLIC

Kirriemuir, J. (2010). UK university and college technical support for second life developers and users. *Educational Research*, 52(2), 215–227. doi:10.1080/00131881.2010.482756

Kuiper, R. A., Heinrich, C., Matthias, A., Graham, M. J., & Bell-Kotwall, L. (2008). Debriefing with the OPT Model of Clinical Reasoning during High Fidelity Patient Simulation. *International Journal of Nursing Education Scholarship*, 5(1), 1–14. doi:10.2202/1548-923X.1466 PMID:18454731

Leong, J., Kinross, J., Taylor, D., & Purkayastha, S. (2008). Surgeons have held conferences in Second Life. *BMJ (Clinical Research Ed.)*, 337(jul08 2), a683. doi:10.1136/bmj.a683 PMID:18614495

Mah, J. W., Bingham, K., Dobkin, E. D., Malchiodi, L., Russell, A., Donahue, S., & Kirton, O. C. et al. (2009). Mannequin simulation identifies common surgical intensive unit teamwork errors long after introduction of sepsis guidelines. *Society of Simulation in Healthcare*, 4(4), 193–199. doi:10.1097/SIH.0b013e3181abe9d6 PMID:21330791

Mayo, P. H., Hackney, J. E., Mueck, J. T., Ribaudo, V., & Schneider, R. (2004). Achieving house staff competence in emergency airway management: Results of a teaching program using a computerized patient simulator. *Critical Care Medicine*, 32(12), 2422–2427. doi:10.1097/01.CCM.0000147768.42813.A2 PMID:15599146

Medley, C. F., & Horne, C. (2005). Using simulation technology for undergraduate nursing education. *Educational Innovations*, 44(1), 31–34. PMID:15673172

Minocha, S., & Reeves, J. (2010). Design of learning spaces in 3D virtual worlds: An empirical investigation of Second Life. *Learning, Media and Technology*, 35(2), 111–137. doi:10.1080/17439884.2010.494419

Nehring, W. M., & Lashley, F. R. (2009). Nursing Simulation: A Review of the Past 40 Years. *Simulation & Gaming*, 40(4), 528–552. doi:10.1177/1046878109332282

Oblinger, D. (2006). *Learning Spaces*. London: EDUCASE.

Pfeil, U., Ang, C. S., & Zaphiris, P. (2009). Issues and challenges of teaching and learning in 3D virtual worlds: Real life case studies. *Educational Media International, 46*(3), 223–238. doi:10.1080/09523980903135368

Rosen, K. R. (2008). The history of medical simulation. *Journal of Critical Care, 23*(2), 157–166. doi:10.1016/j.jcrc.2007.12.004 PMID:18538206

Stephens, M., & Chapman, C. (2009). *The Virtual First Responder: Exploring Virtual Reality in the Context of Medical Education.* Poster Presentation. Presented at Campus Technology. *USC Institute for Creative Technologies* (homepage). Retrieved from: http://ict.usc.edu/

University of Michigan Health Sciences Libraries. (2008). *HSL Videos - Second Life and Public* Health - Video | Health Sciences Libraries | MLibrary.

Wayne, D. B., Didwania, A., Feinglass, J., Fudala, M. J., Barsuk, J. H., & McGaghie, W. C. (2008). Simulation-based education improves quality of care during cardiac arrest team responses at an academic teaching hospital: A case-control study. *Chest, 133*(1), 56–61. doi:10.1378/chest.07-0131 PMID:17573509

KEY TERMS AND DEFINITIONS

Clinical Reasoning: The ability for the learner to use previous knowledge and skills and apply those to a new situation.

Effective Communication: Communication between two or more individuals that results in a good outcome.

Exemplar: An example that highlights the specific action you want the learner to replicate.

Learning Framework: A guide to use when developing learning activities.

Patient Safety: Patients do not suffer any harm during their care.

Simulation: A technique used to re-create a realistic environment for learners to practice skills.

Virtual Simulations: Simulations conducted in an on-line, 3D computer environment.

This work was previously published in the Handbook of Research on Digital Media and Creative Technologies edited by Dew Harrison, pages 265-286 copyright year 2015 by Information Science Reference (an imprint of IGI Global).

APPENDIX

Scenario Storyboard: Nurse-Physician Communication using Crew Resource Management Strategies

- **Key Concepts:**
  - Interpersonal relations.
  - Communication.
  - Teamwork.
- **Prerequisites:** Completion of Crew Resource Management Training.
- **Timeframe:** 15 minute (scenario); 15 minute (de-briefing).
- **Setting (In Second Life):**
  - Participants begin in unit conference room.
  - Patient care to occur in the Patient room.
- **Participants:**
  - RN,
  - Physician,
  - Charge Nurse.

Scenario Design and Timeline

Assign participants to roles within the scenario. Additional participants can be assigned an observer role. Once assignments in roles are complete, pass out the SL notecards, which provide guidance to the roles.

- **Staff Nurse Notecard:** You will be the primary nurse on a general medicine unit, working the night shift. You have been assigned four patients, one of which is Mr. Howard. Further instructions will be given by the facilitator at the beginning of the simulation. Please note that you may speak with the charge nurse or physician at anytime during the scenario.
- **Charge Nurse Notecard:** You will be available as a resource for the staff nurse. If the nurse calls for your assistance, you should recommend calling the physician (based on the patient's current assessment findings).
- **Physician Notecard:** During the course of the scenario, the nurse will contact you with a specific request related to Mr. Howard. If the nurse clearly articulates her concern and wants (e.g. uses the 3Ws…What I see, What I am concerned about, What I want), consider ordering some of her requests (but not all). If the nurse does not clearly articulate her concern and wants, be vague in your response and only order fluids if you see fit. Regardless of the nurse's effectiveness at communicating needs, refuse to come to the unit to assess the patient or transfer the patient to the ICU.

Once roles are assigned and notecards distributed, the facilitator should introduce the simulation and give context to the simulation, including the environment and role-specific instructions (as needed).

- **Facilitator Introduction:** "Hello and welcome. As you know, communication among the health care team is critical for high quality of care. For this reason, we are going to have an opportunity to 'practice' our communication skills. Sometime during the scenario you may find it necessary to communicate to other members of the healthcare team. If the situation arises, consider using the communication strategies you learned in the Crew Resource Management training you recently completed. The scenario begins with shift report on a general medicine unit. Nancy (who is the participant playing the role of the staff nurse), you have just received report on your four patients. One of the patients you will be caring for is Mr. Howard. Mr. Howard is a 55 year old who suffered a stroke 10 days ago, his baseline is oriented to person only, left sided weakness, chronic a-fib (a heart dysrythmia), and hypertension. He has a tracheostomy (a breathing tube in his neck) and has been requiring every four hour suctioning for moderate amounts of secretions. In addition he has had a temperature around 100.2F and oxygen saturation (i.e. level of oxygen in the blood, want above 90%) has been running around 95% on 30% trach mask. It is now 2AM and you are heading into Mr. Howard's room to assess him. Please use your charge nurse and physician as a resource (as needed). Tom and Tracey (who are playing the role of charge nurse and physician, respectively), you can wait in the conference room and be available if Nancy asks for your assistance. Nancy, you may begin."
- **Phase I (Nurse Assessment):** The staff nurse (Nancy) will 'assess' the patient, using the notecard function in SL. Specifically, the notecard will provide current vital signs and assessment findings. Upon review of the assessment data, the Nancy would find Mr. Howard's condition to have deteriorated since the initial report. Specifically, Mr. Howard would have difficulty breathing, increased blood pressure and heart rate, lots of secretions needing to be suctioned, high temperature, and mental status changes. Upon assessment, Nancy would see the need for closer observation and would more than likely identify the need to call the physician. She may also speak with the charge nurse, who has been instructed to mention the need to call the physician.
- **Phase 2 (Nurse-Physician Interaction):** Nancy would contact the physician (Tracey) to describe Mr. Howard's current status. The primary expectation of the staff nurse includes use of the 3 Ws:
  - What I see,
  - What I am concerned about, and
  - What I want (VA National Center for Patient Safety).

The nurse should state her needs clearly without 'hinting' about what she wants (i.e. "Mr. Howard needs to be transferred to the ICU" versus "Mr. Howard is going to require a lot of care"). When the physician does not comply to her wishes (if she sees the need to transfer the patient), she should re-state her needs, using either the 3 W's again or use a more assertive communication strategy:

- State the name or position (to get the individuals attention),
- State concern ('I am uncomfortable with…'),
- Offer an alternative, and
- Pose a question to get a resolution ('Do you agree?') (Sculi, 2010).

This phase may require a couple interactions with the physician, as the initial response from the physician will not be transferring to the ICU. The simulation will continue until the staff nurse uses one of the methods above in an effective manner (e.g. no 'hinting or hoping') to obtain the transfer order as needed or time is up. (maximum timeframe of 15 minutes).

De-Brief Questions

1. What went well during the scenario?
2. How would you describe the interaction between Nancy, the staff nurse, and Tracey, the physician?
3. What might the nurse have done differently?
4. Was the 3W's approach used effectively and if not, how so?
5. How do you believe use of the communication strategies can impact patient care?

Chapter 47
Using a Smartphone as a Track and Fall Detector:
An Intelligent Support System for People with Dementia

Chia-Yin Ko
TungHai University, Taiwan

Fang-Yie Leu
TungHai University, Taiwan

I-Tsen Lin
TungHai University, Taiwan

ABSTRACT

This chapter proposes a smartphone-based system for both indoor and outdoor monitoring of people with dementia. The whole system comprises wandering detection, safety-zone monitoring, fall detection, communication services, alert notifications, and emergency medical services. To effectively track the elderly, the proposed system uses a smartphone camera to take real-time pictures along the user's path as he or she moves about. Those photos, accompanied with time and GPS signals, are delivered to and stored on the Cloud system. When necessary, family caregivers can download those data to quickly find a way to help the elderly individual. Additionally, this study uses tri-axial accelerometers to examine falls. To assure individuals' data is safeguarded appropriately, an RSA method has been adopted by the system to encrypt stored data. This reliable and minimally intrusive system provides people with dementia with an opportunity to maintain their social networks and to improve their quality of lives.

1. INTRODUCTION

Today, people live longer than they did in the past century. Consequently, most countries, from Europe and the United States to Asia, are facing aging problems among their populations. Research indicates that in 2005 about 10% of the world's population was over 60 years old; this proportion will be more than doubled by 2050 (Pollack, 2005). Although recent advances in medical technology

DOI: 10.4018/978-1-4666-8756-1.ch047

greatly extend life expectancy for people, several aging problems such as dementia have been a serious threat to the quality of life for older adults. Research also finds that the prevalence of dementia increases with age (Landau et al., 2010; Hebert et al., 2013). In other words, the older adults have a greater potential for suffering from this disease. In 2010, the United States had 4.7 million individuals aged 65 years or older with Alzheimer's disease (AD) dementia (Hebert et al.). That number is growing rapidly; it is estimated that in 2050 there will be 13.8 million people in the United States with AD dementia.

People with dementia (PwD) usually exhibit a gradual loss of their sense of time and place (Naumann et al., 2011; Wherton & Monk, 2008). They are prone to getting lost when they go out alone. Such a risk not only becomes a source of burden for caregivers, but is also a source of frustration and low self-esteem for the elderly individuals. However, most PwD expect to live independently. They are unwilling to be a burden to others (Naumann et al.). Given those expectations by the elderly, it is vital that our societies learn how to use emerging technologies to support this group of people in their desire to live at home, to be able to maintain their social networks, and to keep their quality of life.

At present, a number of technological devices have been developed to support PwD living at home, for instance, using global positioning systems (GPS) to locate a missing person (Sposaro, Danielson, & Tyson, 2010), using accelerometers and gyroscopes to detect falls (Yavuz et al., 2010), and developing dedicated algorithms to improve the performance of technological devices (Yavuz, Kocak, Ergun, & Alemdar, 2010). However, a critical characteristic of dementia is that recent memories and skills are damaged or lost (Naumann et al., 2011). PwD have difficulty learning how to use new devices or operating complicated tools. Hence, newer technology products developed for this group of people are better than the existing, familiar ones that are already in their daily lives.

It is evident that smartphones are prevalent and popular among various age groups. Their components—such as GPS, accelerometers, gyroscopes, cameras, microphones, and other audio units—can be used to collect data and to support specific events (Moore, Barolli, Xhafa, & Thomas, 2013). Therefore, in this study, we use a smartphone to track and locate a missing elderly individual with dementia. Furthermore, the proposed system is able to detect falls and can automatically provide appropriate alerts and required medical aid for PwD.

In short, the purpose of this study is to design a system, named the Smartphone-based Track and Fall System (STFaS), which tracks a missing elderly individual by taking pictures of his or her walking route and delivering those pictures and relevant information to the Cloud. The system also allows the limits of the individual's safety zones to be set and checks whether the monitored elderly individual is within the established safety zones. Furthermore, the STFaS monitors a fall occurrence for the elderly individual. When necessary, it is capable of issuing an alert to caregivers as well as calling for emergency medical assistance so as to assist the elderly individual in a timely manner.

Additionally, to ensure that all pictures and relevant information are securely protected, in this study, we employ the RSA method as the encryption/decryption algorithm. We believe that all personal data is stored in a very safe and secure manner.

2. BACKGROUND AND RELATED STUDIES

In recent years, dementia has been recognized as a serious threat to most older adults. It is estimated that about 5% of people over 65 and more than 40% of people over 90 have dementia (Moore, Barolli, Xhafa, & Thomas, 2013). How to use technology to assist those groups of people has been a critical challenge for research. This section reviews the approaches used for wandering and fall detection from a series of emerging studies. Encryption concerns for the collected data are also presented at the end of this section.

2.1 Wandering Detection

Researchers note that wandering occurs among most PwD since they feel a compelling urge to walk (Sposaro, Danielson, & Tyson, 2010). When going out, PwD have difficulty finding their way home because of their memory loss. Although GPS is useful for locating the missing person, providing further urgent communication and medical support requires additional strategies. For instance, Sposaro, Danielson, and Tyson (2010) used an Android platform to establish a monitoring device called *iWander*. Along with GPS, the device adopted Bayesian theory to calculate the wandering probability of the monitored person. Based on calculation results, the *iWander* could automatically issue a fall alert and navigate the dementia patient to a safe location. Simultaneously, the device notified caregivers of the current location of the patient and called the local 911 service for further medical aid. In addition, to improve the accuracy of wandering detection, some influential parameters, such as time of day, current weather condition, and length of time outside, were added into the equation. However, there is no evidence to confirm that performance of the system improved as those selected parameters were added. The device is still in its modification stage as a result of researchers having identified that more effort needs to be put into collecting further data to establish a reliable baseline model.

2.2 Fall Detection

Falls are a primary cause of injuries and the leading cause of hospitalizations as well as a major obstacle to independent living for elderly people (Abbate et al., 2012; Sposaro, Danielson, & Tyson, 2009; Yavuz et al., 2010). Quick and effective detection of falls as well as immediate and/or timely medical support can greatly reduce health risks and therefore achieve better quality-of-life outcomes for patients. Therefore, the smartphone-based fall detector normally contains an alert system and medical-support communication capability.

Among all the components of a smartphone, the tri-axial accelerometer is the most frequently adopted unit in building a fall detector. The accelerometer is used for measuring the magnitude of an external force. If an acceleration value significantly exceeds the normal range, then the fall incidence is susceptible to discovery (Sposaro, Danielson, Tyson, 2009; Yavuz et al., 2010). Furthermore, the directional information in tri-axial accelerometer also helps to distinguish the degrees of severity and types of falls.

Current fall detection approaches attempt to incorporate various techniques to enhance their detection accuracy and performances. Yavuz, Kocak, Ergun, and Alemdar (2010), for instance, tried to integrate wavelet transform techniques and thresholding to improve the accuracy of their fall detection system. The results showed that using wavelet transforms achieved better positive performance. The developed device produced an approximately 37% increase in true positives and decreased the false negatives significantly (Yavuz, Kocak, Ergun, & Alemdar). A work by Sposaro and Tyson (2009) utilized an Android-based smartphone to create a fall detection mechanism. The researchers argued that the user's height, weight, and level of activity highly influenced the threshold value; consequently, using adaptive thresholding was more appropriate. Their findings showed that false positives were reduced as expected. However, without reporting any precise data for true positives or false negatives, the method requires more studies for validity.

One line of inquiry addresses the relationship between movements and falls. For example, Bai, Wu, and Tsai (2012) stated that humans' actions could be divided into six types: going upstairs, going downstairs, standing up, sitting down, running, and jumping. Based on the above distinctive activities, falls may present in various postures, such as free fall, body hitting the floor, and overturning of the body. Consequently, the researchers suggested that by using three patterns of acceleration values to recognize normal and abnormal values of threshold, falls probably can be detected accurately.

Abbate et al. (2012) developed a smartphone-based fall detection system that included a request-help service to assist elderly people. They pointed out that the elderly may engage in several fall-like movements, such as sitting on a sofa, lying on a bed, walking or running, and unintentionally hitting the sensor of the monitoring device. Those fall-like behaviors possibly generate an effect in acceleration magnitude which is similar to a real fall. To effectively distinguish fall-like events from real-fall incidents, Abbate et al. employed a "machine learning theory" and incorporated a classification engine to enhance fall-recognition effects. The findings showed that, through the training procedure, the device demonstrated better recognition ability in detecting real-fall occurrences. Also, the experimental results revealed that, when an acceleration value was higher than the 3g threshold, the data set in that study would generate a false alarm, which was distinctive from the results other studies reported. Moreover, the research found that an angle of 60^0 is the minimum variation from the standing position to a real fall. And, finally, it showed that the orientation of the user's waist can be used to determine real-fall occurrences.

Indeed, recent advances in technology, such as artificial intelligence, provide researchers with an alternative solution for fall detection. However, as Abbate et al. (2012) discussed, the fall is an ill-defined event; an effective strategy should not only focus on developing new detection techniques but also highlight the user's perceptions about the tool.

2.3 Security

Current encryption techniques can be classified into symmetric and asymmetric encryption approaches. 'Symmetric-key algorithm' refers to sender and receiver using the same cryptographic key for both encryption and decryption procedures. 'Asymmetric cryptography' uses a pair of keys to encrypt and decrypt messages; one is called a 'public key' and the other, a 'private key.'

Diffie and Hellman proposed asymmetric encryption in 1977. They noted that an asymmetric algorithm is a 'trap door or one-way' function. That means the function is easy to perform in one direction but difficult to reverse. The Diffie-Hellman method is a key-exchange protocol and not utilized for encryption (Huang, Leu, & Wei, 2013; Huang, Leu, You, & Chu, 2014). The concept can be explained by using an example: For instance, Bob and Alice deliver their own public keys to each other. Both public keys are individually derived from their own private keys. Also, Bob and Alice do not allow the transmission of their private keys through wireless channels. Each party can individually obtain the common secret key by using his or her own private key and the other party's public key. As we can see, using the Diffie-Hellman protocol, the decryption is difficult since solving a Diffie-Hellman problem is a very complicated process. Such a case is also known as a 'discrete logarithm problem' (ElGamal, 1985; Huang et al., 2014).

Essentially, a cryptographic technique requires confidentiality, availability, reliability, and integrity characteristics (Romney & Steinbart, 2008).

1. **Confidentiality:** means that encrypted data will not be exposed to unauthorized individuals, entities, or processes.
2. **Availability:** refers to any authorized entities allowed to access the data when necessary.

3. **Integrity:** guarantees data accuracy and security. In fact, integrity can be further divided into three sub-characteristics.
   a. The first is accountability, which assures that the behavior of an entity can be traced back to the entity itself.
   b. The second is authenticity, which guarantees that the identity of an entity or a resource belongs to the one who really issues the identity.
   c. The last characteristic is non-repudiation, which ensures that when a behavior or an event occurs, the behavior or event cannot be repudiated afterward.
4. Digital signature is also a type of security service. It is an electronic signature that can be applied to authenticate the identity of the sender and to ensure that the message or document, once sent, is the original one, not an altered one.

3. RESEARCH STATEMENTS

The purpose of this study is to create a monitoring system which supports elderly with dementia who wish to live independently in their own homes. With the recent increase in computer technology, applying emerging techniques to assist PwD to keep their quality of life becomes a critical issue in the world. This study utilizes the smartphone to design a wandering and falls-detection monitor specifically for the elderly. It is able to periodically and automatically record the monitored individual's walking paths and can detect falls. The system is also capable of issuing adaptive alert messages to notify family caregivers and, further, to call emergency responders by itself when necessary.

The detail functions of current research are as follows:

1. The system will track the PwD by using a smartphone to take photos and send photo time and GPS signals to the Cloud system, from which the family caregivers can download those data and incorporate them into a Google map to develop a search path in a timely manner.
2. The system will set an appropriate safety zone and determine whether the elderly person is within the safety zone. Once the elderly individual walks beyond that zone, the system will issue family members' voice messages to the monitored individual to urge that elderly individual to go home. At the same time, the zone monitor will call an emergency contact list in sequence until one contact answers and is thereby notified of this event. If nobody responds to the phone call, the system then immediately calls emergency medical services to initiate aid as needed for that elderly individual.
3. The system will monitor falls for elderly indoors or outdoors. When a fall incident has been confirmed, the system sends notification messages accompanied by GPS coordinates to all emergency contact persons to inform them of a fall event. If nobody can be reached in this matter, the system will automatically call an ambulance depot for rapid support for that elderly individual.

To begin, the framework of the proposed system is introduced in Section 4. The effects of a smartphone, a wireless system, and Cloud storage are presented to give an overview of the current study. The detail settings and insights about wandering detection, safety-zone monitoring, and falls detection are described in Section 5 for a more comprehensive understanding of the operation of the whole device. Then, Section 6 contains a discussion of a series of experiments performed to simulate several daily movements and to clarify some unclear fall-like events. Also, a discussion of experiments involving real-fall occurrences is provided at the end of Section 6 for further understanding of the threshold concept of this research. Lastly, the conclusions and proposed future studies are presented in Sections 7 and 8, respectively.

4. THE PROPOSED APPROACH

The operation framework of the STFaS system can be divided into three parts: smartphone, wireless system, and Cloud system. The overview of this system is presented in Figure 1. The first part, smartphone, is placed and fixed on the user's front chest, front pocket, or front waist so as to use the embedded camera to take pictures along the street. Those pictures can be utilized to find the most likely location of the smartphone user at any given time. The second part, the wireless system, allows use of the detection system without the user being limited to a specific position for detection purposes. Our wireless system, in other words, is able to recognize any suspect occurrence indoors or outdoors. The last part is the Cloud system, which is the storage of all collected data. The STFaS system provides each user with a 2-GB capacity of Cloud storage.

4.1 Missing Detection

The first function of the STFaS is to automatically take pictures along the monitored individual's route. The pictures of shops or landscapes along the streets, accompanied by GPS coordinates and time, will be delivered to the Cloud system. The three items–pictures, GPS coordinates, and time–are called the *tracing triple*, which are used to rapidly depict a search path when there is a need. More detail settings and descriptions of detection processes will be presented later.

The STFaS system sets five minutes as the default time period for sending a new tracing triple to the Cloud system. The default time can be adjusted to meet individual needs. But a higher frequency for photographing, for instance, photographing at one-minute intervals, may quickly exhaust battery capacity. It is important to note that in such settings, the battery capacity of a mobile phone may be exhausted in five or six hours, depending upon the energy consumption speed of the smartphone.

As mentioned earlier, the system provides each user with a 2-GB capacity of Cloud storage. It is estimated that the total storage space can accommodate approximately 820 photos (i.e., 2.5MB for a picture, 2048 MB for total Cloud capacity, 2048MB / 2.5MB ≒ 820). And the total photographic time is about 68 hours in the system (i.e., 12 pictures for an hour, 816/12 ≒ 68). These carrying capacities should be sufficient to meet detection purposes indoors or outdoors. To reduce Cloud space and wireless delivery time, every tracing triple is compressed before being sent out. Table 1 shows the format of a tracing triple before compression.

The strategy of using photos to strengthen detection performance effectively improves upon the weakness of other systems whose tracking

Table 1. Format of an unencrypted tracing triple

op code	picture	GPS Longitude and Latitude	time

Figure 1. The framework of the STFaS system

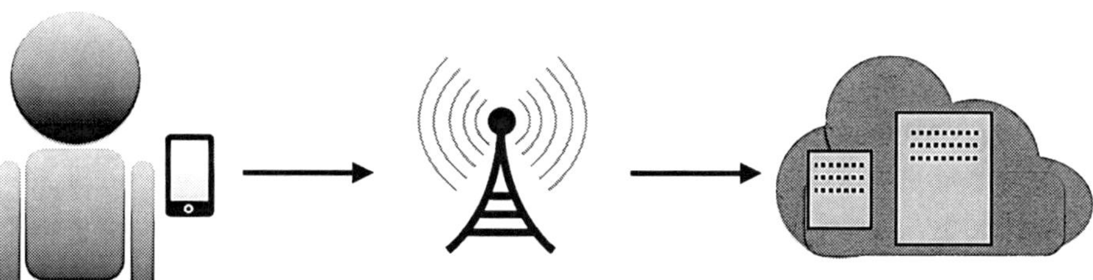

Figure 2. Consecutive photos show a possible path

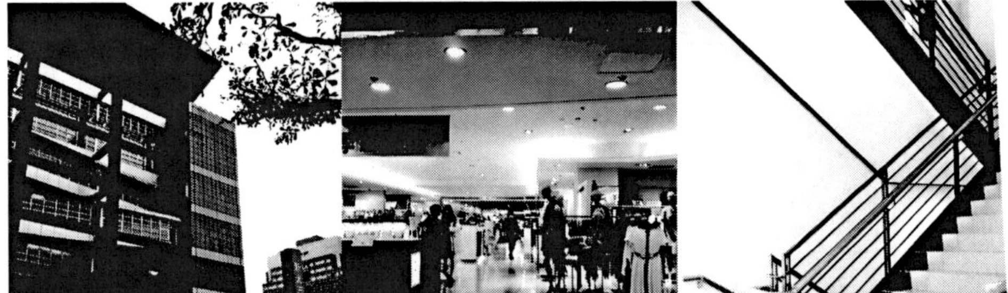

procedures rely heavily on GPS coordinates. When necessary, those large amounts of tracing triples data can be downloaded and linked with Google Maps to display the walking path of the monitored user. Specifically, when family caregivers click those points, the corresponding landscape pictures will be exhibited to illustrate the traversed path of that specific user. If the elderly individual goes indoors, the GPS signals might become weak or lost and potentially produce a null GPS value in the tracing triples. The system still continues to periodically gather pictures and time data. Using only those pictures and the time data in tracing triples, however, still makes it relatively likely that the position of the missing elderly individual can be determined. Figure 2 presents a possible scenario.

As shown, we found an elderly individual who had walked toward a department store (as pic-1), entered the department store (as pic-2), and then approached or went up the stairs (as pic-3). Through these consecutive and real-time pictures, the family members can easily and quickly go to the right place to find the elderly individual.

It is important to note that since each user is provided with 2G cloud capacity, and therefore, the individual's walking history is unable to be stored permanently. As such, a selection menu is offered for family caregivers to input the date or time that they want to inquiry; so that the relevant tracing triples can become a picture-walking route to show on the smartphone's screen.

Moreover, each tracing triples is used lossy compression method to compress data, which is likely to minimize the amount of data capacities but without impacting vision effects.

4.2 Safety Zone Monitor

As we know, regular walking has been recognized as an effective method to reduce the risk of chronic illness. However, for some elderly people, due to the gradual degradation of their cognitive function, a regular walk might become a missing-person occurrence. This study therefore establishes a customized safety area as the second feature to assist this group of people. Normally, the safety region, such as a nearby park, grocery stores, library, bank, or some shops, can be deemed as familiar locations for an elderly individual and can be set as a safety zone. Inside this area, the system will not issue any alert alarm. In the present study, the first layer of the safety zone is set to within a radius of 300 meters. That distance is considered a safe area for the elderly (see Figure 3). However, the safety region for an elderly individual can be customized to meet an individual's personal needs.

Figure 3. Different alert distances provide different levels of alert notifications

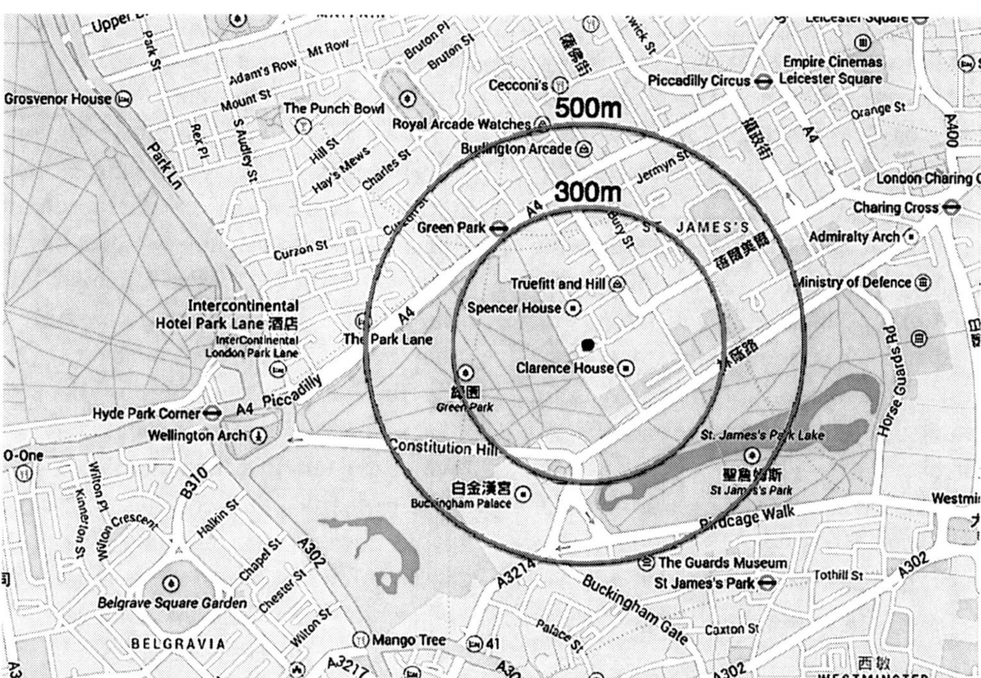

The second layer of the safety zone is set to within a radius of 500 meters. If the elderly individual stays between 300 meters and 500 meters, where he or she will be only slightly outside the safety area, the system will trigger the alert function. The alert system first broadcasts pre-recorded voice files by the elderly individual's family to request the elderly individual not to go too far and to ask that elderly individual to go home soon. The voice messages should be something like, "You are too far away from home; please come back as soon as possible." For those people in early stages of dementia, that message plausibly makes sense. For people in later stages of dementia, although they may have lost the ability to go home by themselves, those pre-recorded voice messages provide opportunities for bystanders or police to better understand what that elderly individual needs. This function can be extended to include such recordings as family members' voice files associated with familiar and pleasant music to comfort elderly patients, or pre-recorded family videos to awaken the elderly individual's memory. Those strategies are meaningful and can be considered to be added in this feature.

When reaching the first alert area (between 300 to 500 meters), the system sends family voice files to remind the elderly individual not to walk too far; it also automatically sends a short message to all emergency family caregivers to notify them of this event. Furthermore, once that the elderly individual goes more than 500 meters, that range is identified as a highly dangerous area; our system will instantly call all emergency contact persons in sequence until at least one person answers the call.

As already noted, the first and second alert distances can be adjusted to meet individual needs. For instance, if the elderly individual lives in suburbs, the distance settings can be lengthened whereas if he or she lives in a metropolitan area, the safety area can be reduced to 100 or 200 meters or even shorter.

4.3 Fall Detection

To detect fall occurrences, our system employs tri-axial accelerometers to measure acceleration values of the smartphone and to examine whether the acceleration magnitude can be identified as a fall incident. The reason for using tri-axial accelerometers is that this sensor, besides showing the magnitude of acceleration, can also display the direction of the x-, y-, and z-axes, which represent the current direction it is facing of the smartphone (see Figure 4). This direction information is useful in determining whether the user has experienced a fall occurrence.

In this study, we adopt the Signal Magnitude Vector (SMV) and Tilt Angle (TA) methods (He, Li, & Yin, 2012) to detect the fall occurrence. The SMV and TA equations are as follows:

$$SMV = \sqrt{x_i^2 + y_i^2 + z_i^2} \tag{1}$$

$$TA = \arcsin\left\{ \frac{y_i}{\sqrt{x_i^2 + y_i^2 + z_i^2}} \right\} \tag{2}$$

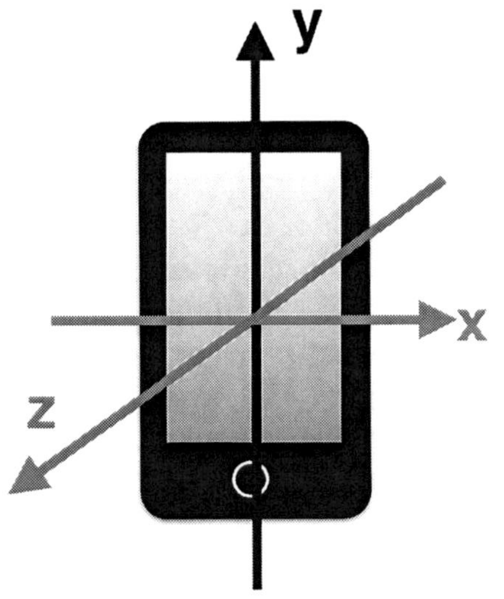

Figure 4. Three-axial directions of a smartphone

The x_i, y_i and z_i in Equation (1) represent the ith samples of the signals on the three axes (i.e., x-, y- and z- axes, respectively).

TA is the angle between $+y_i$ and the gravitational vector g. When the user carries the smartphone, theoretically we can retrieve the accelerations on the three axes from the tri-axial accelerometers. If the calculated SMV value by Equation (1) is greater than a predefined threshold, named 'fall-incident threshold,' the system would possibly recognize that there has been a fall incident.

However, the challenge of fall detection is that several fall-like movements may be confused with a real fall. It is clear that a good performance system should filter out those fall-like events to avoid false alarms. To solve this problem, our system first makes sure there is a real-fall occurrence, and then the alert notification service is started. The procedure for confirming a suspected fall is, first, the system issues a fall-confirmation message to the smartphone user, using both text and voice modes to ask that user whether he or she has fallen onto the ground. If that elderly individual feels that he or she is not experiencing a problem, the user can press the "Not Fall" button to express his or her current status. The system then understands that the elderly individual is all right and simultaneously decides there is no need to issue any alert alarm. Otherwise, the system would recognize that the elderly individual has experienced a fall occurrence. At that moment, the alert system begins to issue notification messages accompanied by GPS coordinates to all emergency contact persons in sequence until one person replies to the system. The alert notification procedure is the same as that described in the safety zone monitor service

After receiving a system alert notification, the family members or caregivers can quickly download the tracing triples from the Cloud system and input them into a Google Map so that they can provide timely support to that elderly individual. Because falls usually cause injury and become primary causes for hospitalizations, our system is able to determine when to call for ambulance service and thus shorten the rescue time. Specifically, if no one answers the phone call, that means there is no contact person who can call the ambulance depot for that elderly individual. In that event, the system evaluates the situation and automatically calls the ambulance depot by itself for rapid support for that fallen elderly individual. It is worth noting that the system calls will be accompanied by both the GPS coordinates and a current picture of the fallen individual's location so that the emergency responders can find that potentially injured elderly individual in a very short time.

In sum, when an elderly individual loses his or her way back home, that event does not instantly endanger the individual. This system therefore does not need to call emergency services at once. The main process, instead, is to begin sending family members' voice messages to comfort the wandering elderly individual and to ask that the elderly individual go home soon. At the same time, all emergency contact persons will receive a short message notifying them of the event. This treatment is used for the walking distance between 300 meters and 500 meters from the user's home base, under the assumption that the elderly individual has not fallen down while walking. If that elderly individual walks more than 500 meters from his home base, our system determines that the individual is in a region where it is easy for him or her to get lost; the alarm system will call all contact persons to ensure that at least one knows of this event. Finally, the system will assume the need for medical support in the worst-case scenario, such as when no one answers the phone call or the elderly has a detected fall incident. As noted, the relevant emergency alert and medical services provided by the STFaS not only avoid issuing a false alert, but greatly decrease unnecessary assistance.

4.4 System Security

In 1977, Rivest, Shamir, and Adleman proposed a cryptosystem method, called RSA, which is an asymmetric-key technique. The idea of RSA is to use a public key to encrypt plaintext into ciphertext. 'Public key' means that the key is known to the public. The designated receiver owns a corresponding 'private key,' and he or she is the only one who can convert the ciphertext into plaintext. In general, this technique is considered to be a secure approach because it uses different keys for each party. In a current study, we employ RSA to encrypt tracing-triple data for elderly individuals. That is, the elderly individual uses a public key, and family caregivers own the corresponding private key. With both keys working together, the tracing triples can be decrypted and shown on a Google map. Through this procedure, the individual's privacy is strongly protected.

Furthermore, to prevent the special-purpose smartphone from being picked up by other people or maliciously used by others, whenever the phone is activated, the system will activate the front camera to take a picture of the current user. This photo is then compared to the owner's pre-stored photo to confirm the identity of the user. Using face recognition for the comparison, the system will determine whether the current user is the legal user; if not, the relevant functions such as tracking and detection will not be triggered. This approach is intended to prevent innocent people from being maliciously monitored.

5. IMPLEMENTATION

This section describes the detail settings of the STFaS system.

5.1 Start Up

The STFaS is displayed as an icon on the smart-phone's screen. The icon, as shown in Figure 5, is a picture of Nan-Ji Xian Wong, who is the god of longevity in Oriental myth. Adopting this picture for the icon of our program expresses our hope that all older adults can achieve a healthy longevity.

5.2 Initial Settings

Several settings in the STFaS– such as for the front-camera face photo, emergency contact list, ambulance service calling, safety zone limits, voice recordings, and daily or travel routes–are presented in the following subsections.

5.2.1 Face Photo Setting

The identity of the legal user has to be confirmed in advance of the each use. The approach adopted in this research is to let the front camera always take a face photo of the current user each time the

Figure 5. The picture of Nan-Ji Xian Wong

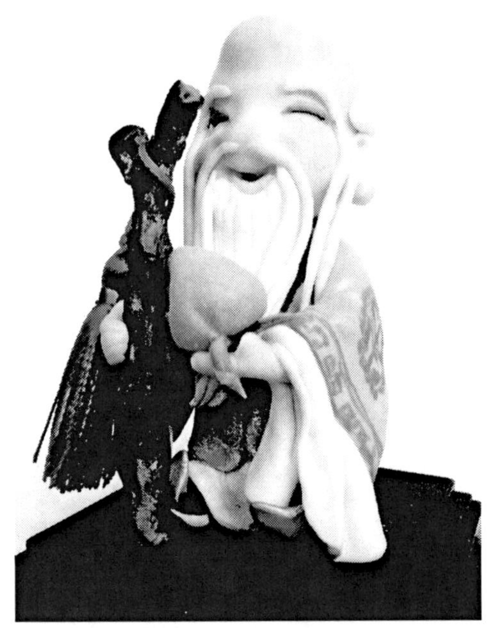

smartphone is started up. As mentioned above, this photo is used to prove to the system that the current user is the legal user. The regular service can be activated to serve this person only when the system confirms that the identity of the current user as the pre-identified phone owner.

5.2.2 Emergency Contact List

This system allows a user to set up 10 emergency contact phone numbers. When an emergency event occurs, as mentioned earlier, the system starts dialing emergency phone numbers in sequence until one of the contacts answers the call and hears about the elderly phone-owner's status. If no one answers the first time, the dialing proce-dure will continue through the list twice more, after which, if the system has not received any replies, it will call a local emergency responder unit. If the user has not set a number for a local emergency ambulance, the system defaults to 119 in Taiwan, 911 in the United States, and 112 for international calls.

5.2.3 Emergency Ambulance Calls

Most countries use three-digit numbers for emer-gency calls, but not all countries use the same numbers. In most Global System for Mobile Com-munication (GSM), 3G (WiMax and LTE), and 4G (LTE-A) systems, mobile users can dial 112, 999, or 911 to call for help. A SIM card usually contains information for emergency calling in various countries.

When a user sets up an emergency number, that number needs to be recognized by GSM, 3G, and 4G systems. The standard operating procedure for an emergency call on a smartphone is that the dialed number is transmitted to the network first, and then the network redirects the emergency call to a local emergency service. Using those prede-termined GSM, 3G, and 4G emergency numbers is the most highly recommended method of call-ing because the majority of operators give those emergency calls the highest priority. Of those emergency numbers, the 112 can be used even when the keypad is locked. However, since 112 is an international emergency number, people call it very often; it may therefore take a longer time for emergency services to answer and consequently may result in unpredictable responder delays. Appendix A lists emergency numbers in several different countries for reference. Users can follow the list to set up their smartphones.

5.2.4 Safety Zone Setting

The system allows the user to set different parameters for the alert region. As mentioned above, in this system a safe area for the elderly is assumed to be within a radius of 300 meters. The distance between 300 meters and 500 meters is considered to be slightly away from home; an elderly individual in that region could become disoriented. The scope of safety feature can utilize the user's home as the setting center to distinguish each region. Some neighborhood features, such as parks, banks, post offices, libraries, and/or supermarkets, can be placed in the safety zone. The GPS coordinates, i.e., the longitude and latitude, of such neighborhood features as are listed above can be set up by inputting those data directly if the user has this information or by using the STFaS to read the GPS coordinates. Also, to make this system operate smoothly, when the system is started up, the smartphone is able to automatically turn on its Bluetooth and WiFi functions to increase the accuracy of positioning. A more detailed description will be presented later.

5.2.5 Voice Recording Setting

It is necessary to record in advance some voice messages by family members for comforting the elderly user when he or she walks beyond the limits of the first alert area (i.e., beyond 500 meters). Voice messages from close family members or caregivers may wake that elderly individual's memory and may be helpful in urging the straying elderly to go home. Also considered to be helpful for the elderly are some further approaches, such as using voice messages associated with familiar music or voice messages accompanied by family members' videos.

5.2.6 Daily or Travel Setting

One special setting in our system is a "travel" or "daily" button. Because people in early stages of dementia still retain some cognitive functions, they may legitimately go beyond the alert zones; they may be out of town for a few days, for example, with their families. In such situations, the user can turn the monitor system to "travel" status. Under that status, the system will suspend the relevant warning function until the "daily" button is pressed again. The purpose of this option is to avoid error detection and erroneous warnings. But, in "travel" mode, the system still offers photographing and GPS-positioning functions to meet some needs in such cases as a missing event or a fall incident.

6. EVALUATION

In this section, we will first discuss the accuracy of the positioning function of a smartphone when a WiFi Access Point (AP) is included or excluded. Several experiments were performed to measure magnitudes of tri-axial accelerometers in daily activities, such as sitting down, standing up, and going up or down stairs. In addition, a real fall was measured and is presented at the end of section 6.3 for further discussion.

6.1 The Positioning Accuracy with/without WiFi

In general, a smartphone is able to collect a set of 3G/4G base stations (BSs) and some WiFi APs, which are helpful in enhancing positioning accuracy, particularly when the GPS signal is weak or blocked by tall buildings, mountains, roofs, or other large objects. Appendix B provides a comparison of results for positioning accuracy in smartphones with and without WiFi support in several locations. For instance, on a university campus, the GPS position error for the smartphone with the support of a WiFi AP was within 5 meters, whereas without WiFi the error was sometimes up to 4000 meters. That is, indeed, a big difference. We also measured positioning accuracy of a smartphone in a university classroom. With a WiFi AP support, the GPS position error was within 65 meters but was up to 1400 meters without the WiFi support. The positioning accuracy in a student dormitory generally was similar to that measured in the classroom. The classroom building and student dormitory had many large buildings around them, which could have block and considerably interfered with the WiFi signals and caused the GPS accuracy to be worse than it would have been in an open area.

6.2 Examining SMV and TA Values in Different Activities

The SMV and TA values and relevant curves in daily activities, such as standing, walking, sitting down, standing up, going upstairs, and going downstairs, are displayed in the following subsections. In addition, a real-fall occurrence is described to further distinguish it from fall-like actions.

6.2.1 Standing

In the following experiments, the initial values of SMVs and TAs as shown in Figure 6 are 1g and -87^0, respectively. Those values imply that the smartphone carrier was standing still, not moving. In this study, the thresholds of the SMVs and TAs of a fall incident were set to 2.3g and 45^0, respectively, which are similar to those in the He et al. (2012) work.

6.2.2 Walking

When the carrier was walking, the values of the SMVs and TAs would change slightly. As shown in Figure 7a, the curve is a little different from that illustrated in Figure 6, indicating that the carrier was walking rather than standing. From the ripples of the curve, we can see that the walking speed of the carrier was about 2 steps per second. In addition, the TA values shown in Figure 7b

Figure 6. Standing

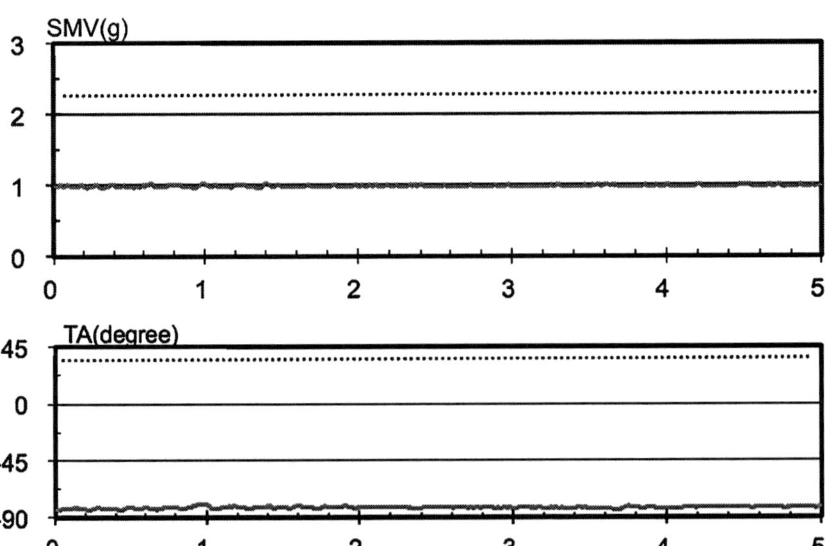

Figure 7. Walking

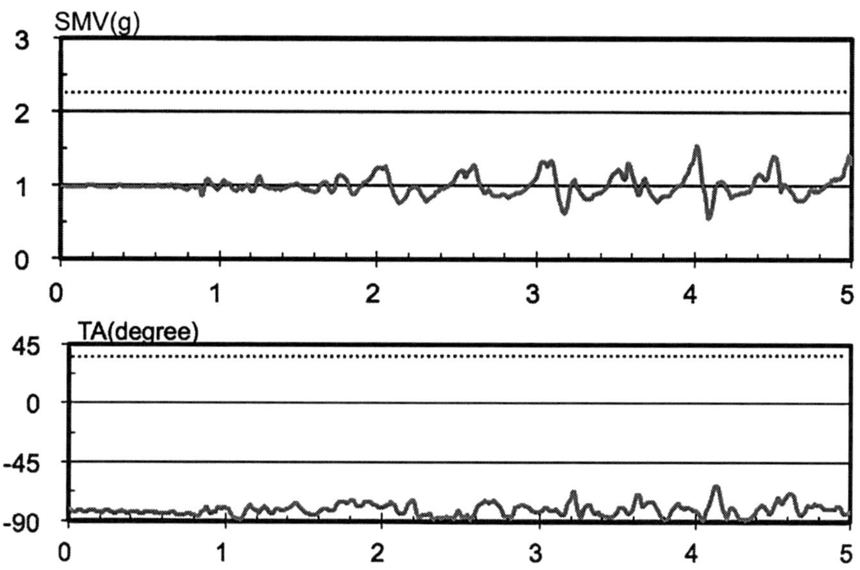

and Figure 6b are also slightly different, implying that the smartphone was not fixed firmly on the front of the user.

6.2.3 Sitting Down

As presented in Figure 8, the values of the SMVs and TAs illustrate that the smartphone carrier was trying to sit on a chair (which was 46 cm high). The first peak of the SMV appeared at about sec 1.8 (see Figure 8a), indicating that the user's buttocks touched the chair. That movement also caused the TAs first to go down a little and then to go up quickly, appearing in the figure as the first peak; that progression reveals that the carrier changed his or her posture. The experiment found that the carrier moved his upper body backward a little, which produced changes in the body-tilt angle, i.e., in the TA (see Figure 8 b). Note that, as described in the above situations, the peak of the SMV curve touches the fall-incident threshold, but the TA curve does not. In such a case, the system will not produce a false alarm.

6.2.4 Sitting Down Very Fast

When the user sits down very fast, that movement usually causes the values of SMVs and TAs to change sharply. Figures 9a and 9b indicate that the values of SMVs and TAs in this experiment were both higher than those shown in Figures 8a and 8b. The duration of this event was also shorter (about 0.85 sec, from sec 0.4 to sec 1.25) than that illustrated in Figure 8 (about 1.3 sec, from sec 1.2 to sec 2.5). Likewise, the SMVs curve went over its fall-incident threshold, but the TAs curve did not go over its threshold. In this case, no false alarm was generated.

6.2.5 Standing Up

When the user stands up or stands up very fast, the different moving speeds may generate distinctive gravities, making SMV and TA values differ greatly. The curves presented in Figure 10 did not go up or down dramatically because the user moved relatively slowly. The experiment recorded that at

Figure 8. Sitting down

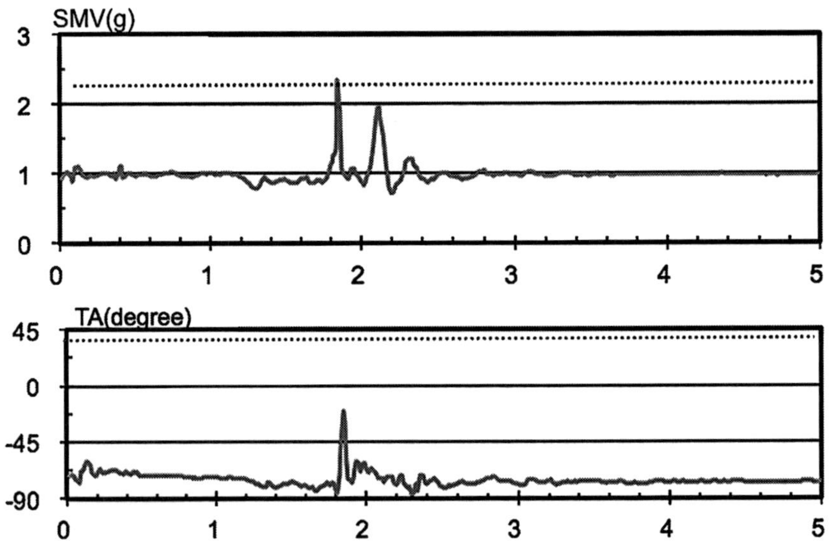

Figure 9. Sitting down very fast

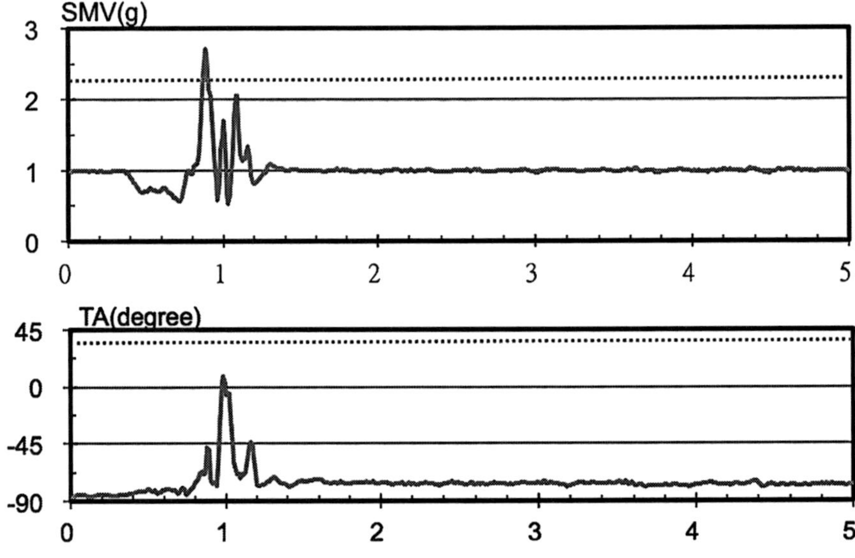

sec 1.4, the smartphone carrier tried to stand up and continued that posture until sec 2.4. During that period, the curve changed a little. But after that movement, the curve became very stable; the SMV value remained 1g, indicating that the user stood very still.

6.2.6 Standing Up Fast

By comparison, when the carrier stands up fast, the movement causes the SMVs curve to change instantly. As shown in Figure 11a, the SMVs curve went down to the bottom of the figure, i.e.,

Figure 10. Standing up

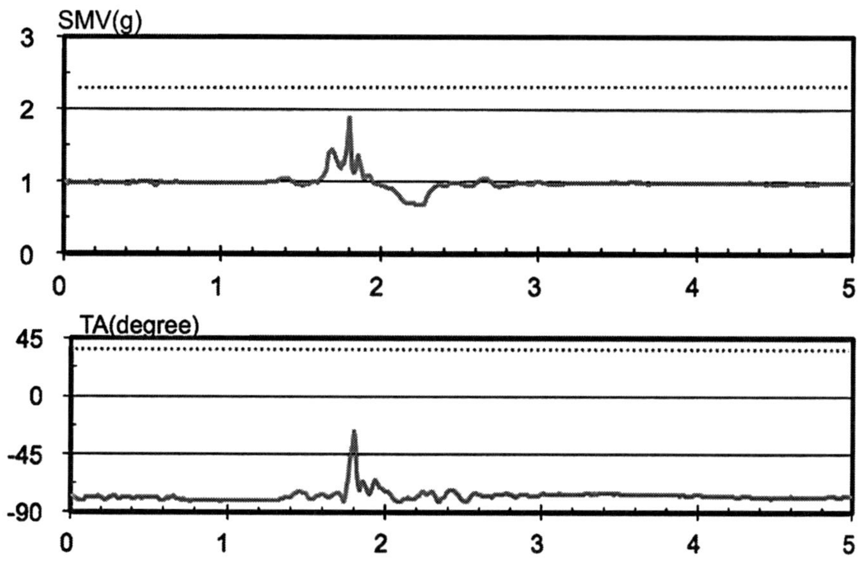

approaching zero. Also, the TAs value reached the fall-incident threshold in Figure 11b, indicating that there was a fall occurrence. Yet, the researchers noted that the carrier's motion was just a fall-like movement. In fact, this situation often is recognized by monitoring systems as a real fall. Because the carrier stood up very fast, the duration of this movement was shorter (about 0.9 sec, from sec 0.6 to sec 1.5) than that in Figure 10 (about 1 sec).

6.2.7 Going Upstairs

The movements of going upstairs are presented in Figure 12. As shown in Figure 12a, the carrier started his motion with his first step at sec 1.2. From the first step to the second, the duration time was between 0.95 and 1 sec. Of interest, after the second step, the remaining steps presented regular shape, indicating that the actions of going upstairs was similar.

Figure 11. Standing up very fast

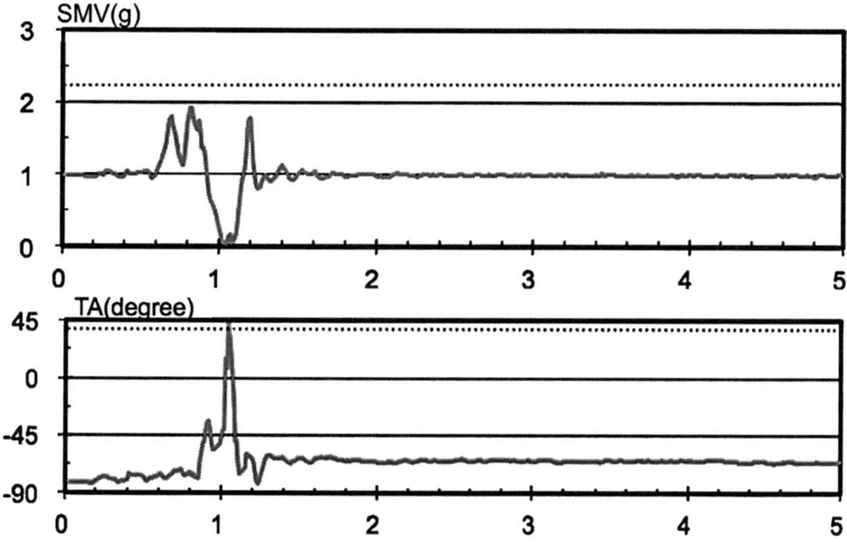

Figure 12. Going upstairs

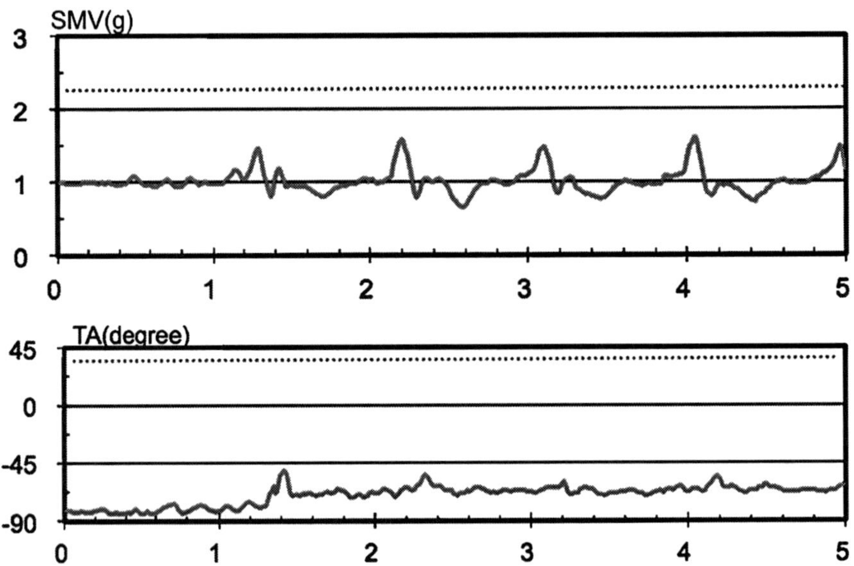

As for the shape of TAs curve, it was approaching the bottom of the figure before sec 1. However, after that time, the curves went up slightly (see Figure 12b), indicating that the carrier intended to climb one stair and the top of body lean forward a little. Likewise, the shape of curve demonstrate a regular shape from sec1 to sec 5, curve demonstrated a regular shape, revealing that the carrier repeated the same consecutive movements. That is a normal posture as people go upstairs.

6.2.8 Going Downstairs

Figure 13 shows that the smartphone carrier is going downstairs. The SMVs graph illustrates that the time period between two consecutive steps was about 0.8 sec. The TAs curve for going downstairs is similar to that as shown in Figure12b. The consecutive movements can be divided into the following steps: leaning the upper body forward a little, then moving one leg forward, impelling the upper body to a proper upright position again to avoid falls, then moving the upper body a little backward again as the other leg moves forward,

and returning the upper body to a proper position to prepare for the next step. These movements are repeated and continue until the last stair has been reached. As can be seen, the TAs curve shown in Figure 13b is not stable since the movement is not fixed but, rather, is varied.

6.3 Real Falls

After performing various experiments in the above-mentioned daily activities, it is clear that the values of SMVs and TAs and their relative curves varied when movements were changed. However, as related research (Abbate et al., 2012) suggests, a real fall must demonstrate different attributes in SMVs and TAs from fall-like movements. The current study, hence, attempted to simulate a real fall and to measure relevant SMV and TA values for further clarification.

Initially, the system assumed that a carrier was standing and then falling down to the ground. In Figure 14, the SMVs curve appears as a consecutive peak, which crosses the fall-incident threshold, but instantly goes down and remains

Figure 13. Going downstairs

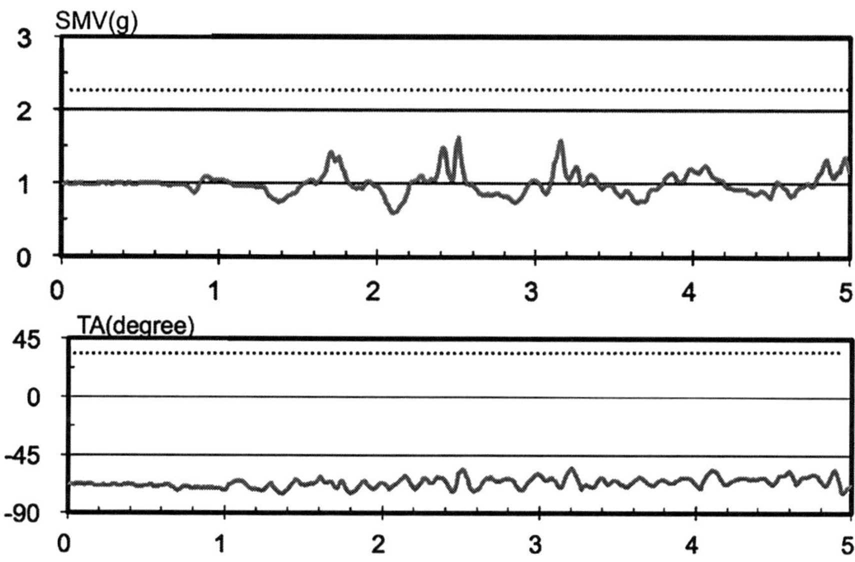

stable at 1g. The TAs value's first peak appears at the same moment as that of the SMVs. That value also reaches the predefined threshold, i.e., the body-tilt angle is 45^0. Since both SMAs and TAs values went across their thresholds, we then claimed that there was a fall incident.

6.3.1 Fall with Face toward the Ground

The above simulation detected several characteristics of a specific fall occurrence. However, falls can be presented in various positions. Figure 15 illustrates the plots from a simulation of a case

Figure 14. Fall simulation as a carrier is falling down on the ground

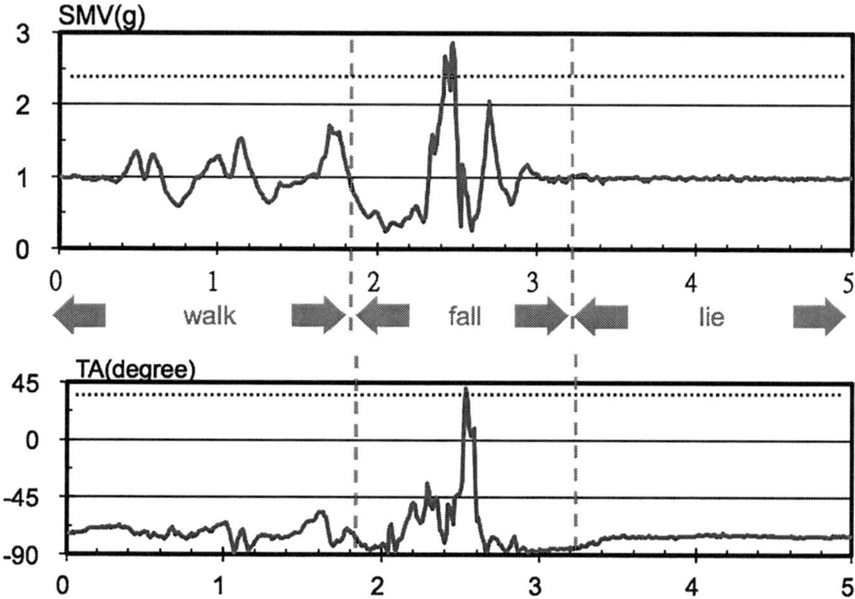

in which the carrier fell with his face toward the ground. The SMVs curve shown in Figure 15a crosses its fall-incident threshold value and then goes down and up again. This part of the curve is quite similar to that shown in Figure 14a. The TAs curve also goes over its threshold. The characteristics in both curves suggest that this case was a fall incident.

7. CONCLUSION

The goal of this study is to provide elderly people with dementia a better living environment in which to maintain their social networks, to improve their quality of life, and to promote their well-being. Wandering and falls are identified as frequent incidents among seniors, particularly for those with dementia. This study uses a smartphone to build the STFaS, which contains wandering and fall detectors, relevant communication services, and emergency medical aid to support elderly indoors and outdoors.

Because the cognitive functions of some people in the early stages of dementia are not completely damaged, those people can live in their own homes independently. The proposed system, hopefully, can assist elderly individuals to reduce the potential risks of engaging in some outdoor activities, such as taking a walk or going shopping, and some indoor activities, such as housekeeping. In addition, this system incorporates the Cloud system to store personal routes, times, and locations; thus the problem of data security cannot be ignored. To ensure that all stored data is protected appropriately, this system uses RSA to encrypt individuals' data. Attempts at unauthorized access to the smartphone or Cloud will not succeed.

The findings in this current research are that

1. False alarms can be effectively decreased by incorporating a user's "confirmed" button,
2. Unnecessary notifications can be reduced by an adaptive communication design, and

Figure 15. Fall simulation as carrier fell with face toward the ground

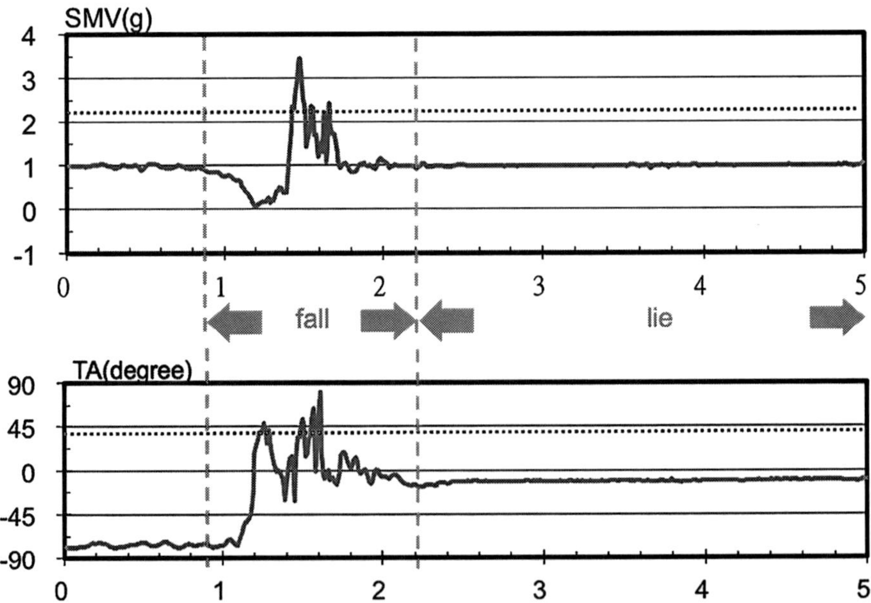

3. Appropriate emergency medical services can be initiated by an intelligent emergency call system as provided in the STFaS.

The sophisticated design in this current research offers a tangible solution to assist people with dementia, specifically those who prefer to live in their own homes independently. In summary, using a smartphone as a system platform, it is possible for this non-intrusive device to support elderly people anytime and anywhere.

8. FUTURE STUDIES AND CHALLENGES

According to a UK report, about one-third of all persons with dementia live in their own homes alone (Mirando-Castillo, Woods, & Orrell, 2010). The proportion increases year by year; it is estimated that between 2008 and 2033 the percentage of people with dementia, aged 75 to 84, who live alone will increase to 38%. Figuring out how to support that group of people to enable them to live independently in a safe and healthy manner is a critical challenge to our society and, as researchers, is our goal as well.

The findings of this study provide useful information for comprehending the operation and effect of a mobile phone monitoring system in an aging society. However, since falls are complicated events, several factors–such as gender, height, weight, and even age, as well as physiological parameters of a person–can confound a real-fall occurrence and, thus, easily lead to an incorrect system response.

In the future, using a gyroscope associated with an accelerometer could possibly enhance accuracy of fall detection. Adding other tri-axial accelerometers at different body locations, such as on shoes, could also potentially improve the accuracy of real-fall recognition. Furthermore, incorporating other algorithms, for instance, machine learning theory or wavelet transform technique, might help to achieve better performance of the system.

A reliable and advanced product should be examined by testers to evaluate the effectiveness of its system. Thus, inviting more potential users to test our proposed monitoring system could be informative and could lead to improved effectiveness. Our system attempts to use a smartphone to build an ideal monitor. The initial endeavors of this study hopefully can advance the knowledge of detection strategy and how best to support persons with dementia with a good quality of life.

REFERENCES

Abbate, S., Avvenuti, M., Bonatesta, F., Cola, G., Corsini, P., & Vecchio, A. (2012). A smartphone-based fall detection system. *Pervasive and Mobile Computing*, *8*(6), 883–899. doi:10.1016/j.pmcj.2012.08.003

Bai, Y.-W., Wu, S.-C., & Tsai, C.-L. (2012, June). Design and implementation of a fall monitor system by using a 3-axis accelerometer in a smart phone. In *Proceedings of Consumer Electronics (ISCE)*. IEEE. doi:10.1109/ISCE.2012.6241717

Demiris, G., & Hensel, B. K. (2008). Technologies for an aging society: A systematic review of "smart home" applications. *IMIA Yearbook of Medical Informatics*, *3*, 33–40. PMID:18660873

Hebert, L. E., Weuve, J., Scherr, P. A., & Evan, D. A. (2013). Alzheimer disease in the United States (2010–2050) estimated using the 2010 census. *Neurology*, *80*(9), 1778–1783. doi:10.1212/WNL.0b013e31828726f5 PMID:23390181

Laudau, R., Auslander, G. K., Werner, S., Shoval, N., & Heinik, J. (2010). Families' and professional caregivers' views of using advanced technology to track people with dementia. *Qualitative Health Research*, *20*(3), 409–419. doi:10.1177/1049732309359171 PMID:20133506

Luxton, D. D., McCann, R. A., Bush, N. E., Mishkind, M. C., & Reger, G. M. (2011). mHealth for mental health: Integrating smartphone technology in behavioral healthcare. *Professional Psychology, Research and Practice*, *42*(6), 505–512. doi:10.1037/a0024485

Mirando-Castillo, C., Woods, B., & Orrell, M. (2010). People with dementia living alone: What are their needs and what kind of support are they receiving? *International Psychogeriatrics*, *22*(4), 607–617. doi:10.1017/S104161021000013X PMID:20214844

Moore, P., Barolli, L., Xhafa, F., & Thomas, A. (2013, October). Monitoring and detection of agitation dementia towards real-time and big-data solutions. In *Proceedings of 8th International Conference on P2P, Parallel, Grid, Cloud and Internet Computing* (pp. 128-135). Academic Press. doi:10.1109/3PGCIC.2013.26

Mubashir, M., Shao, L., & Seed, L. (2013). A survey on fall detection: Principles and approaches. *Neurocomputing*, *100*, 144–152. doi:10.1016/j.neucom.2011.09.037

Naumann, A. B., Hurtienne, J., Gollner, S., Langdon, P. M., & Clarkson, P. J. (2011). Technology supporting the everyday life of people with dementia. In *Proceedings of International Conference on Inclusive Design and Communications*. Academic Press.

Noury, N., Fleury, A., Rumeau, P., Bourke, A. K., Laighin, G. O., Rialle, V., & Lundy, J. E. (2007). Fall detection–Principles and methods. In *Proceedings of the 29th Annual International Conference of the IEEE Engineering in Medicine and Biology Society*. IEEE.

Plaza, I., Martin, L., Martin, S., & Medrano, C. (2011). Mobile applications in an aging society: Status and trends. *Journal of Systems and Software*, *84*(11), 1977–1988. doi:10.1016/j.jss.2011.05.035

Pollack, M. E. (2005). Intelligent technology for an aging population: The use of AI to assist elders with cognitive impairment. *AI Magazine*, *26*(2), 9–24.

Sposaro, F., Danielson, J., & Tyson, G. (2009). iFall: An android application for fall monitoring and response. In *Proceedings of 31st Annual International Conference of the IEEE Engineering in Medicine and Biology Society* (vol. 1, pp. 6119–22). IEEE. doi:10.1109/IEMBS.2009.5334912

Sposaro, F., Danielson, J., & Tyson, G. (2010). iWander: An Android application for dementia patients. In *Proceedings of Annual International Conference of the IEEE Engineering in Medicine and Biology Society* (pp. 3875–3878). IEEE.

Wherton, J. P., & Monk, A. F. (2008). Technological opportunities for supporting people dementia who are living at home. *International Journal of Human-Computer Studies*, *66*(8), 571–586. doi:10.1016/j.ijhcs.2008.03.001

Yavuz, G. R., Kocak, M. E., Ergun, G., Alemdar, H., Yalcin, H., Incel, O. D.,... Ersoy, C. (2010). A smartphone based fall detector with online location support. In *Proceedings of International Workshop on Sensing for App Phone*. Academic Press.

Yu, X. (2008). Approaches and principles of fall detection for elderly and patient. In *Proceedings of 10th IEEE International Conference on e-Health Networking, Applications and Service* (pp. 42–47). IEEE.

KEY TERMS AND DEFINITIONS

Cloud Storage: Cloud storage is a store service approach in which data is maintained, managed and backed up remotely and made available to users over a network.

Cloud: Cloud is the delivery of computing as a service, whereby shared resources and information are provided to computers and other devices as a utility over the Internet.

Decryption: A process that transforms data from unreadable encrypted codes back to its unencrypted form.

Dementia: A symptoms that affects thinking and social abilities such as memory loss, impaired judgment or language, and the incapability to perform some daily activities.

Emergency Ambulance Calls: The phone numbers that people call for ambulance when there is an emergent condition.

Emergency Contact List: A list of contact persons/telephone numbers when there is an emergent condition.

Encryption: A process of using an algorithm to protect sensitive data such as credit card numbers or personal ID numbers by encoding information into unreadable cipher text.

GPS: The Global Positioning System (GPS) is a space-based satellite navigation system that provides location anywhere, moving direction, time information, etc. in all weather conditions of the Earth.

Gyroscope: A gyroscope is a device for measuring or maintaining orientation, based on the principles of angular momentum. It can be used to measure the quantity of rotation of a body, which is the product of its moment of inertia and its angular velocity.

Private Key: A private key also named as secret key is used to decrypt ciphertext or to create a digital signature. In an asymmetric encryption/decryption system, public key is used to encrypt messages and basically only the corresponding private key can decrypt them.

Public Key: A key used in asymmetric cryptography method. The public key is known to everyone and is used to encrypt plaintext or to verify a digital signature.

RSA: RSA is an asymmetric encryption/decryption technique for protecting important data, especially data that's transmitted over wireless or the Internet. RSA stands for the names of creators of the technique, Rivest, Shamir and Adelman.

Safety Zone: An area in which we consider it is safe for people with dementia when he/she stays or wanders in this area.

Smartphone: A smartphone (or smart phone) is a mobile phone (or called cell phone or cellular phone) with more advanced computing capability, features and connectivity than basic feature phones.

SMV: Signal Magnitude Vector (SMV) (some people call it Signal Vector Magnitude (SVM)) is $\dfrac{1}{n}\sum_{i=1}^{n}\sqrt{x_i^2 + y_i^2 + z_i^2}$ where x_i, y_i, and z_i are respectively the ith samples on x-, y- and z-axis and n the number of samples.

TA: Tilt Angle (TA), the angle a moving object makes with the vertical as it curves along its trajectory, is defined as

$$TA = \arcsin\left\{\frac{y_i}{\sqrt{x_i^2 + y_i^2 + z_i^2}}\right\}.$$

Tri-Axial Accelerometer: Accelerometer is a meter that converts acceleration into an electrical signal. A tri-axial accelerometer is a device used to sense the accelerations on X, Y, and Z axes.

Wireless System: A communication technique that can transfer information between two or more points through radio signals and can be applied indoors or outdoors.

This work was previously published in Advanced Technological Solutions for E-Health and Dementia Patient Monitoring edited by Fatos Xhafa, Philip Moore, and George Tadros, pages 272-295 copyright year 2015 by Medical Information Science Reference (an imprint of IGI Global).

APPENDIX A

Table 2. Emergency phone numbers for reference

Country	Police	Ambulance	Fire
China	110	120	119
Brazil	190	192	193
Thailand	191	1669	199
Japan	110	119	
Taiwan	110	119	
England	999 or 112		
Spain	112		
Germany	112		
France	112		
Australia	000		
Canada	911		
United States	911		

Table 3. Smartphone positioning accuracies in different locations (unit: meter)

Measuring Point	Campus		Classroom		Dormitory		Street	
	WiFi On	WiFi Off	WiFi On	WiFi Off	WiFi On	Wifi Off	WiFi On	WiFi Off
1	5.00	4069.95	65.00	1414.00	75.62	1414.00	30.00	1414.00
2	5.00	1579.75	65.00	1414.00	65.00	2121.31	65.00	1414.00
3	65.00	495.19	65.00	1414.00	65.00	1414.00	30.00	30.00
4	10.00	5.00	65.00	1414.00	65.00	1414.00	30.00	30.00
5	5.00	10.00	65.00	1437.05	65.00	1414.00	50.00	50.00

Section 4
Cases and Applications

This section discusses a variety of applications and opportunities available that can be considered by practitioners in developing viable and effective E-Health and Telemedicine programs and processes. This section includes 13 chapters that review topics from case studies to best practices and ongoing research. Further chapters discuss E-Health and Telemedicine in a variety of settings. Contributions included in this section provide excellent coverage of today's IT community and how research into E-Health and Telemedicine is impacting the social fabric of our present-day global village.

Chapter 48

The Role and Use of Telemedicine by Physicians in Developing Countries:
A Case Report from Saudi Arabia

Dana Alajmi
Independent Researcher, Saudi Arabia

Suleiman Alomran
King Saud University, Saudi Arabia

Mohamed Khalifa
King Faisal Specialist Hospital and Research Center, Saudi Arabia

Ashraf El-Metwally
King Saud Bin Abdul Aziz University for Health Sciences, Saudi Arabia

Amr Jamal
King Saud University, Saudi Arabia

Majed Al-Salamah
Independent Researcher, Saudi Arabia

Nasria Zakaria
King Saud University, Saudi Arabia & Universiti Sains Malaysia, Malaysia

Mowafa Househ
King Saud Bin Abdulaziz University for Health Sciences, Saudi Arabia

ABSTRACT

As technological advance leaps into the developing world, telemedicine is expected to significantly grow in many developing countries. It is important to investigate the awareness, preferences, requirements, perceptions and attitudes of physicians in Saudi Arabia towards the use of telemedicine technology. In order to promote the use of telemedicine among physicians, training should be focused on older professionals and those who show lower levels of IT knowledge and experience. This chapter uses the results of a survey that was conducted in the city of Al-Dammam, Saudi Arabia, which gathered information about physicians' awareness and attitude towards telemedicine. Most physicians reported high level of awareness of telemedicine and showed interest in using telemedicine technology in their work. Physicians' preference of using such technology was predicted by their awareness, knowledge and previous experience, using telemedicine and technology affinity. Physicians' willingness to use telemedicine was influenced by age, technology preparedness and practice.

DOI: 10.4018/978-1-4666-8756-1.ch048

INTRODUCTION

Worldwide, the use of information technology and software applications constitutes an integral component of the daily workload in business, banking, industry, education and healthcare settings. Computers and the Internet, as a part of modern information and communication technologies (ICTs), have changed the way of how individuals communicate and exchange information. The development of computer technology and telecommunication services has had a significant impact on quality of health care especially for rural areas where access to quality health care has usually been an obstacle (Bashshur, 2002). Telemedicine is one of those technologies that have brought an opportunity for people who are living in rural areas to gain better accessibility and quality of healthcare services.

Over the past few years, user resistance and acceptance of technology has received more attention in healthcare research (Kim et al., 2010; Chau & Hu, 2002). Schopenhauer, a German philosopher in 1860, suggested that there are three stages for the revelation of each truth. "First, it is ridiculed; in the second, resisted; in the third, it is considered self-evident".

The same situation is applicable with regards to telemedicine technology. Telemedicine in one of the technologies that help facilitate medical care at a distance and have been found useful to reach those patients living in rural and underserved areas (Cox & Towle, 2012; Alajlani, 2010). Telemedicine can include various services ranging from the simplest form as store-and-forward to the highly specialized and sophisticated services, which can be found in academic medical centers. However, telemedicine is still not self-evident because it is still not an integral part of classic healthcare practice (Weiss, 2008). The successful adoption of telemedicine technology relies mainly on the recognizing of barriers to telemedicine. Physicians' attitude and acceptance are considered some of the main challenges for telemedicine. In order to overcome these issues and facilitate the adoption

of innovative technologies, it is very important to understand the factors that affect the acceptance of telemedicine technologies by clinical staff in healthcare (Kim et al., 2010).

Telemedicine is about using information and communication technology (ICT) in order to deliver health care services at a distance (American Telemedicine Association, 2013; Currell et al., 2000). Telemedicine can provide the population in particular who are living in rural areas with the opportunity to gain better-quality healthcare services (Khalifehsoltani & Gerami, 2010; Bashshur, 2002). The industrial countries have had a significant amount of experience with the use of telemedicine during the last 50 years. In 1959, Nebraska Psychiatric Institute was one of the first health organizations that implemented telemedicine in the United States (Ramos, 2010; Jung et al., 2012). It utilized a television link to connect with Norfolk Hospital, which was 12 miles away. Such a link allowed physicians to communicate with both physicians and patients on the other end (Ramos, 2010).

In April of 1968, there were some other early implementations of telemedicine services in Massachusetts General Hospital where a microwave video was used to communicate with Boston Logan airport. With such a link, Massachusetts General Hospital was able to provide instant healthcare services to employees and passengers at the airport. The services provided at the Logan Airport included cardiology, dermatology and radiology services (Ramos, 2010; Adler, 2000). Since then, telemedicine has achieved significant progress in the developed world. In the 1970's, telemedicine became a separate field of study. In the 1990's, the innovation was increased due to the appearance of new technologies like the Internet and mobility services (Wade et al., 2010). Currently, there is a wide range of services already implemented in the industrial countries ranging from basic forms to complicated virtual reality services. These services can be used everywhere mostly in areas whereas a shortage physicians and specialist of specific medical condition. Moreover, there are various successful implemented projects, and plenty of the pilot projects under development that would change the way in which a healthcare is delivered (Bashshur, 2002).

Today, Telemedicine can be classified into three main categories; store-and-forward, live interactive services and hybrid model (Ramos, 2010). Store and Forward (SAF) technology is about capturing the medical data at one time and location and then transmitting the data to another location in convenient time to be assessed offline (Ramos, 2010; Devaraj & Ezra, 2011). SAF is used mostly in Radiology, Dermatology and Pathology (Ramos, 2010). The second model is called synchronous which is a live interactive technology that provides remote real-time communications between the patient and the specialist and it can be used in many activities same to those done in traditional face-to-face appointments such as physical examination, history review, and psychiatric evaluations (Ramos, 2010; Devaraj & Ezra, 2011). The last model is the hybrid which combines both of live interactive and store and forward consultation components which is primarily used for specific conditions, such as heart disease in cardiology specialty (Ramos, 2010).

The implementation of telemedicine might be more effective in developing countries like Saudi Arabia since those countries are being challenged with medical services problems, financial needs, lack of resources and lack of healthcare professionals (Khalifehsoltani & Gerami, 2010; FBA et al., 2010). Telemedicine is one of advanced technologies that attempt to solve the problem related to the provision of quality healthcare. (Bashshur, 2002; Horsch & Balbach, 1999). The key objectives of telemedicine are to provide clinical decision support by sharing information among the healthcare providers, overcome geographical barriers by connecting consumers who are not in the same physical location and improve healthcare outcomes by enabling patients to manage their own healthcare (Bashshur, 2002; Horsch & Balbach, 1999).

The Kingdom of Saudi Arabia is one of the largest countries in the Middle East. It has a population of about thirty million people spread over the entire kingdom's area of more than two million square kilometers with hundreds of cities and villages. Over the past twenty years, Saudi Arabia has made tremendous progress in various sectors through ambitious development plans. Health sector has been given a high priority by heavily investing in building healthcare infrastructure including the latest diagnostic and therapeutic applications (El-Mahalli, El-Khafif & Al-Qahtani, 2012). With great advances of modern medical systems, and growing demand for qualified physicians and surgeons in Saudi Arabia, it becomes a necessity to find new and creative ways to help in achieving healthcare goals. In Saudi Arabia, the idea of telemedicine adoption was introduced as a supportive tool that could promote quality healthcare by enabling residents of remote areas in Saudi Arabia to benefit from the advanced central healthcare services easily and conveniently. The vast zone of Saudi Arabia and widespread population distribution across the country were key elements encouraged the establishment of national telemedicine network (El-Mahalli, El-Khafif & Al-Qahtani, 2012).

Telemedicine in Saudi Arabia was first launched by King Faisal Specialist Hospital and Research Center. The hospital is one of the largest specialist hospitals in the Middle East. It provides free medical care and accommodation for patients' in need of treatment inside and outside Saudi Arabia. Telemedicine services in Saudi Arabia allowed healthcare providers to connect directly with leading specialists around the world. The hospital is connected with George Washington University Hospital for continuing medical education purposes and with Massachusetts General Hospital in Boston for consultation purposes. The consultation telemedicine connect with Massachusetts General hospital included confirming the accuracy of radiology, histopathology reports and also patient management protocols. Nowadays telemedicine consultation between both hospitals is to a large extent limited to patient management protocols.

Some public and private sector hospitals in Riyadh, the capital of Saudi Arabia, and Jeddah, the second largest city, have contracted later with private healthcare services and plans providers to purchase patient management consultations. In 1993, Saudi government established an e-Health Center according to a royal decree. Since that time, the center has been delivering telemedicine services such as medical consultations and continuing medical education through international videoconferencing and fiber optic networks. At the beginning, the signed agreements for the telemedicine services have included only a few hospitals in Saudi Arabia and years later the number of connected sites for the national telemedicine network increased to twenty sites around the Kingdom of Saudi Arabia (Alyemeni, 2010).

Koch (2006) showed in his research that there is a lack of proper guidelines for successful implementation of telemedicine and home telehealth solutions while Broens et al. (2007) found that the patient's' preferences, acceptance and attitude towards telemedicine are key factors that affect the development life cycle of the implementation of telemedicine services. The successful adoption of telemedicine projects is partly depended on the acceptance by both health providers involved and the patients (Chau & Hu, 2002; Kim, Chun & Song, 2009). The acceptance of telemedicine technology in turn can be affected by many factors where physicians' attitude towards telemedicine technologies is one of these factors that influence the meaningful use of telemedicine technology which in turn affect their acceptance towards telemedicine (Kim, Chun & Song, 2009; Eikelboom & Atlas, 2005; Meher, Tyagi & Chaudhry, 2009).

Studies showed that physicians' attitude towards technology is considered as a key predictor of the successful adoption of new technology in healthcare field (Esmaeilzadeh et al., 2011; Straub, 2009). Accordingly, physicians' attitude towards

telemedicine can play a significant role in the successful adoption of telemedicine technology (Bashshur, 2002; Kim, Chun & Song, 2009; Esmaeilzadeh et al., 2011). With the increased use of telemedicine technology in healthcare, there has been resistance, and in some cases acceptance of these technologies as an alternative form of healthcare delivery (Kim et al., 2010), (Xue & Liang, 2007). Physicians find it difficult to adapt to these technologies for fear that such use might have a negative impact on patient/physician communications and adds another layer of complexity to their currently busy work schedule (Kim et al., 2010). Despite the importance of attitude factor in determining and predicting individual's behavior towards technology, many studies about the adoption of technologies have discounted the important role of attitude in predicting individual's acceptance towards technologies (Bashshur, 2002; Kim, Chun & Song, 2009; Ekeland, Bowes & Flottorp, 2010).

From a review of literature, we find a relatively small number of studies that were concerned with the perspective of physicians and patients. Jung et al. (2012) reported that there are several telemedicine services which already have been implemented in Korea and those services are expected to increase in the future. The study presented patients' attitude towards telemedicine services and showed that almost half of the participating patients are aware of telemedicine and 73% of participating patients actually preferred telemedicine (Jung et al., 2012). The study also showed that patient's residence, education and occupation are affecting patient's awareness of telemedicine, while patient's age and income impacted on the patient's preference of telemedicine services (Jung et al., 2012), on the other hand, Terschüren et al. (2012) examined physicians' acceptance of telemedicine services. Researchers of this study found that 36% of physicians are aware of telemedicine devices and 1.8% of them experienced using such technology (Terschüren, Mensing & Mekel, 2012). According to Meher et al. (2009)

most physicians, of all ages, found telemedicine important. Contradictory results were reported by Gaggioli et al. (2004), who documented that some physicians were not interested in telemedicine or convinced with its usefulness in improving the quality of care. Physicians' beliefs of the latter study were mostly apparent with novice and older physicians who showed a lower level of knowledge and prior experience of telemedicine (Gaggioli et al., 2004; Hanson, Calhoun & Smith, 2009).

SAUDI ARABIA AS A CASE EXAMPLE: THE SURVEY STUDY

Despite all potential benefits of telemedicine, it has been slowly adopted in Saudi Arabia emphasizing the need for more studies that explores key factors combating the implementation of telemedicine services. Only few studies were conducted in Saudi Arabia to identify such factors. The objectives of this study were (1) to explore the factors that affect physicians' attitude in Saudi Arabia towards telemedicine technologies such as age, gender and work experience, and (2) to investigate physicians' opinions, requirements and priorities in telemedicine in order to support the meaningful use of telemedicine in Saudi Arabia. The research question guiding this study was "What is the attitude of physicians towards the adoption and use of telemedicine in Saudi Arabia?"

Study Setting

The survey among physicians was conducted in Imam Abdurrahman Bin Faisal Hospital, National Guard Health Affairs. This hospital was selected, as it is one of the leading hospitals in the Eastern Region of Saudi Arabia. The hospital was officially opened in 2002 with a capacity of 112 inpatient beds, over 85,000 outpatients visits annually and around 48,000 ER encounters. The hospital is JCIA accredited.

Study Design

An exploratory cross sectional study was conducted in order to identify the present attitude of physicians towards telemedicine services and to explore the factors that affect their attitude. The study determined the nature of the relationship between these factors and participants' attitude towards telemedicine.

Target Population and Sample Size

All 219 physicians, who work full-time at Imam Abdurrahman Bin Faisal Hospital constituted our target population. Invited physicians worked in nine medical departments: 8 in family medicine, 17 in surgery, 7 in anesthesia, 22 in internal medicine, 13 in obstetrics and gynecology, 12 in pediatrics, 18 in emergency medicine, 6 in medical imaging 4 in dental and 14 locums from different specialties. The study focused on physicians only, so other clinical staffs were excluded. The study used a convenience sampling method. Such sampling technique had been used because only the physicians who were in the hospital during the one-month data collection period were accessible to the research group. According to convenience sampling technique, a total of 121 physicians from all departments were invited to take part in this survey. Informed consent with a clear explanation of the project was distributed first together with the questionnaire. Out of a total of 121 doctors invited 93 completed the questionnaire giving a response rate of 77%.

Data Collection Method

For this cross sectional study, a self-administrated questionnaire was used to collect data from physicians. The survey included a mix of close-ended and open ended questions. The questionnaire assessed the knowledge, attitudes, opinions and perceptions of physicians towards telemedicine. It included 25 questions which were divided into four major categories: (1) Physicians' demographics; (2) Level of awareness about telemedicine services; (3) Accessibilities to telemedicine services; (4) willingness to use telemedicine services; (5) Preferences in telemedicine.

A pilot phase of the study was conducted in order to test the instrument and the survey procedures before the actual survey. The reliability and validity of the survey were both evaluated by distributing the questionnaire to 18 randomly selected physicians from the target population. Of whom 14 physicians replied and completed the survey. This pilot phase gave an initial insight of how the physicians from different medical specialty view and think about telemedicine technology. The pilot survey collected data about clarity of the questions and all required adjustments in the questionnaire were conducted based on such comments.

The survey was conducted in the time period from first of March 2013 to the first of April 2013. participants' responses were kept confidential, while only the investigators could identify individuals participated in the study in order to make people more comfortable in sharing the information. In order to increase the response rate, a contact in advance was established with respondents to let them know about the survey and its purpose. Moreover, a follow-up reminder email was sent to non-responding physicians.

Study Variables

Independent variables included physicians' medical specialty, age, gender, years of practice and technology exposure. In order to detect telemedicine preferences according to specific age, five age groups were designed within the questionnaire. Gender of the participants was also scanned in order to examine different styles and attitudes toward the use of telemedicine for both males and females. Medical specialty was surveyed for investigating differences in attitude in various medical specialties. Technology affinity was measured in order to learn how physician's attitude towards technology influences their preferences in telemedicine. For dependent variables, physicians' awareness was assessed, as well as physicians' confidence of telemedicine were measured Physicians' willingness to use telemedicine was also used as the dependent variable is some parts of the analysis.

Data Analysis

Data were coded and entered into Statistical Package for Social Sciences (SPSS). Descriptive analysis was conducted first and results were depicted in tables. To examine factor that significantly had an effect on physicians' opinions, t-test and ANOVA were used.. Spearman correlation test was also used to determine the relationship between the study's quantitative variables. The level of significance was set to ($P<0.05$). The least squares difference Post hoc analysis was carried out for the factors that significantly influenced physicians' attitude in order to identify the points of differences.

Results

According to the personal demographics data section, as shown in table 1, different specialties participated in different proportions, 95% of participating physicians were between thirty and sixty years old, three quarters of the participants were males, most of the participants had over six years of medical experience and most of participants had moderate technology skills and affinity.

The study also showed the participants' background about telemedicine. As seen from table 2, the majority of the physicians were aware about telemedicine with 72%; 15 physicians (16%) described their knowledge about telemedicine as not knowledgeable, 53 physicians (56.4%) as somewhat knowledge and 24 physicians (24.5%) as knowledgeable. Physicians reported receiving information about telemedicine from different

Table 1. Characteristics of participating physicians According to medical specialty, age group, gender, years of practice and level of technology affinity (N=95)

Characteristic	N=95	Percent
Medical Specialty (N=95)		
Family Medicine or GP	7	7.5
Gynaecology	14	15.0
Internal Medicine	14	15.0
Paediatrics	8	8.6
Neurology	2	2.2
Ophthalmology	2	2.2
Radiology	3	3.2
Others	4	4.3
Anaesthesia	6	6.5
Surgery	17	18.3
Dental	3	3.2
Emergency Medicine	14	15.0
Age Group (N=95)		
Less than 30	1	1.1
30- 39	36	38.7
40-49	29	31.2
50-59	24	25.8
More or equal to 60	4	4.3
Gender (N=95)		
Female	24	25.8
Male	71	76.3
Years of Practicing (N=95)		
Less than 1	2	2.1
1 – 5	6	6.4
6 – 10	29	30.9
11 – 20	36	38.3
More than 20	21	22.3
Level of Technology Affinity (N=95)		
Low	4	4.2
Moderate	84	89.4
High	10	6.4

Table 2. Physicians' awareness about telemedicine

Physicians' Awareness About Telemedicine (N=92)	N	Per cent
No	26	28.3
Yes	66	71.7
Physicians' Knowledge about Telemedicine (N=92)		
Not knowledgeable	15	16.3
Somewhat knowledgeable	53	57.6
Knowledgeable	24	26.1
Source of Knowledge (N= 78)		
Colleagues	34	29.8%
Practicing	22	19.3%
Media	46	40.4%
Survey	8	7.0%
Lectures	2	3.5%

With respect to physicians' accessibility to telemedicine, the study found that 47.3% of physicians have never used telemedicine, 11.8% rarely used it, 28% sometimes used it, 6.5% often used telemedicine and 6.5% have been always using this technology. Those physicians who used telemedicine previously, actually used different types of telemedicine and for different purposes; 29 physicians (36.7%) used interactive video, 12 physicians (15.2%) used store and forward technology, 22 physicians (27.8%) used shared computers, 12 physicians (15.2%) used telemetry and 4 physicians (5.1%) used different types of telemedicine. Table 3 shows that 12 physicians (11.8%) used telemedicine for administrative purposes, 40 physicians (39.2%) used telemedicine for continuous medical education, 14 physicians (13.7%) used telemedicine for second opinion, 7 physicians (11.8%) used telemedicine for diagnosis, 12 physicians (11.8%) used telemedicine for follow up, 2 physicians (7.8%) used telemedicine for emergency cases and 8 physicians (7.8%) used telemedicine for other purposes.

Table 4, describes physicians' willingness to use, their perception and preference of telemedicine. Most physicians were enthusiastic and

sources; 29.8% got information from their colleges, 19.3% from practicing, 40.4% from media, 3.5% from lectures and 7% from survey.

Table 3. Physicians' accessibility to telemedicine technology

How Often Physicians Used Telemedicine	N	Percent
Never	44	47.3%
Rarely	11	11.8%
Sometimes	26	28.0%
Often	6	6.5%
Always	6	6.5%
Common Uses of Telemedicine (N=57)		
Interactive Video	29	36.7%
Store and Forward	12	15.2%
Shared Computer	22	27.8%
Telemetry	12	15.2%
Use Other	4	5.1%
Purpose of Using Telemedicine (N=58)		
Administrative	12	11.8%
CME	40	39.2%
Second Opinion	14	13.7%
Diagnosis	12	11.8%
Follow Up	12	11.8%
Emergency	4	3.9%
Other	8	7.8%

willing to use telemedicine technology, but with the need of further research on the effectiveness of telemedicine. (53.2%) of physicians agreed and (39.4%) strongly agreed that they would use interactive video in their practice if it was available or attend continuing medical education via telemedicine. Additionally, Most of physicians either agreed (56.5%) or strongly agreed (40.2%) that use of telemedicine can enhance the communication process in healthcare either between the physicians themselves, physicians and patients or healthcare centers. With regards to the physicians' preferences in telemedicine, there was a variation in physicians' perspective due to different purposes of telemedicine use. Most physicians agreed and strongly agreed that patient is more likely to receive better quality of care in case they had seen the specialist in person

with 48.2% and 47.1 respectively. Physicians disagreed that telemedicine might be effective in emergency cases and Post-surgical follow-up with 44.9% and 34.5% respectively. On the other hand, 40.4% of sampled physicians agreed that use of telemedicine might be effective for preventive care. Physicians strongly agreed and agreed that use of telemedicine might be effective for second opinion and home health care with 48.9%, 43.5 and 40.2, 47.1 respectively. Additionally, 46.7% of physicians agreed that use of telemedicine might be effective for acute, nonemergency care. Most of physicians 51.1% believed that their specialty can readily be adapted to the use of tele-consultation. Finally, (51.1%) of physicians strongly agreed and 45.7% agreed that telemedicine can enhance educational opportunities.

Table 5 shows the relationship between specific physicians' demographics and physicians' awareness, willingness to use telemedicine and physicians' preferences of telemedicine technology. The statistical significance differences were found between respondents age group and physicians' willingness to use (P=.019) and their preferences of telemedicine (P=.001). Technology affinity of respondents was significantly affecting physicians' willingness to use of telemedicine technology (P=0.19). Additionally, respondents' awareness of telemedicine significantly affected their willingness to use of telemedicine ((P<0.001) and physicians' preferences about telemedicine (P<0.001) (Table 6).

DISCUSSION

Telemedicine in developing countries still needs more consideration in order to improve the efficiency of healthcare accessibility. Despite the potential benefits of telemedicine in Saudi Arabia due to its vast area and widespread population distribution, the availability of telemedicine services is considered low in comparison with developed countries (El-Mahalli, El-Khafif & Al-Qahtani,

Table 4. Physicians' willingness to use, perception and preference of telemedicine

	Strongly Agree		Agree		Disagree		Strongly Disagree		Don't Know		Total
	N	%	N	%	N	%	N	%	N	%	
Willing to use telemedicine	37	39.4	50	53.2	4	4.3	3	3.2	0	0	94
Telemedicine & communications	37	40.2	52	56.5	3	3.2	2	2.1	0	0	94
Telemedicine with Physical Examination	40	47.1	41	48.2	2	2.4	2	2.4	9	9.6	85
Telemedicine with Emergency Medicine	7	7.9	25	28.1	40	44.9	17	19.1	5	5.3	89
Telemedicine with preventive care	24	27	36	40.4	19	21.3	10	11.2	10	10.6	89
Telemedicine with second opinion	45	48.9	40	43.5	5	5.4	2	2.2	7	7.4	92
Telemedicine with post-surgical follow-up	13	15.5	25	29.8	29	34.5	17	20.2	10	10.6	84
Telemedicine with acute, nonemergency care	25	27.8	42	46.7	22	24.4	1	1.1	4	4.3	90
Telemedicine with home health care	35	40.2	41	47.1	9	10.3	2	2.3	7	7.4	87
Telemedicine with physician's specialty	15	17.0	45	51.1	18	20.5	10	11.4	6	6.4	88
Telemedicine with educational	47	51.1	42	45.7	3	3.3	0	0	2	2.1	92

Table 5. Relationship between physicians' characteristics and their awareness, willingness to use and their preferences of telemedicine

	Age Group		Gender		Medical Specialty		Years of Practicing		Technology Affinity	
	F	Sig.	F	Sig.	F	Sig.	F	Sig.	F	Sig.
Telemedicine & Awareness	4.299	.073	.425	.516	1.577	.129	3.544	.401	.034	.855
Willing to use telemedicine	.565	.019	.492	.485	1.470	.165	.947	.441	.047	.019
Telemedicine & Preferences	1.762	.001	.839	.362	.740	.671	1.023	.060	.000	1.000

Table 6. Relationship between awareness and accessibility factors and physician's willingness to use and their preferences of telemedicine

	Awareness		Accessibility	
	F	Sig.	F	Sig.
Willing to use telemedicine	15.836	.000	1.550	.195
Telemedicine & Preferences	25.306	.000	.870	.486

2012). In addition, there are very few studies that had discussed the status, adoption, implementation and patient awareness of telemedicine services in Saudi Arabia, even though there are telemedicine services being provided at both public and private hospitals (El-Mahalli, El-Khafif & Al-Qahtani, 2012; Goldberg et al., 1994). Many of the studies show that the attitude towards telemedicine is one of the key factors that influence adoption, however, not much is known about the attitude towards telemedicine or physicians' willingness to use it in Saudi Arabia. The factors that may influence the use and adoption of telemedicine is still unknown (Kim, Chun & Song, 2009; Ekeland, Bowes & Flottorp, 2010).

The reported findings of the current study revealed that the majority of our surveyed physicians were aware of telemedicine (72 per cent, Table 2) regardless of their personal characteristics, and almost half of them had never experienced the use telemedicine (47.3 per cent, Table 3). This result was consistent with the findings of the study that was conducted in the North Rhine-Westphalia, Germany, which investigated the physicians' awareness and attitude towards home tele-monitoring as one type of telemedicine services. Although the majority of physicians approved the idea of using telemedicine in different healthcare settings, this good attitude is age-determinant. The proportion of the physicians who disliked the use of telemedicine is slightly increased for older physicians with age greater than 50 years. The per cent of opponent is heavily increased with older physicians greater than 60 years. Such result is comparable to the findings of the study by Terschuren et al., 2012 where showed that the most of the resistance of telemedicine is mostly appeared with older physicians. On the other hand, the findings are contradicted by a Saudi study by El-Mahalli et al. (2012) which found that older physicians have strong intension to use telemedicine and the reason is probably because their experience which gave them more insights about the improving the efficiency and quality of healthcare using new technological tools. The findings also showed that physicians' willingness to the use of telemedicine was differed when investigating physicians' technology affinity. Physicians with low and intermediate levels of technology affinity were more enthusiastic and eager to use to telemedicine than the physicians with high level of technology affinity. The study suggested that the reason of those findings is that physicians with high level of technology affinity might be more resistant to telemedicine technology because of their knowledge of technical problems that may occur as a result of the use of these services. In contrast to physicians' age and technology affinity, the gender, medical specialty and years of practicing did not affect the willingness and preferences of telemedicine in study's sample.

The current study also showed that telemedicine was preferred in certain healthcare settings such as second opinion, acute and nonemergency cases. On the other hand, physicians did not prefer telemedicine in healthcare settings that are related to emergency, preventive care and post-surgical follow-up cases. In addition, the study showed that most of the physicians preferred face-to-face consultations for cases related to physical examination. This result is similar to the findings noted by Whitten and Love (2005) which reported face-to-face consultation as an ideal type of medical encounter. Older physicians have been found to dislike telemedicine in emergency cases and home healthcare. Moreover, there was some relationship between physicians' awareness and their preferences of telemedicine. Most of the physicians who did not prefer the use of telemedicine in preventive care, second opinion and education were not aware about telemedicine as others.

FUTURE DIRECTIONS AND WAY FORWARD

In conclusion, telemedicine technology could have bright and promising future in Saudi Arabia when it gets more attention and consideration from decision makers. Telemedicine provide users with promising solutions that could maintain the healthcare in the area-wide of the Kingdom especially with the shortage of medical experts. In the current study, it has been found that physicians' acceptance, preferences and wiliness to use telemedicine technology are influenced by physicians' characteristics such as age and technology affinity. Physicians' knowledge and awareness about telemedicine is also found to be key determinants of physicians' preferences and intention to the use of telemedicine technology. The current study reported a variation of physicians' preferences. This difference in physicians' perspectives occurred mainly because of the diversity of telemedicine models and different services provided by telemedicine technology. For this reason, additional studies should be conduct focusing on physicians' attitude towards each model and service of telemedicine and to explore new avenues of interaction through social media and mhealth, especially in the developing word. (Paton, Househ & Malik, 2013; Aldabbagh, Alsharif & Househ, 2013; Kushniruk et al., 2013; Ababtain, Almulhim & Househ, 2013; Househ, 2013; Borycki et al., 2011; Almutairi et al., 2011; Househ et al., 2012a; Househ et al., 2012b; Househ, Borycki & Kushniruk, 2012; Househ, 2014)

The main recommendations that can shape the way forward includes basically identifying and overcoming the challenges facing the processes of developing, implementing, utilizing the evaluating telemedicine. It is important as much to provide the proper support, promotion and enhancement of telemedicine in Saudi Arabia. Each of these challenges needs to be studied thoroughly and each needs a plan to overcome. Challenges facing telemedicine and many other types of health informatics applications could be classified into human, professional, technical, organizational, financial and legal or regulatory challenges (Khalifa, 2013). Telemedicine development and implementation might remain in the pilot phase and may not succeed in scaling-up to robust products that are used in daily practice. Some studies identified and classified determinants, which would influence the future implementations of telemedicine interventions, into five major categories: (1) Technology, (2) Acceptance, (3) Financing, (4) Organization and (5) Policy and Legislation. Each category contains determinants that are relevant to different stakeholders in different domains. Accordingly, technology challenges need building good technical infrastructure and continuous support, users' training, enhancing systems usability and quality from the patient perspective, while acceptance challenges need improving attitude and usability, from the physicians and other providers' perspectives, being evidence based and the effect

of diffusion and dissemination, the financial challenges needs proper planning of the investment for both initiating projects and maintaining their operations. Organizational challenges need developing managerial awareness and commitments towards such projects while the upper most level of challenges, the policy and legislation need direct intervention of the state, ministry of health and national policy makers. (Broens et al., 2007; Wootton, 2008; van Gemert-Pijnen et al., 2011; Mair et al., 2012; Hendy et al., 2012)

REFERENCES

Ababtain, A. F., Almulhim, D. A., & Househ, M. S. (2013). The state of mobile health in the developing world and the Middle East. *Studies in Health Technology and Informatics, 190*, 300–302. PMID:23823455

Adler, A. T. (2000). A cost-effective portable telemedicine kit for use in Developing countries (Doctoral dissertation, Massachusetts Institute of Technology).

Alajlani, M. (2010). Issues facing the application of telemedicine in developing countries: Hashemite Kingdom of Jordan and Syrian Arab Republic (Doctoral dissertation, Brunel University, School of Information Systems, Computing and Mathematics).

Aldabbagh, D., Alsharif, K., & Househ, M. S. (2013). Health information in the Arab world. *Studies in Health Technology and Informatics, 190*, 297–299. PMID:23823454

Alyemeni, M. (2010). *Five Year Program to Transform Healthcare Delivery in Saudi Arabia.* Saudi Arabia Ministry of Health.

American Telemedicine Association. (2013). *What is telemedicine.* Retrieved form http://www.americantelemed.org/about-telemedicine/what-is-telemedicine

Bashshur, R. L. (2002). Chapter 1: Telemedicine and health care. *Telemedicine Journal and e-Health, 8*(1), 5–12. doi:10.1089/15305620252933365 PMID:12020402

Borycki, E. M., Househ, M. S., Kushniruk, A. W., Nohr, C., & Takeda, H. (2011). Empowering Patients: Making Health Information and Systems Safer for Patients and the Public. Contribution of the IMIA Health Informatics for Patient Safety Working Group. *Yearbook of Medical Informatics, 7*(1), 56–64. PMID:22890342

Broens, T. H., Vollenbroek-Hutten, M. M., Hermens, H. J., van Halteren, A. T., & Nieuwenhuis, L. J. (2007). Determinants of successful telemedicine implementations: A literature study. *Journal of Telemedicine and Telecare, 13*(6), 303–309. doi:10.1258/135763307781644951 PMID:17785027

Chau, P. Y., & Hu, P. J. H. (2002). Investigating healthcare professionals' decisions to accept telemedicine technology: An empirical test of competing theories. *Information & Management, 39*(4), 297–311. doi:10.1016/S0378-7206(01)00098-2

Cox, J. V., & Towle, E. L. (2012). Business and Science: Lessons From the 2011 Cancer Center Business Summit. *Journal of Oncology Practice, 8*(2), 67–68. doi:10.1200/JOP.2012.000584 PMID:23077430

Currell, R., Urquhart, C., Wainwright, P., & Lewis, R. (2000). Telemedicine versus face to face patient care: Effects on professional practice and health care outcomes. *The Cochrane Library.* PMID:10796678

Devaraj, S. J., & Ezra, K. (2011, April). Current trends and future challenges in wireless telemedicine system. In *Electronics Computer Technology (ICECT), 2011 3rd International Conference on* (Vol. 4, pp. 417-421). IEEE. doi:10.1109/ICECTECH.2011.5941933

Eikelboom, R. H., & Atlas, M. D. (2005). Attitude to telemedicine, and willingness to use it, in audiology patients. *Journal of Telemedicine and Telecare, 11*(8suppl 2), 22–25. doi:10.1258/135763305775124920 PMID:16375788

Ekeland, A. G., Bowes, A., & Flottorp, S. (2010). Effectiveness of telemedicine: A systematic review of reviews. *International Journal of Medical Informatics, 79*(11), 736–771. doi:10.1016/j.ijmedinf.2010.08.006 PMID:20884286

El-Mahalli, A. A., El-Khafif, S. H. & Al-Qahtani, M. F. (2012). Successes and Challenges in the Implementation and Application of Telemedicine in the Eastern Province of Saudi Arabia. Perspectives in health information management/AHIMA, American Health Information Management Association, 9(Fall).

Esmaeilzadeh, P., Sambasivan, M., Kumar, N., & Nezakhati, H. (2011). Adoption of technology applications in healthcare: the influence of attitude toward knowledge sharing on technology acceptance in a hospital. In U- and E-Service, Science and Technology (pp. 17-30). Springer Berlin Heidelberg. doi:10.1007/978-3-642-27210-3_3

FBA, A. W., Liddell, K., FBA, S. M., Rose, N., Smith, P. C., FRS, J. S. & Wootton, R. (2010). Medical profiling and online medicine: The ethics of 'personalised healthcare' in a consumer age (Doctoral dissertation, London School of Economics and Political Science).

Gaggioli, A., di Carlo, S., Mantovani, F., Castelnuovo, G., & Riva, G. (2004). A telemedicine survey among Milan doctors. *Journal of Telemedicine and Telecare, 11*(1), 29–34. doi:10.1258/1357633053430476 PMID:15829041

Goldberg, M. A., Sharif, H. S., Rosenthal, D. I., Black-Schaffer, S., Flotte, T. J., Colvin, R. B., & Thrall, J. H. (1994). Making global telemedicine practical and affordable: Demonstrations from the Middle East. *AJR. American Journal of Roentgenology, 163*(6), 1495–1500. doi:10.2214/ajr.163.6.7992754 PMID:7992754

Hanson, D., Calhoun, J., & Smith, D. (2009). Changes in provider attitudes toward telemedicine. *Telemedicine Journal and e-Health, 15*(1), 39–43. doi:10.1089/tmj.2008.0052 PMID:19199846

Hendy, J., Chrysanthaki, T., Barlow, J., Knapp, M., Rogers, A., Sanders, C., & Newman, S. (2012). An organisational analysis of the implementation of telecare and telehealth: The whole systems demonstrator. *BMC Health Services Research, 12*(1), 403. doi:10.1186/1472-6963-12-403 PMID:23153014

Horsch, A., & Balbach, T. (1999). Telemedical information systems. Information Technology in Biomedicine. *IEEE Transactions on, 3*(3), 166–175.

Househ, M. (2013). The use of social media in healthcare: Organizational, clinical, and patient perspectives. *Studies in Health Technology and Informatics, 183*, 244–248. PMID:23388291

Househ, M. (2014). The role of short messaging service in supporting the delivery of healthcare: An umbrella systematic review. *Health Informatics Journal*. PMID:25038203

Househ, M., Ahmad, A., Alshaikh, A., & Alsuweed, F. (2012a). Patient safety perspectives: The impact of CPOE on nursing workflow. *Studies in Health Technology and Informatics, 183*, 367–371. PMID:23388315

Househ, M., Borycki, E., & Kushniruk, A. (2014). Empowering patients through social media: The benefits and challenges. *Health Informatics Journal, 20*(1), 50–58. doi:10.1177/1460458213476969 PMID:24550564

Househ, M., Borycki, E., Kushniruk, A. W., & Alofaysan, S. (2012b). mHealth: a passing fad or here to stay. Telemedicine and E-Health Services, Policies and Applications: Advancements and Developments, 151-173.

Jung, S. G., Kweon, H. J., Kim, E. T., Kim, S. A., Choi, J. K. & Cho, D. Y. (2012). Preference and awareness of telemedicine in primary care patients. *Korean Journal of Family Medicine, 33*(1), 25-33.

Khalifa, M. (2013). Barriers to health information systems and electronic medical records implementation. A field study of Saudi Arabian hospitals. *Procedia Computer Science, 21*, 335–342. doi:10.1016/j.procs.2013.09.044

Khalifehsoltani, S. N., & Gerami, M. R. (2010, January). E-health challenges, opportunities and experiences of developing countries. In *e-Education, e-Business, e-Management, and e-Learning, 2010. IC4E'10. International Conference on* (pp. 264-268). IEEE.

Kim, J., DelliFraine, J. L., Dansky, K. H., & McCleary, K. J. (2010). Physicians' acceptance of telemedicine technology: An empirical test of competing theories. *International Journal of Information Systems and Change Management, 4*(3), 210–225. doi:10.1504/IJISCM.2010.033076

Kim, Y. J., Chun, J. U., & Song, J. (2009). Investigating the role of attitude in technology acceptance from an attitude strength perspective. *International Journal of Information Management, 29*(1), 67–77. doi:10.1016/j.ijinfomgt.2008.01.011

Koch, S. (2006). Home telehealth–current state and future trends. *International Journal of Medical Informatics*, *75*(8), 565–576. doi:10.1016/j.ijmedinf.2005.09.002 PMID:16298545

Kushniruk, A. W., Bates, D. W., Bainbridge, M., Househ, M. S., & Borycki, E. M. (2013). National efforts to improve health information system safety in Canada, the United States of America and England. *International Journal of Medical Informatics*, *82*(5), e149–e160. doi:10.1016/j.ijmedinf.2012.12.006 PMID:23313431

Mair, F. S., May, C., O'Donnell, C., Finch, T., Sullivan, F., & Murray, E. (2012). Factors that promote or inhibit the implementation of e-health systems: An explanatory systematic review. *Bulletin of the World Health Organization*, *90*(5), 357–364. doi:10.2471/BLT.11.099424 PMID:22589569

Meher, S. K., Tyagi, R. S., & Chaudhry, T. (2009). Awareness and attitudes to telemedicine among doctors and patients in India. *Journal of Telemedicine and Telecare*, *15*(3), 139–141. doi:10.1258/jtt.2009.003011 PMID:19364898

Paton, C., Househ, M., & Malik, M. (2013). The challenges of publishing on health informatics in developing countries. *Applied Clinical Informatics*, *4*(3), 428–433. doi:10.4338/ACI-2013-04-IE-0030 PMID:24155794

Ramos, V. (2010, November). Contributions to the history of Telemedicine of the TICs. In Telecommunications Conference (HISTELCON), 2010 Second IEEE Region 8 Conference on the History of (pp. 1-5). IEEE. doi:10.1109/HISTELCON.2010.5735269

Straub, E. T. (2009). Understanding technology adoption: Theory and future directions for informal learning. *Review of Educational Research*, *79*(2), 625–649. doi:10.3102/0034654308325896

Terschüren, C., Mensing, M., & Mekel, O. C. (2012). Is telemonitoring an option against shortage of physicians in rural regions? Attitude towards telemedical devices in the North Rhine-Westphalian health survey, Germany. *BMC Health Services Research*, *12*(1), 95. doi:10.1186/1472-6963-12-95 PMID:22507694

van Gemert-Pijnen, J. E., Nijland, N., van Limburg, M., Ossebaard, H. C., Kelders, S. M., Eysenbach, G., & Seydel, E. R. (2011). A holistic framework to improve the uptake and impact of eHealth technologies. *Journal of Medical Internet Research*, *13*(4), e111. doi:10.2196/jmir.1672 PMID:22155738

Wade, V. A., Karnon, J., Elshaug, A. G., & Hiller, J. E. (2010). A systematic review of economic analyses of telehealth services using real time video communication. *BMC Health Services Research*, *10*(1), 233. doi:10.1186/1472-6963-10-233 PMID:20696073

Weiss, S. (2008). The need for a paradigm shift in addressing privacy risks in social networking applications. In The future of identity in the information society (pp. 161-171). Springer US. doi:10.1007/978-0-387-79026-8_12

Whitten, P., & Love, B. (2005). Patient and provider satisfaction with the use of telemedicine: Overview and rationale for cautious enthusiasm. *Journal of Postgraduate Medicine*, *51*(4), 294. PMID:16388172

Wootton, R. (2008). Telemedicine support for the developing world. *Journal of Telemedicine and Telecare*, *14*(3), 109–114. doi:10.1258/jtt.2008.003001 PMID:18430271

Xue, Y. & Liang, H. (2007). Analysis of telemedicine diffusion: the case of China. IEEE transactions on information technology in biomedicine. *IEEE Engineering in Medicine and Biology Society*, *11*(2), 231-233.

KEY TERMS AND DEFINITIONS

Developing Countries: Are countries with an underdeveloped industrial base, and low Human Development Index (HDI) relative to other countries.

Healthcare: Is the diagnosis, treatment, and prevention of disease, illness, injury, and other physical and mental impairments in human beings.

Information Exchange: Is the bidirectional information transmission/information transfer in telecommunications and computer science.

Information Technology (IT): Is the application of computers and telecommunications equipment to store, retrieve, transmit and manipulate data, often in the context of a business or other enterprise.

Technology Affinity: Is the natural attraction towards and liking of technology, including high acceptance and preference of using technology.

Telemedicine: Is the use of telecommunication and information technologies in order to provide clinical health care at a distance.

User Acceptance: Is the level of accepting or resisting new technologies or changes by users, measured through meeting their requirements and needs.

This work was previously published in Transforming Public Health in Developing Nations edited by Mohamud Sheikh, Aziza Mahamoud, and Mowafa Househ, pages 293-308 copyright year 2015 by Information Science Reference (an imprint of IGI Global).

Chapter 49

Use and Reuse of Electronic Health Records:
Building Information Systems for Improvement of Health Services

Michele Ceruti
University of Turin, Italy

Silvio Geninatti
Catholic University "Sacro Cuore", Italy & Statistics and Epidemiological Research, Italy

Roberta Siliquini
University of Turin, Italy

ABSTRACT

Electronic Health Record (EHR) is a term with several meanings, even if its very definition allows distinguishing it from other electronic records of healthcare interest, such as Electronic Medical Records (EMR) and Personal Health Records (PHR). EMR is the electronic evolution of paper-based medical records, while PHR is mainly the collection of health-related information of a single individual. All of these have many points in common, but the interchangeable use of the terms leads to several misunderstandings and may threaten the validity and reliability of EHR applications. EHRs are more structured and conform to interoperability standards, and include a huge quantity of data of very large populations. Thus, they have proven to be useful for both theoretical and practical purposes, especially for Public Health issues. In this chapter, the authors argue that the appropriate use of EHR requires a realistic comprehensive concept of e-health by all the involved professions. They also show that a change in the "thinking" of e-health is necessary in order to achieve tangible results of improvement in healthcare services through the use of EHR.

DOI: 10.4018/978-1-4666-8756-1.ch049

INTRODUCTION

Electronic records are being produced in several health contexts, mainly hospital, laboratory services, imaging services, insurance claims.

The aim of this chapter is to understand the nature of electronic health records, their subtypes, their expectations, the grey areas, those that need more clarification and disambiguation, the concerns about misuse and misinterpretation, highlighting the real potential for the ethical development of Information technology in healthcare.

As it has been stated (Habib, 2010), EHR technology is an important piece of health information technology infrastructure and is a cornerstone for reform health care systems across the world. EHR is an important tool for the improvement of health care quality, efficiency, and patient safety, diminishing research costs, decreasing the inefficiencies associated with paper based research and aligning research with implementation of new health technology devices. (Weiskopf & Weng, 2012).

Most countries are now focusing healthcare delivery through a health informatics strategy. EHR has been focused as the central power tool in most of the national e-health and HIT strategies, including telemedicine, personalized medicine, and large-scale genome analysis projects (Ruch, 2010).

DEFINITION OF EHR

A semantic problem that researchers, engineers and developers in the field of Health Technology will encounter if they intend to extend the research on the topic both in Biomedical and in Engineering literature is the confusion between EHR and other electronic records. We believe that the core of the correct evolution of such a vision with the patient at the centre of care delivery needs a clear definition of what is and what is not an "electronic health record".

According to the current literature, the definition of EHR is evolving and still confusing (Hayrinen, Saranto & Nykanen, 2008). Electronic health records may include all health-related information on electronic support: Electronic medical record (EMR), Personal health record (PHR) and Electronic personal record (EPR). All these terms are often used interchangeably, although there are huge differences between each of them. This confusion has been propagated not only by the scientific community but by governments, consultants and vendors as well. (Healthcare Information and Management Systems Society [HIMSS] 2006).

It is conceivable to consider "widely" all these as health electronic records but scientists, developers and users are confused by these interchangeable meanings. Electronic health records need first of all to be defined as clearly as possible, in order to avoid any confusion in its interpretation and application. This is the reason for which we call the attention to the following definitions and clarifications.

In 2008 the US National Alliance for Health Information Technology defined EHR, EMR and PHR as separate concepts (National Alliance for Health Information Technology, 2008):

Electronic Medical Record: *An electronic record of health-related information on an individual that can be created, gathered, managed, and consulted by authorized clinicians and staff within one healthcare organization.*

Electronic Health Record: *An electronic record of health-related information on an individual that conforms to nationally recognized interoperability standards and that can be created, managed, and consulted by authorized clinicians and staff across more than one healthcare organization.*

Personal Health Record: *An electronic record of health-related information on an individual that conforms to nationally recognized interoperability standards and that can be drawn from multiple sources while being managed, shared, and controlled by the individual.*

This is the first official precision that allowed not only to distinguish EHR from other codified (or defined) concepts such as EMR and PHR but moreover to define clearly that EHR are not any medical mass of unstructured data stored without standards or rules from any clearinghouse around the world or from user-produced extractions of health data through the web.

Other important health information data, which may be collected as unstructured health records, are the ones directly produced and controlled by Internet users. These data are the information substratum of the so defined e-health 2.0. and are substantially separated from health information produced by technologies within the official care delivery organizations. They might, instead, be integrated within the framework of Health IT in a further evolution of the vision of personal health, care delivery and legal policy for all their challenging and potentially hazardous consequences. Indeed, health information research by Internet customers showed some evidence of measurable effects on health behaviors, such as drug consumption and access to healthcare providers (Siliquini et al., 2011). The comprehensive influence in health behaviors induced by the growing user-generated health information data with the health 2.0 is still uncertain and need further investigations. At moment, it is impossible to merge this health information with the severely structured and controlled data of the official EHRs.

Disambiguation of EHR and EMR

Another important distinction to do in order to allow some clarity among electronic records related to health and health delivery is to clarify more precisely the differences between EHR and EMR.

In 2010, the Office of the National Coordinator for Health Information Technology (ONC) of the United States made an important distinction between the terms *EHR* and *EMR*.

"The EHR is the system that gives patients, physicians and other healthcare providers, employers, and payers or insurers access to a patient's medical records across facilities" (Garrett & Seidman, 2011), thus going beyond the restrictions and the geographical limitations, the mission of the healthcare provider and the possible fit-for-purpose health information technology system. It goes over the interpretation models applied within any single provider, allowing a more comprehensive patient history.

"The EMR is the legal patient record that is created in hospitals and ambulatory environments" (Garrett & Seidman, 2011). It is very important to note that EHR advances in quality, safety and accountability cannot be separated from the ones of EMR, as these are the main data source for EHR. Thus, the more EMR will be performing, well-built and predisposed to sharing, the more the portability and interoperability goals of EHR will be met, with higher quality accuracy of information gathered (The National Alliance for Health Information Technology, 2008). The collection from different EMRs is obviously enriching and depends on the policy of the national or regional EHR promoter.

As the term suggests in itself, EMR may be assumed as the electronic evolution of the "paper medical record". EMR may be unstructured, narrative, codified in several different ways according to the different services, uses and even habits. Clinicians, nurses, and administrative personnel produce EMRs. According to different countries it may be only a collection of clinical data or else a highly protected official legal document (but these differences are legally based on the different interpretation or use of the Medical records, electronic or not).

According to the Australian e-health Standards (2010), EHRs are information repositories that are "collected primarily to support the provision of integrated holistic healthcare to that individual but may also be used, subject to legislation and consent, for secondary purposes that benefit the health of the wider community".

The fundamental concept of a correct EHR is that it may be *sharable* and *comparable* with other collected health information. A further concept of EHR is *interoperability*. All these concepts are possible only if appropriate levels of standardization will be ensured.

EHR, according to official definitions that have been cited might be defined as any structured record that belongs to a official national or regional collector, through direct inputting or by extraction from medical databases. Specific rules must be followed, and data will be collected in information systems built according to official standards, and that may allow interoperability for further interpretation. (Habib, J. L., 2010)

The reason for which EHR models based on hospital information are much more prevalent across the world (rather than on primary care, ambulatory and laboratory settings) can be explained by the pre-existence of several structured EMR systems for hospitals. The transition from Paper Medical record, actually a medico-legal document that has been eminently recognized since a long time, has been much easier than the conception of the process care management taken by General Practitioners or by others health delivery actors. As for the management of in-patient data, formalized paper-based medical records are widely being used across the world, the shift to the electronic version has been less difficult. Actually, there are however quite a few complications that are directly connected with the construction of EHR. Conceptually EHR are indeed the electronic based evolution of a concept that is quite nearer to epidemiology databases and to health delivery management, but it is actually a tool primarily used for accountancy purposes, thus depleting it from its full potential (Hersh et al., 2013). A probable cause of this may be the need of a deeper underlying Public Health strategy. EHR may encourage the use of clinical decision support and for the use and evaluation of technologies. Vice versa the Health Technology Assessment Methodology may be enriched by EHR system.

While EMR models are expression of the health provider's policy or CDO's strategy, EHR seek to meet higher international semantic and architecture standards and aim to put the patient at the centre of data management. EHR data can be created, managed, and consulted by authorized providers across different health care organization. International aims are to build patient-centered EHR models in order to allow health data to move together with the patient whatever the health events he will come upon, such as medical encounters, hospitalization, home care delivery, nursing, etc. The international aspiration of EHR, such as it has been experienced in the US-India cooperation (Government Computer Based Patient Record Project [G-CPR], 1999) and in the EU, (epSOS - European Patients - Smart open Service), is to extend the *portability* (with all the standards concerning language, semantic, messaging, security, privacy) across different countries.

EHR STANDARDS

Standard documentation must guarantee the unique identification of subjects, processes (or even subprocesses), providers, devices, codified diagnosis, treatment and potentially final outcomes.

Very often, clinicians are called to apply to recommendation ensuring all of these standards. Albeit, the compliance to such standard application is not the primarily mission of clinicians. Healthcare practitioners are indeed more and more suffering from an excess of constraining rules in the compilation of electronic records. As it has been suggested above, a frequent bias is that health care personnel is thought to be involved directly with EHR, whereas what there are filling are mainly "Electronic Medical records", more and more frequently through IT systems that may ensure completeness and easiness of compilation. Now it is interesting to note that EMR may not be the simple translation of a paper record to a digital support. There is instead the need of professional development among the involved human resources in order to enhance their own **flexibility** toward the "filling" of electronic records. By such a use, they are also called to be accustomed to a greater rigor in both the identification of concepts that must be filled or transcribed in the EMR, especially in the different phases of the process of care (intermediate diagnosis and procedures) as well as in the identification of the final outcome, that shall be "matching" with logical predetermined fields or checks in templates (final diagnosis, setting the follow-up, etc.). All these are essential competencies that cannot be mastered passively by only applying routine tasks, but need purpose-built vocational training programs. The enhancement of e-health in healthcare services will become crucial in the following years, involving all professionals, especially nurses and health technicians. The capacity building of all these professionals is a core component for an appropriate integration of all e-health applications within healthcare services. The promotion of a new way of thinking health is an essential step for a proper skill acquisition among all involved actors (i.e. health workers) for the approach, the utilization and the management of electronic health information.

In order to promote the *interoperability* of health informatics applications, many frameworks for health informatics standards have been proposed and have been made available. According to Sinha (2013) the essential ones are:

- Structural standards.
- Data content standards.
- Data exchange standards.
- Security standards.

EN 13606 European Standard is the first EU official "structural" proposal for a rigorous and stable *architecture* for the communication

among partner and sharers of EHRs regarding any single subject of care. Through this standard, EHR building systems comprise two fundamental parts: a Root Architecture Component and a Record Component. The standards deal with Architecture, Domain Term Lists, Distribution Rules and Message for Information Exchange. The latter has been since 2006 the one that has influenced more deeply data exchange, through HL7 v3 standard, for the development of reliable and compatible paths for sharing information. This part of the EN 13606 explicitly focuses the possibility of rendering more easy the extraction of data from different environments, in observance of the ISO RM-ODP Information viewpoint for EHR Extract. This standards supports *interoperability* of different systems that need to transfer add or complete interchangeably without losing or overwriting previous messages, notes, preserving the privacy of attended by the health practitioner and the confidentiality of the patient towards data (see below for a WHO proposed distinction between privacy and confidentiality).

This standard is based also on the relatively new paradigm of "object" model for information sharing and does not restrict this modeling in the way the internal architecture and setting can be applied. The intention is to propose a guideline for designing or transforming EHR systems in a way that might not completely overwhelm the already existing health information systems through the building of a common set of external interfaces or communication procedures.

It is worth noting, however, that EN 13606 ignores ISO RM-ODP views towards behavioral aspects of EHR systems (Blobel, Engel & Pharow, 2006).

In the frame of HL7, *open*-EHR defines a method of querying based on archetypes, known as AQL (Archetype Querying Language). This is achieved by the innovation of 'multi-level modeling', whereby clinical content is standardized using a modeling layer known as 'archetypes' that is separate from the data standards layer. The openEHR foundation, integrating threads of R&D in Europe and Australia (openEHR, 2013), is an important example of such an application and implementation evolution of EN 13606. (Weiner, Fowles & Chan, 2012).

APPLICATIONS OF EHR

Databases actually contain both structured and unstructured information such as patient gender, age, diagnosis and treatment or event features, hospital admission, length of stay and, furthermore, social conditions, eating and drinking habits.

Several Institutes and Official Boards have appointed the *reuse* of EHR as the future instrument for clinical research, health delivery management, quality assessment but also decision making for health policy. Research communities in the field of clinical engineering, epidemiology and health management have been actively searching new methodologies for enable secondary use of electronic data, enhancing accuracy and accountability (Hersh et al., 2013).

In the classification of research areas of EHR proposed by Najaftorkaman, Ghapanchi, Talaei-Khoei and Ray (2013), two topics are addressed to application research: impacts in terms of healthcare improvement and medical research.

Healthcare Improvement

EHR for its very definition is already the output of a secondary use of EMR and of other electronic records. The concept that allows defining an EHR is actually the possibility of interoperability and reuse for any purpose. This reutilization may be interpreted both for profit and non-profit purposes.

In HIT (Health information technology) domain, reuse concerns the effort to optimize resources and investments particularly regarding software. High economic investments, performed technological research activities, sharing knowledge aims to support the necessity to assume reuse strategy.

Translating the concept of reuse, EHR availability enables a large opportunity for further interpretation and meta-interpretation in several scientific fields (Hripcsak, Albers, 2012). Health data reuse indeed has been focused as an e-government tool allowing both spending rationalization and more effective services supply (Blobel et al. 2006). Information is gathered in order to sustain adaptability of software development to customer needs, according to the fit-for use paradigm (Weiskopf & Weng, 2007; Hayrinen, Saranto & Nykanen 2008).

A topic that has led particular attention is the possibility to enhance the management and the monitoring of well-known and prevalent chronic diseases. In fact, during the last century the importance of chronic diseases has been expanding dramatically, especially in industrialized countries. Increased life expectancy, improved social and economic status, clinical care systems effective efforts to ensure better conditions, induces an increased risk for the general population to be affected from a chronic disease, thus inducing a continuous increase in health care spending for these conditions. Risk factors are quite known, mainly attributable to lifestyle like unhealthy diet, physical inactivity and tobacco and alcohol use. These causes do not work directly but through intermediate risk factors such as abnormal lipids level, raised blood pressure, impaired glucose levels and obesity. Still, others non-modifiable factors must be included like age and heredity. Moreover, a significant interaction between the major modifiable risk factors and the main chronic diseases has been observed in both low and high income countries and the impact of risk factors increases over the life course. All these information are potentially recordable in Health Information Systems. Acute or chronic complications and death associated to chronic diseases may be monitored through EHR. A valid support for monitoring hospitalization and follow-up of patients may be provided with information about the patient path within the hospital gathering main and secondary diagnoses, medical procedures or surgical interventions submission (according to ICD9-CM or ICD-10 classification according to different countries or to health delivery subset such as Medicare and Medicaid Program in the US).

Estimate occurrence, identify risk factors, evaluate potential determinants and precursors has began a core function of Public Health Institutions (Goldwater et al., 2013). Information related or perceived by patients such as health status, diet, tobacco and alcohol use, and physical activity may be gathered through electronic records together with evident clinical records such as blood pressure, body mass index (BMI), blood lipids level, and so on. Evidence based medicine approach implies the applications of effective procedures in diseases management. Guidelines collect recommendations about clinical management from best evidence based to provide health care through the application of diagnosis and therapeutic steps. EHR implementation may allow a better drug compliance of patients affected by hypertension or diabetes, the frequency of specific check-up, and a better appropriateness of healthcare services. Indeed, any clinical event may been recorded thus allowing the traceability of the whole disease history. Moreover EHR implementation for Public Health may allow the assessment of the impact of actions towards chronic disease monitoring and policies (Albu et al. 2013; Kudyakov et al., 2012; Maylahn, Fleming & Birkhead, 2013).

Medical Research

The most important field of medical research that has been involving actively EHR in the last years is the Comparative Effectiveness Research (CER). Applying an Evidence Based Medicine (EBM) approach through EHR is not incongruous, as Hersh et al (2013) have pointed out. EHR information elaboration may be considered as observational data analysis. In contrast to RCTs and EBM projects designed to focus on specific aspects in selected samples, EHR-based research

may much more reflective or real clinical world, because of the very large size of EHR, and much less expensive.

Use of EHR for Genomic information is under investigations. Several ethical (behavioral) and bioethical issues have been highlighted. Research may be profit of secondary use of existing EHR but it is obvious that fit for purpose model built especially and appropriately for the bimolecular and genomic research will be needed. Experts from the whole world are working together trying to merge all the methodology and the art in a unique apposite network (US eMERGE network -The Electronic Medical Records and Genomics Network).

Another interesting progress of e-health that will lead to evolutions in EHR applications is the implementation of Mobile Health (mHealth) systems, that will apply mobile communication technologies to healthcare delivery more efficiently (Zuehlke, Li, Talaei-Khoei & Ray, 2009). The convergence of progression of telemedicine, mHealth and other emerging health information technologies will make increasingly necessary the homogenization of electronic records both at coding and messaging levels.

CONCERNS AND LIMITS OF EHR

There are albeit increasing concerns about the limits of EHR use (Bernat 2013; Steers 2013). EHR information use is already offering several benefits, but they can also foster errors that would not have been possible with paper based information use. This phenomenon has been termed e-iatrogenesis (Weiner, Kfuri, Chan & Fowles, 2007).

Burnum (1989) stated that the introduction of information technology for health data gathering has allowed disposing to a greater amount of bad data rather than to data of improved quality.

An important statement proposed by van der Lei (1991) is that "data shall be used only for purpose for which they were collected" in order to avoid misuse and misinterpretation. The core of most of this concern is the "processing" of data. Research orientation, epidemiology assumption and public health decision are all based on interpretation of available health information. If this interpretation is human based, it may content several biases. It is obvious, however, that research have always been based not only on information collected through purpose-built investigative systems but often through manual retrieval of useful health information of medical records, claims, registries and so on. For these purposes, the formation of the researcher was very important, as he was called to seize and grasp when and where information are congruent with targets and goals of the research. (Weiskopf et al. 2013; Roukema et al., 2006).

Medication ordering and monitoring seem to be very sensitive to errors (that may be of interest also for the promotion of telemedicine and telecare). Two kind of errors have been highlighted: 1) simple errors such as duplicate medication orders. 2) complex errors due to error in human-EHR interface, mainly errors in data recognition and cognitive errors (Institute of Medicine, 2012; Ash et al., 2011).

These topics are increasingly of interest for risk management in healthcare. The rise of simplicity of collect gather and retrieve data will be accompanied by an increase of the complexity of the "possible" errors as well of the complexity of algorithms, techniques and preventive measures against that risk.

In 1984, Horwitz and Yu reported three kinds of data-recording errors:

- Conflicting data in the source text;
- Information not transcribed;
- Transcription errors (i.e. errors during transcription).

This classification is clear and pragmatic, but is quite old as it does not take into account the possibility of the immediate filling of health records, bypassing the need for transcription to file.

Weiner, Fowles and Chan (2012) have proposed more recently three main electronic record related errors in their e-QM EHR quality measure:

- Incorrect medication ascribable to HIT-related errors in the CPOE/e-prescribing process;
- Erroneous sentinel event impacting in patient management;
- Not received automatically EHR system based e-notification resulting in patient harm.

There is another important distinction between error of omission (lack of completeness) and error of commission (lack of correctness)

As discussed by Weiskopf, Hripcsak, Swaminathan and Weng (2013) the complex issue of EHR completeness overtakes the statistical view of data missing. This is even more considerable because of the heterogeneity of EHR information source.

Lacks of EHRs related to a single patient during a period of time may be actually a error due to one of the following reasons:

1. There may be a lack in the information system of the EHR: for example the patient may have accessed a health provider that is connected with the EHR system.
2. The provider that should have collected the record has not accomplished correctly, partially or totally his mission.
3. There is the actual absence of medical encounter: this is known also as "extrinsic incompleteness" and may be due both to the actual healthy condition of the index subject (there is no reason for a medical encounter) or may be due to:
   a. Objective ignorance of the unhealthy condition;
   b. Subjective misperception of the unhealthy condition;
   c. Objective refusal, impossibility or renounce of the patient to access any health provider (this is possible in case of follow-up or secondary encounter).

This last possibility is much easier in countries where health services are paid for by third parts (Bernat, 2013).

Other dimensions of completeness have been investigated, (Blobel, 2006) but are specific objects of EMRs of healthcare providers, such as granular completeness and task-dependent completeness. As it has been highlighted, granularity and precision of electronic sources of EHRs are an important target for development of EHR consistency and reliability, however there are not specific feature that may be focused at that higher level.

Healthcare systems tend now especially in United Europe to develop platforms of cooperation and networks for which interoperability is highly necessary. EHR systems must meet first of all requirements of *flexibility* and *interoperability* through semantic integration.

The Governmental Computer-based patient Record (G-CPR) has been an important international effort concluded in 2003 that involved the US Department of Defense, the US Department of Veterans Affairs and the Indian Health Service trying to adhere to HL7 standards and to enable bi-directional secure sharing of patient health information among international participating agencies through the implementation of purpose built environments (GPCR, 2001). This is an example of fit for purpose EHR ideation, that has aimed to adhere to international standards and helped to the identification of critical points.

ETHICAL ISSUES

Most of ethical issues raised by EHR use and in implementing strategies involving EMR and health delivery data management as well, were already seen with paper records. Therefore, ease of access, transmission and sharing have elicited more risk of violation of patient confidentiality, privacy and misuse of sharing (Bernat, 2013; Burnum, 1989).

According to what stated by WHO in 2012, the concepts of privacy and confidentiality are defined referring to the way of relationship between the parts involved with a sensitive information.

In particular, EHR *privacy* reflects both the interest of the involved person as well of the public as a stakeholder to keep the information safe, away from any third party view.

EHR *confidentiality* concerns the degree to which the subject allows to share the information with relatives and other people with trusted relationship, as well as the government and application of such a rule, according to different laws and formalized codes.

Research models are focusing the attention on how to enhance patient-centered EHR evolution and amelioration keeping intact the standards improving reliability keeping confidentiality. Practical examples have been developed through problem-oriented approach aiming to a multi-professional electronic patient record (De Clercq, 2008).

In the field of EMR, "copying and pasting" issues have been illustrated by Thielke (2007) that provoked as well ambiguities of authorship with associated medico-legal concerns. There is no doubt that this problem has always existed, has been enlarged by first implementation of electronic records at hospital, primary care and other health providers and might have undermined derived EHR, but may be overcome by templates in which specification are mandatory and by second and third level quality controls. The challenging question is whether it is better to prefer a rigid template or a flexible format. This is the dilemma between *flexibility* and *uniformity* of data, that has been underpinned by Los, Ginneken, Roukema, Moll and van der Lei (2005): the advance of health data information availability may be accompanied by a lost in details, uniformity tending to lower quality data, too schematic and too synthetic with the hazard of artificial information.

Computerized Physician Order Entry (CPOE) users may not be satisfied by the possibility displayed, according to what found in the clinical findings; this issue is obviously more consistent for medical history and physical examination signs. Doctors and nurses may fill directly records of concluding judgment and to be inclined to prefer normal findings. In order to prevent this issue, it has been suggested (and already implemented) to separate rigidly findings from interpretations in separate format of the grid. (Los et al. 2005). Another problem is that checkboxes, very often associated for the filling the EMRs do not conceive all the degrees of subtlety of the clinical information. Indeed rigid templates may induce a more subjective derive and to avoid circumlocutory and bombastic language, not always associated to specific and distinguishable definition or feature. Another EMR-related pitfall is the presence of excess of rigidity built around the chief complaint that is an important voice for EHR. Indeed, some EMR allow automatically generated grid of questions from the selected chief complaint, potentially misleading the patient, especially in the case of multidisciplinary patient management (for example if a nurse or a trainee manage choices a misleading chief complaint according to symptoms and situation to specialty or to diagnostic services in hospitals as well as in primary care centers).

Threats in *pre populated data* have been raised (Bernat, 2005) as they can automatically be inserted, especially for laboratory or image reports if not validated by the health staff, may induce to automatically generated indication to further unnecessary in-depth examinations, exams or consultations or even handovers, sometimes hazardous.

The discharge summary may provide a clear understanding of exactly what has been done, why it has been done, the reasoning of the physicians leading to the formulation of conclusion and the proposal of the treatment plan or the follow-up. EHR purposes of interoperability, especially across countries might be set up, especially for trans-language classification or horizon scanning of archetype model implementation.

As it has been stressed, good EHR presume good EMR. But another limit of current electronic system in health provider, especially the most advanced in granularity, request much more time in front of the computer than in front of the patient. Patient-physician relationship, which is at the heart of good health delivery, may be suffering more deeply from this problem that might be increasing. Possible solutions may be to predispose the dedication of a health worker to the compilation of the Information Technology System (that may be aggregated into EHRs), possibly under dictation of the health practitioner (doctor, nurse or technician) performing the health action; another solution may be the development of advanced interpretation system of the unstructured field. This latter is actually under deep R&D actions, but has till now produced only unsatisfactory results (Weiner et al. 2012; Kahn, Raebel, Glanz, Riedlinger & Steiner, 2012; Spriggs, Arnold, Pearce & Fry, 2012).

It has been raised that attention to EHR may decrease attention to patients (Balka E, Tolar M, 2011). Indeed, well-built electronic records systems may help reminding the user in all the possible granularity, not to forget the parts of the medical history, of the physical examination and the collection of useful preventive medicine information, such as drugs, alcohol consumption, smoke etc (Burnum, 1989). As it was already emphasized, these features are particularly important for EHR-based healthcare improvement, especially for the management of chronic diseases.

There is finally the risk of a gradual evolution of EMR and EHR from being a tool for quality improvement and promotion to becoming a tool for a better compliance to national, mutual fund or assuring reimbursement goals (Bernat, 2013). In other words, a shift of EHR use from quality enhancement tool to performance monitoring tool. This may be a threatening deviance if such a use will not be balanced by a major attention to tempering the conflict between patient and policy regulatory interests, defending the paradigm of time for patients against time consumed in front of the technologies (computer and devices as such).

FUTURE DIRECTIONS AND CONCLUSION

The ability to achieve a wide and correct use of EHR will become increasingly important in both developed and developing countries. (Legal frameworks for e-health, WHO, 2012). The target of a performing use in developed countries is to help with the provision of health through adequate tools for the growing old population, deals with the enhancement of connection with and through health providers, promoting the shift of health delivery outside the hospital, but outside the traditional General Practitioner setting as well, and through the integration of pre existing home-centered services, as support of realistic patient empowerment models, in order to chase in a sustainable way the goals of equity, safety and efficiency.

In developing countries, EHR are actually emerging, sometimes becoming the structural framework of health delivery and of the management of needs according to available resources and in which introduction of e-health solutions are increasingly successful.

Indeed EHR models are more and more connected with pay-for-performance programs, especially where these are more advanced such as in the US for Medicare and Medicaid Program (Health IT Gov, 2013), and in Australia (Australian e-health standards, 2010) where such EHR use is actually under discussion for General Practitioners.

There is wide agreement about the various and growing benefits of EHR for healthcare services, especially in terms of promotion of effectiveness,

quality enhancement, and cost containment. Engineering, Informatics, Biostatics and Public Health Professionals should address these challenges together. An important advance in this direction is the evolving implementation of EHR information in Comparative effectiveness research (Hersh et al, 2013).

As it has been highlighted in the chapter, another very important question, both for theoretical and practical progress, is the consensus for coding and messaging EHR standards. This may facilitate the integration between the different forms of evolution of the e-health, as telemedicine, mHealth and the personalized genomic medicine.

A proper appraisal of the challenges of EHR and of all the electronic data requires a correct interpretation of the e-health. Thus, because of the evolving complexity of Informatics and Electronic applications for healthcare, this appraisal cannot be reached without the promotion of a change in the "thinking" of the e-health among all healthcare practitioners.

ACKNOWLEDGMENT

The authors would like to thank the anonymous reviewers and the editor for their insightful comments and suggestions and are gratefully indebted with the Library of the Department of Public Health and Pediatrics of the University of Turin, for greatly contributing to retrieving bibliographic references for this work.

REFERENCES

Albu, J., Sohler, N., Matti-Orozco, B., Sill, J., Baxter, D., Burke, G., & Young, E. (2013). Expansion of electronic health record-based screening, prevention, and management of diabetes in New York City. *Preventing Chronic Disease*, *10*, E13. doi:10.5888/pcd10.120148 PMID:23369766

Almond, H., Cummings, E., & Turner, P. (2013). Australia's personally controlled electronic health record and primary healthcare: Generating a framework for implementation and evaluation. *Studies in Health Technology and Informatics, 188*, 1–6. PMID:23823280

Ash, J., Kilo, C. M., Shapiro, M., Wasserman, J., McMullen, C., & Hersh, W. (2011). *Roadmap for Provision of Safer Healthcare Information Systems: Preventing e-Iatrogenesis.* Institute of Medicine.

Australian e-health standards. (2010). *Electronic Health Record Interoperability.* Available at http://www.e-health.standards.org.au/IT014SubjectAreas/EHRInteroperability.aspx

Bernat, J. L. (2013). Ethical and quality pitfalls in electronic health records. *Neurology, 80*(11), 1057-61 doi:.10.1212/WNL.0b013e318287288c

Blobel, B. (2005). Advances in secure and architectural EHR approaches. *International Journal of Medical Informatics, 75*(3-4), 185–190. Epub 2005 Aug 19 doi:10.1016/j.ijmedinf.2005.07.017 PMID:16112891

Burnum, J. F. (1989). The misinformation era: The fall of the Medical Record. *Annals of Internal Medicine, 110*, 482–484. doi:10.7326/0003-4819-110-6-482 PMID:2919852

CEN. ISO 13606 standard. The EN 13606 Association. (2009-2011). Retrieved September 29, 2013 from www.en13606.org

De Clerq, E. (2008). Problem-oriented patient record model as a conceptual foundation for a multi-professional electronic patient record. *International Journal of Medical Informatics, 77*(9), 565–575. doi:10.1016/j.ijmedinf.2007.11.002 PMID:18248847

Garets, D., & Davis, M. (2006, January 26). *Electronic medical records vs. electronic health records: yes, there is a difference.* HIMSS Analytics. Retrieved 2013, September 28, from: http://www.himssanalytics.org/docs/wp_emr_ehr.pdf

Garrett, P., & Seidman, J. (2011). US Department of Health & Human Services. *EMR vs EHR – What is the Difference?* Retrieved 2013, September 28, from: http://www.healthit.gov/buzz-blog/electronic-health-and-medical-records/emr-vs-ehr-difference/

Gibbons, P. (2007). Health Level Seven EHR Interoperability Work Group. *Coming to terms: Scoping Interoperability for Health Care.* Retrieved 2013, October 2, from: http://www.hln.com/assets/pdf/Coming-to-Terms-February-2007.pdf

Goldwater, J.C., Kwon, N.J., Nathanson, A., Muckle, A.E., Brown, A., &Cornejo, K. (2013). Open source electronic health records and chronic disease management. *Journal of American Medical Informatics Association.* doi: 11367ami-ajnl-2013-001672

Habib, J. L. (2010). EHRs, meaningful use, and a model EMR. *Drug Benefit Trends, 22*(4), 99–101.

Hayrinen, K., Saranto, K., & Nykanen, P. (2008). Definition, structure, content, use and impacts of electronic health records: A review of the research literature. *International Journal of Medical Informatics, 77*, 291–304. doi:10.1016/j.ijmedinf.2007.09.001 PMID:17951106

Hersh, W. R., Cimino, J., Payne, P. R.O., Embi, P., Logan, J., Weiner, M., Bernstam, E. V., Lehmann, H., Hripcsak, G., Hartzog, T., & Saltz, J. (2013). Recommendations for the use of operational Electronic Health Record data in comparative effectiveness research. *eGEMs, 1*(1), Article 14. DOI: 10.13063/2327-9214.1018

Hripcsak, G., & Albers, D. J. (2012). Next-generation phenotyping of electronic health records. *Journal of the American Medical Informatics Association, 0*, 1–5. doi:10.1136/amiajnl-2012-001145 PMID:22955496

ICD-10. (2010). *International Classification of ICD*. Available at: http://www.who.int/classifications/icd/en/

ICD-9-CM. (2011). International Classification of Diseases, Ninth Revision, Clinical Modification. Available at http://www.cdc.gov/nchs/icd/icd9cm.htm#ftp

Institute of Medicine (IOM). (2012). *Health IT and Patient Safety: Building Safer Systems for Better Care*. Washington, DC: The National Academies Press.

ISO 18308 Conformance. (n.d.). *OpenEHR Foundation*. Retrieved September 29, 2013 from http://www.openehr.org

Joellenbeck, L. M., Russell, P. K., & Guze, S. B. (Eds.), *Strategies to Protect the Health of Deployed US Forces* (pp. 79–82). Washington, DC: National Academy Press.

Kahn, M. G., Raebel, M. A., Glanz, J. M., Riedlinger, K., & Steiner, J. F. (2012). A pragmatic framework for single-site and multisite data quality assessment in electronic health record-based clinical research. *Medical Care, 50*, S21–S29. doi:10.1097/MLR.0b013e318257dd67 PMID:22692254

Kalra, D. (2006). Electronic Health Standards. *IMIA Yearbook of Medical Informatics, 45*(Suppl1), S136–S144.

Kudyakov, R., Bowen, J., Ewen, E., West, S. 1., Daoud, Y., Fleming, N., & Masica, A. (2012). Electronic health record use to classify patients with newly diagnosed versus preexisting type 2 diabetes: infrastructure for comparative effectiveness research and population health management. *Population Health Management, 15*(1), 3–11. doi:10.1089/pop.2010.0084 PMID:21877923

Los, R. K., van Ginneken, A. M., Roukema, J., Moll, H. A., & van der Lei, J. (2005)... *Medical Informatics and the Internet in Medicine, 30*(4), 267–276. doi:10.1080/14639230500367563 PMID:16531353

Maylahn, C., Fleming, D., & Birkhead, G. (2013). Health departments in a brave new world. *Preventing Chronic Disease, 10*, E41. doi:10.5888/pcd10.130003 PMID:23517584

Medicare and Medicaid EHR Incentive Programs. (2013). Available at http://www.healthit.gov/providers-professionals/ehr-incentive-programs

Najaftorkaman, M., Ghapanchi, A. H., Talaei-Khoei, A., & Ray, P. (2013). Recent research areas and grand challenges in Electronic Health Record: A Literature survey approach. *The International Technology Management Review, 3*(1), 12–21. doi:10.2991/itmr.2013.3.1.2

Office of the National Coordinator for Health Information Technology (ONC). (2013). *Health IT Policy Committee: Recommendations to the National Coordinator for Health IT*. Retrieved September 12, 2013 from http://www.healthit.gov/policy-researchers-implementers/health-it-policy-committee-recommendations-national-coordinator-heal

Ruch, P. (2010). Section Editor for the IMIA Yearbook Section on Decision Support Systems. Findings from the yearbook 2010 section on decision support systems. *IMIA Yearbook of Medical Information, 2010*, 55–57.

Siliquini, R. (2011). Surfing the internet for health information: an italian survey on use and population choices. *BMC Medical Informatics and Decision Making*, (11), 21. doi:10.1186/1472-6947-11-21 PMID:21470435

Sinha, P. K., Sunder, G., Bendale, P., Mantri, M. D., & Dande, A. C. (2013). *Electronic Health Record. Standards, Coding Systems, Frameworks, and Infrastructure. Wiley*. IEEE Press.

Steers, W. D. (2013). The Electronic Medical Record: How Not to Communicate. *The Journal of Urology, 190*(5), 1636–1637. doi:10.1016/j.juro.2013.08.003 PMID:23933460

The National Alliance for Health Information Technology. (2008). *Report to the Office of the National Coordinator for Health Information Technology on Defining Key Health Information Technology Terms*. Retrieved September 12, 2013 at http://hitechanswers.wpengine.netdna-cdn.com/wp-content/uploads/2013/05/NAHIT-Definitions2008.pdf

US eMERGE network The Electronic Medical Records and Genomics (eMERGE) Network. (n.d.). Retrieved from http://emerge.mc.vanderbilt.edu/

Weiner, J. P., Fowles, J., & Chan, K. S. (2012). New paradigms for measuring clinical performance using electronic health records. *International Journal for Quality in Health Care, 24*(3), 200–205. doi:10.1093/intqhc/mzs011 PMID:22490301

Weiskopf, N. G., Hripcsak, G., Swaminathan, S., & Weng, C. (2013). Defining and measuring completeness of electronic health records for secondary use. *Journal of Biomedical Informatics, 46*, 830–836. doi:10.1016/j.jbi.2013.06.010 PMID:23820016

Weiskopf, N. G., & Weng, C. (2013). Methods and dimensions of electronic health record data quality assessment: enabling reuse for clinical research. *Journal of the American Medical Informatics Association, 20*(1), 144–151. doi:10.1136/amiajnl-2011-000681 PMID:22733976

WHO. (2012). Legal frameworks for e-health. Global observatory for ehealth series – Vol.5.

Zuehlke, P., Li, J. H., Talaei-Khoei, A., & Ray, P. (2009). A functional specification for mobile eHealth (mHealth) systems. In *Proceedings of E-Health Networking, Applications and Services*. IEEE.

KEY TERMS AND DEFINITIONS

Data Reuse: Use of data for purpose other than the one for which it was originally created.

Electronic Health Record: An electronic record of health-related information that conforms to interoperability standards allowing its creation, gathering and management across different healthcare organizations.

Electronic Medical Record: The electronic version of the paper-based medical record containing health information about a patient in one healthcare organization.

Health Information Technology: The technology for the creation, management and secure exchange of health information in an electronic environment across computerized systems for healthcare settings.

Healthcare Services: Services delivered to patients for the diagnosis and treatment of diseases and the maintenance of health.

Interoperability: The ability of a system to work together with other systems through a successful interpretation of the exchanged data.

Medical Confidentiality: The privacy and protection against unauthorized disclosure of information arising from any contact with healthcare services or professionals.

Public Health: The science and art of preventing diseases, promoting health and prolonging healthy life in a population through health education, directions for health policy and research.

This work was previously published in Healthcare Informatics and Analytics edited by Madjid Tavana, Amir Hossein Ghapanchi, and Amir Talaei-Khoei, pages 212-226 copyright year 2015 by Medical Information Science Reference (an imprint of IGI Global).

Chapter 50

Nurses Using Social Media and Mobile Technology for Continuing Professional Development:
Case Studies from Australia

Carey Mather
University of Tasmania, Australia

Elizabeth Cummings
University of Tasmania, Australia

ABSTRACT

Continuing professional development is mandatory for all healthcare professionals in Australia. This chapter explores how the expectations of the regulatory and professional organisations of nursing and midwifery can be integrated within the profession by enrolled and registered nurses and midwives to meet the requirements and maintain their registrations. Using actual case studies as a basis, the chapter demonstrates how continuing professional development can be delivered as mobile or m-learning using social media or mobile technologies within this health profession. This chapter focuses on case studies from the Australian healthcare sector; however, it appears that similar issues arise in other countries and so the challenges and solutions described in the case studies can inform practice in other countries. It concludes by discussing the potential for continuing professional development m-learning into the future.

INTRODUCTION

Health professionals use a complex network of communication strategies to share important information within professions and multidisciplinary teams to improve patient or client outcomes and ensure high quality care is safely delivered. Building on the ubiquitous use of a variety of communication strategies can transform how continuing professional development (CPD) is delivered and accessed. By extending communication beyond the borders of the workplace it is

DOI: 10.4018/978-1-4666-8756-1.ch050

possible to improve access and enable a flexibility that is unprecedented. Regulatory authorities have provided direction and scope regarding what CPD is and how it can be achieved.

Social media and the use of mobile technologies is the way of the future for CPD of health professionals. CPD is mandatory for the 580,000 health professionals registered by the Australian Health Practitioner Regulation Agency (AHPRA). Annual evidence of compliance with the CPD Standard for each health profession is required to ensure competence is maintained. CPD is essential for health professionals to be contemporary in their knowledge and use best practice to ensure high quality and safe care. Additionally, it provides opportunities for practitioners to be exposed to innovation within their field. There are other less tangible benefits that include opportunities for interdisciplinary collaboration and networking with colleagues.

CONTINUING PROFESSIONAL DEVELOPMENT

In Australia, AHPRA regulates the practice of 15 health professional bodies, all members of which are required to undertake CPD on an annual basis. Each profession has its own standards, codes, guidelines and policies that describe the requirements necessary to meet AHPRA requirements for maintaining registration within the profession (AHPRA, 2013).

The Nursing and Midwifery Board of Australia (NMBA) is the professional body for nurses and midwives and they define continuing professional development or CPD as:

...the means by which members of the profession maintain, improve and broaden their knowledge, expertise and competence, and develop personal and professional qualities required through their professional lives. (NMBA, 2013, p1)

The NMBA CPD Registration Standard prescribes that there must be documented evidence of a minimum number of hours of CPD undertaken each year or per triennium, in areas relevant to the health professional (NMBA, 2013). It describes acceptable CPD activities that may be undertaken. CPD may include formal courses, conferences, or online learning. Self-directed programs that are planned and developed by individuals are acceptable provided they include reflection. Nurses are required to keep written documentation and verified evidence of compliance within a personal portfolio (NMBA, 2013).

The NMBA CPD Registration Standard supports a range of activities that can be undertaken as e-learning, using social media or mobile technologies (NMBA, 2013). The development of a range of digital technologies and the growth of social media ensure mobile technologies are well positioned over time to replace traditional learning and teaching models of CPD. Development and delivery of CPD opportunities to health professionals is only limited by imagination about the utility of social media and mobile technology as a strategy for achieving CPD requirements.

CPD is embedded within each of the Australian Nursing and Midwifery Council (ANMC, now NMBA) competency domains (ANMC, 2006). It is encapsulated in critical thinking and analysis (Domain 3, Element 4) that states nurses will "participate in ongoing professional development of self and others" (ANMC, 2006: p4).

Health informatics and health technology competency is now included in Standard 4 about program content of the Australian Nursing and Midwifery Council (ANMAC) Standards (ANMAC, 2012). ANMAC is the independent accrediting authority responsible for monitoring education providers and nursing and midwifery programs of study leading to registration or professional endorsement in Australia. There are accreditation assessment standards that must be attained to be authorised to develop curricula and assess student performance (ANMAC,

2012). Information communication technology (ICT) competency is now embedded in each of the nine standards. They were written with the expectation that stakeholders will facilitate and provide the means to support the development of ICT literacy of student nurses. Additionally, ICT competency standards for Australia are currently being developed (Borycki, Foster, Sahama, Frisch, & Kushniruk, 2013; Staggers, Gassert, & Curran, 2002). The inclusion of health informatics and health technology has major implications for delivery of CPD using social media and mobile technologies with the current enrolled and registered nurse and midwifery workforce. CPD using m-learning approaches will need to focus on developing appropriate knowledge and skills of the current workforce in using this technology. Whereas the focus for new graduates will be ensuring they understand the legal and ethical implications of embedding these emerging technologies into their career and professional development.

Whilst the requirement for CPD is mandatory for all Australian healthcare professionals, this chapter is limited to discussion of the possibilities for enrolled and registered nurses, and midwives – referred to as healthcare professionals. It explores how the expectations of the regulatory and professional organisations of nursing and midwifery can be integrated within the profession by enrolled and registered nurses and midwives to meet the requirements and maintain their registrations. Furthermore, this chapter discusses the background to the current situation and using case studies from Australia will demonstrate how CPD can be delivered as m-learning using social media or mobile technologies within this health profession. It appears that similar issues arise in other countries and so the challenges and solutions of using social media and mobile technologies within health care settings may be transferrable.

TERMINOLOGY CONSIDERATIONS

There is a lack of standard definitions for describing terminology in informatics that enables easy discussion about using social media and mobile technology for CPD (Georgiev, Georgieva, & Smrikarov, 2004; Ruiz, Mintzer, & Leipzig, 2006). For the purpose of this chapter information communication technology is used to describe all branches of informatics and digital media. Sub-groupings of health informatics also known as e-health and refers to clinical and health service delivery hardware, middleware and software. Health technology refers to web-based software and mobile applications to diagnose, monitor, treat or educate end-users. Kaplan and Haenlein (2010; 60) define Social media as "a group of internet-based applications that build on ideological and technological foundations of Web 2.0. and that allow the creation and exchange of User Generated Content". This definition encompasses a range of applications that include Facebook, YouTube, Flickr, Twitter and Instagram. New applications are constantly being created that include varying levels of social presence, media richness, self presentation and self-disclosure (Kaplan and Haenlein 2010). These classifications impact on the way social media is viewed in the literature. This description satisfactorily defines social media in this chapter.

M-health is a sub-grouping of e-health that relates to any mobile technology or computing used to interface with any stakeholder group involved with digital health service delivery or care (WHO, 2011). E-learning encompasses pedagogical frameworks that use the digital mediums for delivery and interaction. M-learning refers specifically to learning and teaching interaction that uses mobile hand-held devices such as electronic notebooks, tablets or smartphones (Traxler, 2007). The use of the term connected health to describe digitally mediated healthcare by Wicklund (2013) has merit. Over time there will no longer be the need to distinguish ICT in health from mobile technology used to as a platform to learn in this environment.

The current lack of standard definitions to describe social media and mobile technologies requires further exploration. Consideration of the terms used and standardisation of terminology would improve communication and clarify meaning for researchers, health service providers, educators and other end-users of this emerging technology.

AUSTRALIAN POLICY DEVELOPMENT

There has been a significant increase in the development and use of ICT in healthcare at individual and systems levels (Abbott & Coenen, 2008; Smedley, 2005; While & Dewsberry, 2011). The rapid change in healthcare delivery and communication models has implications for different healthcare settings. A number of challenges and potential solutions in relation to meeting the needs of stakeholders within the healthcare sector in Australia have been outlined in the Australian National E-Health Strategy (Australian Health Ministers' Conference, 2008). An ICT skilled health workforce was identified as a key resource required to drive change and the adoption of technological solutions.

There is a requirement for the higher education sector and professional bodies to encourage and support their students and health professionals in gaining high quality educational experiences that support this changing environment (Bembridge, Levett-Jones, & Yeun-Sim Jeong, 2011; MacKay & Harding, 2009). Therefore, the development and provision of educational programs that meet and extend the demand and transference of ICT skills in the Australian workplace is imperative. Additionally, digital platforms provide flexibil-

ity and e-learning CPD opportunities that were unavailable before the advent of the Australian Government's 'Digital Education Revolution' (DEEWR, 2008).

The introduction of the Australian Government's 'Digital Education Revolution' policy (2008) is particularly relevant to e-learning, CPD and the use of social media and mobile technologies (DEEWR, 2008). The policy reorientated secondary school students for post-secondary education and training, by routinely introducing them to digital media technologies (DEEWR, 2008; White, 2008). Literature regarding the use of digital technology in tertiary institutions, especially universities, suggests introducing students to the technology prior to attending the experiential environment (ALTC, 2008; Kenny, Neste-Kenny, Park, Burton, & Meiers, 2009; Mather, 2012b). By enabling the current nursing workforce to develop knowledge and skills in the use of social media and mobile technologies it is possible to foster collaboration and create opportunities to integrate student knowledge, skills and expectations to promote collegiality. Furthermore, offering m-learning CPD opportunities that are accessible within the clinical workplace can be used as a vehicle to model and engender life-long learning required by the profession (ACN, 2013a).

The capacity for health professionals to use digital platforms for CPD is mixed. There are a number of factors that currently impede or improve the likelihood of engagement of health professional use of mobile technologies for CPD (Mather, Marlow, & Cummings, 2013a). Reducing or minimising the barriers to using mobile platforms has the potential to globalise the health professions and create unprecedented inter-professional collaboration and CPD opportunities. By harnessing the capacity of digital technologies for CPD has the ability to accelerate the implementation of the national digital E-health strategy, meet the aims of ANMAC and support the aims and philosophy of the ANMC competency standards.

If the tertiary nursing education curriculum is to remain responsive to the changing clinical workplace environment and meet the needs of current and future nurses there is a need to develop, monitor and evaluate the usefulness of these emerging technologies within the clinical nursing environment. Furthermore, CPD opportunities must match current needs and plan for future requirements of nurses who work in a variety of urban and rural settings within Australia.

SPECIFIC CPD REQUIREMENTS FOR NURSES

The Nursing and Midwifery Board of Australia (NMBA, 2013) mandates that nurses and midwives registered in Australia will participate in at least 20 hours of CPD per year in each category. The NMBA CPD Registration Standard also prescribes that one hour of active learning will equal one hour of CPD. The CPD must be relevant to the nurse's context of practice. The standard also provides detailed information about the documentation required to enable it to be used as evidence. There is recommendation of the use of a portfolio for capturing elements required for completion of the CPD cycle (NMBA, 2013).

As clinical informatics becomes widespread within nursing environments there is an expectation that nurses are already, or will become familiar with e-health and m-health technologies as they are developed and implemented in the workplace. The personally controlled electronic health record (PCEHR) is an example of the Australian e-health strategy initiative (DoHA, 2013) that requires clinicians and consumers to have a functional understanding of computer and internet use. Nurses are expected to be advocates and assist potential registrants in becoming part of this user-centric mobile technology assisted initiative.

CPD in relation to the use of digital technologies is paramount to support clinicians in developing the necessary technical skills to undertake their role and function as nurses. Developing digitally supported CPD meets both the process and content requirements to be competent in decision-making regarding the use of digital technology. Digital technology, especially mobile platforms are easily accessible and can be used to meet CPD registration requirements. While accessing digital technology to complete CPD is not new, using mobile technology to deliver m-learning CPD through this media channel will become more popular. It will be multimedia supported, easily accessible, with flexible modes of delivery in real-time at workplaces.

IMPACT ON CPD OPPORTUNITIES

Workforce Considerations

Currently, CPD may be initiated by an individual health professional, facilitated by a supervisor or provided by an institution and undertaken or delivered at different levels (Lorenzo & Ittelson, 2005; Mason, Pegler, & Weller, 2004). Ownership of CPD can be invested with individuals, supervisors or companies (Lorenzo & Ittelson, 2005). However, within this framework there are workplace factors that impede CPD using traditional delivery models. These limitations include shift work, part-time employment, recreation leave, staffing skill mix and patient or client workload that make consistent, flexible or easy delivery of learning and teaching to support CPD difficult in the workplace (Mather, 2011, 2012b; Mather & Marlow, 2012). Additionally, geographic isolation can compound equity of access to CPD opportunities (Mather & Marlow, 2012). The advent of digital technologies and the growth of m-learning technologies is an attractive alternative for the development of e-learning CPD opportunities.

The expansion of CPD opportunities using social media and mobile technologies provides opportunities for health professionals bridge gaps of health technology knowledge and skills in the workplace. Use of social media and mobile technologies could enable health professionals to learn in situ, without the need for face-to-face tuition. Instruction on how to use new equipment or software could be undertaken remotely. Health professionals could obtain instructions from a supervisor as required, while learning how to master new skills or behaviour or gain feedback about performance (Kuiz et al., 2006). Additionally, the availability for browsing multimedia information for learning or being reminded about a topic could occur quickly and easily if access was provided by an organisation. Point and shoot collection of objects and artefacts could facilitate access to expert advice or opinion rapidly on a global scale. Observation or recording of activities could be undertaken for discussion, reflection or peer review after completion (Ruiz et al., 2006; While & Dewsberry, 2011). Mobile technology offers learners the opportunity to have control over the content, pace of learning and enable them to individualise their learning objectives. There is also potential for collaborative learning with health professionals from the same and different fields. Encouragement to collaborate to meet CPD requirements could be facilitated by organisations by supporting access to mobile devices and provision of easy access to data delivery (Kenny et al., 2009; Ruiz et al., 2006).

Generational Cohort Considerations

Brunetto, Farr-Wharton and Shacklock (2012) describe generational cohort differences that may influence the use of the digital media strategies for CPD. The average age of registered nurses in Australia, as with many countries, is increasing to the extent that in 2011 the average age was 44.4 years and 22% of all nurses were aged over 55 years (HWA, 2013a). Experienced registered nurses are more likely to be Baby Boomers or Generation X clinicians. These generations are acknowledged to be less likely to use digital technology for communication (Brunetto et al.,

2012; Windham, 2005) which may limit their uptake of e-learning opportunities. Mather et al. (2013b) identified that registered nurses need to be educationally prepared in ICT skills to be able to confidently engage in sharing information that would facilitate CPD.

Nelsey and Brownie (2012) describe the values and needs of Baby Boomers, X and Y generations that represent a large component of the nursing workforce (HWA, 2013a). Career aspirations of these groups are important when considering CPD opportunities and how social media or mobile technology could be adopted and integrated into their learning culture. Baby Boomers value learning and training opportunities while Generation X enjoy working independently and have a tendency to be self-reliant. Generation Y pursue life-long learning and are technologically advanced (Nelsey & Brownie, 2012).

Oblinger (2003), Oblinger and Oblinger (2005) and Skiba and Barton (2006) defined the age range of the 'digital native' or millennial generation described by Prensky (2001) as born between 1980 and the mid 1990s and are known as the Net generation or Millenials (Epstein & Howes, 2006). Millenials are accustomed to active, rather than passive, learning, preferring flexible and multi-faceted approaches than previous generations (ALTC, 2008). They tend to prefer online learning rather than the formal classroom approach but they need an interactive multimedia and multi-faceted approach to online educational delivery (Dede, 2005; Windham, 2005). Millenials are comfortable using computers for social networking and web interfacing, but that does not translate into them having the appropriate ICT skills required for use in the workplace (ALTC, 2008; Mather, 2012a). Additionally, this generation of nurses want information immediately and will seek answers through their computers or mobile phones rather than use other sources of media such as newspapers (Windham, 2005). These nurses are considered to be able to engage effectively and more widely through social networking and global communication services, than earlier generations. For them the notion of 'friendship' extends further than the geographical boundaries of where they live. The Internet opens networks beyond any local or national boundary, and enables a connectedness that was not available to previous generations of nurses (Dede, 2005).

Australian workplaces are increasingly an intergenerational mix of health professionals so it can be advantageous to harness the characteristics of generational cohorts to enhance or strengthen opportunities for undertaking CPD that uses m-learning technology in the workplace. This approach also provides secondary advantages that include improving collegiality, team work and mentoring within healthcare settings (Nelsey & Brownie, 2012).

Educational Considerations

Use of traditional models of punctuated access to learning opportunities to meet CPD can stifle the opportunities provided by real-time learning. Mobile computing offers multimedia access in real-time (Kenny et al., 2009; Kovachev, Aksakali, & Klamma, 2012; Lupton, 2012; Ruiz et al., 2006). Self-directed learning can be completed on the job as desired, rather than being completed later, away from the workplace. While it is not possible to complete more structured modules or courses during usual daily activities, by using mobile technologies, it is possible to collect and collate artefacts or learning objects as evidence that can be reviewed or reflected on once the shift is completed (Van der Rijt & Hoffman, 2013). Strategic use of mobile devices or software and applications will require re-orientation of learning behaviour and habits to change the culture of how CPD is undertaken. How and what evidence is accumulated has the opportunity to create a constant and consistent updating of knowledge and skills which can augment reflective processes that is a key behaviour required for e-learning to be effective (Kenny et al., 2009; Phillips, Kennedy, &

McNaught, 2012). This change in behaviour has the opportunity to revolutionise the workplace, create learning organisations (Senge, 1990) that are globally connected to best practice and expert opinion.

Technology Considerations

The availability of m-learning opportunities for CPD using social media and mobile technologies will continue to increase in parallel with the commercialisation of this technology. There will be a burgeoning increase in access to platforms to meet user demand. The main barrier to continued growth will be missing regulations regarding security, privacy and ownership of data issues (Treuer & Jenson, 2003). Similarly, issues of copyright, authenticity and access still need to be addressed and incorporated into any standards that are developed (ALTC, 2008; Treuer & Jenson, 2003). Potential users may lack the confidence, understanding or knowledge and skills to embark on using these platforms through fear of making mistakes that breach professional or workplace policies and guidelines (Mather, Marlow, & Cummings, 2013b). Additionally, some users may have concerns about data security and privacy issues associated with data storage and retrieval (ALTC, 2008). Lack of standardisation of terminology to describe use of these technologies, may also create issues that could impede uptake of m-learning by health professionals (Burgess, Bruns, & Hjort, 2013).

Access to mobile data services that provide sufficient bandwidth to support multimedia resources, sharing and storage of files need to be considered (Mather, 2011). Delivery support for m-learning may be problematic in some settings where healthcare facility policies and guidelines or geographic isolation may render access to data difficult (Mather et al., 2013b).

At an individual level, m-learning for CPD requires clinicians to have access to a mobile device, data support services, formal m-learning modules or a self-directed plan. The current choice of operating system, device, screen size, data storage, memory and battery life impact on the access to the type of m-learning users will choose. Furthermore as multimedia content delivery and creation becomes more complex so will the pressure for being competent with management of mobile learning interfaces. End users, such as health professionals, will be required to understand how keyboard, touch screen, stylus use and speech recognition assisted software operates as well as an understanding of the importance of data security.

Funding Considerations

The cost of investment to develop the infrastructure to support mobile technology is well recognised (Pagan, Higgs, & Cunningham, 2008). Pagan, Higgs and Cunningham (2008) reported that 3% of total Australian healthcare costs, or about $1-2 billion annually was spent on ICT. These estimates exclude expenditure specifically related to learning and teaching in the tertiary sector. The report stated that software based technologies will need to be developed to assist healthcare providers with understanding complex systems including educating and skilling medical professionals individually and in teams (Pagan et al., 2008).

Prior to embarking on m-learning CPD health professionals will need to consider the cost of any chosen mobile device, data support services, formal m-learning modules or a self-directed plan. They will need to consider their choice of operating system, screen size of the device, amount of data storage, memory and battery life that will impact on the access to the type of m-learning they can utilise. Furthermore, users will need to consider whether they are required to purchase a pre-paid or a data management contract from a commercial provider or whether their organisation will allow them to use the organisational data delivery provider.

THE NEXUS OF DIGITAL TECHNOLOGY AND EDUCATION TO SUPPORT CPD OPPORTUNITIES

Currently digital technology is used as a platform to offer a range of online CPD opportunities. Professional bodies such as the Australian Federation of Nurses (ANF) and the Australian College of Nursing (ACN) offer CPD portals to their members (ACN, 2013a; ANF, 2013). Commercial companies and education providers also offer a range of stand-alone digital educational opportunities for purchase that are endorsed by the ACN as meeting the CPD requirements (ACN, 2013b). Regardless of the supplier of e-learning to nurses, the majority of the digital CPD available is delivered as self-paced online modules that may include asynchronous discussion and submission of online assessments (ACN, 2013a; ANF, 2013). There are also national initiatives such as the Health Workforce Australia NHET-Sim program that utilises both face to face and online modules for completion of the program (HWA, 2013b). The majority of these fee-paying programs are yet to be adapted for tablet or smart phone use. Additionally these forms of CPD do not utilise social media or mobile technologies that could provide a level of connection that has previously been untapped.

Recently there has been an emergence of digital media research (Burgess et al., 2013), including a number of studies of undergraduate students (Kocoglu, 2008; MacKay & Harding, 2009; Mather, 2011, 2012b; Twomey, 2004) or health professional behaviour (Mather et al., 2013a, 2013b). Studies directly relating to the use of m-learning for CPD within a healthcare context are scant. The following case studies provide insights into the strengths and limitations of delivering m-learning for CPD in the clinical setting. The first relates to the implementation of e-portfolios to the experiential environment (Mather, 2011). The second describes the use of a social media platform to disseminate and share information (Mather et al., 2013a). The final case study demonstrates how the use of more than one m-learning platform can create a collaborative and connected learning community (Mather et al., 2013a).

Case Study 1. Use of Mobile Technology: E-Portfolios

One key factor in CPD is maintaining evidence of competence. Collation of evidence to meet the ANMC competency standards (ANMC, 2006) recognised by AHPRA can be facilitated through the use of an e-portfolio. Mobile technologies support a range of e-portfolio software that can be used as a repository and for documenting self-directed CPD (NMBA, 2013). Case study 1 demonstrates how the implementation and experience of e-portfolios as a user-centric mobile technology can be used to support learning outcomes.

E-portfolios are a function of the 'knowledge economy' with relevance across all industry sectors (ALTC, 2008). The technology is considered useful as increasing nurses' skills and competencies in ICT thereby better preparing them for the workplace to be more work ready at registration (Wade, Abrami, & Sclater, 2005). Used effectively e-portfolios can be an excellent tool for creating meaning and relevance to nurses exploring their professional interests and potential while in practice (ALTC, 2008). Capturing personal and professional development in an easily accessible format can enable individuals to make stronger links between their own aspirations and the within professional opportunities available (ALTC, 2008) A critical element for implementing the use of an e-portfolio is relevance throughout the learning and professional development of an individual and their portability, flexibility and adaptability that make them a usable tool in the workplace (Madden, 2007). An evaluation of the implementation of an e-portfolio into the experiential environment of a foundation unit of a Bachelor of Nursing

program in Australia was undertaken during 2010. The study provided valuable insights and uncovered assumptions about user understanding about ICT use.

This study was conducted across four campuses in two states of Australia. Students were allocated to approximately 250 placement agencies that included a range of healthcare environments. These were tertiary and district acute care services in hospitals, residential aged care facilities, multi-purpose health centres, general practice surgeries and community based health service settings. Organisations took one or up to 60 students depending on its size and the capacity to provide high quality supervision experience for students.

Prior to implementation of the technology there was the development of a range of learner support artefacts including face-to-face tutorials, web conferencing, media vignettes, narrated slide presentations, a user manual and fact sheets. Technical support was also provided prior and during the implementation phase.

Online surveys completed by students resulted in a response rate of 60% (311/511). Pre-implementation findings indicated that approximately half the students had not used a portfolio before. It was found that 82% of students used social media even though only 15% of respondents indicated they used file sharing sites such as Flickr, YouTube, Tumblr or Picasa. Eight percent of participants had their own website and only 2% had used an e-portfolio before.

The post-use findings indicated that 66% of students strongly agreed or agreed they liked the e-portfolio blog tool for reflection and 78% strongly agreed or agreed or the use of blogs enabled them to feel connected with peers. Furthermore, 65% of respondents strongly agreed or agreed that e-portfolios supported integration of knowledge and skills. Qualitative responses from students also indicated that more training in the use of the technology was required. Others indicated that security of data was cause for concern.

The findings of the evaluation indicated the assumption that students could utilise learning and teaching software was flawed. Furthermore the notion that students had a base-line understanding of computing and software terminology was ill-founded. Although the use of computers is ubiquitous in the environment it became apparent that although students used digital media for a variety of uses, it did not translate into understanding about the purpose of an e-portfolio.

This case study also demonstrated that lead-time and appropriate technical support were paramount for enabling appropriate use of the software within the clinical environment. Additionally, the development of applications suitable for tablet and smartphones have been developed since this study was completed (Mather, 2012b). Adaptation of e-portfolios with mobile technology has improved access and the development of native applications will enhance usability.

The implications from this study for using m-learning for CPD include ensuring that health professionals have the opportunity to become familiar with the device and software to be used for delivery of the m-learning CPD. An e-portfolio is a recommended method for collection and collation of evidence. Therefore it is imperative that current practitioners gain understanding and access to this platform to support their CPD journey. The collection and storage of artefacts and objects in this repository will further increase the possibilities for collaboration and sharing of multimedia information. As millennial generation professionals embark on CPD, they will build on their digital knowledge and skills to create content that will be disseminated and shared using mobile technologies. It will be imperative that this generation of nurses are provided with a sound understanding of privacy and security issues surrounding any content captured or developed using mobile technology (Van der Rijt & Hoffman, 2013). As m-learning for CPD diffuses into the workplace repurposing artefacts and objects for peer learning will also be enabled. Health professionals will be able to demonstrate their commitment to

Figure 1. Mobile technology supports the use of an e-portfolio for mobile learning

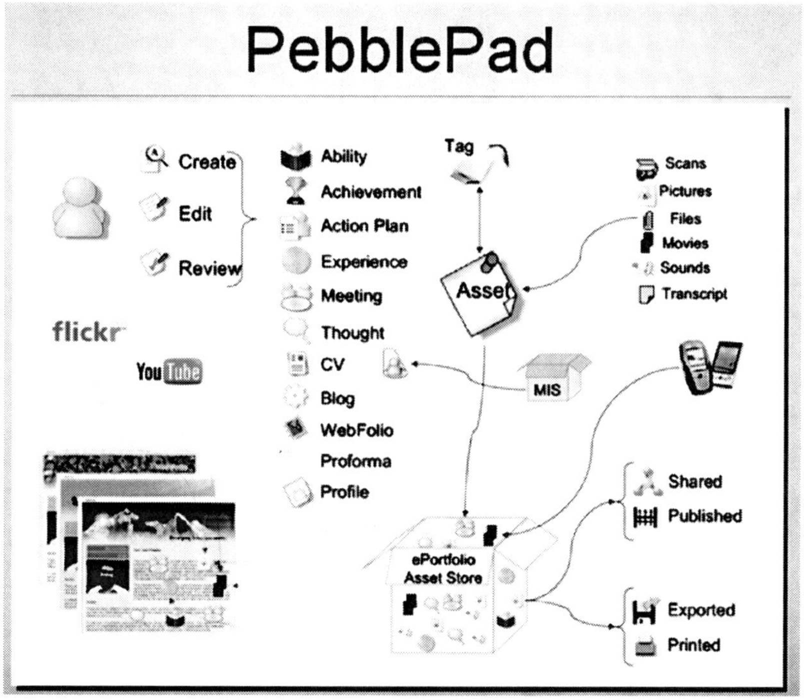

maintaining their registration by documentation of their CPD plan, storage of artefacts and objects and inclusion of their learning through using a reflective practice within their e-portfolio.

Case Study 2. Use of Social Media: Micro Blogging

Self-directed learning is an acceptable method of CPD (NMBA, 2013). An evaluation of the implementation of using micro blogging for m-learning about clinical supervision for health professionals as self-directed CPD was undertaken during 2012. Initially 12 clinicians who undertook clinical supervision of students were identified and were offered the opportunity to attend workshops aimed at up-skilling and building confidence in the use of ICT. These clinically based practitioners were orientated to mobile technology and supplied with a tablet computer. They undertook workshops to

learn how to use the micro blogging social media platform known as Twitter.

Twitter was chosen as it was free, easy to set up and use. Importantly this form of connection was limited to information transfer of 140 characters per interaction making it useful as a text message on any smartphone. These short messages were advantageous to users in rural areas where internet connectivity could be unreliable or slow (Mather & Marlow, 2012). Clinicians could choose to have messages directly pushed to their mobile telephone or accessed at an appropriate time via their hand held device or by computer. Depending on the settings, this software enabled the development of public or private communities and users could search or follow topics, individuals or organisations of interest. Participants could choose whether they wanted to contribute or ignore any conversations or tweets. They could also disseminate information by sending or retweeting messages to

Figure 2. @PEPCommunity microblog showing information feed or 'tweets'

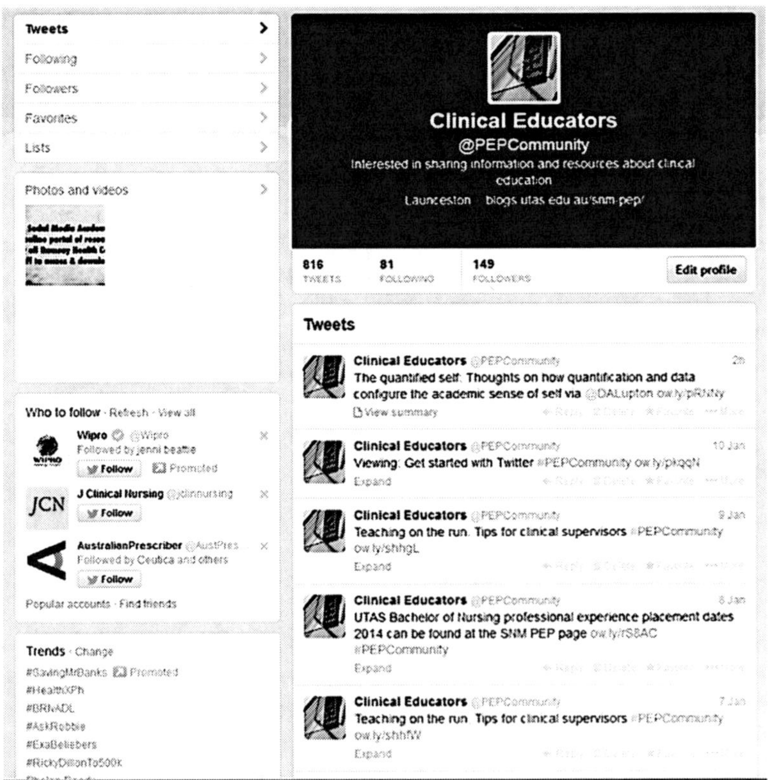

others. The @PEPCommunity account was managed using a social media management tool known as Hootesuite. This software enabled scheduling dissemination of information of interest to clinical supervisors.

The micro blog data tweeted by participants was limited to sharing information about clinical supervision. The digital strategy focused on improving connectedness and increasing communication flow among group members. Discussion relating to personal data was not a focus of the strategy and no personal or sensitive data or information about patients, clients or health professionals was shared using this software platform.

The security of these data relied on the privacy controls provided and updated by the owners of the digital communication platform. However, participants could customise their own accounts to control the level of visibility that suited their needs. Participants from this University or its partner organizations were expected to adhere to the social media guidelines that outlined appropriate use and consequences of breaching confidentiality (RCNA, 2011; University of Tasmania, 2010).

Baseline data about current digital media use by clinicians was obtained by online questionnaire. These clinicians became key change agents for disseminating information about this digital communication strategy in their clinical environments. Additionally, two personal capture vignettes and four fact sheets about the digital communication strategy and how to join were developed and hosted on the clinical supervision webpage within the University website. Technical support was provided by an ICT consultant throughout the study. It was intended that these clinicians would promote cultural change by modelling the communication strategy in the clinical environment. The digital media survey attracted 29 respondents and although numbers were low, it provided useful feedback about the clinicians that were prepared to be involved with the study. Over 66% of participants indicated they were aged over 46 years. Furthermore, 72% of

respondents indicated they were from regional or rural areas. The remaining participants (24%) were from urban environments. The majority of respondents (93%) indicated they had used the internet for more than 5 years.

During the study the micro blog @PEPCommunity account attracted 103 members or followers. The group consisted of 25 nurses known to be associated with the University and 18 other nurses. There were 16 academics involved of which 11 were identified as nurse academics. The remainder of participants were medical and allied health personnel involved with higher education or health organisations (n=27). There were 6 participants that were unidentified. TweetReach software indicated that the account content posted reached an average of 5000 accounts and 10 000 impressions per week. Of the 447 micro blogs posted or tweeted the content was evenly distributed between learning and teaching; students; practice tips; education; social media and clinical supervision.

Qualitative feedback about using this methodology was mixed. The majority of respondents indicated they liked receiving information from the micro blog few felt competent or comfortable with commenting or providing information. There were a small group (n=4) that were familiar with using Twitter. At interview they were enthusiastic about the potential reach of the platform. One respondent indicated it provided a connectedness to the University that was previously lacking. This respondent indicated they followed up the information posted on the micro blog and retweeted information to their own networks.

Case Study 3. Use of Social Media and Mobile Technology to Support a Community of Practice for Peer Learning

As previously stated, self-directed learning is an acceptable method for accumulation of CPD hours (NMBA, 2013). An evaluation of the use of a blog

Figure 3. Summary of micro blog key words by Vizify (Source: https://www.vizify.com/clinical-educators)

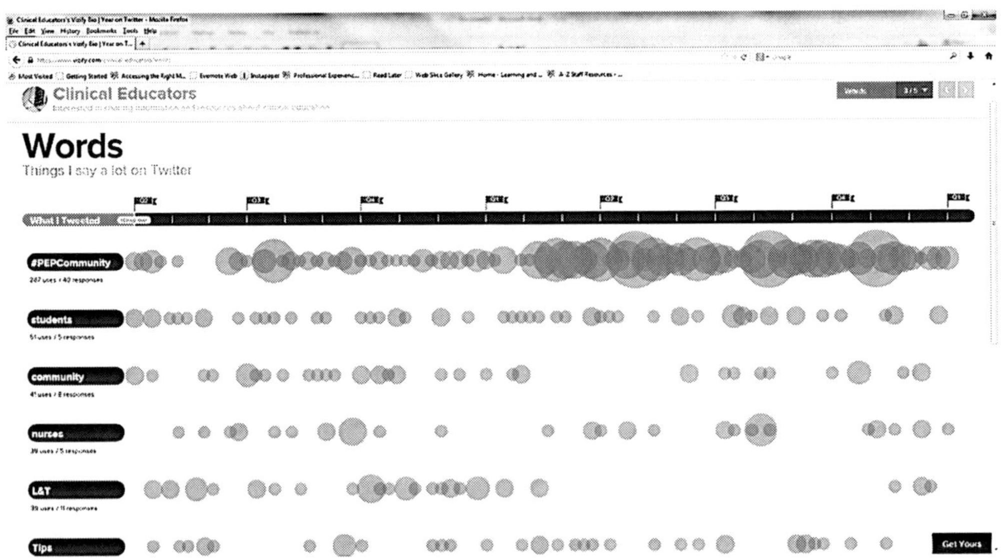

and micro blogging to support and disseminate contemporary clinical supervision information as self-directed CPD was undertaken during 2012. It also provided a conduit to promote connectedness among this group of health professionals. The development of this Web 2.0 enhanced digital media strategy was to support the development of a community of practice of clinical supervisors. It was implemented to strengthen partnerships by information sharing and access to resources between the University, organizations, facilities and registered nurses who supervise students. The use of an asynchronous or synchronous digital methodology enabled feedback or information sharing to occur at the users' convenience.

The Professional Experience Placement blog was hosted by the University web service and Google Analytics were used to track visits to the blog content. Clinical supervisors were provided with a weekly précis of contemporary clinical supervision information via the blog. These updates matched the cycle of students attending the experiential environment during their course. Blogs were approximately 300-400 words each and provided contemporary information about clinical supervision. Topics spanned the role,

function and student-supervisor interface. It included scholarly discussion about orientation; preparedness; belongingness; or giving and receiving feedback. There was capacity to provide comment on the blogs and it also displayed a web link to the micro blog. Now, rather than relying on receiving information via their organization, registered nurses had the opportunity to choose to receive the information directly from the University through engaging with the blog or micro blog activity. Additionally, it enabled registered nurses to have access to information such as key dates that previously may have been sent to managers at organizations rather than the clinicians responsible for nurses. Registered nurses were able to access updates about changes within the BN curriculum that may impact on learning and teaching of students (Mather et al., 2013b).

During the first 12 months of the implementation of the blog, 67 blogs were published. Each new blog was announced on the micro blog, with a resulting spike in views recorded in the 24 hours after the broadcast. The blog page attracted an average of 60 page views per week; with an average viewing time of three minutes per visit. Visitors to the blog were global, however, the

Figure 4. Blog showing information posted about clinical supervision

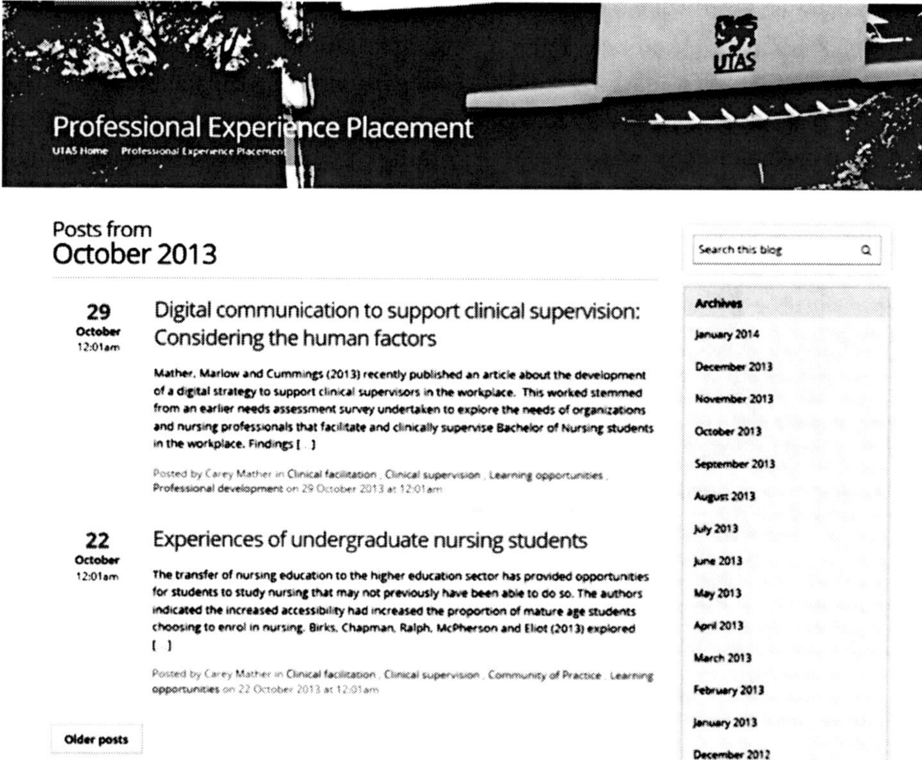

Figure 5. Google analytics captured information about blog use

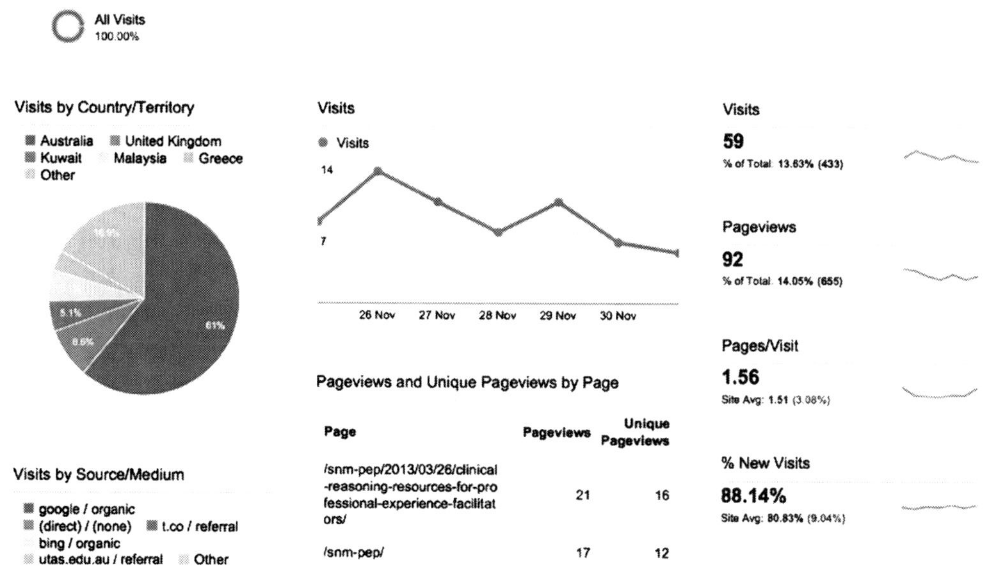

majority (70%) originated in Australia. Other regular visitors registered from Canada, United Kingdom, India, Philippines, Vietnam, Spain and Malaysia. Access to the micro blog was also available via a widget link on the blog web page.

Eighteen face-to-face interviews were conducted to elicit qualitative information about the development of the community of practice using Web 2.0 technology. Findings from this evaluation highlighted a number of structural barriers for CPD that will need to be addressed prior to the large scale inception of CPD within the workplace. It was found that clinicians at some sites were unable to access the internet while at work. Hospital policy precluded the use of mobile technology during work time. Staff at other facilities reported that using mobile technology while working with patients or clients was considered poor role modelling and was discouraged as it demonstrated a lack of social presence in the workplace (Condon, 2013). Further discussion with regarding the issue uncovered a perception by a few of the community of practice members that some of their peers did not understand the capacity of the technology. Colleagues were unaware they could learn about clinical conditions or receive feedback and suggestions about patient or client care from peers or an expert external to the organisation, while in the workplace. Some practitioners identified they lacked confidence in how to respond using the software platform while other practitioners reported they were satisfied with 'lurking' or being passive members of the group. They did not perceive they needed to post comments or messages to feel part of the group. There was a core group of participants that found the community of practice was beneficial for their learning. One respondent indicated they waited for the blog to be published each week. It was the only CPD they undertook regularly. They stated that as it was relevant to their role and function it was all they needed to remain contemporary in their practice as a nurse.

To increase equity of access to m-learning opportunities to augment and facilitate CPD opportunities, a change in organisational policy regarding Web 2.0 technology is required. Additionally, a cultural shift by health professionals in the perception of the uses of this technology needs to occur to enable legitimisation of its use for CPD in the workplace or in real-time. Ironically, to develop understanding about the capacity and capability of using social media and mobile technology, there needs to be professional development to understand it. Further research on the use of Web 2.0 technology in the clinical environment is necessary to ensure it is systematically developed and appropriately resourced.

CONCERNS AND LIMITATIONS

As the growth in commercialisation and development of native applications for mobile health continues, there will need to be the development of new regulations and standards that reflect this changing environment. The expansion of social media and mobile technology will create pressure on health organisations to meet the current challenges associated with the lack of standards, regulations or policy regarding the use of these technologies in the workplace.

In response there is a need for technology planning, enabling education, and fostering cultural change of health professionals, and empowerment of their staff to enable those organizations that do allow the personal use of m-learning supported devices, to be easily accessible and reliable. There needs to be parallel development of social etiquette and conduct within organisations that promote the potential of developing learning organisations. Educational institutions, professional bodies, CPD providers and health professionals need to become involved and fully conversant with policy development regarding security, privacy, ownership of data and copyright issues. All stakeholders have an important role in guiding current and future health professionals on effective and responsible use of social media and mobile technology use in the workplace, with control, access and standards for use being a major challenge (Lorenzo & Ittelson, 2005; Treuer & Jenson, 2003). It is therefore incumbent on educational institutions to introduce foundation information in their courses about ethical and legal issues surrounding this technology. They are vested with ensuring that health professionals gain a thorough understanding of legal, ethical and safe use of m-learning artefacts and objects. Curriculum design needs to include security, privacy, ownership of data and copyright issues (ALTC, 2008; Lorenzo & Ittelson, 2005; Madden, 2007). Furthermore, student health professionals would benefit from simulation opportunities to explore appropriate integration of m-learning and the ramifications of illegitimate use.

As evidenced by the case study 3, the use of social media and mobile technology for CPD in some organisations is limited by lack of regulation or outmoded policies that dissuade m-learning opportunities (Mather et al., 2013b). Currently, the growth of m-learning within Australian workplaces has been organic and without coordination. Conversely, other healthcare environments and health professions have embraced social media and mobile technology to capitalise on this expanding area of communication and interest in participatory healthcare by patients or clients (iHealthBeat, 2011; Ramsay Health Care, 2012). Case study 3 demonstrates there are opportunities for interested groups to develop discourse regarding a global or national approach to self-directed CPD opportunities using Web 2.0 technology. Once social media and m-learning is embedded as an accepted form of CPD there will be opportunities to develop novel and innovative approaches for a more structured approach for CPD that can attract formal recognition as acceptable m-learning in situ, in the workplace in real-time.

There are challenges that have been identified for preparing health professionals in developing understanding and skills in social media and mobile technology use. These factors included cost, maintenance and lack of training (Russin & Davis, 1990). An ageing workforce may initially impede the pace of integration of m-learning into the workplace. However, for the successful introduction of m-learning platforms, nurses must first acquire the necessary information, communication and technology program skills. One of the inherent dangers of embedding social media and mobile technology into the workplace for m-learning is that the technological novelty of the product could overshadow the purpose its introduction, resulting in the learning opportunities being subsumed by the technology itself (Kenny et al., 2009; Woodward & Nanlohy, 2004). Furthermore, as the pace for contemporary information increases and new information is rapidly available there will be a need for health professionals to filter information, and also demonstrate maintenance of currency in their area of specialisation.

FORMAL AND INFORMAL METHODS OF CPD

There are opportunities to undertake massive open online courses (MOOCs) (WDREC, 2013). These modules may be undertaken as web-based activities or can be adapted for mobile computing. Similarly there has been rapid development of mobile educational gaming opportunities (DiPietro, Ferdig, Boyer, & Black, 2007; Sánchez & Olivares, 2011). Completion of these formal courses or objects can be used as evidence to demonstrate CPD. This formal approach enables demonstration of evidence to meet the annual requirements for CPD.

Informal self-directed CPD may initially be more difficult to set-up, however there are advantages to using local context opportunities to learn in situ. Development of the knowledge and skills to develop a learning plan, documentation and recording evidence of learning will facilitate health professionals to create artefacts and objects using a range of Web 2.0 technologies will require commitment by health professionals. The use of point and shoot learning using mobile device embedded cameras will enable artefact creation. The generation of content to facilitate learning artefacts that can be shared and repurposed to maximise their use will become more popular. This informal strategy to promote learning opportunities that can be used for obtaining CPD hours may become more acceptable as mobile technology becomes more embedded in the workplace.

THE FUTURE OF M-LEARNING IN CPD

The nature and scope of the potential reach of human interface technology is being explored, however, there is much work to be undertaken if they are to become widely used or accepted (Davis, 2009). Growth and commercialisation within these digital technology fields is occurring more rapidly than incumbent 'mature' or Baby Boomer educators from the health sciences or education fields can innovate within the curriculum before further advances render it is superseded (Kurzweil, 2001; Moore, 1965; Skiba & Barton, 2006).

Simulation has been used to teach a range of skills such as beginning nurse communication and skills competency, at undergraduate and graduate levels (Nehring & Lashley, 2009). The scope of using mobile hosted human interface technology applications is broad. For example augmented reality technology can be used to support fundamental anatomy and physiology and complex skill development in the simulation skills laboratory or the experiential environment (Rolland, Wright, & Kancherla, 1996; Sherstyuk, Vincent, & Berg, 2008; Vilkoniene, 2009). As the development of applications that support augmented

reality increase, so will the number of healthcare professionals who benefit from the learning and teaching opportunities the mobile augmented reality technology can provide (Mather, 2010). This technology can be used as an adjunct to traditional CPD and to enhance accepted technologies such as mannequin simulation or in situ learning in the practice environment (Mather, 2010). There is an urgency for educational providers to respond creatively in the development of m-learning artefacts and objects to engage current and future health professionals with m-learning opportunities that challenge and inspire them to remain contemporary and competent in their chosen fields (Kenny et al., 2009; Skiba & Barton, 2006).

Ausburn and Ausburn (2004) discuss the use of human interface technology within the industrial, technical instruction education environment. They critique the capabilities, limitations and effectiveness of human interface technology maintaining it is an important emerging technology where competence with complex technical skills is required. They state the technology has the capacity to re-orientate the m-learning environment (Ausburn & Ausburn, 2004). Human interface technology can enable healthcare professionals to gain an understanding of complex concepts and develop competence in cognitive and behavioural attributes that are desirable in their chosen profession (Ausburn & Ausburn, 2004; Georgiev et al., 2004; Ruiz et al., 2006).

By CPD becoming more embedded within the workplace, in situ learning in real-time will become faster and more collaborative. The creation of self-directed content that is shared between colleagues or interested others will be possible (Kenny et al., 2009). Increased opportunity for increased connectivity between nurses with similar interests will enable the use of social media to develop and sustain communities of practice. The rapid evolution of ideas and concepts will become more commonplace and feedback from experts and peers about performance support and knowledge will become possible (Mather et al., 2013a). Content creation and sharing between interested practitioners will encourage diffusion of information and innovations (Rogers, 1995; Sanson-Fisher, 2004). Collation of evidence, owned by the user, stored in e-repositories external to workplace and allowing access or sharing with colleagues and peers as necessary will be popular. Repurposing of artefacts and objects as learning tools among members will be widespread as m-learning for CPD will become more accessible and flexible.

CONCLUSION

In conclusion, social media and mobile technology will become embedded in healthcare and become part of what will be known as connected health, rather than remain with the fragmented terminology currently used to differentiate between the fields (Wicklund, 2013).

Recent Australian policy development regarding accountability and responsibility of health professionals to maintain their registration by demonstration of evidence of competency has provided opportunities to reorientate the CPD landscape. In conjunction with these changes has been the rapid expansion of social media and mobile technology that is now becoming embedded within healthcare. There are currently gaps in the knowledge and skills of health professionals to maximise the integration of this technology, to include CPD in the workplace. The lag in the development of standards, policies and guidelines related to legal and ethical issues, may be an advantage as there remains sufficient time to explore opportunities to reorientate CPD using this technology. Human interface technology, including wearable computing sensors and accelerometers, will be developed and will be used for feedback and provide mobile performance support (Lupton, 2012).

The introduction of mobile technology based CPD could promote life-long learning opportunities at the beginning of a nurse's career. Over time it will promote a cultural shift in how CPD is viewed and undertaken. The development and adaptation of mobile applications to facilitate reflective practice and enable the collation of a repository for storage of artefacts as evidence to demonstrate competency will become more refined. There will be further integration of CPD in real-time, rather than as an asynchronous entity conducted outside the workplace. M-learning using social media and mobile technology will become ubiquitous in the workplace.

Connected health is possible through the success of market penetration of mobile technology within healthcare and will exert pressure on healthcare professionals to adopt and keep up with the changing trends of digital technology use both within and external to the workplace. During the next 5 years it is predicted that commercialisation of e-health and m-health tools will become embedded within the healthcare settings (Walsh, 2013). To meet the demand for competent use of this technology, CPD providers will rapidly adapt to deliver e-learning opportunities through a range of mobile technology including tablet and smartphone applications rather than web-based software. To maintain competency in the workplace health professionals will need to embrace new ways of undertaking CPD. Learning in situ, in real-time with the assistance of augmented reality applications will be possible.

The possibilities of m-learning using social media and mobile technologies for CPD are bounded only by the limits of current technology and the pace of acceptance by health professionals and regulatory bodies as a legitimate strategy for learning.

REFERENCES

Abbott, P., & Coenen, A. (2008). Globalisation and advances in information and communication technologies: The impact of nursing and health. *Nursing Outlook*, *56*(5), 238–246, 246.e2. doi:10.1016/j.outlook.2008.06.009 PMID:18922277

ACN. (2013a). *Continuing Professional Development*. Retrieved 23 July 2013, from http://www.nursing.edu.au/CPDh

ACN. (2013b). *External CPD providers*. Retrieved 23 July, from http://www.nursing.edu.au/CPDh

AHPRA. (2013). *Australian Health Practitioner Regulation Agency Registration Standards*. Retrieved 24 July 2013, from http://www.ahpra.gov.au/Registration/Registration-Standards.aspx

ALTC. (2008). *e-Portfolio use by university students in Australia: Informing excellence in policy and practice*. Australian E-Portfolio Project final Report. Retrieved 20 July 2011, from http://www.altc.edu.au/resources?text=Australian+E-Portfolio+Project

ANF. (2013). *Continuing Professional Education*. Retrieved 25 July 2013, from http://anf.org.au/pages/cpe

ANMAC. (2012). *Australian Nursing and Midwifery Accreditation Council Registered Nurse Accreditation Standards*. Retrieved 23 July 2013, from http://www.anmac.org.au/sites/default/files/documents/ANMAC_RN_Accreditation_Standards_2012.pdf

ANMC. (2006). *Australian Nursing and Midwifery Competency Standards for Nurses and Midwives*. Retrieved 26 February 2011, from http://www.nursingmidwiferyboard.gov.au/Codes-and-Guidelines.aspx

Ausburn, L., & Ausburn, F. (2004). Desktop Virtual Reality: A Powerful New Technology for Teaching and Research in Industrial Teacher Education. *Journal of Industrial Teacher Education*, *41*(4), 33–58.

Australian Health Ministers' Conference. (2008). *National E-Health Strategy*. Author.

Bembridge, E., Levett-Jones, T., & Yeun-Sim Jeong, S. (2011). The transferability of information and communication technology skills from university to the workplace: A qualitative descriptive study. *Nurse Education Today*, *31*(3), 245–252. doi:10.1016/j.nedt.2010.10.020 PMID:21093125

Borycki, E., Foster, J., Sahama, T., Frisch, N., & Kushniruk, A. (2013). Developing national level informatics competencies for undergraduate nurses: Methodological approaches from Australia and Canada. *Studies in Health Technology and Informatics*, *183*, 345–349. PMID:23388312

Brunetto, Y., Farr-Wharton, R., & Shacklock, K. (2012). Communication, Training, wellbeing and commitment across generations. *Nursing Outlook*, *60*(1), 7–15. doi:10.1016/j.outlook.2011.04.004 PMID:21703652

Burgess, J., Bruns, A., & Hjort, L. (2013). Emerging methods for digital research: An introduction. *Journal of Broadcasting & Electronic Media*, *57*(1), 1–3. doi:10.1080/08838151.2012.761706

Condon, B. (2013). The present state of presence in technology. *Nursing Science Quarterly*, *26*(1), 24–28. doi:10.1177/0894318412466738 PMID:23247344

Davis, R. (2009). Exploring Possibilities: Virtual Reality in Nursing Research. *Research and Theory for Nursing Practice: An International Journal*, *23*(2), 133–147. doi:10.1891/1541-6577.23.2.133 PMID:19558028

Dede, C. (2005). *Planning for Neomillennial Learning Styles: Implications for Investments in Technology and Faculty.* Retrieved 30 July 2013, from www.educause.edu/educatingthenetgen

DEEWR. (2008). *Digital education revolution: Overview.* Retrieved 20 June 2013, from http://www.digitaleducationrevolution.gov.au/about.htm

DiPietro, M., Ferdig, R. E., Boyer, J., & Black, E. W. (2007). Towards a Framework for Understanding Electronic Educational Gaming. *Journal of Educational Multimedia and Hypermedia, 16*(3), 225–248.

DoHA. (2013). *Welcome to eHealth.gov.au.* Retrieved 25 July, from http://www.ehealth.gov.au/internet/ehealth/publishing.nsf/Content/home

Epstein, M., & Howes, P. (2006, September-October). The Millennial Generation: Recruiting, Retaining and Managing. *Today's CPA,* 66-75.

Georgiev, T., Georgieva, E., & Smrikarov, A. (2004). *M-Learning - A New Stage of E- Learning.* Paper presented at the ComSysTech'2004. New York, NY.

HWA. (2013a). Nurses in focus. *Australia's Health Workforce Series.* Retrieved 23 July 2013, from https://www.hwa.gov.au/sites/uploads/Nurses-in-Focus-FINAL.pdf

HWA. (2013b). NHETsim. *Training the Healthcare simulation community.* Retrieved 23 July, from http://www.nhet-sim.edu.au/

iHealthBeat. (2011). Mayo Clinic launches social networking site on health care issues. *iHealthBeat, 15.* Retrieved 17 August 2011, from http://www.ihealthbeat.org/articles/2011/7/15/mayo-clinic-launches-social-networking-site-on-health-care-issues.aspx

Kaplan, A. M., & Haenlein, M. (2010). Users of the world, unite! The challenges and opportunities of social media. *Business Horizons, 53*(1), 59–68. doi:10.1016/j.bushor.2009.09.003

Kenny, R., Neste-Kenny, J., Park, C., Burton, P., & Meiers, J. (2009). Mobile learning in Nursing practice education: Applying Koole's FRAME model. *Journal of Distance Education, 23*(3), 75–96.

Kocoglu, Z. (2008). Turkish EFL student teachers' perceptions on the role of Electronic portfolios in their professional development. *The Turkish Online Journal of Educational Technology, 7,* Article 8,

Kovachev, D., Aksakali, G., & Klamma, R. (2012). *A real-time collaboration-enabled Mobile Augmented Reality system with semantic multimedia.* Paper presented at the Collaborative Computing: Networking, Applications and Worksharing (CollaborateCom), 8th International Conference. Pittsburgh, PA. doi:10.4108/icst.collaboratecom.2012.250436

Kurzweil, R. (2001). Law of Accelerating returns. *KurzweilAI.net.* Retrieved 23 July 2013, from http://www.kurzweilai.net/articles/art0134.html?printable=1

Lorenzo, G., & Ittelson, G. (2005). An overview of e-portfolios. *Educause Learning Initiative.* Retrieved 14 February 2010, from www.educause.edu

Lupton, D. (2012). M-health and health promotion: The digital cyborg and surveillance society. *Social Theory & Health, 10*(3), 229–244. doi:10.1057/sth.2012.6

MacKay, B., & Harding, T. (2009). M-support: Keeping in touch on placement in primary health care settings. *Nursing Praxis in New Zealand Inc, 25*(2), 30–40. PMID:19928649

Madden, T. (2007). *Supporting student e-Portfolios: A physical sciences practice guide.* Hull, UK: Higher Education Academy Physical Sciences Centre.

Mason, R., Pegler, C., & Weller, M. (2004). E-portfolios: An assessment tool for online courses. *British Journal of Educational Technology, 35*(6), 717–727. doi:10.1111/j.1467-8535.2004.00429.x

Mather, C. A. (2010). *Human interface technology: Enhancing tertiary nursing education to ensure workplace readiness.* Paper presented at the International Technology, Education and Development Conference. New York, NY.

Mather, C. A. (2011). *E-portfolios: Lessons from an interdisciplinary collaboration: The School of nursing and Midwifery experience abstract.* Paper presented at the EDULEARN11 (3rd International Conference on Education and New Learning Technologies). Barcelona, Spain.

Mather, C. A. (2012a). An Interdisciplinary evaluation of an e-portfolio: WIL at the University of Tasmania. In C. Simmons, W. Sher, A. Williams, & T. Levett-Jones (Eds.), *Workready. E-portfolios to support professional placements in nursing and construction management degrees in Australia* (pp. 73–88). Sydney: Office for Learning and Teaching.

Mather, C. A. (2012b). *Embedding an e-portfolio into a work Integrated learning environment: The School of Nursing and Midwifery experience.* Paper presented at the EDULEARN12 (4th International Conference on Education and New Learning Technologies). Barcelona, Spain.

Mather, C. A., & Marlow, A. (2012). Audio teleconferencing: Creative use of a forgotten innovation. *Contemporary Nurse, 41*(2), 177–183. doi:10.5172/conu.2012.41.2.177 PMID:22800383

Mather, C. A., Marlow, A., & Cummings, E. (2013a). Digital communication to support clinical supervision: Considering the human factors. *Studies in Health Technology and Informatics, 194*, 160–165. PMID:23941949

Mather, C. A., Marlow, A., & Cummings, E. (2013b). *Web 2.0 strategies to enhance support of clinical supervisors of undergraduate nursing students: An Australian experience.* Paper presented at the EDULEARN13 (5th International Conference on Education and New Learning Technologies). New York, NY.

Moore, G. (1965). Cramming more components into integrated circuits. *Electronics, 38*(8), 114.

Nehring, W., & Lashley, F. (2009). Nursing Simulation: A Review of the Past 40 Years. *Simulation & Gaming, 40*(4), 528–552. doi:10.1177/1046878109332282

Nelsey, L., & Brownie, S. (2012). Effective leadership, teamwork and mentoring – Essential elements in promoting generational cohesion in the nursing workforce and retaining nurses. *Collegian (Royal College of Nursing, Australia), 19*(4), 197–202. doi:10.1016/j.colegn.2012.03.002 PMID:23362605

NMBA. (2013). *Nursing and Midwifery Continuing Professional Development Registration Standard.* Retrieved 23 July 2013, from http://www.nursingmidwiferyboard.gov.au/Registration-Standards.aspx

Oblinger, D. (2003). Boomers, Gen-Xers and Millenials: Understanding the New Students. *Educause Review.* Retrieved 14 February 2010, from www.educause.edu/educatingthenetgen

Oblinger, D., & Oblinger, J. (2005). *Educating the Net Generation.* Retrieved 23 December 2009, from http://www.educause.edu/educatingthenetgen

Pagan, J., Higgs, P., & Cunningham, S. (2008). *Getting Creative in Healthcare: The contribution of creative activities to Australian Healthcare.* Retrieved 23 july 2013, from http://eprints.qut.edu.au/14757/

Phillips, R., Kennedy, G., & McNaught, C. (2012). The role of theory in learning technology evaluation research. *Australasian Journal of Educational Technology, 28*(7), 1103–1118.

Prensky, M. (2001). Digital Natives, Digital Immigrants On the Horizon. MCB University Press, 9(5).

Ramsay Health Care. (2012). *Ramsay Health Care's Social Media Policy.* Retrieved 6 May 2013, from http://www.youtube.com/watch?v=f-xo0237n6U

RCNA. (2011). *RCNA Social Media Guidelines for Nurses.* Canberra, Australia: Royal College of Nursing Australia.

Rogers, E. (1995). *Diffusion of Innovations* (5th ed.). New York: Free Press.

Rolland, J., Wright, D., & Kancherla, A. (1996). Towards a Novel Augmented-Reality Tool to Visualise Dynamic 3-D Anatomy. In J. Westwood, S. Westwood, L. Felländer-Tsai, R. Haluck, R. Robb, S. Senger, & K. Vosburgh (Eds.), *Medicine Meets Virtual Reality: Global healthcare grid* (pp. 337–348). Washington, DC: IOS Press.

Ruiz, J., Mintzer, M., & Leipzig, R. (2006). The impact of E-learning in medical education. *Academic Medicine, 81*(3), 207–212. doi:10.1097/00001888-200603000-00002 PMID:16501260

Russin, M., & Davis, J. (1990). Continuing education electronic bulletin board system: Provider readiness and interest. *Journal of Continuing Education in Nursing, 21*(1), 23–27. PMID:2106537

Sánchez, J., & Olivares, R. (2011). Problem solving and collaboration using mobile serious games. *Computers & Education, 57*(3), 1943–1952. doi:10.1016/j.compedu.2011.04.012

Sanson-Fisher, R. (2004). Diffusion of innovation theory for clinical change. *The Medical Journal of Australia, 180*, S55–S56. PMID:15012582

Senge, P. M. (1990). *The Fifth Discipline.* New York: Doubleday/Currency.

Sherstyuk, A., Vincent, D., & Berg, B. (2008). *Creating Mixed Reality Manikins for Medical Education.* Paper presented at the Artificial Reality and Telexistance (ICAT, 2008). Yokohoma, Japan.

Skiba, D., & Barton, A. (2006). Adapting your Teaching to Accommodate the Net Generation of Learners. *The Online Journal of Issues in Nursing, 11*(2), Manuscript 4.

Smedley, A. (2005). The importance of informatics competencies in Nursing: An Australian Perspective. *Computers, Informatics, Nursing. CIN, 23*(2), 106–110. PMID:15772512

Staggers, N., Gassert, C., & Curran, C. (2002). A Delphi study to determine Informatics competencies for nurses at four levels of practice. *Nursing Research, 51*(6), 383–390. doi:10.1097/00006199-200211000-00006 PMID:12464758

Traxler, J. (2007). Defining, discussing and evaluating mobile learning: The moving Finger writes and having writ. *International Review of Research in Open and Distance Learning, 8*(2), 67–75.

Treuer, P., & Jenson, J. (2003). Electronic Portfolios Need Standards to Thrive: The proliferation of e-portfolio applications requires compatible software and design standards to support lifelong learning. *EDUCAUSE Quarterly, 2*, 34–42.

Twomey, A. (2004). Web-based teaching in nursing: Lessons from the literature. *Nurse Education Today, 24*(6), 452–458. doi:10.1016/j.nedt.2004.04.010 PMID:15312954

University of Tasmania. (2010). *Social Media Guidelines.* Retrieved 15 January 2013, from http://www.utas.edu.au/__data/assets/pdf_file/0007/82843/Social-Media-Guidelines.pdf

Van der Rijt, R., & Hoffman, S. (2013). Ethical considerations of clinical photography in an area of emerging technology and smartphones. *Journal of Medical Ethics.* PMID:23800451

Vilkoniene, M. (2009). Influence of augmented reality technology upon pupils' knowledge about human digestive system: The results of the experiment. *US-China Education Review, 6*(1), 36–43.

Wade, A., Abrami, P., & Sclater, J. (2005). An Electronic Portfolio to Support Learning. *Canadian Journal of Learning and Technology, 31*(3).

Walsh, B. (2013). *mHealth market poised for explosive growth.* Retrieved 25 July, from http://www.clinical-innovation.com/topics/mobile-tele-health/mhealth-market-poised-explosive-growth

WDREC. (2013). *Understanding Dementia Free online course.* Retrieved 23 July 2013, from http://www.utas.edu.au/wicking/wca/mooc

While, A., & Dewsberry, G. (2011). Nursing and information and communication technology (ICT), A discussion of trends and future directions. *International Journal of Nursing Studies, 48*(10), 1302–1310. doi:10.1016/j.ijnurstu.2011.02.020 PMID:21474135

White, G. (2008). *Digital learning: An Australian research agenda.* Retrieved 24 July 2013, from www.acer.edu.au/documents/TLL_DigitalLearningResearch.doc

WHO. (2011). *mHealth: New Horizons for health through mobile technologies: Second survey on ehealth.* Retrieved 23 July 2013, from http://www.who.int/goe/publications/goe_mhealth_web.pdf

Wicklund, R. (2013). When mhealth and telehealth become just healthcare. *Government Health IT.* Retrieved 26 July 2013, from http://www.govhealthit.com/news/when-mhealth-and-telehealth-become-just-healthcare

Windham, C. (2005). The Student's Perspective. *Educating the Net Generation, Educause.* Retrieved 14 February 2010, from www.educause.edu/educatingthenetgen

Woodward, H., & Nanlohy, P. (2004). Digital portfolios: Fact or fashion? *Assessment & Evaluation in Higher Education, 29*(2), 228–238. doi:10.1080/0260293042000188492

ADDITIONAL READING

Abbott, P., & Coenen, A. (2008). Globalisation and advances in information and communication technologies: The impact of nursing and health. *Nursing Outlook, 56*(5), 238–246, 246.e2. doi:10.1016/j.outlook.2008.06.009 PMID:18922277

Bembridge, E., Levett-Jones, T., & Yeun-Sim Jeong, S. (2011). The transferability of information and communication technology skills from university to the workplace: A qualitative descriptive study. *Nurse Education Today, 31*(3), 245–252. doi:10.1016/j.nedt.2010.10.020 PMID:21093125

Borycki, E., Foster, J., Sahama, T., Frisch, N., & Kushniruk, A. (2013). Developing national level informatics competencies for undergraduate nurses: methodological approaches from Australia and Canada. *Studies in Health Technology and Informatics, 183*, 345–349. PMID:23388312

Brunetto, Y., Farr-Wharton, R., & Shacklock, K. (2012). Communication, Training, wellbeing and commitment across generations. *Nursing Outlook, 60*(1), 7–15. doi:10.1016/j.outlook.2011.04.004 PMID:21703652

Condon, B. (2013). The present state of presence in technology. *Nursing Science Quarterly*, 26(1), 24–28. doi:10.1177/0894318412466738 PMID:23247344

Davis, R. (2009). Exploring Possibilities: Virtual Reality in Nursing Research. *Research and Theory for Nursing Practice: An International Journal*, 23(2), 133–147. doi:10.1891/1541-6577.23.2.133 PMID:19558028

Dede, C. (2005). Planning for Neomillennial Learning Styles: Implications for Investments in Technology and Faculty Retrieved 30 July 2013, from www.educause.edu/educatingthenetgen

Duncan, I., Yarwood-Ross, L., & Haigh, C. (2013). YouTube as a source of clinical skills education. Nurse Education Today. In Press Available online 14 January 2013.

Farr-Wharton, R., Brunetto, Y., & Shacklock, K. (2012). The use of intuition nurse-supervisor relationships and the impact on empowerment and affective commitment. *Journal of Advanced Nursing*, 68(6), 1391–1401. doi:10.1111/j.1365-2648.2011.05852.x PMID:22032539

Househ, M. (2013). The use of Social media in healthcare: organisational, clinical and patient perspectives. *Studies in Health Technology and Informatics*, 183, 244–248. PMID:23388291

Kaplan, A. M., & Haenlein, M. (2010). Users of the world, unite! The challenges and opportunities of social media. *Business Horizons*, 53(1), 59–68. doi:10.1016/j.bushor.2009.09.003

Kenny, R., Neste-Kenny, J., Park, C., Burton, P., & Meiers, J. (2009). Mobile learning in Nursing practice education: Applying Koole's FRAME model. *Journal of Distance Education*, 23(3), 75–96.

Lupton, D. (2012). M-health and health promotion: The digital cyborg and surveillance society. *Social Theory & Health*, 10(3), 229–244. doi:10.1057/sth.2012.6

MacKay, B., & Harding, T. (2009). M-support: Keeping in touch on placement in primary health care settings. *Nursing Praxis in New Zealand Inc*, 25(2), 30–40. PMID:19928649

Mather, C. A., & Marlow, A. (2012). Audio teleconferencing: Creative use of a forgotten innovation. *Contemporary Nurse*, 41(2), 177–183. doi:10.5172/conu.2012.41.2.177 PMID:22800383

Mather, C. A., Marlow, A., & Cummings, E. (2013). Web 2.0 strategies to enhance support of clinical supervisors of undergraduate nursing students: An Australian experience. Paper presented at the EDULEARN13 (5th International Conference on Education and New Learning Technologies).

McLean, R., Richards, B. H., & Wardman, J. (2007). The effect of Web 2.0 on the future of medical practice and education: Darwinian evolution or folksonomic revolution. *The Medical Journal of Australia*, 187, 174–177. PMID:17680746

Periera, R., Baranauskas, M. C., & da Silva, S. R. P. (2010). A discussion on social software: Concepts, building blocks and challenges. *International Journal for Informatics*, 3(4), 382–391.

Phillips, R., Kennedy, G., & McNaught, C. (2012). The role of theory in learning technology evaluation research. *Australasian Journal of Educational Technology*, 28(7), 1103–1118.

Salminen, L., Stolt, M., Saarikoski, M., Suikkala, A., Vaartio, H., & Leino-Kilpi, H. (2010). Future challenges for nursing education - A European perspective. *Nurse Education Today*, 30(3), 233–238. doi:10.1016/j.nedt.2009.11.004 PMID:20005606

Sharples, M., Taylor, J., & Vavoula, G. (2005). *Towards a theory of Mobile learning* Paper presented at the mLearn 2005, Cape Town, South Africa.

Sherstyuk, A., Vincent, D., & Berg, B. (2008, December 01-03). Creating Mixed Reality Manikins for Medical Education. Paper presented at the Artificial Reality and Telexistance (ICAT, 2008), Yokohoma, Japan.

Skiba, D., & Barton, A. (2006). Adapting your Teaching to Accommodate the Net Generation of Learners. *The Online Journal of Issues in Nursing, 11*(2), Manuscript 4.

Smedley, A. (2005). The importance of informatics competencies in Nursing: An Australian Perspective. Computers, Informatics, Nursing. *CIN, 23*(2), 106–110. PMID:15772512

Strickland, K., Adamson, E., McInally, W., Tiittanen, H., & Metcalfe, S. (2013, Oct). Developing global citizenship online: An authentic alternative to overseas clinical placement. *Nurse Education Today, 33*(10), 1160–1165. doi:10.1016/j.nedt.2012.11.016 PMID:23260621

Traxler, J. (2007). Defining, discussing and evaluating mobile learning: The moving Finger writes and having writ. *International Review of Research in Open and Distance Learning, 8*(2), 67–75.

Treuer, P., & Jenson, J. (2003). Electronic Portfolios Need Standards to Thrive: The proliferation of e-portfolio applications requires compatible software and design standards to support lifelong learning. *EDUCAUSE Quarterly, 2*, 34–42.

Van der Rijt, R., & Hoffman, S. (2013). Ethical considerations of clinical photography in an area of emerging technology and smartphones. Journal of Medical Ethics, Published Online First 25 June 2013

WHO. (2011). mHealth: New Horizons for health through mobile technologies: second survey on ehealth [Electronic Version]. Retrieved 23 July 2013, from http://www.who.int/goe/publications/goe_mhealth_web.pdf

Wicklund, R. (2013). When mhealth and telehealth become just healthcare [Electronic Version]. Government Health IT. Retrieved 26 July 2013, from http://www.govhealthit.com/news/when-mhealth-and-telehealth-become-just-healthcare

Wilson, R., Ranse, J., Cashin, A., & McNamara, P. (2013). Nurses and Twitter: The Good, the bad and the reluctant. Collegian, Early Online 1 November 2013.

KEY TERMS AND DEFINITIONS

Health Technology Competency: As for technology competency but with a specific focus on the health industry.

M-Health: Relates to any mobile technology or computing used to interface with any stakeholder group involved with digital health service delivery or care.

Micro Blogging: Allows subscribers to use a web service to broadcast short posts to other subscribers.

M-Learning: Refers specifically to learning and teaching interaction that uses mobile handheld devices such as electronic notebooks, tablets or smartphones.

Technology Competency: Observable and measurable factors representing the knowledge and skills in relation to the use of technology that are required for performing and supporting the underlying required work processes.

Chapter 51
Implementation of Electronic Health Record (EHR) System in the Healthcare Industry

Robert P Schumaker
Central Connecticut State University, USA

Kavya P. Reganti
Central Connecticut State University, USA

ABSTRACT

The purpose of this research is to demonstrate the efficiency of the Electronic Health Record (EHR) software that is adopted in the healthcare industry to provide better patient care. The authors examine the impact of EHRs on the efficient delivery of healthcare services. More specifically, they detail the origin of EHR, its significance in modern healthcare delivery along with the selection and implementation criteria for EHR software. They present a survey on the extent of adoption of EHR by clinicians. They also highlight the challenges and barriers faced by organizations in adopting EHR software such as cost, workflow impact and data security. Finally, the authors contemplate the future of EHR, its role in the implementation of health information exchange and its implementation in the cloud. They conclude that the implementation of EHR in the cloud is an important step towards better health management across the population with the end-goal of better health outcomes.

1. INTRODUCTION

Historically, health records of a patient are managed using paper charts. Overtime, the benefits to patient safety and quality of care by upgrading paper records to electronic charts are realized. With the advent of electronic storage and importance given to patient-centered healthcare, the concept of the electronic health record was born (Hoerbst and Ammenwerth, 2010). The purpose of this research is to evaluate the efficiency of adopted EHR software in a medical practice.

EHR provides the potential to improve effectiveness and efficiency by maintaining the privacy of health information, minimizing medical record errors and having health information immediately available to healthcare professionals at all times (Razzaque and Jalal-Karim, 2010). EHR supports

DOI: 10.4018/978-1-4666-8756-1.ch051

clinical decision, physician order entry, capture and query information relevant to health care quality, and exchange electronic health information with authorized sources (U.S. Department of Health and Human Services, 2009). Despite its advantages, adoption of EHR in the US healthcare system experiences several barriers with respect to the rising costs and inconsistent quality (Zeng, 2008). Technological advancements and research in vendor applications categorized according to the user groups are crucial for wide spread implementation of EHR and to overcome those barriers.

In the future, cloud computing has the potential to greatly increase the availability of EHRs to small practices at an affordable cost and recent congressional policies also have the potential to positively impact the adoption of EHR by small practices. This paper will discuss the possible impact of such technological and congressional changes to EHR and contemplates its future being in the efficient delivery of healthcare.

While several surveys have targeted large hospitals, there is little to no surveys targeting small practices. Our research aims to explore the challenges and hurdles in the adoption of EHR by small health care practices. We will present a survey of physicians and staff members of small practices regarding the adoption, usage and problems with EHR software.

Further sections are categorized into literature review section with a focus on processes involved in adoption of software; system and experimental design section gives the description of the system and the methodology used for conducting the survey; survey results are presented under results and discussion. Finally, the paper concludes by suggesting enhancements along with future directions.

2. LITERATURE REVIEW

The Electronic Health Record (EHR) System emerged as a result of a combination of information communications technology and knowledge management to capture, code, and disseminate health information in the form of electronic health record systems that enhance care, not simply replace paper. Electronic health records have enormous potential to improve the flow of information across healthcare systems, and information is critical in the effective management of patient care (Mason, 2013).

In this section we will discuss several aspects of EHR software. Section 2.1 describes the importance of software, section 2.2 gives the details right from the selection of software to its adoption. Section 2.3 focuses on future of EHR.

2.1. Importance of EHR

The idea behind converting the paper-based records into digital form is to provide patients health records to healthcare professionals which are easily accessible from multiple facilities. Electronic health records are crucial considering the frequency with which people move for economic reasons, change physicians, and when healthcare problems arise during business trips and vacations (Mason, 2013).

In conjunction with efforts to adopt EHRs, hospitals are actively seeking to convert their paper-based work environments into paperless work environments and transform their Health Information Management (HIM) resources. The reasons for this conversion are many, including more centralized patient records management, the move toward Computerized Physician Order Entry (CPOE), and the need for timely access to medical history, improved data privacy and security, regulatory compliance, and more generally, improved operational effectiveness and reduced costs (Hanover, 2011).

Moreover with the paper based health records, tracking updates, sending the records to other offices happens either manually or by fax which is not as fast and reliable as EHR. Paper based medical records have several disadvantages like illegible handwriting, ambiguous and incomplete data, and data fragmentation. In addition, paper records often become bulky with time, hence maintaining and tracking paper based health records would be complex. All these weaknesses could obstruct the continuity and quality of care (Roukema et. al., 2006).

2.2. All about EHR Software

It is important for EHR health providers to have an idea regarding how to select software that works best for the practice considering the size of the practice. Prior to selection, problems should be identified and proper planning should be done in order to design a solution. Once the preliminary stages are done we can move to examining the adoption process and security features supported by the software.

2.2.1. Selecting EHR Software

Software providers need to plan, prepare, and budget for record conversion during EHR deployment. Topics such as cleanup of the master patient database and eliminating duplicate records need to be tackled before the transition to the EHR (Hanover, 2011).

EHR software should bring in significant advances in the quality of patient care by enhancing readability, availability, and data quality. The software should support comprehensive, reliable, relevant, accessible, and timely patient information to each member of the healthcare team, whether in primary or secondary care and whether a doctor, nurse, allied health professional, or patient. The updated medical record should be available concurrently for use everywhere.

The EHR also provides medical alerts and reminders. EHR systems have some built-in intelligence capabilities, such as recognizing abnormal lab results or potential life-threatening drug interactions. Research findings supporting diagnostic tests and the EHR can link the clinician to protocols, care plans, critical paths, literature

databases, pharmaceutical information and other databases of healthcare knowledge (Gurley, 2004).

2.2.2. Implementation

The implementation of EHR depends on mainly three T's, which are Team, Tactics and Technology. Team refers to the people in the organization who will be using the software. The entire team should be aware of the functionalities of the software. Tactics includes the discussion of techniques used in design and setup. The term Technology is related to the software, hardware and network choices made. This section will provide an in-depth review of the three aspects of EHR implementation (Adler, 2007).

2.2.2.1. Team

Effective implementation of EHR requires a sound team with one or more EHR professionals. The team must include the organization's senior executive who fully supports the implementation. In addition, an experienced, skilled project manager with sound change management principles is needed. For the EHR implementation to succeed, the team must have clear, measurable, and achievable goals.

2.2.2.2. Tactics

Implementation of EHR software involves a set of decisions that determine the outcome of the implementation. The workflow design plays an important role in answering questions that arise during the implementation phase. Workflow redesign is a way to conceptually redesign the current paper based information workflow in order to reconfigure, automate and improve less efficient processes. As a starting point each major office process should be identified along with the current paper processes under it. The current paper processes should be schematically documented. Next, the process should be streamlined in order to improve its efficiency and reduce process redundancy. Office processes that must be examined include medication refilling, telephone messaging, appointment requesting, lab reviewing, other test reviewing, prescription writing, patient check-in, health maintenance tracking, referral making, lab and test ordering, communicating test results to patients, interoffice messaging, and note charting (Adler, 2007).

2.2.2.3. Technology

Technology also plays an important role in the success of EHR software implementation. Technological problems such as poorly written software or inadequate server memory can cripple EHR implementation. Therefore, selecting and spending on IT infrastructure is a critical component in EHR software's overall success. For smaller practices, selecting a good application service provider is an added critical step. Adequate testing and utilization of expert IT advice allows the implementation to be executed smoothly. Daily backups and a sound disaster recovery plan allow the organization to effectively tackle the worst case scenario (Adler, 2007).

Mistakes in EHR implementation may affect patient satisfaction. The impacts of several problems are explained in Table 1 (Dolan, 2012).

2.2.3. Adopting EHR Software

The major stages of adopting EHR software are investigate, create, plan and evaluation phases (O'Hare, 2009).The key points specified at every phase are crucial for the successful adoption of EHR.

2.2.3.1. Investigate

The key points involved in this phase are identify the problem, develop the design brief, and formulate a design specification. The role of Information Technology (IT) in the health care industry varies according to the requirement of the practice. The problems like paper-based patient records, no computerized clinical operations, and a lack of long term IT strategies are identified. According to the problem, outline design should be prepared. Understanding specified requirements like how far the practice should avail the benefits of IT is helpful in the selection of an EHR system.

2.2.3.2. Plan

The key point involved in this phase is to plan a product or solution. Planning is very important for any successful accomplishment. A project

Table 1. Impact of problems (Dolan, 2012)

Problem	Impact
Lack of necessary infrastructure	Computers could be knocked offline or run slowly, resulting in a patient backlog.
Lack of workflow assessment	Important steps in the patient encounter could be missed or not documented.
Lack of training	Disgruntled employees will become unhappy and affect the entire implementation process. Mistakes are possible, or the practice could run more slowly because employees can't do their jobs.
Not preparing patients	Long wait times will become a bigger problem as patients are not informed as to what is wrong. Patients used to a certain work flow may notice unexplained changes.
Computer not integrated into patient encounter	Patient will view the computer as an intrusion as opposed to a useful tool.
Lack of employee buy-in	Negative feelings from employees could rub off on patients. Employees also will be less willing to learn the new system.
Lack of privacy and security policies	The practice will be at a higher risk of a data breach

plan should include all the important activities and major updates reflecting the progress and inevitable changes until the end. Timelines and policies should be discussed with the vendor. The vendor should ensure proactive, responsive and available support as per needed. Planning should be done carefully for the implementation period that reduces the risk of loss of productivity during installation of hardware or software.

2.2.3.3. Create

The key points to be considered in this phase are to create a product or solution, follow the plan, and to use appropriate technology and equipment. Before transitioning to EHR a baseline for the technology should be established. Choosing the technology according to the size of the practice plays a crucial role. The selection of EHR should be done considering whether the practice needs basic functionality like billing, scheduling and office operations to be computerized. If the practice needs value added services, it can go forward and select the software that could support integrated systems, and improve operational efficiency and digital diagnostics etc. If a practice wants to deliver significant benefits, the software selected should enhance current system handling all the aspects of practice operations and management, clinical, and administrative benefits.

To summarize, a practice that is new to EHR may start with basic functions like creating and maintaining electronic records and enhance the components later. In order to support functions such as creating, maintaining, and transmitting electronic health records securely and reliably, hardware is a must. Selected hardware should ensure consistent performance, advanced features, mobility, and networking features.

2.2.3.4. Evaluate

The key point in this phase is to evaluate the product or solution. Evaluating EHR software should consider questions such as does the tech-nology have the functionality that is essential? Does the vendor meet the needs of practice? The software should identify key workflows and be able to address the challenges and problems encountered. Evaluation can be done best when a physician-led team effort and administrative needs are taken into account. At least one member of clinical staff, representatives of the office staff, and the practice administrator should be involved in implementing the product that was chosen.

Adopting software is not just a single step process. Before moving our discussion to challenges and barriers involved in adopting EHR software, we shall review the functionality model of EHR software.

The EHR system is software that provides functionality to manage and maintain the health record, and accomplish various clinical research and business requirements. It may be a monolithic system or a combination of systems.

The software adopted promises better care to the patients with several functionalities embedded in it. The functional model of EHR describes the functions of EHR software divided into three categories as shown in Figure 1.

Physicians' EHR adoption is slowed by a reimbursement system that rewards the volume of services more than it does their quality. Though EHRs have the potential to improve quality, many practices, especially solo or small group practices, face many challenges in successfully using EHRs thus leading to slow pace of Health Information Technology (HIT) adoption (Miller, et.al, 2005). The following sections focus on the challenges, barriers and security aspects of EHR software.

2.2.3.5. Challenges

When the adopted EHR system achieves optimal benefits, it's a success. Through creativity, commitment, and with trial and error methods, the hospital should successfully address most of the

Figure 1. The functional model of EHR (HL7, 2004)

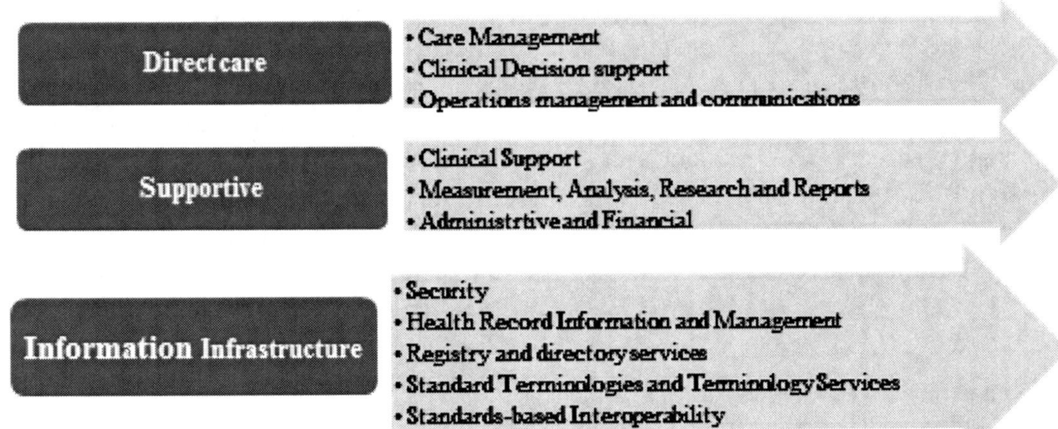

challenges. The challenges will be discussed along with the derived solutions from set of strategies that play a crucial role in achieving success (Carroll et. al., 2012).

The successful implementation of EHR lowers the burden of the physicians by helping in documenting more patient encounters in less time followed by accurate coding and higher reimbursement levels. EHR also makes billing simple by uploading the patient encounter information into the billing system which in turn electronically transports it to a clearinghouse (Dolan, 2008).

2.2.3.6. Barriers

The greatest barrier to adopting EHR in hospitals is a lack of financial resources. The cost of integrating patient access to existing EHR is unclear, but it seems likely that 'retrofitting' systems not originally designed for lay use would entail significant costs. Predictive or operational modeling could provide estimates of some of these potential cost implications (Beard et al., 2011).

According to the article published by Prognosis Health Information Systems, EHR deployments are not about technology. They are about equipping organizations to achieve critical business objectives by providing people with technical capabilities that make new innovations possible and by educating people in changing their behavior so that they can use the new capabilities to generate results (Matthews, 2012).

The current concerns of EHR are about its ongoing maintenance costs, loss of productivity, and increased time to document clinical information in digital format when compared to paper charts. Physicians who have adopted EHR generally make the transition process smoother by taking advantage of readily available technical support. Training and the support from the vendor are the most important things in the EHR adoption at a practice (Glenn, 2012). Many studies reveal cost as the biggest barrier for EHR adoption; in addition to cost other barriers are explained in the Table 2 (Markle Foundation, 2004).

2.2.3.7. Security

The Health Insurance Portability and Accountability Act of 1996 (HIPAA), privacy rule, Public Law 104-191, provides federal protections for personal health information held by covered entities and gives patients an array of rights with respect to that information. At the same time, the Privacy rule is balanced so that it permits the disclosure of personal health information needed for patient care and other important purposes.

Table 2. Barriers of EHR (Markle Foundation, 2004)

Barrier to Adoption	Explanation
Cost	The cost of software can vary significantly depending upon the system's features such as a problem list, messaging, personal digital assistant with wireless capabilities, and medical record interface, which can add significantly to the cost. While some vendors offer inexpensive systems, many practices are finding that these systems lack desired functionality.
Workflow impact	Clinicians may resist the additional time it takes to load initial patient data into the e-prescribing tool and the time it takes to use the tool, which can be longer than it takes to write a prescription by hand.
Lack of benefits	The reimbursement benefits often flow through to other stakeholders, such as health plans and employers, and not to the physician's practice that purchases the system.
Integration	The lack of integration of these systems with others that contain more comprehensive patient information is a key barrier to the seamless treatment of a patient.
Business impact	The costs of installation such as process re-engineering, including the planning and change management cycles are required to ensure transition from paper systems to the EHRs and related systems.

The HIPAA privacy rule establishes national standards to protect individuals' medical records and other personal health information and applies to health plans, health care clearinghouses, and those health care providers that conduct certain health care transactions electronically. The rule requires appropriate safeguards to protect the privacy of personal health information, and sets limits and conditions on the uses and disclosures that may be made of such information without patient authorization. The rule also gives patients' rights over their health information, including rights to examine and obtain a copy of their health records, and to request corrections (U.S. Department of Health and Human Services, 2009).

According to the HIPAA security rule, health care providers are meant to set up physical, administrative, and technical safeguards to protect electronic health information. The software should ensure techniques like access controls (ex: passwords, PIN numbers) that limit access to information and as well as encryption techniques for the safety. An audit trail should be maintained to monitor the changes recorded and by whom they were done (Rodriguez, 2011).

Privacy of patient data is a significant concern, particularly if the data are accessible outside healthcare institutions and are available on the internet. Leaked clinical data could compromise patients on a variety of levels and expose medical practitioners to lawsuits related to negligence in the care of patient's data. The US Department of Health and Human Services, which enforces national standards for confidentiality and security of electronic health information (the HIPAA security rule), has received 445 claims since 2009 that the security rule was violated. In response to security concerns, new security architecture for EHR, including multiple data-protection features, such as encryption, remote and protected data storage, monitored exchanges between computer systems, digital signatures, authentication processes and usage audits, have been created (Beard et.al., 2011).

2.3. The Future of EHR

Recent studies have revealed that EHR usage by clinicians and healthcare organizations are continuing to proliferate across the country due to the federal incentives. While EHRs have been transformational for some large corporations, majority of the medicine is mostly practiced by small medical groups, with limited finances and IT support. Therefore, there is scope for growth in this area and several technological and bureaucratic factors will play a key role in its proliferation in the future (Schoen et. al., 2012).

In addition, the meaningful use requirement of the Health Information Technology for Economic and Clinical Health (HITECH) act will also be another primary force in determining the future of EHR in the health care industry. Congress enacted the HITECH act in order to move towards an outcome based model to improve the overall efficiency of the health care system and thereby reduce its costs. HITECH authorized incentive payments through Medicare and Medicaid to clinicians and hospitals when they use EHR privately and securely to achieve specified improvements in healthcare delivery (Classen and Bates, 2011).

Several companies are already updating their clinical processes using cloud-based software in order to provide faster and more accurate billing to individuals, shortening the average time to create a bill from seven days to less than 24 hours, reducing transcription costs by 80%. In addition, associations are developing e-Health cloud to host healthcare applications including clinical software, decision support tools for diagnosis and management, care plans, referral tools, prescriptions, training, and other administrative clinical services (Kuo, 2011).

2.3.1. Other Information Technology Based Innovations

There is also some evidence that the future might include some change of large shared databases for comparative prescription and use of natural language processing, improved clinical decision support, and greater use and integration of wireless remote outpatient monitoring of patients (Navathe and Conway, 2010).

However, the current systems are not multifunctional. While such systems may involve compromising the privacy and security of the data, they also provide systems for the next generation of healthcare computing (Cerrato, 2012).

2.3.2. Health Information Exchange and Publishing

Health information exchange and publishing is another area that most likely will have a place in EHR implementation and usage. However, with the breadth of competitors in this space, the exchange of data will be a challenge and standardization of data will be key. Notwithstanding, one of the most promising advantages for health information exchange and publishing is improved patient safety. Up to 18% of the patient safety errors and 70% of adverse drug events can be eliminated if right information about the right patient is available at the right time. Health information exchange makes this possible. EHR will allow improved patient safety, medication information processing, laboratory information processing, radiology information processing and communication among providers, communication between patients and providers, and public health information processing (Kaelber and Bates, 2007).

3. RESEARCH QUESTIONS

To answer the challenges of EHR adoption in small healthcare practices, we focus on evaluating efficiency and quality of care provided by the hospitals by adopting EHR system; analyzing the requirements that were met by the EHR system and the requirements that were not fulfilled and barriers and challenges of the current system:

1.   How does Electronic Health Record (EHR) software improve efficiency and provide better care to the patients?

The structures of the record that are stored electronically are compared to the paper-based system. Advantages such as readability, sharing the information among multiple facilities and smart phones access by physicians are examined.

2. What are the essential financial and technical capabilities that the physician's office is required to afford for the implementation of EHR system?

To answer this question, estimated financial budgets that are planned by the physician's practice are discussed. The estimated budget varies according to the size of the practice and requirements as well. Training offered by the vendor to the team and support given by the vendor are also discussed.

3. What factors are considered as barriers for the adoption or implementation of EHR in a physician's practice and how can they overcome the barriers?

The barriers such as cost, lack of proper training are keeping hospitals from moving forward with implementing and using electronic health records. The possible solutions for overcoming these barriers are also discussed.

4. How does the EHR system influence in terms of cost and time when compared to the past paper-based records?

Returns on investment, the maintenance costs, and loss of revenue during transition to the new system are discussed. The time required for the data entry when using electronic records in comparison to the paper-based are discussed.

4. SYSTEM AND EXPERIMENTAL DESIGN

Evaluation is performed to measure the actual user performance to judge whether the system can meet its requirements. Performance is examined by collecting user performance data on aspects such as successful task completion, performance difficulties and failures to complete the task successfully or in proper sequence.

We have developed a questionnaire to conduct survey on EHR software. The main objective of the survey is to assess the performance of the software adopted in small healthcare practices. The results of the survey act as an input to enhance the software. It is designed to complement existing functionalities of the system that support the physicians to provide better patient care. The survey addresses barriers for the wide spread of EHR, examines the possible reasons leading physicians to switch to different vendor from current one, and compares present system in terms of cost and time to the paper-based records. Questionnaire also asks the participants to rate the current software. Survey is conducted by distributing questionnaire forms to several practices and some by online.

Participants for this survey are the users of EHR. We have surveyed 43 users. Among them, 30% of participants are physicians, 46% of them are medical assistants, 20% of them are administrative staff, and 4% of them are business analysts who are using EHR software. Some of the results are categorized according to their job role. None of the questions elicit personal data outside of the broad demographics on age and background. Received responses are kept confidential and data retrieved from the survey is reported in the research only as a combined total.

We surveyed a representative sample of physicians in Connecticut and Massachusetts regarding adoption and use of EHRs. After excluding ineligible practices, the remaining sample included 60 participants, of whom 43 (71%) responded to the survey. We believe that these results can provide an insight on performance of the software which might be helpful for other small health practices that are considering EHR adoption.

5. EXPERIMENTAL RESULTS AND DISCUSSION

Results are based on the responses from physicians, medical assistants, administrative staff and business analysts at small practices working with EHR. Addressing our first research question:

1.   How does Electronic Health Record (EHR) software improve efficiency and provide better care to the patients?

Results emphasize that the ability to share the medical records across the providers and organizations as a huge advantage of EHR. The adopted EHR software is expected to achieve quick record retrieval; data entry should be easier and reduce errors.

Out of forty three respondents, 86% of them stated record retrieval is faster when the health records of a patient are stored electronically. Searching, tracking and analyzing information is easy with EHRs. Though 51% stated easier data entry, majority of physicians' response reveal that entering data through EHR is time consuming as difficulties include having too many free-text fields or a mismatch between the reporting requirements and data storage formats, necessitating data abstraction and manual translation.

EHR is most useful when the data needed exist in discrete fields, so that they can be aggregated, sorted, and manipulated. Data that exist only in free-text fields require manual intervention to extract and analyze. Some hospitals have been deliberate in structuring data fields to maximize their use and avoid text fields. Others have deferred to their physicians' preferences for free-text fields, and rely on quality review staff to read through clinicians' notes to manually extract usable information. Even those hospitals that use manual chart review report that the EHR is an improvement because it eliminates the need to track down paper charts.

Regarding features of EHR, 55% responded that their EHR has the copy/paste feature and 60% of them responded that their EHR has search feature and 65% of them uses templates to enter patient's data. When we asked about how the physician maintains progress notes, responses are as follows.

62% of them maintains as a hard copy, 79% of them scans directly into the EHR, 74% of them transcripts into the EHR, 74% of them types directly into EHR as free text, 79% of them enter data into EHR using templates, 13% of the participants responded that EHR can help to reduce errors. Few medical assistants and administrative staff responded that physician's handwriting which was a problem in the past is now solved by the EHR enabling physicians to type notes directly into EHR as free text or by using templates. Table 3 provides results regarding the features and advantages of EHR that are categorized according to the job role.

The results in Table 3 reveal an interesting point. Though reducing errors is stated as one of the advantages of EHR, only 13% of participants agree on it. It implies that software did not deliver the results as expected on the feature 'reducing errors'. If the progress notes are scanned into EHR or if they are entered into the EHR by using templates errors can be reduced and using templates may also save time.

2.   What are the essential financial and technical capabilities that the physician's office is required to afford for the implementation of EHR system?

Forty-one percent of the participants replied that the type of their EHR software is one or more commercial vendors, 28% of them are using from one vendor, and 30% of them are using as a combination of vendors and internally developed products.

Table 3. Features and advantages of EHR

Features and Advantages	Physicians	Staff
Record retrieval is faster	12	25
Data entry is easier	6	16
Copy/Paste	10	14
Templates	10	18
Search	9	17
Reduce errors	4	2

Nine percent of participants have been using EHR since last year, 63% of participants have been using EHR since three years, 7% of participants have been using since five years, and 26% of participants have been using since more than five years. Thirty percent of them responded that they switched to different vendors' software. Majority of the physicians have started using EHR since three years and they did not switch to other vendor yet but the physicians who have been using EHR since more than five years have switched to different vendor. Some practices must be switching to other vendors as they wanted to adopt software that supports enhanced features than the current one and some may be switching due to the problems related to performance. This is the area where vendors have to work.

When we filtered the results among physicians and staff regarding training criteria, 37.5% of physicians and 41.1% of staff responded that they were offered training for a period of less than a week; 50% of physicians and 35.2% of staff responded that they were offered training for a period of one-two weeks; 12.5% of physicians and 5.8% of staff responded that they were offered training for a period of two-four weeks; 17.6% of staff responded that they were offered training for a period of greater than four weeks. None of the physicians got training for a period of greater than four weeks.

To gain knowledge on software and to accustom with the new environment, training period of less than a week may not be enough. At least one-two weeks of training should be provided. Results imply that physicians cannot afford their time on training more than a week as there will be an impact on their day to day activities. But if physicians could manage enough time to train themselves, EHR could be utilized more efficiently.

3. What factors are considered as barriers for the adoption or implementation of EHR in a physician's practice? How can they overcome the barriers?

Sixty-seven percent of the participants answered that cost as major barrier of adoption. The biggest barrier in adopting EHR is start up and maintenance cost. Small and medium-sized practices have significantly fewer opportunities to achieve financial gain through IT. The cost of software varies upon the system's features. Apart from procuring the software it is a burden for a small practice to bear the costs of installation such as process re-engineering, and change management cycles that during transition from paper systems to the EHRs and related systems. Moreover, several physicians have complained that their system frequently freezes which leads to loss of productivity.

Forty four percent of them responded that learning and transition is hard. Better implementation procedures can overcome this barrier. Implementing a new technology demands modifications in clinical practice, so the hospitals have to staff the process to keep their systems current and running. The transition will be smooth, when the entire team has better coordination, and aware of the anticipated upheaval changes in their day-to-day activities.

Thirty percent of them responded that it is not user friendly software. Adequate training can help to overcome this barrier. Vendors need to come up with improvised applications that could turn the software more friendly.

Survey results related to barriers in the adoption of EHR are shown in Figure 2.

4. How does the EHR system influence in terms of cost and time when compared to the past paper-based records?

Paper records are bulky, they take up space and require labor-intensive methods to maintain, retrieve and file. Unlike paper records, EHR provide easier access at times of emergency and can be backed up easily to avoid loss during times of disaster, especially when linked into a health information network.

Figure 2. Barriers in the adoption of EHR

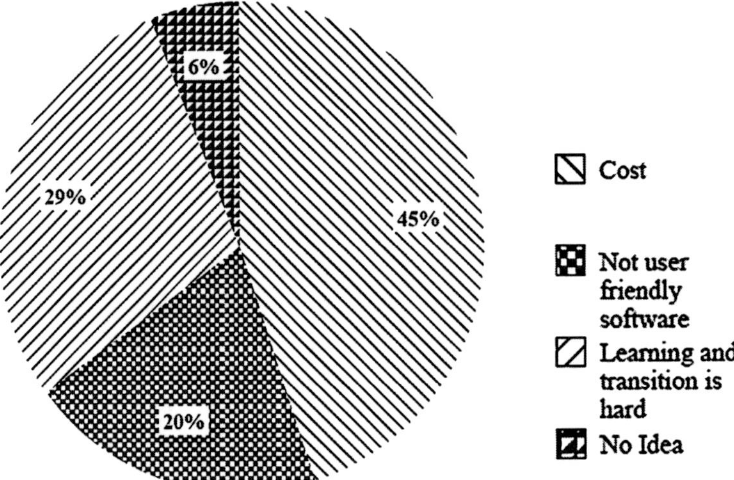

Further results found that 77% are using I.D. and password for user authentication. Just like paper records, electronic health records must comply with the federal Health Insurance Portability and Accountability Act (HIPAA) in regard to protecting patient privacy. Electronic Health Records can be encoded so that only authorized individuals can view them. So, we have collected some information regarding features related to security that were accomplished by their current software. The results are shown in Table 4.

In the event of power outage or damage to the system where it is inoperable, 33% of participants responded that they have planned backup and 65% of participants responded that they will wait till the system gets fixed.

Fifty percent of participants responded that the hospitals allow outside entities access to the EHR technology remotely and 39% of participants responded that the hospitals allow outside entities access to the EHR technology on-site. Forty six percent of participants responded that EHR users have limitations to electronically export, transfer or print EHR documents.

To test regarding usability of the current EHR software, we have focused on learnability, data entry, accessibility and satisfaction. These features

Table 4. Features related to security

Security Features of EHR	
Automatic user log-off/ session time-out	37
Minimum password configuration rules	39
Regular changing of password	37
User awareness on password non-sharing policy	38

convey efficiency of software considering, how easy it is to learn, how the users could enter data using its applications, how fast a record can be retrieved and the overall user satisfaction respectively. We have obtained the ratings on each of them and then we categorized the results based on the role physicians and staff. Data entry is rated below 3 on scale of 5 by physicians. But when we observe the ratings given by staff on data entry, it comes to 3.45 (p-value 0.15). Other than data entry ratings for rest of the features given by physicians and staff does not show much difference.

Figure 3 shows the further details on rating given by physicians and staff on these four areas.

If the physicians are properly trained on EHR best practices and providing resources such as voice recognition software that facilitates documentation may help to improve data entry methods.

Figure 3. Ratings given by physicians and staff

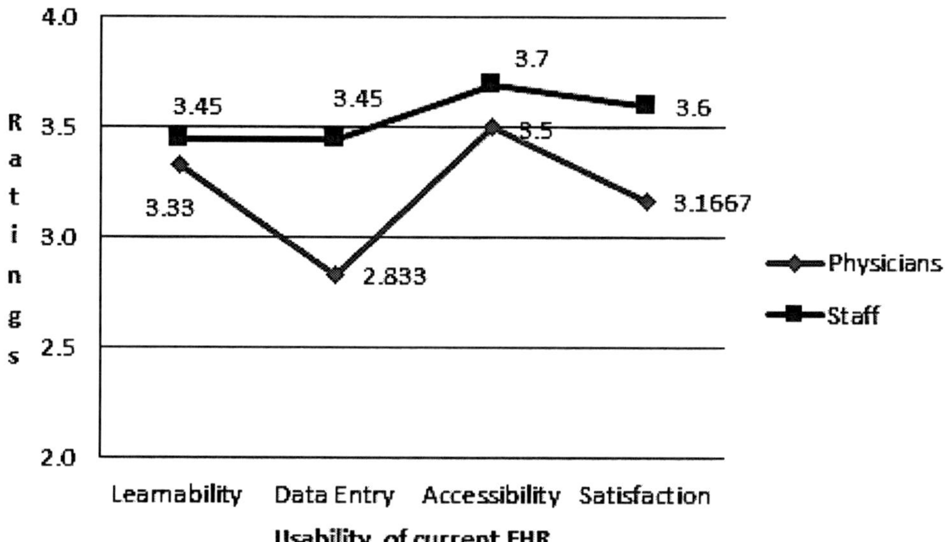

On a final note, when we asked them how well they like their current EHR software, the average rating given by the physicians is 2.92 and the average rating given by the administrative staff is 3.7 on a scale of 5.

These results clearly show that the importance of EHR is realized by the physicians' and they support for its adoption all over the country. Future EHR software design should focus on turning reluctant users to willing with its enhancements for user friendly features. To reduce the reluctance level among physicians, Government should help small providers by facilitating a virtual linkage so that they can access EHR systems at a reasonable price (Bates, 2005).

6. CONCLUSION AND FUTURE DIRECTIONS

Though EHRs have potential benefits to patients, caregivers and organizations, it needs some enhancements. Widespread adoption and use of EHRs will not be possible unless the software can provide perceptible value to the users. Survey results show non interoperability, software being not user friendly, and complex data entry as three major problems.

Interoperability within an EHR is crucial as it needs to connect patients, providers, referral providers and other key personnel and it should support synchronized view of the patient health history that is shared among the multiple facilities. Benefits can be realized if and only if the government and medical device manufacturers join together to promote the development and adoption of interoperable devices. Devices have to interoperate with each other and also should be able to accept data from IT systems for safety and efficiency gains (Versel, 2013). In order to achieve interoperability, the Office of Standards & Interoperability (OSI) at the U.S. Department of Health and Human Services is encouraging to develop health IT standards and move toward the seamless exchange of health data across all stakeholders.

Many physicians in our survey responded that data entry is not quick and software is not user friendly. Physicians often use keyboard shortcuts to save time when charting. Sometimes this may lead to medical errors and improper billing and when that erroneous data is carried from one progress note to other, medical records lose clarity. Adequate staff training and interoperable technology together can help prevent adverse events and data entry errors (Guerrero, 2013).

Future EHR implementations will probably involve vendor applications that are more focused on flexible system architecture and patient-directed functions based on each user group's specific task-oriented requirements. Vendors will have to add new features and functionality, and health care organizations are changing their implementations to focus on achieving meaningful use. To help vendors understand how to improve the design of their products, post marketing surveillance could be used.

In future, EHRs may come into practice using cloud technology. The main advantage of cloud computing is its low cost which is at present treated as a major barrier in adopting EHR software in the hospitals. As cloud is capable of rapid elasticity and ubiquitous access to health resources, as demand changes, hospitals and other health care providers do not need to adjust their infrastructures to accommodate the changes. Cloud offers potential opportunities for improving EHR adoption, but there are still many challenges to fostering the new model in health care such as data security and legal issue.

REFERENCES

Adler, K. (2007). How to Successfully Navigate Your EHR Implementation. *Family Practice Medicine, 14*(2), 33–39. PMID:17330715

Bates, D. (2005). Physicians and Ambulatory Electronic Health Records. *Health Affairs, 24*(5), 1180–1189. doi:10.1377/hlthaff.24.5.1180 PMID:16162561

Beard, L., Schein, R., Morra, D., Wilson, K., & Keelan, J. (2011). The challenges in making electronic health records accessible to patients. *Journal of the American Medical Informatics Association, 19*(1), 116–120. doi:10.1136/amiajnl-2011-000261 PMID:22120207

Carroll, S., Edwards, J., & Rodin, D. (2012). Using Electronic Health Records to Improve Quality and Efficiency: The Experiences of Leading Hospitals. Retrieved on February 09, 2013, from http://www.commonwealthfund.org/~/media/Files/Publications/Issue%20Brief/2012/Jul/1608_SilowCarroll_using_EHRs_improve_quality.pdf

Cerrato, P. (2012). 5 Healthcare IT Resolutions for 2013. Retrieved on March 01, 2013, from http://www.informationweek.com/healthcare/cpoe/5-healthcare-it-resolutions-for-2013/240144068

Classen, D., & Bates, D. (2011). Finding the Meaning in Meaningful Use. *The New England Journal of Medicine, 365*(9), 855–858. doi:10.1056/NEJMsb1103659 PMID:21879906

Dolan, P. (2008). Practices that are thriving after the changeover. Retrieved on February 08, 2013, from http://www.ama-assn.org/amednews/2008/05/05/bisa0505.htm

Dolan, P. (2012). EHR implementation: How common blunders can alienate your patients. Retrieved on February 08, 2013, from http://www.amednews.com/article/20120924/business/309249969/4/

Glenn, B. (2012). Barriers to EHR adoption determined more by provider type than patient population served Retrieved on February 08, 2013, from http://medicaleconomics.modernmedicine.com/news/barriers-ehr-adoption-determined-more-provider-type-patient-population-served

Guerrero, A. (2013). Cloning Persistent Problem in EHR Data Entry. Retrieved on March 26, 2013, from http://www.hitechanswers.net/ehr-software-usage-study/

Gurley, L. (2004). Advantages and Disadvantages of the Electronic Medical Record. Retrieved on March 10, 2013, from http://www.aameda. org/MemberServices/Exec/Articles/spg04/Gurley%20article.pdf

HL7. (2004). EHR System Functional Model: A Major Development Towards Consensus on Electronic Health Record System Functionality. Retrieved on March 01, 2013, from http://www. hl7.org/documentcenter/public_temp_C0208297-1C23-BA17-0C15421DF7C2DDFB/wg/ehr/EHR-SWhitePaper.pdf

Hanover, J. (2011). Moving from Paper to Electronic Health Records: Optimizing the Transition Retrieved on March 10, 2013, from http://www.ironmountain.com/~/media/Files/Iron%20Mountain/Knowledge%20Center/Reference%20Library/White%20Paper/Sponsored/IDC/Moving%20from%20Paper%20to%20Electronic%20Health%20Records%20IDC%20Whitepaper.pdf

Hoerbst, A., & Ammenwerth, E. (2010). Electronic Health Records: A Systematic Review on Quality Requirements. *Methods of Information in Medicine, 49*(4), 320–336. doi:10.3414/ME10-01-0038 PMID:20603687

Kaelber, D., & Bates, D. (2007). Health information exchange and patient safety. *Journal of Biomedical Informatics, 40*(6), 40–45. doi:10.1016/j.jbi.2007.08.011 PMID:17950041

Kuo, M. (2011). Opportunities and challenges of cloud computing to improve health care services. *Journal of Internet medical research* 13(3), e67.

Markle Foundation. (2004). Financial, Legal and Organizational Approaches to Achieving Electronic Connectivity in Healthcare. Retrieved on March 10th, 2013, from http://www.markle.org/sites/default/files/flo_sustain_healtcare_rpt.pdf

Mason, M. (2013). What Can We Learn from the Rest of the World? A Look at International Electronic Health Record Best Practices. Retrieved on March 10th, 2013, from http://www.moyak.com/papers/best-practices-ehr.html

Matthews, T. (2012). Overcoming the Top Five Barriers to EHR Implementation. Retrieved on February 08, 2013, from http://www.prognosishis.com/pdf/Overcoming%20Barriers%20Whitepaper.pdf

Miller, R., West, C., Brown, T., Sim, I., & Ganchoff, C. (2005). The Value Of Electronic Health Records In Solo Or Small Group Practices. *Health Affairs, 24*(5), 1127–1137. doi:10.1377/hlthaff.24.5.1127 PMID:16162555

Navathe, A., & Conway, P. (2010). Optimizing health information technology's role in enabling comparative effectiveness research. *The American Journal of Managed Care, 16*(12), 44–47. PMID:21314220

O'Hare, H. (2009). Status Update on The HL7 Project -EHR System Design Reference Model. SOA in Healthcare: Value in a Time of Change, Chicago, IL USA.

Razzaque, A., & Jalal-Karim, A. (2010). Conceptual Healthcare Knowledge Management Model For Adaptability and Interoperability Of EHR. *European, Mediterranean & Middle Eastern Conference on Information Systems,* Abu Dhabi, UAE.

Rodriguez, L. (2011). Privacy, Security, and Electronic Health Records. Retrieved on February 09, 2013, from http://www.healthit.gov/buzz-blog/privacy-and-security-of-ehrs/privacy-security-electronic-health-records/

Roukema, J., Los, R., Bleeker, S., Gineeken, A., Lei, J., & Moll, H. (2006). Paper Versus Computer: Feasibility of an Electronic Medical Record in General Pediatrics. *Pediatrics, 117*(1), 15–21. doi:10.1542/peds.2004-2741 PMID:16396855

Schoen, C., Osbron, R., Squires, D., Doty, M., Rasmussen, P., & Applebaum, S. (2012). A Survey Of Primary Care Doctors In Ten Countries Shows Progress In Use Of Health Information Technology. *Health Affairs*, *31*(12), 2805–2816. doi:10.1377/hlthaff.2012.0884 PMID:23154997

U.S. Department of Health and Human Services. (2009). Understanding Health Information Privacy. Retrieved on March 05, 2013, from http://www.hhs.gov/ocr/privacy/hipaa/understanding/coveredentities/hitechact.pdf

Versel, N. (2013). West: Device interoperability with EHRs could save $30B annually. Retrieved on March 27, 2013, from http://mobihealthnews.com/21120/west-device-interoperability-with-ehrs-could-save-30b-annually/

Zeng, X. (2008). Electronic Records in Health care. *North Carolina Medical Journal*, *69*(2), 108–111. PMID:18605159

Chapter 52
Employing Opportunistic Networks in Dementia Patient Monitoring

Radu-Ioan Ciobanu
University Politehnica of Bucharest, Romania

Ciprian Dobre
University Politehnica of Bucharest, Romania

ABSTRACT

By 2050, 135.5 million people will suffer from dementia worldwide. Ambient Assisted Living (AAL) technologies can help dementia patients enjoy an independent life. In particular, communication is vital to any AAL system. Opportunistic networking uses low-cost wearable devices to exchange packets at a close range in cases where there is limited or no infrastructure. In this chapter, the authors propose and describe an autonomous patient monitoring support system based on opportunistic communication. The monitored patient wears non-intrusive sensors, computing devices and actuators, forming a Body Area Network (BAN). The BAN can provide memory impairment support services for the patient and is used to construct personalized condition-monitoring patient models to evaluate against a set of potential life-threatening events. The authors present two data transfer algorithms and show that they are able to offer good hit rates while decreasing congestion and overhead when compared to other existing solutions.

1. INTRODUCTION

In recent years, mobile devices have become ever-present all around us. Ranging from simple sensors, smartphones and tablets, to high-range mobile access points, mobile devices can be found everywhere. A way of organizing these heterogeneous devices into a coherent unit that serves well-defined purposes is by creating an opportunistic network (ON) where they act as nodes. ONs are generally composed exclusively of mobile devices that wish to communicate between each other, although there may be no direct route between them at any time. Nodes in opportunistic networks are not aware of the topology of the network and of the other participating nodes. The only information they have is learned from encounters with other devices, through short-range proximity

DOI: 10.4018/978-1-4666-8756-1.ch052

communication. Opportunistic networks are based on a paradigm entitled store-carry-and-forward. It implies that a node wishing to send a message to another node starts by storing the data and carrying it around the network, until it finds a suitable destination for it. Such a destination is not necessarily the message's destination, but it can also be another node that has a better chance of delivering the message to the destination than the current carrier. Thus, through collaboration and altruism, ON nodes end up delivering data even when there is no direct connectivity between two nodes.

There are many real-life use cases where opportunistic networks can or have already been employed successfully, because not only can they help ease communication in situations where two nodes may never be connected, but they can also decrease the costs of communication. This can be done, for example, by using short-range data exchanges (such as Bluetooth or WiFi Direct) instead of cellular communication (such as 3G or LTE). One of the first ever real-life applications for ONs was wildlife tracking, i.e., recording the movement and behavior of animals in their natural habitat without being intrusive. Special tags containing GPS sensors and close-range communication capabilities are attached to the animals, and fixed or mobile access points are set up in key places in the animals' habitats. Whenever two tagged animals encounter each other, information is exchanged between the devices. When a tagged animal comes in range of an access point, it uploads all available information, which may include data gathered not only from the carrier, but also from other encountered animals. Another situation where opportunistic networks have been successfully employed is in offering Internet access in limited conditions, where no infrastructure exists, such as rural areas where the deployment of Internet is not feasible or cost-effective (e.g., Indian villages). Kiosks are built in the village centers, equipped with digital storage and wireless communication devices, which interact periodically with mobile base stations mounted on buses, motorcycles or bicycles. These mobile stations collect the data from the kiosks and deliver it to Internet access points located in the larger cities, and vice versa.

Opportunistic networks are also appropriate for disaster management, when a natural disaster such as an earthquake, a tsunami or an explosion might disrupt the physical components of the network, such as switches and cables. In these situations, the cellular infrastructure cannot be used, so there is a need for ensuring more efficient and dependable solutions for the rescue missions, by using the unaffected components of the static infrastructures as nodes in an ON, along with mobile devices (such as smartphones) belonging to nearby citizens or survivors of the disaster, with the purpose of offering connectivity where otherwise there would be none, or simply decreasing congestion. Congestion problems may also appear in very crowded areas such as concerts, sporting events, amusement parks, where cellular communication is spread very thin by the large number of open connections from the same geographical location. Opportunistic networks can thus be employed to reduce the cellular communication to fewer nodes and access points, which are then able to spread the data to the other network participants.

Another situation where opportunistic networks could prove useful is in smart cities, which monitor and integrate the conditions of all their critical infrastructures (such as roads, rails, airports, power, water, etc.) in order to optimize resource usage and to plan preventive maintenance activities. By using opportunistic networks, every sensor in a smart city can be leveraged in order to have a big picture of the entire town, without the need of long-range communication capabilities. Sensors simply communicate with any device in range, which can then transport the data to access points that can communicate faster and with a longer range. Other opportunities for ONs exist, such as advertising, geographical area-based floating content, context-aware platforms or distributed social networks.

Although there are multiple advantages in using opportunistic networks, as seen above, there are several challenges that have to be taken into consideration when deploying ONs in real-life situations. The first of these challenges is the very premise of ONs itself, namely that the lack of connectivity at all times leads to a potential lack of end-to-end paths. Thus, if the network is very sparse (i.e., there are few nodes spread on a large area), contact opportunities are very low and so not all nodes may receive the messages destined for them. Moreover, in sparse networks, large delays in message delivery may be incurred. Closely related to this challenge is the decision of selecting a message's next hop. Ideally, content should be spread epidemically in the network, so whenever two nodes meet, they should exchange all data between each other. However, this may lead to congestion issues in the network, as well as on a node level, since the devices have relatively low storage capabilities. Moreover, if the nodes travel at high speeds, the duration of a contact might not be sufficient for exchanging all the content between the encountering nodes. Thus, informed decisions should be made in order to decide if an encountered node is a suitable carrier for a given message. Various routing and dissemination algorithms have been proposed over the years, which take advantage of a node's encounter history, its social relationships with other nodes, or its interests, in deciding whether an encountered device is a suitable forwarder. Furthermore, the nodes from an opportunistic network are mobile devices that generally have limited battery capacity, so this information should also be taken into consideration when performing routing decisions, in order to optimize a node's lifetime.

We believe that opportunistic networks can be successfully applied to the area of dementia patient monitoring. We envision an infrastructure where the patients are being monitored by various sensors, each of them offering different types of readings. These sensors would have short-range communication capabilities, so they can exchange information with data-collecting devices that are carried around the wards by the nurses or the doctors which visit the patients on a regular basis. When two doctors meet, their devices can also exchange the collected data, which is uploaded to the main processing and storage units whenever the doctors are in their proximity. If the patients are mobile (e.g., they have a daily routine which requires them to move to different rooms or wards), they could also be equipped with data-collecting devices. These devices would not only collect data from their sensors, but they would also be able to perform individual computations based on the sensors' readings, in order to potentially alert the doctors if critical situations arise. For such critical situations, the hospital's cellular or WiFi infrastructure can be used, but our proposed solution would drastically reduce the costs of maintaining such an infrastructure. Moreover, opportunistic networks can also be used to disseminate information among the hospital staff, based on their interests, area of expertise, patient list, etc. Opportunistic networks can also be used to track patients suffering from dementia, in order to autonomously detect and alert competent authorities when the patients deviate from their usual walking routes and might get potentially lost. Thus, they are perfect candidates to construct middleware support for services designed to offer a decent quality of life, and perceived health and well-being, for dementia patients.

2. PROBLEM STATEMENT

Human memory is notoriously faulty. We constantly forget important dates, meetings, names, and, let's not forget, the proverbial car keys. It is probably safe to predict that this is only going to get worse: the world is becoming more complex and information-driven, while the human memory is not improving, but in fact is probably becoming worse, due to this information overload. Thus, it is no wonder that human memory has been the subject of various studies in biology, cognitive science, and in psychology. Today, we have studies that relate stress to the difficulty of transferring information from short-term memory to medium-term memory. This difficulty is often the root of a reduction in personal every day's efficiency as things to do tend to come to mind unordered and unplanned. When it comes to medical problems, dementia is the term used to describe various symptoms of cognitive decline such as forgetfulness[1].

For memory-related medical problems such as dementia, Information and Communication Technology (ICT) has an important role in patient monitoring and even for treatment support. More and more people see ICTs as part of their everyday lives, and this includes people with dementia. For example, offering activities that use technology can encourage people to engage better with medical services. ICTs open up avenues for intellectual stimulation for everyone, regardless of their interests and capabilities. The Internet puts a world of knowledge at one's fingertips. Encouraging staff to use ICTs with people with dementia means they will improve their own ICT knowledge and skills. It also means the working day can be made more varied, which improves morale for staff and people with dementia alike.

While the likelihood of having dementia increases with age, it is not a normal part of aging. Before we had today's understanding of specific disorders, "going senile" used to be a common phrase for dementia (sometimes also referred by the term "senility"), which was misunderstood as a standard part of getting old (Ninds, 2013; ALZ, 2013). Dementia describes a number of brain disorders that are severe enough to affect daily activities. Alzheimer's disease is probably among the most known and most common[2].

According to an analysis of the most recent census, 4.7 million people aged 65 years or older, in US alone, were living with Alzheimer's disease in 2010 (Hebert et al, 2013). The Alzheimer's Association estimates in its 2013 report (ALZ, 2013) that over a tenth of people aged 65 years or

more have Alzheimer's disease, and this proportion rises to about a third of people aged 85 and older. The organization indicates that Alzheimer accounts for between 60% and 80% of all cases of dementia, with vascular dementia caused by stroke being the second most common type.

3. APPLICATIONS FOR MOBILE NETWORKS IN DEMENTIA PATIENT MONITORING

Technologies related to multi-hop (mobile) ad-hoc networking emerged in the 1990s, when off-the-shelf wireless devices became able to provide direct network connections among mobile devices: Bluetooth (IEEE 802.15.1) for personal area networks, and the 802.11 standards family for high-speed wireless LAN. Wireless Sensor Networks (WSNs), in particular, are a special class of multi-hop ad-hoc networks developed to control and monitor a wide range of events and phenomena. In WSNs, a number of sensor nodes are typically deployed (in a dense and possibly random manner) inside a monitoring area. The information collected by the sensor nodes is delivered, by following the multi-hop paradigm, to a sink node and through this to nodes connected to the Internet.

WSNs were long seen as perfect candidates for health monitoring systems (i.e., wireless mobile sensors can be worn by the patient). With an increasing cost of healthcare and a growing population of seniors in nursing homes and hospitals worldwide, patient monitoring using wireless technologies is considered as a solution to both improving the quality of healthcare and reducing the rate of increase for healthcare services (Akyildiz et al, 2002; Gieras, 2003). Physiological sensors (e.g., to measure EKG, blood pressure, and temperature) can be used to automatically collect physiological parameters to be delivered via a body-area network to devices that can be worn and for real-time processing and/or storing for future use (long-term observation) (Varshney, 2008). For example, the CodeBlue system developed at Harvard University exploits a WSN to raise an alert when vital signs fall outside of the normal parameters (Malan et al, 2004). The system monitors heart rate, oxygen saturation, and EKG data and relays the data over a short-range wireless network to a set of devices, including ambulance-based terminals. However, as developers and practitioners alike remarked, WSNs are not necessarily ideal technological support for patient monitoring, as they face a difficult challenge: they represent an engineering approach designed to hide node mobility by constructing "stable" end-to-end paths as in the Internet. When the patient is moving around, as in real-world hospital environments, coping seamlessly with mobility is not so easy to handle in traditional WSNs - possibly, due to interferences or lack of wireless coverage, there is simply no support to form a path between the sensor (patient) to its data sink (doctor) in one single session.

In general, patient monitoring involves periodically transmitting routine vital signs of patients across certain boundaries (and, in some cases, alerting signals when vital signs cross a threshold; in other cases, the data processing of vital signs is moved on a specialized in-the-Cloud platform). As one might think, there are many challenges in wireless monitoring of patients, including the coverage, reliability and quality of monitoring (Varshney, 2008). The current work done in patient monitoring includes, among others, home monitoring (Lee et al, 2000), wireless systems for digitized EKGs (Khoor et al, 2001), hospital-wide mobile monitoring systems (Pollard et al, 2001), mobile telemedicine (Hung & Zhang, 2003; Pattichis et al, 2002), or real-time home monitoring of patients (Mendoza & Tran, 2002).

A variety of approaches previously made attempts to address the issues of reliable and efficient message delivery from deployed sensors to central processing units (for an analysis we refer the reader to Braem et al, 2008). The problem is finding a trade-off between reliability and energy efficiency, because any patient monitoring system will need to maximize the amount of delivered messages, with minimum energy consumption. In an ad-hoc environment, the success of message delivery is not only related to the consumed power, but also depends on the cooperation of neighboring devices. As specified in (Varshney, 2007), it is impossible to use a single method to coordinate multiple entities in a dynamic and complex environment. Apparently, patient monitoring has become an interdisciplinary topic and needs more intelligent technologies than other subjects (e.g., artificial intelligence). The Ambient Cardiac Expert (ACE) monitoring system (Sehgal et al, 2007) is a cardiac patient monitoring system which collects physiological data observed by sensor networks (together with gene expression data) to predict the heart failure rate. Clinical data monitored by attached sensors on patients' bodies is used to generate training data to predict the odds of heart failure.

Elderly dementia patient monitoring is on the other side of mobile healthcare systems. Unlike cardiac-assistance, in dementia patient monitoring delays can in some cases be tolerated (i.e., when monitoring the location of the patient, and in cases where the social interaction with the patient surroundings is actually encouraged). For example, (Lin et al, 2008) presents an indoor and outdoor active safety monitoring mechanism, built based on radio frequency identification (RFID) technology. The monitoring system can automatically remind caregivers once an elderly patient is close to a dangerous area or too far from caregivers. During the information exchange process, the Tame Transformation Signatures (TTS) algorithm is applied to encrypt tag IDs and protect patients' privacy. Here, and in other similar systems, opportunistic networks can easily find applicability. As seen, patients with dementia are generally monitored in terms of changes in their behavior (i.e., alerts are sent if the patient forgets his whereabouts).

Opportunistic networking brings an interesting evolution of the multi-hop networking paradigm. With ONs, node mobility is not a problem anymore, but rather an opportunity to be exploited. In this case, the mobility of nodes creates contact opportunities among nodes, which can be used to connect parts of the network that are otherwise disconnected. Dementia patient monitoring is one case study where ONs can be easily integrated with other health monitoring techniques. ONs can offer support for alerting people in the location-based proximity when a patient deviates from his normal path and is potentially lost (i.e., in a hospital, the nearby nurse could be more easily alerted by an opportunistically-disseminated message, if the dementia-suffering patient exits a particular critical zone). WSNs can still be used for disseminating life-critical messages (and, even better, they can be extended with capabilities for short-time delay tolerance to better cope with the loss of transmission path, for example), but for collecting information about the state-of-mind and habits of patients, we believe ONs to be perfect candidates. Wireless patient monitoring and mobile healthcare can benefit a lot from this. Inside the house, the dementia-suffering patient can be conditioned through external stimuli to remember doing a specific activity (i.e., through turning a light bulb on, or starting the TV, ringing the doorbell, etc.). Outside, a GPS-enabled device carried by the patient can prevent him from being lost (i.e., by monitoring the patient's activity and location, and triggering automatic alarms when he deviates far from his usual routine), or support him by triggering memory reactions through specific stimuli (e.g., triggering a specific alarm or small voltage on the device the user is carrying around his wrist). For such applications, ad-hoc networking techniques can provide the necessary technological base and support.

4. A DEMENTIA PATIENT MONITORING SYSTEM USING OPPORTUNISTIC NETWORKS

Living assistance systems focusing on the support of dementia-suffering patients in their own environments are generally referred to as patient-care systems. Elderly people, in particular, have a high risk of suffering from typical high-age diseases, dementia (including Alzheimer's) being one of them. The costs of providing care for this population increases with a decreasing age-dependency ratio defined by the number of working individuals divided by the number of handicapped people of a country. Experts predict this ratio will dramatically approach 1 in the next 10 to 20 years. Thus, it is obvious that society has to react somehow to this dramatic process. Therefore, innovative solutions for living assistance systems must be envisioned in order to cope with this development. Automated patient-care systems based on ambient intelligence technology are a promising approach. They aim at the prolongation of a self-conducted life of assisted persons, reducing the dependency on intensive personal care to a minimum and thereby increasing the quality of life for the affected group while substantially decreasing the costs for society.

The ultimate goals of any patient monitoring system are high recall in detecting every real emergency immediately, and high precision, to prevent invalid emergency detections and alerts as a consequence of misinterpretations. The first requirement is mandatory to provide a trustworthy service quality to the affected persons in case of emergency situations that should be much safer than anything else they experienced before. The second requirement is essential for economic reasons, since invalid emergency alerts may unacceptably increase care costs and decrease trustworthiness. It is highly desirable to extend a pure emergency detection service by an emergency prediction service, which attempts to recognize a critical health condition before it escalates into an emergency. As a reaction to the detection of such critical situations, the service may assist the person in preventing the emergency, e.g., by suggesting appropriate medication.

Generally, memory has been an extensively studied topic in psychology, cognitive sciences and biology. Of course, regarding the process of passing information from short-term memory into long-term memory, we can say that it is a very complex one that requires a high amount of energy from a person, being a stress factor in the cognitive level.

Migliardi et al. performed a study on efficient software on smart devices and how they influence the short and long-term memory (Migliardi & Gaudina, 2011), and concluded that the system developed by them, in which some sensors that vibrated were placed on a jacket, improves memory and prevents user frustration that comes from the inability to remember the time and place in which they communicated. Another important discovery made by the authors is that the communication through the use of a vibrant jacket does not distract from the important things and does not phonically affect the environment. Regarding the dynamics of today's technology and all stimuli which one faces in daily life, implementing techniques to improve memory has become a necessary way for man to be able to function at full capacity anytime anywhere. The development of the robotics industries in the last 25 years has seen a remarkable progress. Although industrialization has brought upon the streamlining of productivity and quality, the human factor had a significant decline as these technologies are quite advanced for workers who until recent years used to work manually. Based on this problem, the software technology and robotic equipment developers focus on the human factor problem.

Improving the lives of people who have memory problems can be done by designing systems to assist them in daily activities. To do this, these systems need to study and analyze the life context of people to see what kind of problems occurs because of memory. The quality of life of older people can be improved by using new technologies. Wireless technology and the increasing computational power have brought upon new solutions for health monitoring systems in real-time (real-time monitoring). Lindeberg et al. (2010) state that users of such techniques, like patients or medical staff, enjoy two advantages. Firstly, wireless technology reduces the number of cables involved in the monitoring system, resulting in a better mobility of patients within the hospital. Moreover, wireless technology may collect data from sensors connected to the patient's body, while they are at home or in places where cables would prevent this possibility. The second advantage is that wireless systems allow data collection and processing at any time. Older people should get accustomed with an active lifestyle. This requires strategies to improve the quality of their life. They must participate in society through citizen initiatives in which they use their time, experience and energy in various organizations.

Active participation of the elderly people in society can bring economic and social benefits to society through activities that older people do and the opportunities they create as workers or volunteers. Also, the motivation and usefulness feeling of elderly people can be maintained and enhanced, thus avoiding the risk of social isolation and many of the risks associated with this. Elderly people face many obstacles in trying to still be active in society. They are often faced with restricted access to certain social, political or infrastructure activities. The results of these limitations are observed by their inability to keep up with technology, lack of information, few social communities and low self-esteem. Local authorities play an important role in the process of keeping the elderly involved in society. The authorities should create and promote social inclusion programs for seniors. Examples of such programs are: senior volunteering, active citizenship, social networks.

In today's society there was a simultaneous increase of elderly population and technology development (Bouwhuis et al, 2007). Among the goals of technology, solving the problems that society is facing is one of the most important. The new assistance systems that technology provides enable elderly people to be independent, thereby enhancing their quality of life. Society relies increasingly on technology, so the need to use ICT always increases. Therefore, these systems must be constructed so as to demonstrate ergonomics and be intuitive and easy to use by seniors.

Although those who design new technological systems have this in mind, the elderly often face problems when choosing to use technology due to the increased complexity that characterizes new technologies. Caprani et al. (2012) believe that, in order to prevent and mitigate this aspect, it is necessary to conduct research aimed at ways of understanding the lifestyle of the elderly, the way they use technology and how to build new systems and devices that can be more easily used by them.

One way to find these things is provided in (Caprani et al, 2012), and consists of using a questionnaire to collect data on elderly people's attitudes about technology and about how they use technology. The questionnaire also investigates where elders use technology, how often they use it, as well as lifestyle issues that prevent their access to technology. Therefore, in designing new technological products, experts must take into account the available information about the elderly, so that future products can be used by them, thereby helping improve the lives of older people.

Emphasis on video and audio sensing technology allows the development of a new branch of technology, the smart home systems and automated home care. This system is based on recording and reading information collected from sensors that are placed in the house. Søberg et al. (2010) state that data obtained from the sensors is processed through CEP (complex event processing). The concept of smart homes based on sensors can be useful especially for the elderly. For old people it can be a significant improvement in the quality of life, by reducing the effort that they have to submit in performing certain daily activities requiring a significant amount of energy on their part. However, the challenge for the designers of these types of sensor systems is to take into account the difficulties faced by the elderly in the use of technology. Thus, given the complexity of such a system, it may seem difficult to understand and use even by persons for whom technology is an important part of life and moreso for the elderly.

Considering this aspect, the systems must include a user-friendly and easy to access interface for any group of people and show increased ergonomics. Besides, the design of such systems must take into account the needs that older people have, given that they may represent an important segment of the population that will use sensor systems and the concept of smart homes. Søberg et al. (2010) created such a sensor system for homes, which they named CommonSens. Their solution introduces a complex event processing system for automated home care, that provides personalization between core concepts like Locations of Interest (LoIs - a set of coordinates describing the boundaries of an interesting location in the environment) and the monitored persons at home through complex event processing. Such awareness applications have received significant attention from researchers lately. Most of them were extruded on studying the improvement of human functioning in some contexts and difficult environmental situations by increasing the state of awareness with the help of computers. With CommonSens, the improvement in the memory of elderly people was tested by designing an application which receives verbal commands regarding the needs of people, translating those needs into queries to a GIS and building a map of the locations where these needs can be satisfied when the environment in which the person exists allows this.

This system is based on three separate models: an identifier model that monitors events and state changes that occur in the home environment and are of interest, a model that describes the physical and logical sensors possibilities, the coverage they have and the type of used signal, and an environment model that describes the physical environment and the impact that it has on the signal. What is new compared to the existing systems is the ability to identify events that indicate that something is not right. This ability is called deviation detection and is based on lists of words and phrases that are entered into the software that can notify contacts when one signals that something is not right. The system perceives the existence of a problem, and emergency contacts are announced. An advantage of the system is that it does not come with a standard list of problematic events, leaving them to be implemented by the user. Thus, each user can create their own list of possible problems that may occur depending on the difficulties that one may face.

The CommonSens system may be beneficial in increasing the safety of any person. But, if we consider the difficulties faced by the elderly, we believe that CommonSens is the biggest help for them. Such a system is especially necessary for people who live alone when something happens in their own homes. In such a situation, a sensor monitoring program instantly contacts the designated contact person. Thus, one can avoid unpleasant events, especially regarding older people who are usually more exposed to risk than the general population.

Chernbumroong identified three major features that a support sensor system has to meet so as to be considered optimum for the elderly (Chernbumroong et al, 2013): high level of acceptance (the system must be environmental and discreet), high degree of adaptation (the system must be able to adapt to situational changes or possible changes of the elderly so as to serve their needs), and ease of use (the system must be in an accessible form so as to be easily used by the user)

The Social Care Institute for Excellence discussed the usefulness of information and communication technology (ICT) in helping and supporting people with dementia (Ciobanu et al, 2014). It is known that among the problems faced by people with dementia, communication problems are very often encountered. Computers (PCs, laptops, smartphones), the Internet and the digital world (audio, photo, video) can stimulate and improve the lives of sufferers. Activities which include ICT in the lives of people with dementia should be conducted in appropriate frameworks and adequate staff should be used so as to maintain the safety of persons. Thus, the realization of a high quality dementia monitoring system requires a sound model of the assisted people, which has a precise notion for critical situations and emergency cases. Such a model must allow personalizing the service, i.e., customizing it by taking into account the existing memory problems associated with each person. The idea of such a model is illustrated in Figure 1.

Figure 1 shows several intervals: the first one defines the normal parameters for good living conditions for a monitored patient, the second one defines boundaries of living conditions, considering the particular person's memory condition, and the last one defines the borderline between normal and critical health conditions. This model is similar to the Event Model proposed in CommonSens. Considering the existing memory impairments of a person, it is mandatory for any monitoring system related to catastrophic events (e.g., a person is lost in a park) to recognize boundary conditions in order to prevent misinterpretation of situations. This can be used to cope with situations where a person deviates from the usual route because of a municipality-operated scheduled detour (e.g., maintenance work to replace an underground pipe in the park), which otherwise might be wrongly recognized as a catastrophic event (i.e., alerting units of potential lost person in the park). Also, the context parameters could be used to formulate user-centric boundaries, considering personalized health conditions. For instance, a person with locomotor disturbance will move slower than a person who does not suffer from this disability.

Figure 1. A condition-monitoring patient model

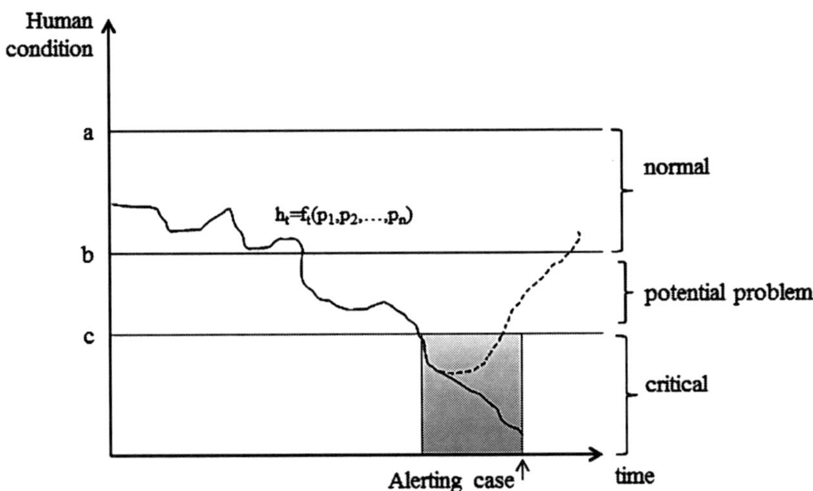

Slow movement of such a person must again not be misinterpreted as a critical situation resulting in a false emergency alert.

The fictive curve in Figure 1 defines the overall condition of a monitored person as a function over time. The function depends on a large, unknown number of parameters and is virtually impossible to describe in a precise mathematical sense. The ultimate goal of any patient monitoring system is to detect the entering of the shadowed area in Figure 1. In such a case, the monitoring system must undertake all possible actions to prevent the emergency (e.g., if the person is detected as having a heart stroke, the system might use animations to remind the patient of medication, drinking, etc.), thereby bringing the health and status condition of the person back to normal (i.e., the dotted line).

An approximation of this model may be achieved by continuously acquiring data about a person's body functions such as temperature, blood pressure, and pulse frequency, together with data on his short-term, medium-term and long-term behavior (including tracking the person in space and time). This data is then evaluated and condensed. Logical predicates (called situations) can be further used to identify states or state transitions of the person under observation.

Examples for such situations are: "Person X forgot to take medicine M", "Person X has fallen down" or "Person X has a blood pressure of 178". Several situations may also be combined in logical expressions, resulting in more complex situations, as in "(Person X has fallen down) AND (Person X forgot to take medicine M) AND (Person X has not responded to call for S seconds)". If such a critical situation occurs, it is taken as evidence that a person's health condition has entered the shadowed region in Figure 1, which now requires appropriate system actions.

The patient monitoring system thus operates by evaluating each situation individually. Whenever the system moves from situation s_i to s_{i+1}, the evaluation cycle is triggered, taking the logical predicates of the actual situation as input for the test against the critical situation indicators in the database. If one or more critical situation indicators are evaluated to be true, a critical situation is concluded and the appropriate system action is initiated.

It is obvious that any living assistance system in the described domain will fail if it requires special skills by the monitored patients for using and handling it. Instead, the assistance system should be completely invisible to those persons.

This also means that the physical condition of the assisted person has to be sensed in an unobtrusive manner. Environmental sensors must be preferred to sensors directly attached to the body, even if this results in a lower precision of the measured values. The system has to compensate this by taking several environmental measurements into account and drawing conclusions from them. This is, of course, a challenging task, but this is the way monitored systems should work.

Based on the identified situations, the system should operate proactively and do its job automatically with minimal human intervention. It would interact with humans by speech, gestures, and other forms of natural communication. It would provide its service in a stable, robust and reliable way, even in the presence of component malfunctions, power/battery breakdown, or other exceptional conditions. Software release changes and maintenance actions will be performed remotely without interrupting the system operation and with minimal intervention by maintenance personnel.

We present a patient monitoring system composed of several subsystems (see Figure 2): the body area network (BAN), the home network, and the central processing node, which also acts as a gateway to the Internet and other external services like the telephone network. We assume sensors, computing devices and actuators are used to provide memory impairment support services

for the patients. Sensors can also be used to (semi-) automatically collect data about the lifestyle of the subjects. As specified before, this can enrich the data collected in the traditional way (i.e., currently the health/mental status for the dementia patients is monitored mostly through interviews and observation).

The body area network is composed of special sensors that monitor vital body functions like blood pressure, temperature, pulse frequency, etc., together with location, acceleration and other environmental parameters, and transmit their results via a wireless connection. The body network is invisibly embedded in clothes, in watches and glasses, so that the patient does not have to put on those sensors explicitly. In fact, they should not even be aware that sensors exist. The system collects the measurements from the different sensors, on-body and also external sensors where available (i.e., for indoors, located inside the house, and for outdoors, possibly provided by persons in the wireless proximity), aggregates the provided sensing data, and periodically transmits it toward a central station for further processing. When there is a direct Internet connection, this will be the preferred means to transmit the data. For indoor scenarios, it is more likely that a wired connection is available. However, things are different for outdoor scenarios. Consider the patient walking around the park. In the absence of an all-

Figure 2. The patient monitoring system

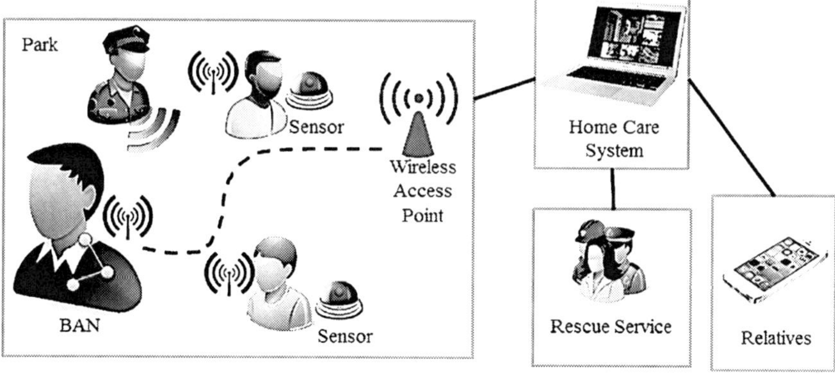

available Internet connection, the system might use ad-hoc networking alternatives to send the data to the Wireless Access Point provided inside the park by the municipality. Here, we employ the use of opportunistic networking techniques. These techniques will be used to also collect sensing data from the environment. For example, while the patient is walking by, he can connect to other mobile devices, carried by other people, and collect valuable sensing data (e.g., location data can be used to certify the whereabouts of the user). The nearby devices are also able to track the patient, so when they are placed together, rescuers can use the tracking data to reconstruct the path followed by the dementia patient. Thus, the monitoring system uses opportunistic networking to connect to nearby devices for at least two causes: support for communication, and support for human tracking and sensor data sharing. Last but not least, when a critical event occurs, the Home Care System can use opportunistic dissemination to send an alert message to people walking in the park (i.e., for asking about the whereabouts of the patient, for finding him, or for sending request for assistance messages, such as "please remind this person, if you see him, to take the medication").

The home network is particularly useful to monitor the patient indoors, and it consists of sensors attached to walls in rooms and their equipment for collecting data about the behavior of the person under observation. Part of the home network might also include loudspeakers, microphones, and video cameras for communicating with the person. It is assumed that video cameras are usually switched off, and they will be activated only after the detection of an emergency, in order to provide external medical personnel the option of looking at the person. This constraint guarantees privacy for the persons under observation.

For the outdoor living assistance, the monitoring system may acquire additional context information that describes unforeseen situations (traffic jams, etc.). Of course, for outdoor living assistance, the monitoring systems may never rely on a stable communication infrastructure, i.e., the quality (bandwidth, transmission delay, etc.) and the reachability of services may dynamically change by orders of magnitude. For tracking, in particular, opportunistic networking techniques described next can provide valuable monitoring applications.

Since full wireless coverage is not easy to find at all times in outdoor environments, network communications can be inevitably intermittent and thus very challenging. To overcome this difficulty, we propose applying a delay/disruption-tolerant network technique to tracking patients, making use of opportunistic, ad-hoc, and short-range wireless communications to disseminate data over the network in a store-carry-and-forward fashion. More precisely, each patient is required to carry a device with a GPS receiver, a Zigbee (or other short- or medium-range) wireless radio. When patients encounter other persons on their trails, their BAN motes (see Figure 2) automatically exchange their IDs and record the encounter information (i.e., the time and location) in their respective memories. The devices continue exchanging their stored data as long as possible (i.e., depending on the encounter time and the wireless bandwidth). Then, when a patient reaches one of the base-stations installed at frequently visited spots in the park, all the information stored in his device is uploaded to an Internet server from the base station via GPRS or Wi-Fi.

An important concern that arises regarding a system such as the one we propose here is related to privacy. Since opportunistic networking uses encountered nodes as relays for data, privacy must be ensured so that the collected data cannot be read by anyone except the intended recipient. Thus, a node that carries a data object for another node must not be able to decipher it for its own personal use. Private sensitive information such as social security number, medical records, or current geographical position might be contained in such a data object, so it is of the utmost importance that the proposed system doesn't permit malicious nodes to read and use the data. For this reason, we propose using an asymmetric cryptography mechanism. This way, the medical facility (i.e., hospital, medical ward, etc.) that a patient is associated with has a pair of public and private keys. Data generated by the patient's BAN and various other sensors is encrypted with the corresponding public key, since it is only of use and relevance to the medical facility. When the data is uploaded to the facility (using a wireless access point or opportunistic contacts), it can be decrypted with the public key and analyzed accordingly. Less sensitive information (that might be used to assess the current condition of the patient in more general terms) does not necessarily have to be encrypted, since it might be used to signal an alarm that something is wrong. This is the type of decision that should be taken as soon as possible, i.e., even before the aggregated data reaches the medical facility. As an example, if the patient's sensors show abnormal conditions in the patient's vital signs, the data should be interpreted by any node that can do so, in order to alert the necessary entities (i.e., an ambulance, the police, etc.) that can respond to the emergency in a timely fashion.

Even if messages might, hypothetically, be still compromised, privacy is further enforced by the fact that a communication can be decomposed into several messages, each traveling on a completely different path to its destination. Given its specifics, in an opportunistic network between any two nodes messages can, in fact, travel on completely different paths, making the process of capturing messages belonging to one single session an impossible task.

It is also important to address the issue of opportunistic network reliability. Since ONs do not assume the existence of paths between nodes (instead relying on contacts), a path between two nodes might simply not exist, so these two nodes will never be connected and/or able to communicate. Thus, minimum requirements regarding the number of nodes running the system proposed here should be set and enforced if possible. There

are various factors that should be taken into account in order to define these requirements. For example, the wireless communication distance of each node should be considered (it depends on the wireless communication protocols assumed), since it specifies how close two nodes must be in order to exchange information. Moreover, the closer two nodes are, the stronger the wireless signal between them is, so the density of the opportunistic network is also an important factor. This has to be balanced against the problem of channel interference: since wireless communication uses air media, there is a huge possibility of having more than one communicating pair within one-hop range, leading to possible congestion at medium access control. Reliability should also be ensured, but this only happens if the correct carriers are selected at each step (but, as we show later on, flooding the network with all the messages is not feasible, since it leads to congestion and messages being dropped). The system we propose assumes the existence of wireless access points where the dementia patient roams (e.g., a park), so requirements might be addressed to the municipality to ensure that these are in place according to predefined distances. Moreover, since the system proposed here might have to deal with emergency situations, it is able to use cellular networks when such situations arise, ensuring another degree of reliability (through the WSN layer, as previously shown).

5. OPPORTUNISTIC ALGORITHMS FOR THE PROPOSED FRAMEWORK

The dementia patient monitoring framework proposed above can be used with various ON-specific algorithms at the data transfer level, depending on the requirements. For example, if certain data should be spread to all the nodes in the ON (such as information about the timely location of a patient walking in the park), then a dissemination algorithm should be employed. If, on the other hand, a node wants to send a message to a specific node (e.g., a monitoring system needs to notify a doctor or a caretaker that they need to attend to a certain patient), then a routing algorithm should be used, which opportunistically moves the message node by node until it reaches the intended destination.

In this Section, we present a dissemination and a routing algorithm that we have previously proposed, and which can be employed in the dementia patient monitoring system presented in Section IV. We also explain why we believe that our solutions can be successfully employed. In Section VI, we show the results obtained when running our algorithms in simulations based on existing mobility traces.

SPRINT: Opportunistic Routing

SPRINT (Social PRedIction-based routing in opportunistic NeTworks) (Ciobanu et al, 2013) is an opportunistic routing algorithm that combines socially-aware routing, including both learned and offline social information about nodes, with a module capable to predict node behavior. Its purpose is to improve the hit rate (i.e., number of messages that successfully reach their destinations) when compared to other algorithms, while also keeping the overhead and delivery latency as low as possible. It is based on the knowledge (proven in Ciobanu & Dobre, 2012) that opportunistic nodes belonging to humans are inherently predictable, since the behavior of their owners is predictable. If we are talking about a situation such as a hospital wing, this is even truer, since doctors and nurses generally follow the same mobility patterns daily, while doing their rounds and visiting the patients they are responsible of. The social aspect assumes that nodes have previous information regarding the social connection between nodes, such as online social network friendship (e.g., Facebook or Google+). When talking about (for example) a hospital or medical care environment, we believe it is better to group nodes socially based on the function and rank of each node in the ON. Thus,

nodes may be first and foremost split into patients and medical staff, each belonging to their own social community. Inside communities, nodes might also be split according to various other criteria, such as nurses and doctors, patients with severe disorders and patients with lesser disorders, etc. In a situation similar to what we have presented in Section IV, the nodes might be split according to the relationship with the monitored patient (for example, family members that visit daily should be socially connected to the patient). These social communities are then used in improving the prediction mechanism of the SPRINT algorithm, since nodes that belong to the same community tend to meet each other more often (e.g., nurses have a higher chance of meeting each other than they do of meeting a doctor). Moreover, connections between members of different communities can also be created. For example, a doctor would be socially connected to all the patients in his care, since they interact on a regular basis.

The memory of a node running SPRINT is split into two sections: a data memory and a cache memory. The former is used to store data objects (which have either been generated by the current node, or are just being stored and carried for future forwarding), while the cache memory contains information about the node's previous encounters with other participants in the network. When two nodes meet, they exchange information about each message in their data memory, based on which each node computes utility values for the messages in its own memory, as well as for the ones advertised by the encountered node. It then sorts them according to their utility values. If some of the messages with high utility values belong to the encountered node, a download request is sent for each of them. The node then starts transferring these messages in utility order, until it has finished downloading all the required messages or the two encountering nodes are not in range anymore. Thus, the formula used by a SPRINT node A to compute the utility of a message M is:

$$u(M, A) = w_1 \times U_1(M, A) + w_2 \times U_2(M, A)$$

$u(M, A)$ is the utility of message M as computed by node A, while w_1 and w_2 are weight values which follow the conditions that $w_1 + w_2 = 1$ and $w_1 > w_2$. U_1 and U_2 are utility components computed according to the following formulas:

$$U_1(M, A) = freshness(M) + p(M, A) \times (1 - \frac{enc(M, A)}{24})$$

$$U_2(M, A) = c_c(M, A) \times \frac{s_n(M) + hop(M) + pop(A) + time(M, A)}{4}$$

Since we want the newly-generated messages to start traveling through the opportunistic network as fast as possible, the $freshness(M)$ component favors new messages. The value is set to 0.5 if the message has been created less than a day ago, and to 0 otherwise. This means that in the beginning, when new messages are created, they are spread to several nodes (the utility value is high). As messages travel along the network, they are forwarded only to other nodes that maximize the changes of successful delivery.

$p(M, A)$ is the probability of node A being able to deliver a message M closer to its destination. The term is based on predicting a node's behavior, combined with the idea that a node has a higher chance of interacting with nodes it is socially connected with and/or has encountered before. It is an environment-specific function that can be configured according to the contact distribution of the network SPRINT is used in. For the environments we are testing with, we compute it based on the assumption that the node contacts follow a Poisson distribution. We have shown this to be true for academic environments, but we also believe the results stand for medical environments, since the members of a hospital generally have fixed schedules and follow the same movement patterns daily. A prediction is thus made using the Poisson distribution and social knowledge, and the first N nodes in the order of encounter probability are picked as potential future contacts. This is done for each of the next 24 hours (sorted by probability), while for the rest of the nodes, $p(M, A)$ is set to 0.

U_1 also uses $enc(M, A)$, which is the hour of the day when the destination of message M will be met according to the probabilities previously computed. If the destination will never be encountered, then $enc(M, A)$ is set to 24 (so the product is 0). We multiply $p(M, A)$ by $1 - \dfrac{enc(M, A)}{24}$ because the sooner a good target for a message is met, the sooner the node can delete the message from its memory and have room for others.

The second component of the utility function is U_2. Its first member - $c_c(M, A)$ - is set to 1 if node A is in the same community as the destination of message M or if node A will ever encounter a node that has a social relationship with M, and 0 otherwise. Again, the prediction information computed for U_1 is used to analyze the potential future encounters of a node.

The $s_n(M)$ component is set to 1 if the source and destination of M do not have a social connection, because if a message does not have the source and destination in the same community, the chance of it being delivered by the source is low since it will mostly meet nodes belonging to its own community. Therefore, the messages should be given to a different node that has the chance of reaching the destination community. If M's source and destination are in the same community, $s_n(M)$ is 0.

$hop(M)$ represents the normalized number of nodes that M has visited, $pop(A)$ is the normalized popularity value of A according to its social network information (i.e., number of friends in the opportunistic network), and finally $time(M, A)$ is the total time spent by node A in contact with M's destination. The $hop(M)$ and

$time(M, A)$ values are used because nodes should travel as little as possible before reaching their destination.

ONSIDE: Opportunistic Dissemination

ONSIDE (OpportuNistic Socially-aware and Interest-based DissEmination) (Ciobanu et al, 2014) is a publish/subscribe-based algorithm that disseminates data in opportunistic networks based on nodes' interests, together with social information about the nodes in the ON. Its goal is to reduce the overhead of spreading the data, while not affecting the hit rate and the delivery latency.

It is based on several assumptions, the first of them being that nodes which have common interests tend to meet each other more often than nodes that do not. The second assumption that ONSIDE is based on is similar to SPRINT's condition that connections from online social networks are valid in an ON node's encounters. Not only do nodes tend to encounter socially connected neighbors more often, but there is also a high chance that a node encounters a second-degree neighbor (i.e., a node that it has at least one friend in common with).

The functionality of ONSIDE when two nodes meet is very similar to SPRINT's, the main difference being the way the utility of a message is computed. Thus, the function used by a node A to analyze a message M from a node B and to decide whether it should be downloaded is:

$$Exchange(A, B, M) = (CommonInterests(A, B) \geq 1)$$
$$\& Interested(A, M.topic)$$
$$\& (InterestedFriends(A, M.topic) \geq thr_f)$$
$$\& (InterestsEncountered(A, M.topic) \geq thr_i)$$

The result of the *Exchange* function is a Boolean value that specifies whether a download request should be made to B for message M. The

CommonInterests function returns the number of topics that both A and B are interested in. This way, data transfers are only performed between nodes with at least one common interest, based on the previous assumption that these nodes encounter each other often and are thus able to successfully deliver channel data to all subscribed nodes.

The second component of the *Exchange* function is *Interested*, which returns true if node A is subscribed to the channel that generated message M (i.e., if it is interested in M's topic). By using this function, a node will not only download a message for itself and then drop it after use, but will also store it for others, since it is highly likely to encounter other nodes that have similar interests to its own.

The *InterestedFriends* function returns the number of online social network friends of node A that are subscribed to the channel that generated M. By using this component, we assume that a node has access to its social network at any time, which contains at least interest information about the connected nodes. This component has the role of further reducing the amount of messages exchanged in the network, by only requesting a message if a node's social network friends (i.e., nodes that it has a high chance of encountering) are also interested in it. This not only reduces the congestion, but also has the role of speeding up the message's delivery. thr_f is a threshold that can be varied according to the density of the ON and of the social network.

Finally, the last component of the *Exchange* function, *InterestsEncountered*, is computed based on node A's history of encounters. It returns the percentage of encounters with nodes that are interested in messages similar to M, in terms of channel subscriptions. This function is based on the assumption that a node's behavior in an ON is predictable, so that if it encountered many nodes subscribed to a certain channel, it is likely to encounter others in the future as well. thr_i is a threshold between 0 and 1 that can be varied depending on the number of channels in the ON.

When talking about channels and subscriptions in a dementia patient monitoring environment, we envision various sources of information, both for the medical staff, as well as for the patients. Each node subscribes to the channel it is interested in, such as doctors and nurses for feeds regarding the status of certain patients, or said patients for channels that publish information about the visiting hours for the ward they are in, etc. Thus, nodes that are subscribed to the same channel (like a nurse and a doctor that take care of a specific patient) have a higher chance of encountering each other than two nodes without common interests (such as two nurses working in different wards). Similarly, for the solution proposed in Section IV, we envision that proximity police officers subscribe to information generated by the known dementia patients located in their assigned area. This way, they can be notified whenever an alert generated by the sensors that belong to the patient's BAN signal a potential problem, and may thus respond in a timely fashion. Consequently, ONSIDE takes advantage of subscription information to reduce the quantity of messages exchanged in the ON, which leads to a quicker and more efficient delivery.

6. EVALUATION OF OPPORTUNISTIC NETWORKS AS A RELIABLE INFRASTRUCTURE

When employing opportunistic networks for dementia patient monitoring, we need to ensure that the underlying algorithms are viable for the environment where they are being applied. Since ONs are based on contacts between nodes, it is relatively difficult to employ ONs in sparse networks, since there are few nodes and thus the encounters between nodes are rare. However, in a situation such as the one we described in Sec-

tion IV, there are many nodes spread on a small surface, so both the number of contacts, as well as ON nodes, are high. Thus, there are many opportunities for data to be exchanged, leading to high hit rates. However, in such a situation there may appear node congestion, especially if there are many messages in the network, and if the nodes have low data memories. For this reason, the algorithms employed should be able to reduce congestion by carefully selecting the next hop at each step.

In this Section, we present the results obtained by running SPRINT and ONSIDE on several well-known mobility traces using the MobEmu emulator (Ciobanu et al, 2012). Most of the traces used were taken in academic environments, but we believe that a medical environment is similar: the contacts are many and occur often, during a short time span. The traces we tested with are UPB 2011 (Ciobanu et al, 2012), UPB 2012 (Marin et al, 2012), St. Andrews (Bigwood et al, 2008), Content (Scott et al, 2006), Infocom 2006 (Hui & Crowcroft, 2007) and Sigcomm 2009 (Pietilainen et al, 2009). We tried to select traces for various environments, which contained the information needed for the deployment of our solutions (such as social and interest information).

The first metric we analyze is hit rate, defined as the ratio between successfully delivered messages and the total number of generated messages. Next, the delivery latency is defined as the time passed between the generation of a message and its eventual delivery to the destination. Another metric we use is the delivery cost, defined as the ratio between the total number of messages exchanged during the course of the test and the number of generated messages, which shows the congestion of the network. Finally, the hop count is the number of nodes that carried a message until it reached the destination on the shortest path, and should be as low as possible in order to avoid node congestion.

SPRINT

When presenting the results obtained by SPRINT on the mobility traces, we compare it to BUBBLE Rap (Hui et al, 2008), which is one of the most efficient and well-known data dissemination algorithms for ONs. Furthermore, we also compare SPRINT to the Epidemic routing algorithm (Vahdat & Becker, 2006), which is a simple but impractical algorithm that we use in order to find out the maximum possible hit rate that can be achieved in our tests. When two nodes running Epidemic routing meet, they simply download all the messages from each other, so a maximum hit rate is surely to be achieved. However, this happens at the expense of storage space, and in a large real-life network it would be impossible to implement such an algorithm since the data memory required would be extremely large. We only use the hit rate data obtained by Epidemic, since it is the only information relevant to us.

Additional information about the experimental setup and a thorough analysis of the results obtained by running SPRINT can be found in (Ciobanu et al, 2013). Here we present a summary of the results, in order to show that SPRINT is a viable option for the system presented in Section IV.

Figure 3 shows the results obtained when running SPRINT, Epidemic and BUBBLE Rap on the UPB 2011 trace. It can be seen that the hit rate for SPRINT is better than the hit rate obtained by BUBBLE Rap for most of the cases. The figure shows that SPRINT can achieve maximum hit rate, whereas BUBBLE Rap cannot, even for a data memory of 4500 messages. Other improvements brought by SPRINT can be seen when looking at the delivery cost and average hop count charts, where SPRINT outperforms BUBBLE Rap as well. Finally, SPRINT manages to improve latency by up to seven hours, which can prove to be the difference between life and death in certain situ-

Figure 3. SPRINT results for UPB 2011

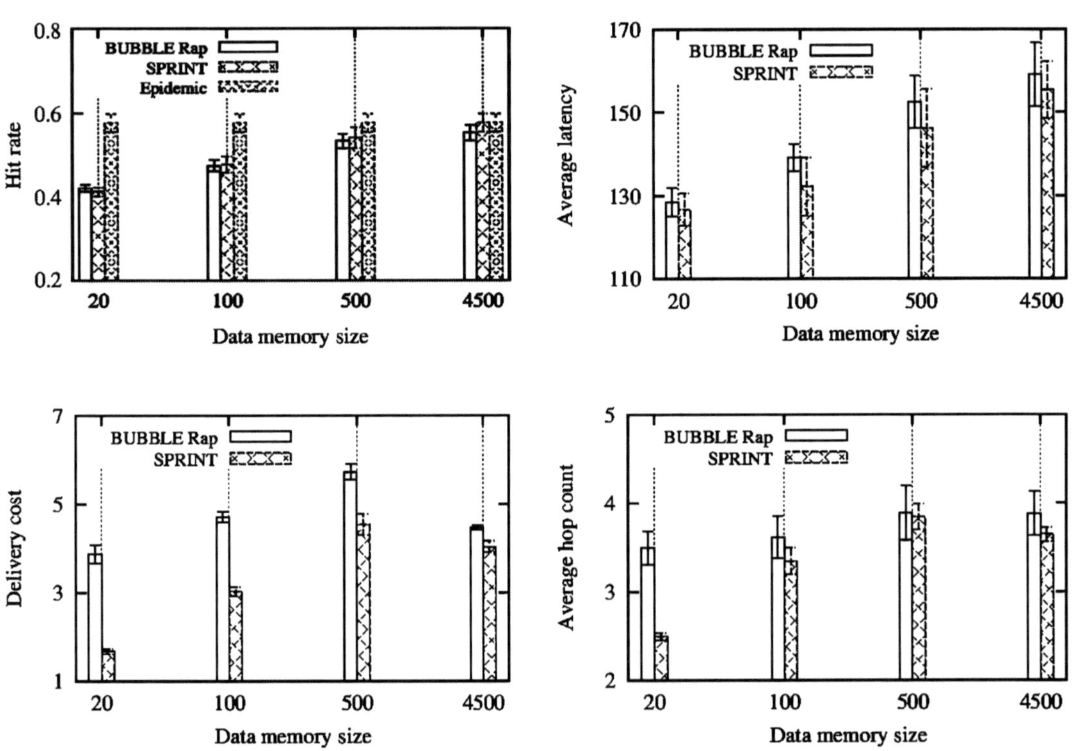

ations. The situation is similar for UPB 2012, as the traces were performed in similar conditions.

Another trace where SPRINT uses contact prediction when performing routing decisions is St. Andrews, and results are shown in Figure 4. This time, SPRINT does not manage to achieve maximum hit rate. Nonetheless, SPRINT's hit rate is better than BUBBLE Rap's, irrespective of the data memory size. The delivery cost and average hop count situation is similar to the one observed at UPB 2012: for small data memory values, they are improved. However, because a larger data memory helps the algorithm distribute more messages to remote nodes, the overall delivery cost and hop count are increased. For large data memory values, SPRINT improves the average latency.

Although Content and Infocom 2006 do not contain social information and the U_1 component of a message's utility for SPRINT is 0, our proposed algorithm still behaves well, as it still uses social and context information to assign utility values to messages.

Figure 5 shows the results for Content and it can be seen that, although SPRINT does not manage to achieve maximum hit rate (because it lacks the prediction component), it still outperforms BUBBLE Rap in terms of hit rate by as much as 3%. However, the important results for this trace concern congestion, namely delivery cost and average hop count. SPRINT manages to decrease the delivery cost by as much as 146, so the total number of messages exchanged in the ON is five times lower when using SPRINT. The hop count is also reduced dramatically by SPRINT. Most importantly, delivery latency is also decreased by as much as 8 hours when using SPRINT. The Infocom 2006 results look very much alike to what was obtained for Content: SPRINT outperforms BUBBLE Rap in terms of hit rate, delivery cost, hop count, as well as average latency.

Figure 4. SPRINT results for St. Andrews

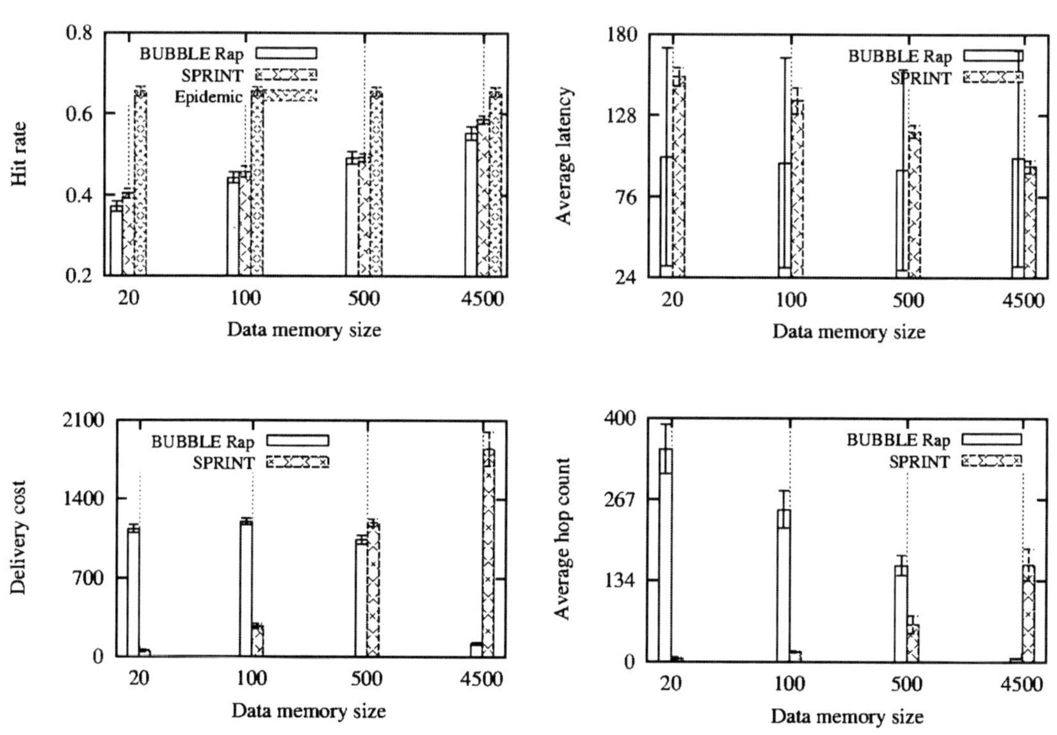

Figure 5. SPRINT results for Content

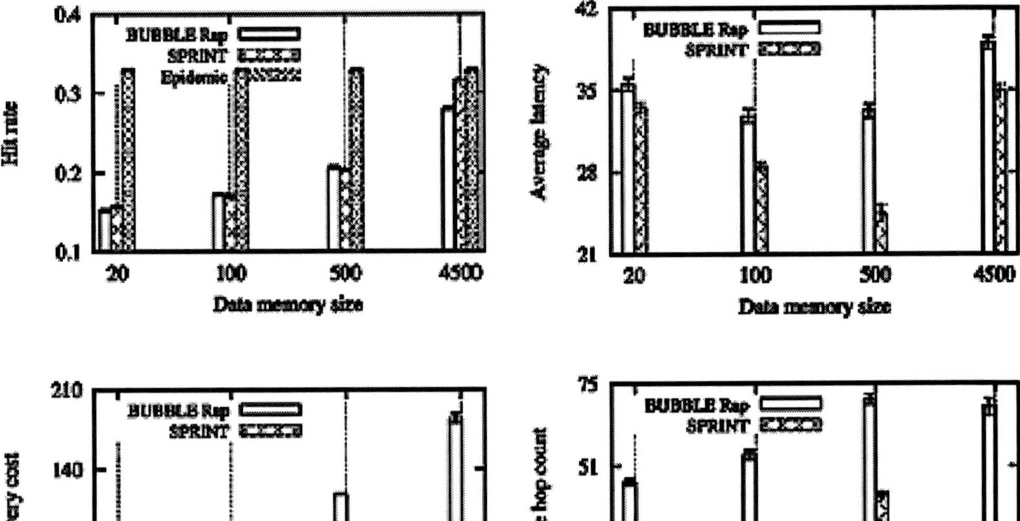

ONSIDE

Information about the way the experiments were run for ONSIDE and more detailed results analysis can be found in (Ciobanu et al, 2014). Similar to SPRINT, in order to highlight the benefits of ONSIDE, we compare it to Epidemic. However, since the classic Epidemic algorithm is not entirely feasible in real life (given that it assumes an unlimited data memory), we also compare ONSIDE to a limited-memory version of Epidemic, that behaves exactly like the original implementation, except that, when the data memory is full and a new message should be downloaded, an existing message must be deleted from memory. We refer to this Epidemic version as Limited Epidemic. Aside from Epidemic, we also compare ONSIDE to a dissemination-modified version of ML-SOR (Socievole et al, 2013). We have chosen this algorithm since it is also interest-based and socially-aware like ONSIDE.

Figure 6 shows the results obtained by applying Epidemic, Limited Epidemic, ML-SOR, and ONSIDE on the Sigcomm 2009 trace. It can be seen that ONSIDE generally performs better than both ML-SOR, as well as Limited Epidemic. For a data memory that can store 4500 messages, ONSIDE yields a hit rate that is very close to the maximum value obtained when running Epidemic and Limited Epidemic. Limited Epidemic is able to achieve maximum hit rate because the memory size is large enough to fit all the messages generated in the trace, since Sigcomm 2009's duration is only three days. The delivery latency chart shows similar results: ONSIDE is able to achieve a better delivery latency than ML-SOR regardless of the data memory size (with a maximum improvement of up to 1.7 hours), whereas Limited Epidemic only outperforms our algorithm when the data memory is large enough to store all the messages generated in the trace. However, the downside of Epidemic-based algorithms is evident from the

Figure 6. ONSIDE results for Sigcomm 2009

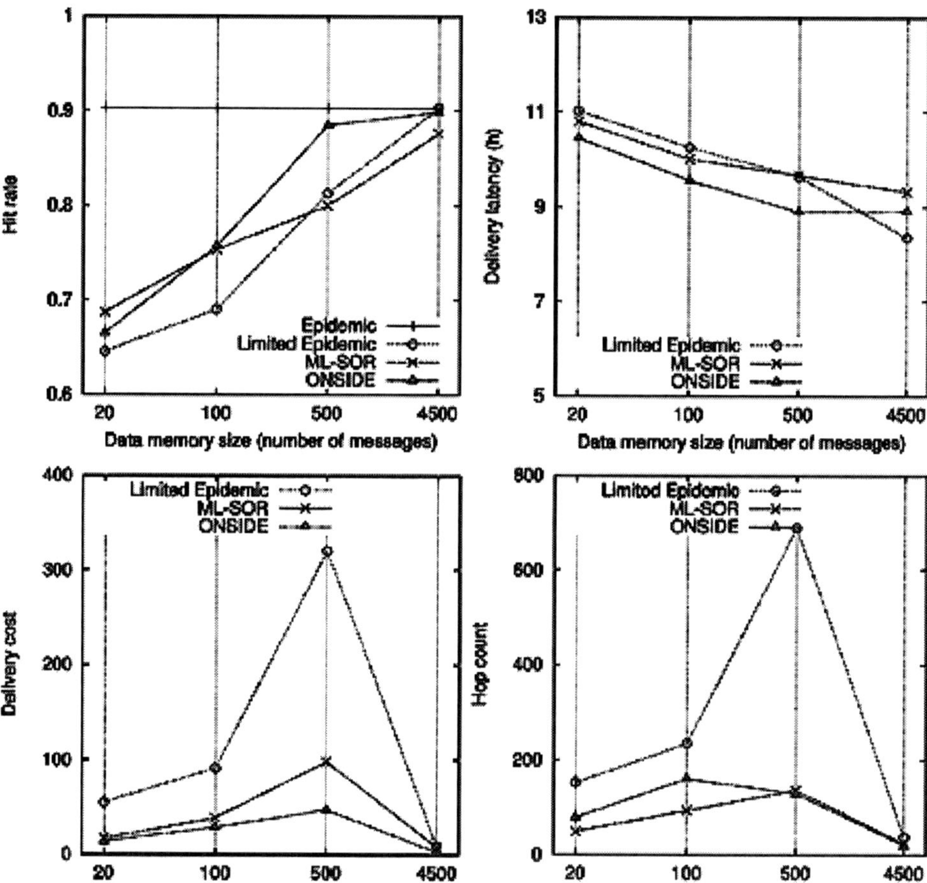

delivery cost and hop count results, where it can be seen that the bandwidth used and the network and node congestion are really high. ONSIDE's delivery cost is lower than the ones obtained by Limited Epidemic and ML-SOR for all data memory sizes. Regarding hop count, ONSIDE again clearly outperforms Limited Epidemic for all data memory sizes, but it does achieve a higher hop count than ML-SOR for lower data memory sizes (like 20 and 100).

The UPB 2012 results are shown in Figure 7. Since the duration of the trace is much higher than Sigcomm 2009's, there are a lot more messages generated in the network, so the maximum hit rate is harder to achieve with a limited data memory. The ONSIDE algorithm performs similarly to both Limited Epidemic, as well as ML-SOR. Because this trace has a much longer duration that Sigcomm 2009 and the network is relatively sparse (with not many contacts), the delivery latency values are very high. Regardless of this, the values are similar for all three algorithms, with a slight edge for Limited Epidemic for higher data memory sizes. However, this comes with the cost of increased congestion and overhead, where Limited Epidemic performs much worse than ONSIDE and ML-SOR. Regarding delivery cost, ONSIDE performs the best out of all three algorithms for data memory sizes of 500 and 4500.

Finally, the results for the Infocom 2006 trace are presented in Figure 8. Infocom 2006 has the disadvantage of not containing social information

Figure 7. ONSIDE results for UPB 2012

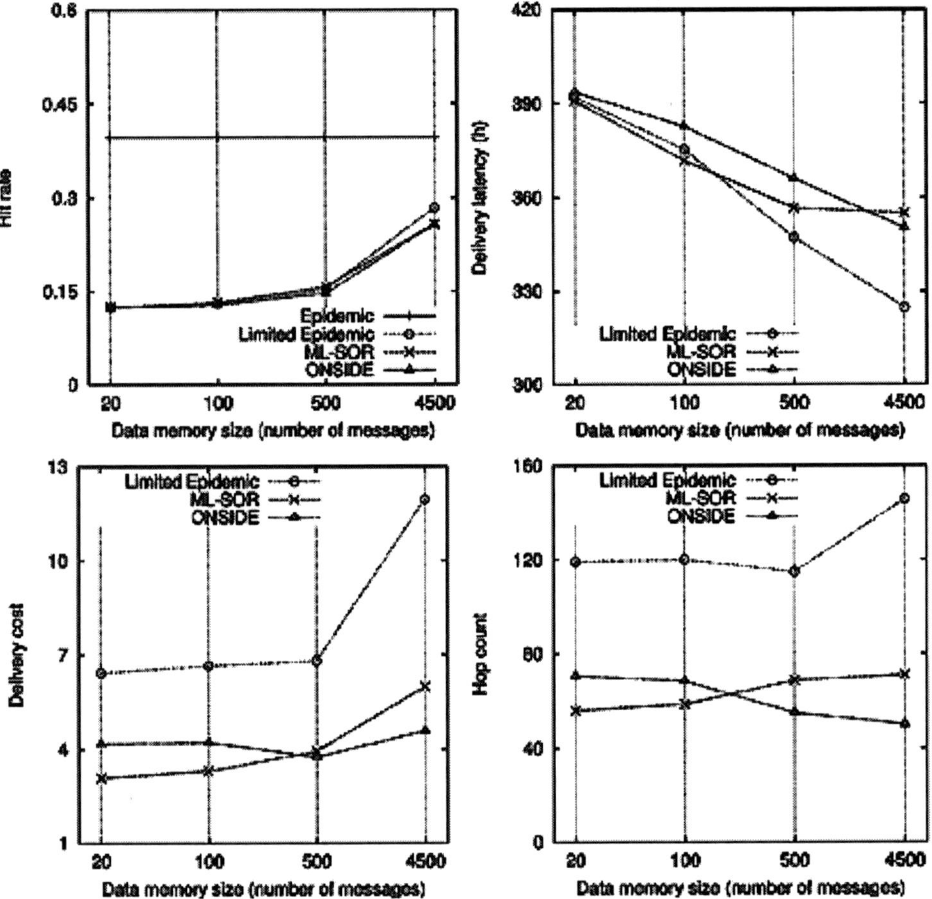

about the participating nodes, so the TSS component from ML-SOR will always be 0. Similarly, ONSIDE does not use the *InterestedFriends* component, since thr_f is set to 0. The results show that ONSIDE yields better hit rates than ML-SOR for all data memory sizes except 20, keeping close to the two Epidemic versions, especially when the data memory size is higher. Regarding delivery latency, ONSIDE fares better than ML-SOR for large memory sizes. Limited Epidemic has the best behavior in terms of latency, but it pays for it with a higher degree of congestion. The hop count obtained by Limited Epidemic is extremely large, about three times larger than the one ONSIDE yields. However, ML-SOR performs better in terms of hop count than both the other two solutions. The delivery cost is lower for ML-SOR and ONSIDE, with our solution faring much better when the data memory size is higher.

Therefore, the results show that, generally, both ONSIDE and ML-SOR barely affect the overall hit rate (with a slight advantage for ONSIDE), while decreasing the congestion and overhead. For most of the situations, ML-SOR seems to work better for lower data memory sizes, while ONSIDE fares well for nodes that are able to store more messages.

7. CONCLUSION

As of 2013, there were an estimated 44.4 million people with dementia worldwide. This number

Figure 8. ONSIDE results for Infocom 2006

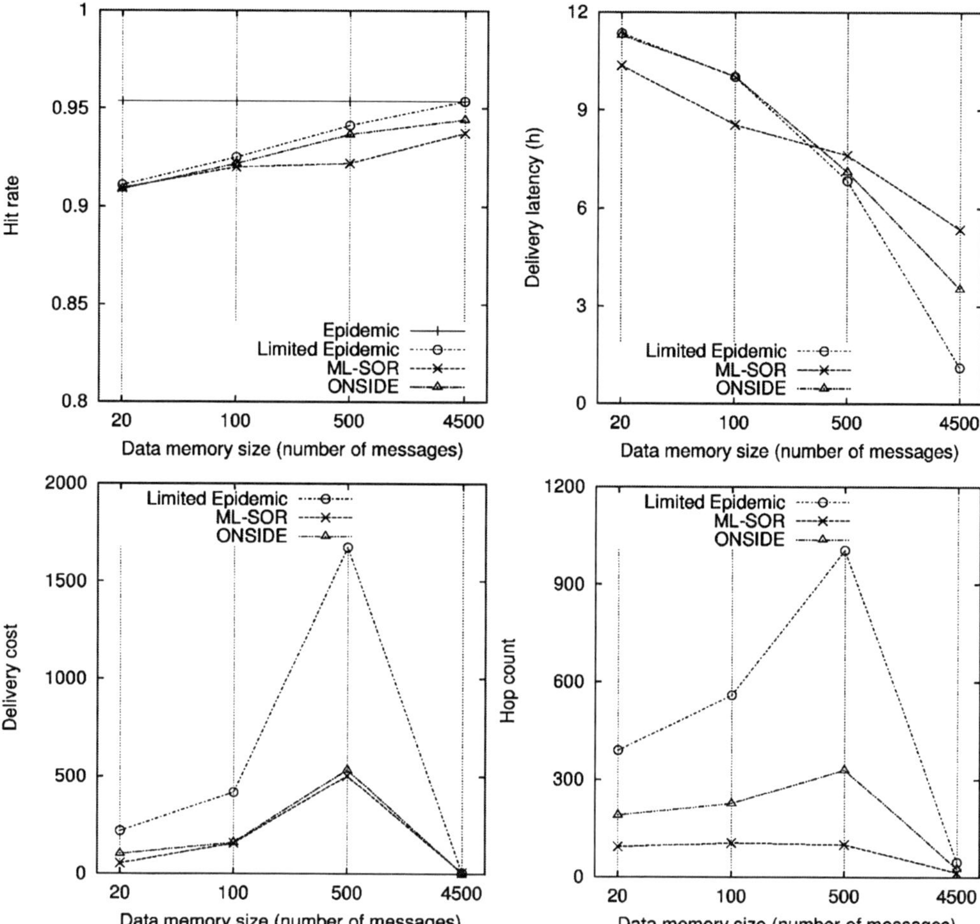

will increase to an estimated 75.6 million in 2030, and 135.5 million in 2050. Much of the increase will be in developing countries. Already 62% of people with dementia live in developing countries, but by 2050 this will rise to 71%. The fastest growth in the elderly population is taking place in China, India, and their South Asian and Western Pacific neighbors. Thus, a change in care for people with dementia is today necessary more than ever. Ambient Assisted Living (AAL) can provide an answer to this.

AALs are system designed to help, through the active use of Information and Communication Technologies (ICT), patients, caregivers and professionals alike. Such systems are designed to provide an ecosystem of medical sensors, computers, wireless networks and software applications for healthcare monitoring, and are designed to meet the personal healthcare challenges. Thus, it is no wonder that, presently, there is a huge demand for AAL systems, applications and devices for personal health monitoring and tele-health services.

Opportunistic communications use low-cost human wearable mobile nodes allowing the exchange of packets at a close range of a few to some tens of meters with limited or no infrastructure. Typically, cheap pocket devices which are IEEE 802.15.4-2006 compliant can be used and they can communicate at a 2-10 meters range, with local computational capabilities and local memory. Here we have proposed and described an autonomous patient monitoring support system based on opportunistic communications. The monitored patient wears non-intrusive sensors, and potentially computing devices and actuators, forming a body area network (BAN). This on-patient network can provide memory impairment support services for the patient, and is used to construct the personalized condition-monitoring patient model used to evaluate against a set of potential life-threatening events.

The system collects the measurements from the different sensors, on-body and also external sensors where available, aggregates the sensing data provided, and periodically transmits it toward a central station for further processing. When there is a direct Internet connection, this will be the preferred means to transmit the data. For indoor scenarios, it is more likely that a wired connection is available. However, things are different for outdoor scenarios. In the absence of an Internet connection, the patient might use ad-hoc networking alternatives to send the data to the Wireless Access Point located in his surroundings. Here, we employ the use of opportunistic networking techniques. These techniques will be used to also collect sensing data from the environment. For example, while the patient is walking by, he can connect to other mobile devices, carried by other people, and collect valuable sensing data. The nearby devices are also able to track the patient, so when they are placed together rescuers can use the tracking data to reconstruct the path followed by the dementia patient. Thus, the monitoring system uses opportunistic networking to connect to nearby devices for at least two causes: support for communication, and support for human tracking and sensor data sharing. Last but not least, when a critical event occurs, the Home Care System can use opportunistic dissemination to send an alert message to nearby people.

For outdoor living assistance in particular, this monitoring system may acquire additional context information, describing unforeseen situations.

Since for outdoor living assistance the monitoring systems may never rely on a stable communication infrastructure, opportunistic networking techniques can provide valuable monitoring applications. To overcome the lack of connectivity, we propose applying a delay/disruption-tolerant network technique for tracking patients, making use of opportunistic, ad-hoc, and short-range wireless communications to disseminate data over the network in a store-carry-and-forward fashion.

To better illustrate what kind of solutions can work in such conditions, we have presented our dissemination and our routing algorithms that we have previously proposed, and that can be employed in the dementia patient monitoring system. SPRINT is an opportunistic routing algorithm that combines socially-aware routing, including both learned and offline social information about nodes, with a module capable to predict node behavior. Its purpose is to improve the hit rate when compared to other algorithms, while also keeping the overhead and delivery latency as low as possible. It is based on the knowledge that opportunistic nodes belonging to humans are inherently predictable, since the behavior of their owners is predictable (which is particularly true in case of dementia-suffering patients, where AAL systems are generally designed to support learning their predictable daily habits and to try to support them as best as possible through augmented memory-triggering support services). ONSIDE, our proposed solution, is a publish/subscribe-based algorithm that disseminates data in opportunistic networks based on nodes' interests, together with social information about the nodes in the ON. Its goal is to reduce the overhead of spreading the data, while not affecting the hit rate and the delivery latency. Such a dissemination opportunistic solution can be employed in the finding or tracking of patients in outdoor scenarios, or to support personalized memory-reminding services (such as sending data to interested volunteers in the park, who might help the patient and remind him to take his medication, or helping a patient suffering a memory loss get in contact with someone who can help).

We have also explained why we believe that our solutions can be successfully employed, and showed a set of results obtained when running our algorithms in simulations based on existing mobility traces. The results prove that both our opportunistic networking solutions can deliver good hit rates, while decreasing the congestion and overhead associated with data transmissions (an important aspect to consider when the system is used to concurrently monitor many different patients, each one generating different independent sensing messages).

8. FUTURE WORK AND CHALLENGES

In the near future, we aim to develop a prototype of the proposed patient monitoring system, to better illustrate how it can be applied to real-world conditions. This system will use opportunistic means of establishing connections with social participants in the environment whenever possible (for the benefits illustrated throughout this chapter). Of course, there are also several challenges we first need to consider in the near future.

Interoperability and integration of medical devices in healthcare systems processing citizens' vital signs are the most frequently addressed attributes in AAL systems and platforms. This is very important if the tele-monitoring system for dementia-suffering patients is to be integrated with various medical support systems already in use today (for example, with the medical systems available on hospital grounds). For monitoring of daily living activities, we could integrate with the Open Service Gateway Initiative (OSGi) platform. The Continua Alliance has also proposed its own reference architecture to construct an ecosystem of interoperable and connected medical devices for personal healthcare and well-being. We could integrate with this through their proposed Peripheral

Area Network Interface (PAN-IF). Similarly, the Assisted Living Platform (ALIP) in the DALLAS (Delivering Assisted Living Lifestyles at Scale) program addresses interoperability as the major concern to achieve scalability in medical device communication. The Interoperability Toolkit (ITK) in DALLAS helps integrate systems based on standardizing technologies and interoperability specifications. More research in the ALIP reference architecture solves interoperability issues by using the DALLAS Interoperability Layer, which extends the ALIP platform with security features for user and component authentication. And there are several other standardization efforts that we aim to consider further.

The second important challenge relates to security, privacy and data protection for the monitored patient. Security and data protection are critical issues in healthcare systems, which exchange and store citizens' medical data. All monitored medical data is, of course, security-sensitive. Therefore, legislation provides guidelines to design authorization policies regarding access and usage of the medical data to avoid intentional misuse or accidental disclosure. Security is an important aspect to consider here, and we aim to further investigate the use of a Public Key Infrastructure-based data encryption and digital certificate infrastructure for ensuring confidentiality and integrity of the medical data. The solution might consist of collecting medical data from mobile/wearable sensors, and cataloging it depending on the level of privacy/protection needed. For example, the most critical data will be securely transmitted for access only to the caregivers and family members of the citizens. A photo of the patient (without references to the actual illness) might be disseminated to trustful users only when needed to support (track, add) the patient (as in the park scenario previously described).

Another challenge relates to the quality of the sensing data. Quality attributes have a greater impact on the usability of AAL systems. Sensors might read imprecise data, or the sensing data might be completely unavailable (e.g., the GPS sensing might be wrongly affected by the weather conditions, or it might not work at all indoors). In such cases, we aim to explore mechanisms to augment the sensing with external sensors (for example, indoors we will superimpose the sensing data from the BAN mote with the data collected from the sensors within the house premises, and for outdoor conditions, as described, the quality of the sensing data will be re-enforced against the set of sensing data obtained opportunistically whenever available for nearby mobile devices). This, of course, will need further research in the establishment of trust models for aggregating the sensing data.

ACKNOWLEDGMENT

The research presented in this paper is partially supported by national project MobiWay, Project PN-II-PT-PCCA-2013-4-0321. The work is aligned with the COST Action IC1303: "Algorithms, Architectures, and Platforms for Enhanced Living Environments (AAPELE)".

REFERENCES

Akyildiz, I. F., Su, W., Sankarasubramaniam, Y., & Cayirci, E. (2002). Wireless sensor networks: A survey. *Computer Networks*, *38*(4), 393–422. doi:10.1016/S1389-1286(01)00302-4

ALZ. (2013). *2013 Alzheimer Disease: Facts and figures*. Retrieved from http://www.alz.org/downloads/factsfigures 2013.pdf

Bigwood, G., Rehunathan, D., Bateman, M., Henderson, T., & Bhatti, S. (2008). Exploiting self-reported social networks for routing in ubiquitous computing environments. In *Proceedings of the 2008 IEEE International Conference on Wireless & Mobile Computing, Networking & Communication* (pp. 484–489). Washington, DC: IEEE. doi:10.1109/WiMob.2008.86

Bouwhuis, D. G., Taipale, V. T., Bouma, H., & Fozard, J. L. (2007). Gerontechnology in perspective. *Gerontechnology (Valkenswaard)*, *6*(4), 190–216.

Braem, B., Latre, B., Blondia, C., Moerman, I., & Demeester, P. (2008). Improving reliability in multi-hop body sensor networks. In *Proceedings of the 2nd International Conference on Sensor Technologies and Applications* (pp. 342–347). IEEE. doi:10.1109/SENSORCOMM.2008.47

Caprani, N., Doyle, J., O'Grady, M., Gurrin, C., O'Connor, N., Caufield, B., & O'Hare, G. (2012). Technology use in everyday life: Implications for designing for older users. In *Proceedings of 6th Annual Irish Human Computer Interaction (HCI) Conference* (iHCI 2012). NUI Galway.

Chernbumroong, S., Cang, S., Atkins, A., & Yu, H. (2013). Elderly activities recognition and classification for applications in assisted living. *Expert Systems with Applications*, *40*(5), 1662–1674. doi:10.1016/j.eswa.2012.09.004

Ciobanu, R.-I., & Dobre, C. (2012). Predicting encounters in opportunistic networks. In *Proceedings of the 1st ACM Workshop on High Performance Mobile Opportunistic Systems* (pp. 9–14). Paphos, Cyprus: ACM. doi:10.1145/2386980.2386983

Ciobanu, R.-I., Dobre, C., & Cristea, V. (2012). Social aspects to support opportunistic networks in an academic environment. In *Proceedings of the 11th international conference on Ad-hoc, Mobile, and Wireless Networks* (pp. 69–82). Berlin: Springer-Verlag. doi:10.1007/978-3-642-31638-8_6

Ciobanu, R.-I., Dobre, C., & Cristea, V. (2013). SPRINT: Social prediction-based opportunistic routing. In *Proceedings of 2013 IEEE 14th International Symposium and Workshops on a World of Wireless, Mobile and Multimedia Networks* (WoWMoM 2013, pp. 1–7). IEEE.

Ciobanu, R.-I., Marin, R.-C., Dobre, C., Cristea, V., & Mavromoustakis, C. X. (2014). ONSIDE: Socially-aware and interest-based dissemination in opportunistic networks. In *Proceedings of 6th IEEE/IFIP International Workshop on Management of the Future Internet* (ManFI 2014, pp. 1-6). Krakow, Poland: IEEE.

Gieras, I. A. (2003). The proliferation of patient-worn wireless telemetry technologies within the us healthcare environment. In *Proceedings of 4th International IEEE Conference on Information Technology* (pp. 295–298). IEEE.

Hebert, L. E., Weuve, J., Scherr, P. A., & Denis, A. (2013). Alzheimer disease in the United States (2010–2050) estimated using the 2010 census. *Neurology, 80*(19), 1778–1783. doi:10.1212/WNL.0b013e31828726f5 PMID:23390181

Hui, P., & Crowcroft, J. (2007). *Bubble Rap: Forwarding in small world DTNs in ever decreasing circles.* Technical Report UCAM-CL-TR-684. University of Cambridge Computer Laboratory.

Hui, P., Crowcroft, J., & Yoneki, E. (2008). Bubble rap: Social-based forwarding in delay tolerant networks. In *Proceedings of the 9th ACM International Symposium on Mobile Ad Hoc Networking and Computing* (pp. 241–250). New York: ACM. doi:10.1145/1374618.1374652

Hung, K., & Zhang, Y.-T. (2003). Implementation of a WAP-based telemedicine system for patient monitoring. *IEEE Transactions on Information Technology in Biomedicine, 7*(2), 101–107. doi:10.1109/TITB.2003.811870 PMID:12834165

Khoor, S., Nieberl, J., Fugedi, K., & Kail, E. (2001). Telemedicine ecg-telemetry with bluetooth technology. In *Proceedings of computers in cardiology* (pp. 585–588). IEEE.

Lee, R.-G., Chen, H.-S., Lin, C.-C., Chang, K.-C., & Chen, J.-H. (2000). Home telecare system using cable television plants-an experimental field trial. *IEEE Transactions on Information Technology in Biomedicine, 4*(1), 37–44. doi:10.1109/4233.826857 PMID:10761772

Lin, C.-C., Lin, P.-Y., Lu, P.-K., Hsieh, G.-Y., Lee, W.-L., & Lee, R.-G. (2008). A healthcare integration system for disease assessment and safety monitoring of dementia patients. *IEEE Transactions on Information Technology in Biomedicine, 12*(5), 579–586. doi:10.1109/TITB.2008.917914 PMID:18779072

Lindeberg, M., Goebel, V., & Plagemann, T. (2010). Adaptive sized windows to improve real-time health monitoring: A case study on heart attack prediction. In *Proceedings of the International Conference on Multimedia Information Retrieval* (pp. 459–468). New York: Academic Press. doi:10.1145/1743384.1743466

Malan, D., Fulford-Jones, T., Welsh, M., & Moulton, S. (2004). Codeblue: An ad hoc sensor network infrastructure for emergency medical care. In *Proceedings of International Workshop on Wearable and Implantable Body Sensor Networks* (*vol. 5*). Imperial College London.

Marin, R.-C., Dobre, C., & Xhafa, F. (2012). Exploring predictability in mobile interaction. In *Proceedings of 2012 Third International Conference on Emerging Intelligent Data and Web Technologies* (EIDWT, pp. 133–139). Bucharest, Romania: Academic Press. doi:10.1109/EIDWT.2012.29

Mendoza, G. G., & Tran, B. Q. (2002). In-home wireless monitoring of physiological data for heart failure patients. In *Proceedings of 24th Annual Conference and the Annual Fall Meeting of the Biomedical Engineering Society Engineering in medicine and biology* (EMBS/BMES 2002, vol. 3, pp. 1849–1850). IEEE. doi:10.1109/IEMBS.2002.1053058

Migliardi, M., & Gaudina, M. (2011). A context aware, mobile system providing memory support for ageing people. In *Proceedings of the 34th International Convention* (MIPRO, pp. 535–540). Opatija, Croatia: Academic Press.

NINDS. (2013). *Dementia: Hope through research*. Available at http://www.ninds.nih.gov/disorders/dementias/detaildementia.htm

Pattichis, C. S., Kyriacou, E., Voskarides, S., Pattichis, M. S., Istepanian, R., & Schizas, C. N. (2002). Wireless telemedicine systems: An overview. *IEEE Antennas and Propagation Magazine*, *44*(2), 143–153. doi:10.1109/MAP.2002.1003651

Pietilainen, A.-K., Oliver, E., LeBrun, J., Varghese, G., & Diot, C. (2009). MobiClique: middleware for mobile social networking. In *Proceedings of the 2nd ACM Workshop on Online Social Networks* (WOSN '09, pp. 49–54). New York: ACM. doi:10.1145/1592665.1592678

Pollard, J. K., Rohman, S., & Fry, M. E. (2001). A web-based mobile medical monitoring system. In *Proceedings of International Workshop on Intelligent Data Acquisition and Advanced Computing Systems: Technology and Applications* (pp. 32–35). IEEE.

SCIE. (2012), Social care institute for excellence. In *Using ICT in activities for people with dementia: A short guide for social care providers.* Available at http://www.scie.org.uk/publications/ictfordementia/

Scott, J., Gass, R., Crowcroft, J., Hui, P., Diot, C., & Chaintreau, A. (2006). *CRAWDAD data set cambridge/haggle (v. 2006-01-31)*. Available at http://crawdad.org/cambridge/haggle/

Sehgal, S., Iqbal, M., & Kamruzzaman, J. (2007). Ambient cardiac expert: a cardiac patient monitoring system using genetic and clinical a cardiac patient monitoring system using genetic and clinical knowledge fusion. In *Proceedings of 6th IEEE/ACIS International Conference on Computer and Information Science* (ICIS 2007, pp. 496–501). IEEE.

Søberg, J., Goebel, V., & Plagemann, T. (2010). Detection of spatial events in commonsens. In *Proceedings of the 2nd ACM International Workshop on Events in Multimedia* (EiMM '10, pp. 53–58). New York, NY: ACM. doi:10.1145/1877937.1877952

Socievole, A., Yoneki, E., De Rango, F., & Crowcroft, J. (2013). Opportunistic message routing using multi-layer social networks. In *Proceedings of the 2nd ACM Workshop on High Performance Mobile Opportunistic Systems* (HP-MOSys '13, pp. 39–46). Barcelona, Spain: ACM. doi:10.1145/2507908.2507923

Vahdat, A., & Becker, D. (2006). *Epidemic routing for partially connected ad hoc networks.* Technical Report CS-200006. Duke University.

Varshney, U. (2007). Pervasive healthcare and wireless health monitoring. *Mobile Networks and Applications*, *12*(2-3), 113–127. doi:10.1007/s11036-007-0017-1

Varshney, U. (2008). A framework for supporting emergency messages in wireless patient monitoring. *Decision Support Systems*, *45*(4), 981–996. doi:10.1016/j.dss.2008.03.006

KEY TERMS AND DEFINITIONS

Ambient Assisted Living: Predominately an European term, that describes technologies aiming to enhance the quality of life of older people through the use of Information and Communication Technologies (ICT). The term ambient relates to the use of non-invasive sensors, such as motion detectors, which help understand how people live their lives and hence detect when things change possibly showing a negative decline. This area may also be referred to by many other names such as: ageing in place, independent living, telemedicine, tele-monitoring, or tele-surveillance.

Delivery Cost: Represents by the ratio between the total number of exchanged messages during the course of the experiment and the number of generated messages. The metric should be as low as possible and it shows the congestion of the network.

Dementia: Not typically a specific disease, but rather is a term that describes a group of symptoms affecting thinking and social abilities severely enough to interfere with daily functioning. Many causes of dementia symptoms exist. Alzheimer's disease is the most common cause of a progressive dementia. Memory loss generally occurs in dementia. However, memory loss alone doesn't mean you have dementia. Dementia indicates problems with at least two brain functions, such as memory loss and impaired judgment or language, and the inability to perform some daily activities such as paying bills or becoming lost driving.

Hit Rate: Computed as the ratio between successfully delivered and total messages, is a metric that suggests the efficiency of a routing algorithm, and ideally it would be 100%. It shows the fraction of requests that can be served by a routing algorithm.

Hop Count: Metric describes the number of nodes that carried a message until it reached the destination on the shortest path.

Latency: Show the time (in seconds) passed between generating a message and delivering it to the destination. In an opportunistic network, which is a type of delay tolerant network (DTN), delivery latency should be improved when possible.

ONSIDE: (OpportuNistic Socially-aware and Interest-based DissEmination) (Ciobanu et al, 2014) is a publish/subscribe-based algorithm that disseminates data in opportunistic networks based on nodes' interests, together with social information about the nodes in the ON. Its goal is to reduce the overhead of spreading the data, while not affecting the hit rate and the delivery latency.

Opportunistic Mobile Networks: Consist of human-carried mobile devices that communicate with each other in a store-carry-and-forward fashion, without any infrastructure. Compared to the classical networks, they present distinct challenges. In opportunistic networks, disconnections and highly variable delays caused by human mobility are the norm rather than an exception. The solution consists of dynamically building routes, as each node acts according to the store-carry-and-forward paradigm. Thus, contacts between nodes are viewed as opportunities to move data closer to the destination. Such networks are therefore formed between nodes spread across the environment, without any knowledge of a network topology. The routes between nodes are dynamically created, and nodes can be opportunistically used as a next hop for bringing each message closer to the destination. Nodes may store a message, carry it around, and forward it when they encounter the destination or a node that is more likely to reach the destination.

SPRINT: (Social PRedIction-based routing in opportunistic NeTworks) (Ciobanu et al, 2013) is an opportunistic routing algorithm that combines socially-aware routing, including both learned and offline social information about nodes, with a module capable to predict node behavior.

ENDNOTES

[1]   We acknowledge that dementia is not a clinical diagnosis itself, unless an underlying disease or disorder has been identified.

[2]   Light cognitive impairments, by contrast, such as poorer short-term memory, can happen as a normal part of aging (we slowly start to lose brain cells after around the age of 20). This is known as age-related cognitive decline, not dementia, because it does not cause the person or the people around them any problems (NINDS, 2013).

This work was previously published in Advanced Technological Solutions for E-Health and Dementia Patient Monitoring edited by Fatos Xhafa, Philip Moore, and George Tadros, pages 106-136 copyright year 2015 by Medical Information Science Reference (an imprint of IGI Global).

APPENDIX: LIST OF ACRONYMS

AAL: Ambient Assisted Living

ACE: Ambient Cardiac Expert

ALIP: Assisted Living Platform

BAN: Body Area Network

CEP: Complex Event Processing

DALLAS: Delivering Assisted Living Lifestyles at Scale

EKG: Electrocardiogram

GIS: Geographic Information System

GPRS: General Packet Radio Service

GPS: Global Positioning System

ICT: Information and Communication Technology

ITK: Interoperability Toolkit

LTE: Long-Term Evolution

LoI: Location of Interest

ON: Opportunistic Network

ONSIDE: OpportuNistic Socially-aware and Interest-based DissEmination

OSGi: Open Service Gateway initiative

PAN-IF: Peripheral Area Network Interface

RFID: Radio Frequency Identification

SPRINT: Social PRedIction-based routing in opportunistic NeTworks

TTS: Tame Transformation Signatures

WSN: Wireless Sensor Network.

Chapter 53

Applying Social Aspects in Home Telecare Design to Improve the Safety of Users and Quality of Service

Lawrence Chidzambwa
Vancouver, BC, Canada

ABSTRACT

Telecare enables remote and cost-effective home treatment of patients, improving the safety and quality of life of frail individuals. However, despite increased availability of telecare devices, many are not fully used and often ignored due to poor social perception and experience. The research suggests the social aspects of quality and safety related to user experience have not been considered. This can lead to misuse or non-use of telecare devices, reducing patient safety and quality of life. This chapter explores the implications for the lack of social considerations in telecare and develops a series of models and methodologies to integrate the social dimension with the traditional medical intervention focus. By applying semiotics and normative behavioural theory, the authors show how a Normative Home Telecare Framework can improve telecare solution design and ensure take up and use of the devices and increase patient safety and life quality.

1. INTRODUCTION

Telecare and telehealth safety issues are adverse events, errors and near misses that compromise the wellbeing of users and service provider staff. Safety issues include emotional and social issues of providing service into the home besides the physical and clinical issues prevalent in telecare. It is stressing enough for a user to cope with aging, illness or a condition the limits one's function. The stress may increase by the introduction of technology into the homecare as the care of an increasing number of conditions is moved from the hospital into the home. Safety risks can be introduced by the system, equipment or human beings. Patient safety in acute and hospital environment is viewed as an issue occurring in a controlled environment where the provider controls the standards and culture

DOI: 10.4018/978-1-4666-8756-1.ch053

that prevail. In home environments things become different and in some ways difficult as homes are designed to suite the taste of the occupants and not for care. A review of literature on telecare revealed that there were few articles that specifically address safety and quality issues in telecare although there are more articles on these aspects in telehealth. The technical aspects of safety and quality can be measured and metrics have been proposed for this (Brook, McGlynn et al., 2000). However the social aspects of quality and safety, which are also related to user experience, have not been given much consideration. The need to capture and structure individual social context led to the framework proposed in this article as a telecare solution design guideline.

Telecare services monitor individuals in their homes from a distance by linking emergency and care professionals directly to a residence using electronic, computing and communication technologies that are dispersed in the individual's home. Emergency "trigger events" can be detected via electronic devices distributed about the home (Porteous and Brownsell, 2000). Telecare operators decide on the appropriate response to the raised alarm. The range of people who receive home care is very diverse and the numbers of users are growing (Sethi, Azzi et al. 2011). This poses challenges of increased safety and quality of service to the providers.

The application of technology in home care will mostly be evaluated from a social perspective by the users. The social perspective includes ethics, privacy, security and the cultural perspective (Perry and Beyer, 2010; Sethi, Azzi et al., 2011) which are linked to user safety and quality of service. It is therefore important to understand the social issues that surround implementation of technology in the home. There is a realisation that the nature of services to which technologies are being applied are very personal and present a range of ethical and social challenges to the service providers and the users alike. This raises the need

to develop methods of designing and implementing telecare that respect the choices of the individual, improve acceptance and minimises unintended injury. In order to understand the social aspects of telecare quality and user safety the following section will give a brief background to telecare. The background will end with a narrative of the current telecare approach using a pilot study. Section 3 looks at the social aspects of quality in telecare followed by a section on patient safety. Section 5 discusses a proposed home normative home telecare framework and section 6 discusses the validation of the framework before a conclusion is made.

2. TELECARE BACKGROUND

The United Nations predicts that 40% of the world population will be over 60 years old in 2050 (UN, 2009). The same report shows that between the years of 2009 to 2050 the ratio of dependent people will double in Africa, Europe, North America and Oceania. The ratio will triple in Asia and Latin America and the Caribbean. Dependent people are calculated as those people under the age of 15 and over the age of 65 who are expected to need some sort of support in order to survive. The significance of this and other reports is that governments will have a decreasing tax base as a source of revenue and this will impact on the social programmes that they provide like the support for the elderly and vulnerable groups. The increase in the number of elderly needing care is partly attributed to improved living conditions. Another contributing factor to the decrease in the working population is the decreasing births rate especially in developed countries. These trends have led to the search for new ways to provide care and the use of technology as advocated in telecare has been identified as one of those with the biggest potential.

2.1 The Generations of Telecare

The beginnings of telecare can be traced back to the introduction of community alarms in the 1960s. Community alarms were introduced to reduce anxiety and provide security for users in sheltered accommodation. The devices transmit radio signals when activated by pressing a button or pulling a chord. They are still used in a variety of forms (Porteous and Brownsell 2000). They are cost effective although they have a limited range and applicability. They are regarded as the first generation of telecare systems (Chidzambwa 2013). The second generation of telecare systems use sensors which continuously transmit information on the vital signs and data on the environment like extreme temperature sensors or flood detectors. The third generation of telecare is a move from reactive approaches to pre-emptive approaches in that they aim to predict risk and summon help to pre-empt that risk like the body worn blood sugar monitors or the heart monitors. The second generation devices are the most common devices particularly with telecare providers. Although the technology for the third generation has been validated the costs have been a constraint in its wide scale adoption.

The application of technology in telecare ranges from the aged (Lawson and Nutter 2008), people with learning disability to the disabled where it is applied as assistive technologies. In UK the Whole System Demonstrator programme provided data on three million users of telecare applications in several locations (DoH 2011) with some projects providing evidence of great potential. For example biosensors, devices that are used to measure minute concentration of substances which are converted into an electrical signal (Chaplin and Bucke 1990), are being introduced to telecare. An example of a wearable bisosensor is shown in Figure 1. Applying this device together with mobile technology enables the recording of data throughout the day wherever the user maybe. Advances in technology like these are improving the quality of telecare.

With a large variety of technology available the important thing is to ensure devices match the identified needs and that they are reliable in order to limit errors. A mismatch of needs and devices causes distress and raises anxiety instead of providing the expected support and the prevelence of device errors erodes confidence in the application of technology as well as putting the users at risk. Challenges with compatibility between devices from different manufactures, lack of awareness,

Figure 1. Wearable biosensor measuring ECG

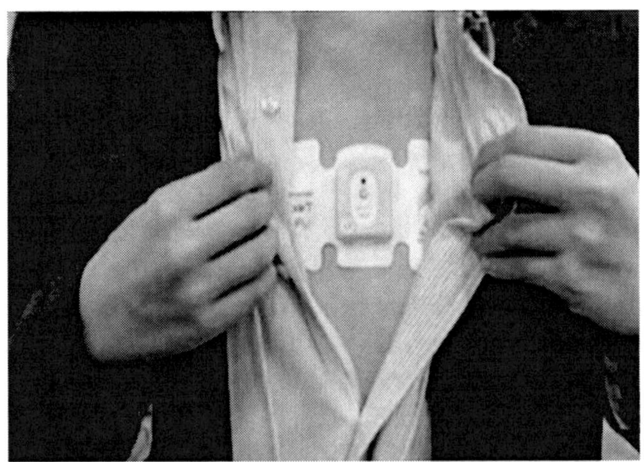

lack of guidelines in the implementation of telecare and funding are still being experienced in making telecare a mainstream product (Sethi and Khusainov 2012) and these are often the source of application errors and poor quality of service.

Examples of telecare devices that were compiled from literature are given in Table 1 (Chan, Esteve et al. 2008). The table shows the category of device and the usual condition that the device is applied to in the second column. The third column shows the example of the device and in the fourth column some social aspects that are considered in the application

of the device. There are far more devices in the market than the ones given in the table. Quality issues that emerge from this kind of list relate to how the devices carry out their function and what effect these devices have on the users when they are installed in the home including the effect of mulfunction. Some devices require human intervention and issues of interactivity and complexity of the device come into consideration. These issues have to be considered in relation to the condition of the user and the the social environment surrounding that particular installation. Safety issues like reliability, installation points and accidental

Table 1. Examples of telecare devices

Category	Condition	Device	Social Aspects
Wellbeing	Wandering	Occupancy sensor/ monitor	Privacy, trust, ethical, safety, control, independence, acceptance
	Incontinence	Enuresis sensor	Privacy, stigma, attitudes, control, ethics, comfort, safety
	Epileptic attack	Epilepsy sensor	Safety, quality of life, independence, stigma, control
	Falling	Fall detector	Safety, quality of life, control, intrusion, independence, easy of mind
Environmental	Detecting floods under the sink and in bathroom	Flood detector	Security, trust, expectation, acceptance, easy of mind, disruption
	Cuts off gas when a leak is detected	Gas shut off valve	Safety, trust, expectation, easy of mind, acceptance, disruption, interactivity
	Detecting leakage of natural gas	Natural gas detector	Safety, trust, expectation, easy of mind, disruption, interactivity
Security	Identifying callers before opening the door	Bogus caller button	Security, safety, policy
	Protecting property on leaving	Arm/Disarm trigger	Integrity, suspicion, control, interactivity
	Setting alarm by zones	Zoning button	Safety, disruption, ADL, policy, user preferences
Sensory impairments	Alerts wearer of activation of sensor	Vibrating pager for deaf people	User preference, intrusion, safety, security, data integrity, expectation, suspicion, trust, easy of mind
	Flashes to indicate a sensor has been activated	Flashing beacon	Disruption, interactivity, stigma
	Notifies carer of an alarm	Carer alert	Intrusion, disruption, privacy, user preference, ADL, policy, easy of mind
Support devices	Allows compatible devices to connect	Radio output module	Security, integrity, trust, expectation, privacy
	Enables devices to raise an alarm wirelessly using Plug and Play functionality to the base unit	Universal sensor	Integrity, security, trust, easy of mind, interactivity, control

switching off devices have also to be considered in addition to the facts that each installation is different and user environments and conditions are different. The reliability of devices is increasing resulting in more confidence on their applications.

The right technology for the identified need is known to empower and raise the self-esteem of the user (Percival and Hanson 2006). It improves the ability of users to cope with conditions that would be depressing. If a person cannot perform a certain function that they really want to do for themselves they get frustrated. That frustration can lead to stress which in the end might lead to depression (Lords 2005). Finding a way to cope with a condition can be uplifting even if that method is not eliminating the condition. A case was quoted during a pilot study of a couple who went to bed with their epileptic son for eighteen years because of the risk of injury to their son. The introduction of an epileptic sensor was very liberating for the family as the son could sleep in his bedroom. There are several advantages of automating some daily activities especially for the physically challenged groups like the automatic switching on of lights when someone gets up to use the toilet at night (Edge, Taylor et al. 2000). Using the enuresis sensor, which detects moisture on the individual and alerts the carer to change the user into dry linen has big advantages. It eliminates the embarrassing physical checks or the verbal inquisitions that have to be made on the person to determine if they are still dry. This promotes dignity, which is an important social value.

Safety issues might result from incorrect installations or inappropriate use of a device. Understanding the technology becomes crucial in the proper handling and use of devices in order to minimise the safety risks. Quality issues become relevant in relation to the objectives set for the service. Despite the advances in technology social aspects still play an important part in providing telecare service in relation to the quality of service and user experience. It is important to understand the social aspects encountered and how they are being applied. In this research a pilot study was conducted to understand the approaches being applied at the time.

2.2 The Pilot Study

It has been argued that the failure of systems is responsible for the increase in safety issues rather than humans (Lang, Edwards et al. 2007). This was one of the reasons a study was carried out to determine how telecare devices are applied. The pilot study was conducted in one of the inner district of London in UK. The study consisted of observations, semi-structured interviews and an analysis of assessment documents as shown in the breakdown in Table 2. No users were interviewed because of patient data protection reasons. Observations were used to provide an independent view of the activities instead of relying on narratives from staff or manuals. This enabled the collection of accurate data on what was taking place including the non-verbal communication that was taking place and its context. Observations of tasks were done more than once in order to capture the repeatable behaviours. There was more attention put on determining how the social aspects relating to the user were handled or discussed. After each observation session clarifications were requested on some issues observed from the assessor or technician after leaving the user's premises. This was in the form of semi-structured interviews.

Semi-structured interviews were conducted using a guide of questions in order to ensure important points were not left out in the study. This approach provided the interviewee opportunities to state things in their own way using the language comfortable to them. Some of the interviews were recorded on audiotape whilst some were recorded in notes.

2.2.1 Findings from Observations

During assessments user details were filled in the spaces provided in the assessment form

Table 2. Breakdown description of observations, semi-structured interviews and analysis

Activity	Tasks	Details
7 Observations	Initial assessments on prospective users and new system installations	Initial assessments and new installations
7 Observations	Device maintenance visits	Maintenance and call out visits
10 Interviews	Questions on all aspects of the telecare service provided	All aspects of telecare service
Document analysis	25 User assessment forms from different service providers	Analysing Initial assessment forms

mainly focussing on the reasons for referring the individual for telecare service. User assessments mainly looked at clinical risks that are linked to home care clients like falling, mobility, cooking and medication risks. Details of family carers and their roles were collected to help in planning the responses to any call out as normally done. At some assessment sessions the recommendations from the assessor were not accepted. This was highlighted in one instance where despite the recommendations from the medical doctor the user refused the recommended monitoring equipment. The assessor tried to convince the individual but only by explaining why the doctor had referred the person for telecare and also the risks highlighted by the doctor. No effort was made to understand the decision from the client's point of view.

During installation the configuration for devices was done as per instruction sheet. In some instances, where alternative device could be offered, the technician made the decision on which device to install. The assumption was that users knew little about the devices and therefore cannot make any meaningful decision to the decisions. There was an evident absence of collecting user opinions and preferences during assessments and installation. These observations affect the user experience and may lead to a service different from the user's expectations. A sample of the observations data is shown in Table 3. In the tables the following coding is used to identify the different tasks;

A0#: Indicates an assessment observation case number

IO#: Indicates a device installation observation case number

MO#: Indicates a device maintenance observation case number

In summary the observations of assessments revealed that;

- Assessors focused on reducing or eliminating risks that were either the reasons of the referral or their interpretation of user needs.
- Some users were not wearing pendants on their necks and the issue was not pursued by the technician. Misuse, wrong usage and non-use of devices were surprisingly not treated with the same importance as technical errors.
- Devices malfunction at times. When a technical fault was detected all effort was put into resolving the aspect and log the maintenance in the system however, observing non-use was not being treated with the same urgency. This was mainly because of the need to maintain an impressive maintenance record for audit purposes, a technical issue, rather than raising the quality of life.
- Most of the devices installed did not require functional configuration, they were single state devices. This reduces errors

Table 3. A sample of observations

Case No:	Personal Details	User Condition	Activity	Observations
AO1	Age: 82 Gender: Male Location: Home	High blood pressure problems, high cholesterol level, four heart-bypass surgeries before, lives alone.	Objective: New Assessment Result: Only accepted son as key-holder. Accepted environmental monitoring devices. Main objective of enabling the user to call for help was not met.	Reluctant to give personal information and did not believe there were risks about his health that required monitoring Refused alarm panic button that would be used to call for help. Refused key holder to anyone close by but accepted one 15 minutes away. Was informed that all costs are covered except for a small rental fee on the equipment. Said very little about social life when he was asked if anyone can check on him. Flat was partly owned by housing association but there were no problems about installing devices. Discussion was centred on the clinical risks pointed out by the doctor. No discussion was held on user's perception about telecare.
MO2	Age: Over 75yrs Gender: Female Location Home	Bed bound. No clinical condition disposed	Objective: Scheduled Maintenance Result: Maintenance carried out. Nothing was discussed about the use of telecare or any concerns with the system	Scheduled maintenance visit. Visit timed with arrival of English speaking day carer because of language problems. Keypad, smoke detector, heat sensor, pendant and base unit installed. Checked location of units and recorded serial numbers. The user has a 24 hour carer who, like the user, did not speak English well. Telecare was installed in addition to the carers. The second carer only comes in at specific times, twice a day, to help.
IO1	Age: Over 80yrs Gender: Male Location: Home	Fully mobile but lives alone. Cautious about security especially between his flat and neighbour who shares entrance door to property	Objective: New installation Result: Installation of the telecare package was completed and devices tested. It appeared like the user had been supplied with devices that he did not understand which meant they were not used as expected.	Keysafe, 3xflood detectors, fall detector, pendant (panic) button and base unit. User had questions on how fall detector works and from what range. Pendant wearing options both offered. Pendant type option not offered but one chose for him by technician. Brief explanation of how equipment works, Welcome visit appointment booked The assessment had already been done and the devices selected but the user showed that he did not understand the operation of some of the devices. The user was asked if he wanted a welcome visit after the installation and said he did. User was eager for someone to go through all the devices again with them. There was no clinical condition but just that he was 80 yrs old and lived alone so social services had referred telecare to minimise risk.

in current devices but configurable multifunction devices being introduced have higher risks.

- The choice of installation sites was made by technicians although in some instances users expressed the risk of pets and children being causes of malfunctioning devices.
- Users were expected to fit within the operation boundaries of the devices. This was a source of frustration as indicated in the interviews. This impacts the quality of service.
- All devices issued by the provider were from a single supplier. The provider was tied to a contract. This limited device selection options and is a constraint in providing the best service and utilising more reliable devices.

2.2.1 Findings from Interviews

Only staff members of the organisation were included in the semi-structured interviews. The interviewees were selected from all the levels of the department running the telecare service. Interviews were deliberately started from the lower levels of the organisation up so that clarifications can be inquired about at higher levels. Open-ended questions were prepared in order to guide the interviews but they were only a guide so that important parts of information would not be omitted. Questions were asked on every stage of the solution design process. Issues that had been observed during the observations were also clarified. Interviews were conducted in environments where there would be no interruption and comfortable as much as possible. Care was taken to keep within the interview time allocated. A sample of interviews conducted is given in Table 4. The questions were compiled to collect information on the following aspects.

1. **From Assessors:**
   a. The procedures followed in assessing a prospective user
   b. Objectives of assessment
   c. The format of assessment and the structure of the assessment form
   d. Any challenges encountered during assessment
2. **From the team leaders and the managers all the issues inquired from assessors as above and:**
   a. Training of assessors
   b. Information provided to the user about telecare

c. The influence of social issues like culture on the assessment and telecare in general
d. Whether user preferences are considered in the solution design
e. Any examples of behaviour or attitude that affect acceptance

The following is a brief description of the process of implementing telecare as given by the telecare manager shown in Figure 2.

As shown in the diagram clinicians e.g. General Practitioners or Social Workers refer clients for telecare service quoting the reasons of the referral. The telecare department carries out an assessment on how to provide for the clinical recommendations. The assessor makes a decision on devices to be installed following the department guidelines and the devices available to the provider. A technician then installs and tests the recommended devices. Commissioning the service is officially linking the installed devices to the call centre, which will start monitoring the user.

It was evident from the responses that the information captured on the assessment form is the information used for decision-making. It was also strongly believed by the interviewees that the procedure was user centred.

Figure 2. Telecare solution design process in Newham

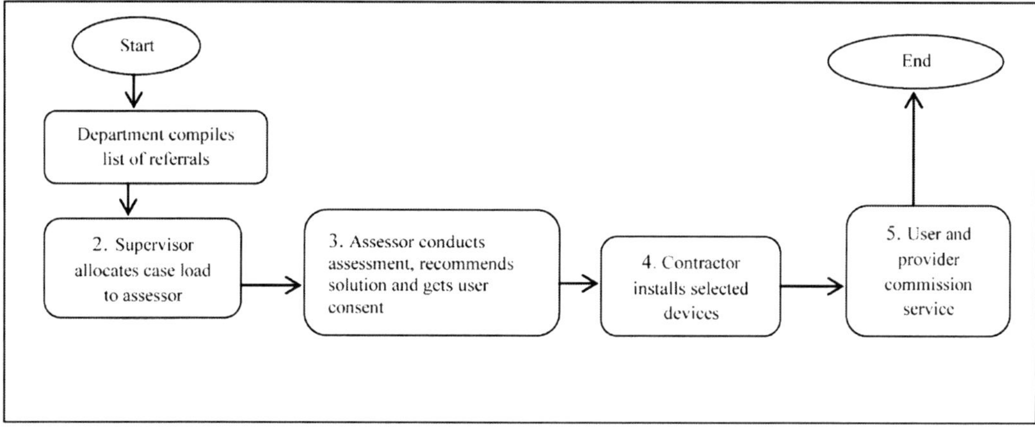

Table 4. Selected interview questions and responses

Case Details	Issues Raised	Responses
ID: I1 Role: Assessor Activity: Assessment	1. How is an assessment conducted? 2. What kind of training have you received? 3. What objectives does an assessment aim to achieve? 4. What are the challenges in achieving the aim? 5. How relevant is the assessment form? 6. What are the limitations of the assessment form? 7. What other information besides that collected on the form do you use to make decisions about what to provide? 8. How do you deal with language/cultural aspects? 9. In which ways is the user involved on the decisions about the choice of devices to install? 10. What other challenges have you encountered in assessing people and how have you overcome them. 11. Give an example of the most outstanding assessment that you have had and how you dealt with it	• Assessment follows the structure of assessment form • Received training from device supplier and in house. • Form covers all the basics although might need more information because of each circumstance • I don't think there is anything the form leaves out • It is important to know what other support the user has and that the family understands how telecare works. • We do not have many problems with language, when we do we always assess in the presence of a family member of carer, it helps • Users do not know much about telecare. In most cases it is the first time that they have heard someone explain it so they normally go along with whatever we recommend • Only use one device supplier • Users asked for preferences e.g. chord or wrist strap • Normally configure at installation if possible e.g. exit sensor for time, chair sensor for weight, pill dispenser, time but they are few. • There are no major problems that arise during assessment maybe because the service is free for most people.

ID: I5
Role: Supervisor
Activity: Assessment procedure
	Question in I1
	+
	1. How have the assessors been trained for telecare?
	2. What information is given to the user about the need for assessment?
	3. How much information do users already have about telecare?
	4. What issues have been identified during assessments that affect decision making?
	a. Culture
	b. Family etc.
	5. How have cultural issues been resolved or how would they be resolved?
	6. Is there any attention given to user preferences and how or how are they applied?
	7. If preferences are not currently captured, how would they be used if they were captured?
	8. What types of issues have been identified as behavioural in assessments?
	9. What perceptions of telecare have been identified among service users?
	10. What are the user perceptions on usefulness?
	a. Trustworthiness perception
	b. Perceived control
	11. What common behaviours have been identified amongst prospective users or among current telecare users?
	12. What attitudes have been identified towards the technology and towards its application?
	13. How are response to device alarms assigned?
	14. What differentiation is there in response levels?
	15. How is the data on numbers and nature of calls/ responses used if any reports are produced about this?
	16. Do you always ask all the questions in the form and if not, when do you select which ones to ask?
	17. What is the relevance of each section on of the form?
		• Only assess for telecare and not any other social needs because of two reasons
		  o Only deal with telecare issues and need information for emergency response
		  o To help in selecting the equipment that can be installed
		• Sometimes we prefill some information on forms but use the form to decide on what solution to provide.
		• Users do not have information about telecare except what they have been told by social services/OT. Most of the information on telecare they get it with the welcome pack
		• Some Jewish orthodox do not touch anything electronic on Sabbath day, For language problems we use interpreters but not often.
		• Users are more open with those who speak the same language
		• There are sensory problems with the elderly especially hearing
		• The main incentives for take up seems to be its free for some and very cheap for the rest.
		• Some preferences that have been given by users are
		  o They like equipment to be hidden
		  o Users are not in favour of wearing pendants around the neck
		  o Some users want the sound of alarms changed
		  o Use of visual alarm or large print where necessary and equipment can be changed which is rare
		• Some pendants are not worn because users are not comfortable. Some users forget and some think they do not need it but it is supplied as a package
		• Some habits that interfere with telecare are erratic sleeping patterns, smoky cooking, changing routines. Some users contact the call centre just to talk to someone yet it is set up for emergencies.
		• The provider does not monitor eating habits
		• The provider has a check in service for someone who has been out but other people forget
		• Assessment is done along devices that the provider can provide, the ones the supplier can give "That's our line really"
		• There is no specific arrangements for dementia or any other complex needs "No specification, no"
		• Duplication of service e.g. smoke detectors is unavoidable because council devices are not connected to telecare
		• Service numbers declined after the first roll out
		• Users are mainly older but diverse
		• Data is not used as live data but audited, it highlights high users of service, identify who needs to be checked because there is no activity. There is no information sharing with other services. Standards required for audit seem to drive how data is captured and stored not the need to use the data.
		• Perceptions are sceptical before but supportive after. Education for users is required on a large scale. Manual surveys are normally conducted among users and the results are very positive
		• An outstanding incident that occurred was when during an assessment a prospective user was asked to produce some benefits documentation. She went back to the bedroom and did not come back. When the assessors went to check on her they found her sitting and watching television in her bedroom. Apparently she had forgotten about the assessment.

2.2.2 Conclusions from the Pilot Study

The observations and interviews revealed the following;

- The assessments are biased towards the equipment that the borough can supply. This means they were not user centred but technology centred. Some conditions for which there were no devices from their supplier were not covered at all for example dementia. One of the answers to a question on how much of complex needs they cover for example dementia the answers was *"Not specifically, no"*. Related to that was a follow up question to a team leader: "It looks like you are capturing preferences relating to the devices that you install" and the answer was *"That's our line really"*. This showed that the assessment is actually technology driven rather than user needs driven which excludes emotional safety and social safety aspects.

- Whilst users had accepted the installation of devices and given consent, adoption, which is the actual usage of some devices, was observed to be low especially for body warn pendants. Expectations mismatch resulted in reduced quality of service.

- The data collected are not shared with other services e.g. social services. One of the interviewees explained that they inform the referrer about what has been installed but they do not have set procedures of feedback. There was no consideration on how the collected data could be used to improve user experience.

- It was observed that some people are not willing to give personal information freely because of confidentiality concerns, which may result in none or a poor risk assessment and installation of an unsuitable solution.

- Solution design was not comprehensive enough to address all safety issues and the application of social factors to improve quality of service and user experience.

3. THE SOCIAL SIDE OF TELECARE QUALITY AND RELATED THEORIES

The wellbeing of an individual is influenced by their physical condition as well as the psychological and social aspects such as relationships, emotions, expectations, perceptions and fears (Kane 2001). These non-clinical aspects of health become more important when a person is cared from home where a clinical condition may become a lower priority to other needs faced in the house like cooking and personal care (Mattke, Klautzer et al. 2010). They become more important as the home has developed into a place which does not only provide shelter and storage but a range of personalised services like business, education, leisure and health services among others can be provided (Dewsbury 2001) which invade social space. However current home telecare models have seen people adjusting their lives in order to suit the telecare devices which can be frustrating or even irritating (Baxter and Monk 2006). The current requirements gathering process mainly considers functions that the technology can provide and pays little attention to personal preferences and cultural needs (Baxter and Monk 2006). Such techniques have proved inadequate in terms of making telecare more acceptable and developing it into a mainstream product (von Niman, Rodriguez-Ascaso et al. 2006). Lack of attention to social and cultural aspects, has been identified as some of the factors influencing the slow adoption of home telecare and increase in costs and waste resulting from inappropriate telecare solutions (Barlow, Bayer et al. 2006). Social aspects include beliefs, expectations, obligations, fears, culture, commitments, associations and communities that one belongs to and even leisure activities (Liu 2000). These issues influence the day to day activities and decision making in the home and will influence the adoption of telecare and user experience. In the majority of cases these social aspects are the ones the user can articulate well and not the technological aspects. The user will therefore use the social aspects to evaluate the service provided.

Home telecare is a complex field because of the wide variety of stakeholders like doctors, social workers, family and friends who have direct input and might have different and at times conflicting expectations on the service (McGee-Lennon and Gray 2007) (Barlow, Bayer et al. 2006). It is important for the stakeholders to have a shared vision and their social factors have to be considered at all stages starting from research up to service deployment (von Niman, Rodriguez-Ascaso et al. 2006). Their values need to be structured in a way that makes it possible to configure them to devices. This research will show how to capture structure and configure social aspects to devices where possible.

3.1 Identifying the Social Aspects

Personal norms are built from a person's general value system and differ from general attitudes as they focus on specific actions and feelings of obligation (Schwartz and Fleishman 1978). Norms are patterns of behaviours. This suggests the need to detect personal norms impacting telecare by identifying specific personal behaviours that are obligated to something or someone in the user's life. Wenzel in his paper on tax compliance behaviour (Wenzel 2002) defines personal norms as peoples own moral standards that are acquired for instance through the internalisation of social norms. From the two definitions above personal norms appear to be the combination of a selective subset of environmental norms and norms developed from personal experience. This is especially true where the potential personal

gain outweighs the sanction. Personal norms refer to self-expectations for behaviour backed by the anticipation of self-enhancement. The key is that personal norms concern the "what is in it for me' rule. They are intrinsically linked to personal gain or loss. Clearly identifying the benefit of telecare adoption to telecare users and appealing to personal norms may significantly impact acceptance levels and correct use of the telecare solution. It is important to note that what appeals to the person is not what telecare does for others but rather how it benefits the particular individual although other people's experience will enhance insight. Their particular circumstances, therefore, warrants proper investigation. In some cases individuals develop unconscious personal behaviours. For example, always switching certain lights off, going to the same restaurant, seeing friends every Thursday. These living habits may often be deeply engrained and provide security and familiarity for the individual. A medical condition and an intrusive telecare solution may greatly impact, displace or alter these living habits. In some cases if the benefit of the telecare provision e.g. in the case of fall monitoring, alarms and sensors, may not be appreciated and valued enough to be included within their current habits then telecare is discarded although it might have been accepted at first when the telecare assessor was present. The individual decision to or not to fully embrace telecare is probably the focal point for any intervention. There has to be enough motivation for an individual to adjust or change the habits that might be impacted by the adoption of telecare in a non-compatible way. In other words the motivations that have been identified are weighed against the comfort or discomfort of changing the habits (Klockner and Matthies 2004). While service providers aim to minimise injury by providing fall detectors, users may be concerned with the risk that if they are known to be falling they lose self-image and be labelled frail. They might be moved to a nursing home and lose their house so even if they are given a fall detector they might not use it (Percival and Hanson 2006). Personal norms play an important part in users' decision making. It is important therefore to determine the social aspects and the personal norm affecting habits during assessment as this puts the user at the centre of the design process, enabling a 'user centred design approach'.

This research applies social constructivism to capture the ideas from the different stakeholders in the design process. Social constructivism is the use of a set of beliefs and mental models by people in a given community to interpret actions and events and arrive at an agreed meaning (Walshman 1995; Jackson and Klobas 2001). It is a sociological theory of knowledge in which groups collaboratively create a culture of shared artefacts with shared meanings. It extends constructivism by including the role of other actors and culture in meaning construction. The underlying assumptions of social constructivism are reality, knowledge and learning. On reality social constructivists believe that members of a community invent the properties of their world which means reality does not exist before its invention. In telecare environments this means that when assessors go to assess an individual, they should not have a pre-conceived assumption of what solution needs to be provided.

3.2 Capturing Social Aspects

User centred design (UCD) approach has been advocated for in order to improve user buy-in. One variation of UCD is participatory design (Baek, Cagiltay et al. 2008). Differences in technical knowledge can be a challenge in this approach but advocates have suggested the use of simplified versions of the artefact or prototyping as a method to overcome some of these issues. User issues can be as simple as filling in a form to complicated interactive applications that require instant update in the system (Baek, Cagiltay et al. 2008).

Koch (2006) noted in a review of telehealth that there is a migration from a purely technical approach to a user-centric one in telecare and telehealth designs. This shift involves coordinating the service users, carers and family members, clinicians and other stakeholders into the decision making process. This is encouraging but seems to be missing from telecare design proposals and is the motivation of this research. Changes in society and organisations are leading to changes from a provider driven service approach to a patient-centred approach. The increase awareness of health issues providers to adopt the much needed personalisation of service by including users and carers to help identify service redesign opportunities. In some programmes carers and social workers are receiving specific training for this role (Clark and Goodwin 2010). The challenge is in defining these non-specific issues in a way that enables application in design.

In this research norm analysis, an organisational semiotics tool is applied in structuring the identified social aspects. In organisational semiotics (OS), norms are defined as socially accepted rules by a community to govern the behaviour of the members within that community (Liu 2000). Norms are attributed to agents as in OS there is no knowledge without a knower and there is no knowing without action. The norm specification will take the context into consideration and a norm will be specified in the format below.

Whenever *<context>* **if** *<condition>* **then** *< some agent>* **is** *<deontic operator>* **to do** *<action> (Salter and Liu 2002).*

While the constructivist approach is used in clarifying the meaning that the service users, clinicians and the service provider attach to the statements that they make on the requirements, norm analysis ensures that the designer comes up with the required details that specify how the desired action is going to be carried out and by whom. The details form the constraints and behaviours that will impact the solution that emerges. The following section will show how these concepts are applied in designing telecare solutions.

3.3 Applying Social Aspects in Telecare Solution Design

Information systems have social as well as technical dimensions (Liu 2000). The reason social aspects are now being given attention in systems design is the recognition that computers are employed within natural environments of human interaction and collaboration (Crabtree 2003). As Crabtree observes the home adds different set of challenges from those found in structured environments like organisations. It exposes designers to new user groups including the elderly, disabled and those mentally impaired. Bringing in tools and conceptual models from work environments into domestic settings emphasises on values like productivity and efficiency at the expense of understanding the values that make home life unique. These values while important in organisations are seen in a different light as domestic life is not organised in the same way as organisations. The challenge for designers is to find how technologies can be fitted in the home environment whilst maintaining its uniqueness. Some researchers suggest a need to study and document the rich and sometimes complex routines or patterns of activities in domestic environments just like the studies that were done to enable office automation (Tolmie, Pycock et al. 2002). The problem with this is that each home differs from the next and within each home things are not always done the same way. However, capturing the patterns serves as a resource for the articulation and coordination of intended action. Some behaviour that might not seem related at all might actually originate from a set of deep-seated internal or even social values. Determining the reasons for the observable

behaviour patterns is important in understanding influences to decision making.

Unlike the traditional perception of viewing information systems as tools to solve problems external to people e.g. budgets, the modern applications are multi user environments that are used to mediate social interactions (Whitworth and de Moor 2003). This means that the user is an active part of the software rather than being regarded as external to the application. Performing only technical evaluations becomes meaningless outside the social context or the norms or forces that dictate how the technical elements have to be applied (Stockdale and Standing 2006). Designers need to begin by identifying social needs and then translate them into socio-technical system design requirements in order to make systems more social.

3.4 The Need for Improved Care Quality

One of the main objectives of implementing telecare is the improvement of quality of care (Koch 2006) as in some instances technology can do a better job than humans. There are also concerns about the quality of service provided in institutions and by home carers (Mattke, Klautzer et al. 2010). From a user point of view the indicators of quality are subjective. There are variations in the definition of quality of care with some definitions preferring the use of outcomes (Kane 2001) and others emphasising on the processes (Campbell, Roland et al. 2000). Whilst certain outcomes are regarded as important by providers it does not follow that the user places the same importance on those outcomes or indicators. It becomes important to determine and include those aspects that are regarded important by the users in order for the telecare solution to remain relevant.

There is some agreement that some elements of quality in care are not easily measurable. Donabedian (1997) explains that in measuring quality of care the performance of a practitioner has to be taken from two different perspectives, technical and personal, in order to arrive at a better assessment as shown in Figure 3. Technical performance depends on the knowledge that is used to arrive at the appropriate strategies of care and also the skills used to implement those strategies (Donabedian 1997; Brook, McGlynn et al. 2000). Privacy, confidentiality, empathy and sensitivity are some of the components that make up the interpersonal relationship and home telecare service utilises these more than institutions because of the social environment found in homes. In general the social aspects of quality emerge from a need by people to be treated humanely and in a culturally appropriate way (Brook, McGlynn et al. 2000). The condition of the individual and their value system determines the importance that they place on the aspects of care quality. The interpersonal process acts as the vehicle by which technical care is implemented and is therefore vital for the success of technical care. The challenge of system designers is on how to include the values of the interpersonal elements in the operation of the device in a technical system. Emphasising on the technical aspects of quality only has resulted in the slow adoption of telecare. It is important therefore to find a method in which the user can contribute to the setting of care objectives that are truly important to them. Emphasising on either technical quality or interpersonal quality issues at

the expense of the other will be detrimental to the overall objective of care quality. The consideration of human factors will play an important role in improving quality by enabling personalisation of service (von Niman, Rodriguez-Ascaso et al. 2006).

Personalisation of the service offers an opportunity to install only the required and approved devices thereby improving user experience and reducing the installation and running costs. For example in cases where the elderly have risks of falling, telecare provides piece of mind and reassurance of quick response. This has a psychological effect of enabling the user to perform their daily activities without anxiety thereby raising their quality of life. Falls can result in serious injury that will lead to hospitalisation. The consequences of falling will increase if the person is not able to get up as a result of the fall and does not get assistance in time. This may lead to dehydration or even hypothermia in extreme temperatures leading to the user spending time in hospital. Additionally the loss of confidence in the individual may limit their mobility because of fear and thereby reduce the quality of life. Hip replacements cost between $24000 to $28000 in Canada (BC-Government; 2004). Broken bones can result in the person having to use a

Figure 3. Quality assessment based on technical and personal perspectives

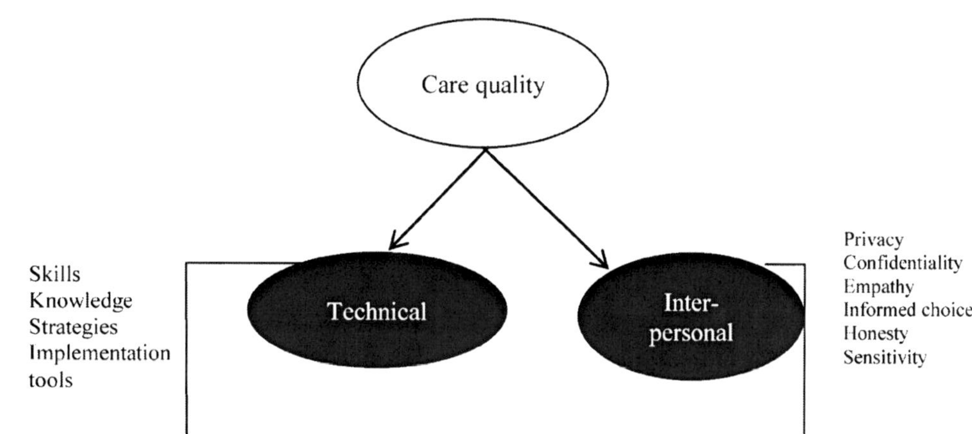

wheelchair for the rest of their life. The quality of service is linked to the user's expectations and the user experience therefore user input in setting service objectives is important.

4. PATIENT SAFETY IN TELECARE

The safety of telecare has to be approached from the service user and the provider point of view. From the service provider point of view safety issues relate to device selection, setup, configuration and maintenance, response times and user procedures which include respecting the user's preferences. These are mainly technical aspects and providers have the means to deal with them. From the user's point of view the safety issues relate to the user's condition, ability to use the device, device familiarity and culture issues. The diversity of these issues indicate that not one stakeholder can be able to articulate all of them if a good understanding is to be obtained. Researchers agree that if the benefits of telecare are to be realised then accurate requirements capturing needs to be done for each case not the one size fits all approach used by some providers (Hanson, Percival et al. 2007).

4.1 Provider Responsibility on Safety Issues

The underlying safety responsibility of telecare providers is that of non-maleficence or the obligation to cause no harm. The ethical responsibility comes from the principle of "first, do no harm" which means that if there is any chance of causing any harm to the user by introducing telecare then it may be better to eliminate the risk or even not introduce the device that might cause harm. Experts in a study that was conducted in UK confirmed that this was an important issue as implementation of telecare is done mainly to reduce or eliminate risks to the user (Perry, Beyer et al. 2010).

Social aspects that have an influence on safety from a provider's point of view are issue like communication barriers, breach of privacy and user intimidation. On communication, the majority of users receiving home care have carer contact on a daily basis. Some concern has been raised that because the communication by telecare devices is now impersonal some issues that would have been noticed on a visit by a carer will go unnoticed. User interaction with the system or device has been identified as an area of concern (Lang, Edwards et al. 2007). While devices used in telecare do not require user calibration or constant user interaction, human-device interaction especially with users whose conditions are deteriorating can be a cause of risk to user safety. In one case quoted in the pilot study the users removed the devices because the constant flashing was making them more paranoid and in another case the constant reminders were viewed as an irritation and the user put the device in a freezer to shut it up. These details are hard to pick if a single approach is applied and instead of providing peace of mind devices can be a source of frustration.

Intimidation of users is an issue that relates to the users being coerced to accept telecare even though they do not understand or they have some misgivings. Users and the carers whether family or the allocated nurses are the experts of the tasks to which the devices are being applied. User opinion needs to be respected and the user be given all the opportunity to participate in the decision-making. That way the user will buy into the decisions, which will translate into a commitment to minimise errors of use which will improve safety. If decisions are made for the user, then the responsibility on safety will not be on the user. These needs are captured during the assessment. There should be a deliberate attempt from a provider's point of view to capture these social aspects as proposed in the proposed framework.

On the technical aspects the provider needs to ensure that the devices selected do not affect the user negatively as was quoted in one of the interviews in the pilot study. There should be a smooth fit between the devices applied and the task to which the user agrees. The knowledge gap between providers and users on technical features of the devices can be reduced by applying conceptual models of the telecare solution that can be understood by the user. Technology should only be applied to the tasks that are required by the user. Issues like power source, interactivity, reliability, and reducing interference on signal transmission are issues that are improving and a responsibility of the device manufacturer. However the responsibility of the telecare provider is to select the devices that offer the user the best service which address the user needs and preferences. This issue has been addressed in the framework proposed. The installation points of devices are in some instances influenced by the device operation however the provider needs to get the consent of the user on device installation points and explain the reasons why some points are mandatory. The most important thing is the user routine must not be dependent on the device where possible. This will minimise operation errors and false alarms and accidental switching off of devices. Response times and response methods need to be discussed and agreed upon. Backup procedures agreed to by the user need to be in place when devices fail. Good maintenance procedures help to minimise device malfunction. Thresholds, language, type of message or alarm raised are all issues that need to be considered in order to improve safety measures and avoid misuse of equipment.

4.2 User Related Safety Issues

Safety issues relating to the user are mainly social aspects although some technical aspects might be made relevant by the condition of the user. The majority of devices are set to operate independent of the user. For devices that are operated by the user, the ability of the user is an important factor in order to minimise malfunction or accidental

switching off. The pilot study found out that the majority of users are elderly and are not familiar with the technology being applied. For instance some pendants were left on the window seal instead of being worn on the individual. In one instance the user was cooking in a very hot and misty kitchen which is considered a high risk yet the user had taken off the device in order to cook. More information on how to use devices will reduce these cases of misuse. Cultural issues and religious considerations can impact on how devices are applied and this misuse can lead to user harm as the provider maybe under the impression that all is well. Identification of these issues during the assessment procedure is important and user participation in decision making will minimise the risks. To address patient safety and provide high-quality care, a normative home telecare is proposed to assist providers in designing personalised solutions.

5. THE NORMATIVE HOME TELECARE FRAMEWORK

There is no single solution or process that applies to all cases and environments in providing telecare. However there are common procedures that are present in most design processes that need to be refined in order to produce acceptable solutions to users. A framework provides this guide without being prescriptive. It provides guidance in a way that is easy to understand and also fosters open communication between the stakeholders. This helps the stakeholders to work towards a shared vision. The framework empowers the team members and allows flexibility in the design of solutions. It raises the quality of the design as stakeholders learn from shared experiences and knowledge. Because all the major stakeholders participate in the solution design, responsibility is shared and all stakeholders get committed to the success of the solution.

5.1 The Framework Components

The proposed components of the Normative Home Telecare Framework on a high level are;

1. User defined care profile helping to understand the prospective user from user point of view. Everything in the solution needs to be centred on the user needs. However the current procedures have had these needs referred from a clinical point of view paying little attention to the social aspects. This aspect was identified during the literature review and at the conclusion of the pilot study.
2. User approved care specification. The care specification is an extension to care plans that are currently drafted by applying norm analysis concept. It provides more details on how the specific tasks are executed whilst considering the prevailing social aspects. This component brings together the clinical needs and social needs as identified by the user.
3. User approved telecare specification. This component provides a method of selecting the care tasks where technology can be applied and applies norm analysis in defining how those tasks are performed in a manner that is approved by the user. The methodical selection of devices was an issue that was observed to be missing during the pilot study section.

4. Device specification component. This stage applies the identified user preferences and home social factors in the configuration of devices. The component links the technology acceptance factors to device attributes and enables the application of social aspects to device operation.

Figure 4 shows the components and their relationships. Each of these components is broken down further in order to clearly show the thought process behind the selection. The procedure of designing a home telecare solution will follow the deliverables in the numeric order shown in the diagram. The double arrows indicate that the processes are iterative and one may need to go to the previous stage to clarify inconsistences before they can continue to the next stage. The dashed arrows show the central role that is played by the user defined care profile at all the stages of the framework. As shown in the diagram, this framework encourages the application of telecare in combination with other care initiatives. This has the advantage of a holistic approach that eliminates some of the duplication of services that was identified within some providers.

5.2 Including Social Aspects in Telecare Design

This section describes the steps taken to compile a user care profile and the reasons behind those

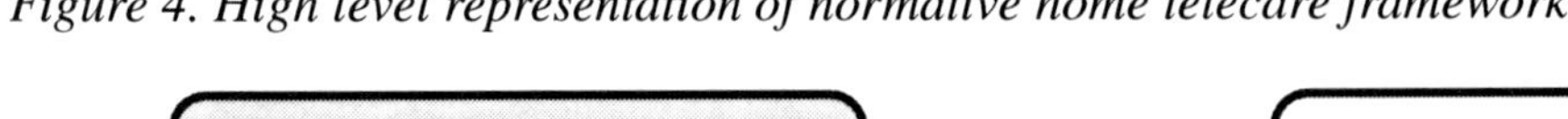

Figure 4. High level representation of normative home telecare framework

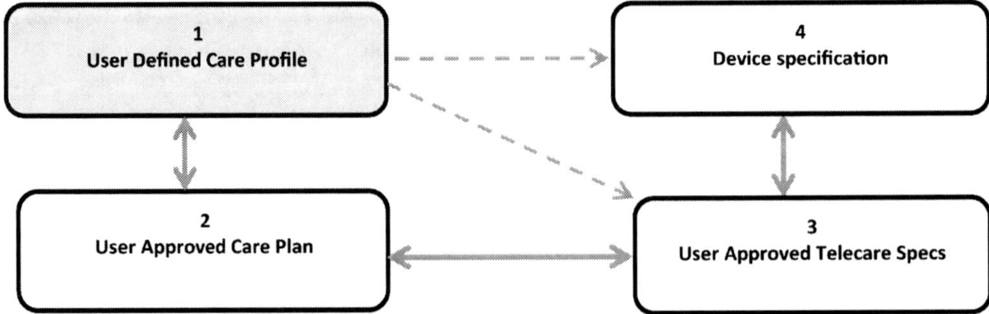

steps. The user defined care profile is what the user expects to be done to support them. The provider will need to confirm that the preferences requested are practical and within their means. This approach emphasises on what the user considers as important aspects of their care in light of what they are capable of doing for themselves as observed by Bandura that "Self-percepts of efficacy influence thought patterns, actions and emotional arousal" (Bandura 1982)(p 122). This means that what one judges one's self to be capable of will influence how they think, act and self – motivate. It is not only what the user is capable of but what they think they should get that will have an effect on how they perceive the support they get. Capturing the beliefs and expectations help tailor the service to their expectation within the capabilities of the provider. Perceptions about one's self have a lot to do with how an individual behaves under different conditions and also how they psychologically cope with the ever-changing circumstances according to Bandura. This stage of the framework uses the concepts on personal choice and self-awareness as its basis. Determining these aspects is done during the assessment process. Perceptual norms are guided by evaluative norms as indicated by the Epistemic, Deontic and Axiological (EDA) model. How an individual perceives an environment or object determines how they describe it, i.e. what signs they attach to the object as shown in Figure 5. Epistemic norms relate to beliefs and justification, axiological norms determine value and deontic norms, which relate to the disposition to act as shown in Figure 5 and an example applying the EDA model is given in Table 5. The framework diagram is given in Figure 6. The contributions of the NHTF are:

- Identifying and collectively defining the care objectives. This would minimise misunderstanding and manage expectations.
- Applying the identified social aspects in the telecare solution design. This leads to an acceptable solution and improved quality of service.
- Correctly configured devices would increase the safety of the users.
- Caring for people at home would reduce visits to the hospital and reduce the risk of further infection.
- The reduced number of hospitalized patients would reduce the pressure on clinicians, which would translate in fewer clinical errors and increase in patient safety.

Care needs can be satisfied at different levels of intensity and within different contexts. Some needs are satisfied in regard to the individual's inner world (Eigenwelt), while others can be satisfied with regards to a social group or what surrounds the individual (Mitwelt) and still others are best satisfied within the influence of the broader environment (Umwelt) (Max-Neef 1992). A better understanding of what influences the individual to

Table 5. Example to show the application of EDA model

Norm Type	Application Example
Epistemic: To adopt a degree of belief or disbelief	The user requested a pill dispenser that would remind him of medication time because he believed he needed it
Axiological: To be disposed in favour or against something in value terms	The assessor inquired if the user had ever been diagnosed of memory problems. The user said he had not. The assessor then told the user he would not be provided the discounted price. He asked for the full price and was given and he immediately said he did not have the money and would have to leave it.
Deontic: To be disposed to act in some way	The user said he will settle for a blister pack which had days of the week marked and medication separated into morning afternoon and evening medication because he could not afford the dispenser

Figure 5. Compiling user care profile and norms applied

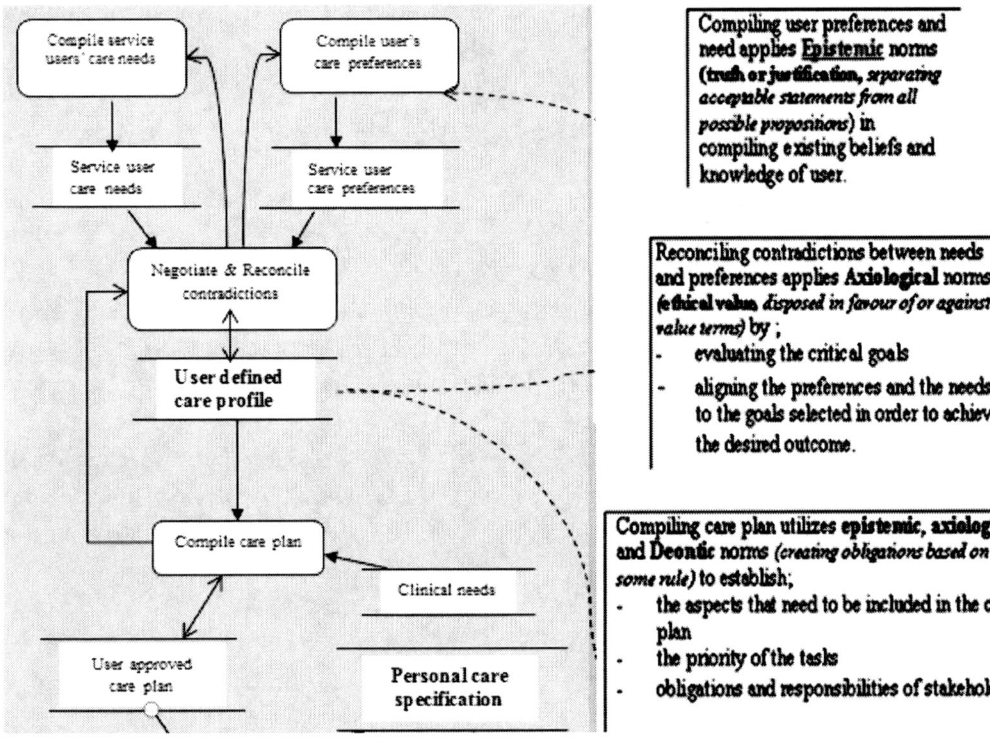

act or make certain decisions can provide a basis of prediction of future behaviour. Therefore the quality and intensity of the satisfier or preference will depend on the context and circumstances of the particular user. The ranking of the preferred care methods helps to remind the stakeholders that there is more than one way of satisfying a need.

5.3 Raising Telecare Quality and User Safety Using the Framework

Two aspects of the framework improve the quality and safety of telecare service. These are the participation of the user at all the stages of solution design and the configuration of the devices with user preferences. To deal with the ambiguity of social aspects, the framework applies norm analysis to structure the identified social aspects in a way that enables them to be applied into a solution. In the second stage of the framework the care plan is a communication tool which at best shows how tasks are to be performed and by whom. Norm analysis is applied to care tasks to show under which conditions the activities are performed. The norms that emerge are not norms in the same sense of what is actually taking place but are a proposal for the future action based on the verbalised user preferences. They will be referred to in this research as design norms to differentiate them from the current norms as they have not been tested but are a highly probable way of future system behaviour.

6. FRAMEWORK VALIDATION

Validity checks aim to determine whether the research or design artefact produces what it is intended to produce.(Golafshani 2003). Telecare managers, assessors, social workers, occupational therapists, researchers, heads of academic departments, supervisors and team leaders took part in

Figure 6. A normative home telecare framework

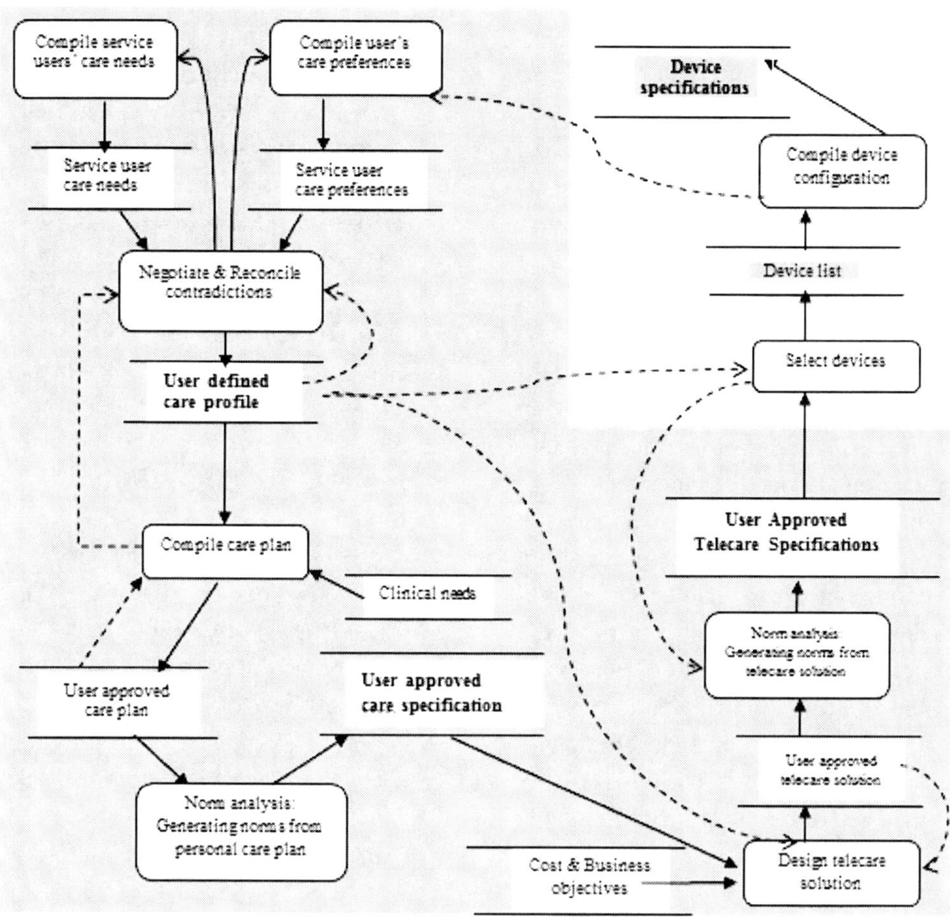

Table 6. Validation objectives and tools applied in validation

Validation Objective	Questions to be Answered	Participants	Tools Applied
Validating framework design & structure	a. Are the components selected for the framework relevant? b. Are the components logically arranged to enable achievement of the intended results? c. Is there consistency between and within the components?	**Telecare experts** People with high degree of knowledge and experience in design and implementation from academic, telecare and related fields	Delphi study questionnaires Follow-up interviews
Validating framework usefulness	a. Whether the underlying concept of identifying and applying user preferences would contribute to improved telecare acceptance b. Whether user participation in solution design would improve telecare acceptance c. Whether service providers would be able to implement the proposed framework	**Telecare assessors** People who were actively involved with assessing of prospective users and dealing with user issues	Questionnaire Follow-up interviews

the validation exercise. They came from England, Wales, Scotland and British Columbia in Canada. Their experience with telecare ranged from assessing prospective users, managing telecare departments, setting policy, researching in and evaluating telecare and related projects (Table 6).

Structural effectiveness validation was approached from the point of determining whether the individual components of the construct are contributing to designing a user centred solution by applying the social aspects of each user efficiently. Efficiency of design here refers to telecare solutions that have acceptable performance and are designed with less cost and in less time. Structure validation checks that the arrangement of components in the framework is logical and leads to the attainment of the set objectives and that there is enough inputs to enable the required deliverables. Usefulness of the components in the framework is validated by whether the framework deliverable, the solution, contributes to the aim of improving quality and acceptance of telecare in a visible way. The second issue in usefulness validation was whether the framework helps the service providers to design better solutions. It was therefore important to determine the opinion of participants on how practical the framework is. If the structural and usefulness aspects are validated then usefulness of the framework was validated. Table 6 shows the validation objectives and the tools applied.

6.1 Structural Validation

1. **Objective 1a:** According to the people who participated, the proposed framework is built from useful components. The degree of confidence that stakeholders have on these components may be a subject for further research.

2. **Objective 1b:** On whether the arrangement of the components is logical, the response to this question was that the components are logically arranged with responses like "the

solution appears logical and easy to follow" "Yes, it appears the framework does a good job of taking into account a variety of inputs and rationalising them".

3. **Objective 1c:** On whether there is internal consistency in the framework, the responses indicated that the inputs and outputs of the components are useful and are utilised in the solution design. Examples of answers are "With the right questions a useful profile can be obtained" and "The care plan is an important document which is used for reviews like the annual review".

6.2 Usefulness Validation

- **Objective 2a:** The question was whether the concepts applied in the framework are relevant to improving telecare acceptance. Some of the comments that were received were "Gathering user requirements is important in the application and development of assistive technologies", "They increase the level of acceptability and usability in the home environment" and "Anything that includes the user in design stands a better chance of being acceptable". Identifying, capturing and structuring of social aspects are important to raise the quality of service and mitigate safety issues in the operation of devices.

- **Objective 2b:** On whether the framework provides the intended improved, comments like "I do believe that if people are engaged in giving their opinions on individual needs and goals they are more invested in the outcomes and more accepting of services" were received from experts. The reasons the assessors gave for saying the framework would increase acceptance were;
  - It instils user confidence on solutions
  - It helps users take ownership of devices

- ○ Users would feel the solutions are not imposed
- ○ Users would feel in control of what is taking place about their care
- ○ It would keep costs down as devices are linked to user needs
- ○ It will save time for those responding to alarms because there are less false alarms

These opinions give confidence in the design. It is the conclusion from the validation participants that the framework can contribute to the improvement of telecare acceptance.

- **Objective 2c:** On whether it is feasible to implement the Normative Home Telecare Framework, the research established that it is feasible. The responses from both the Delphi study and the assessors' questionnaire showed that those that responded are of the opinion that service providers, which were represented by the various assessors, would be able to apply the framework if it was adopted. There were some who had comments on the competence of assessors and some who indicated that they might need to see the actual assessment form compiled using the framework. Those who were very positive provided comments like "Yes, I believe it is simple enough to follow and takes a number of things into consideration". This indicates that the framework is a solid construct and can be applied to many types of cases although there might be a need to customise the framework in some.

7. CONCLUSION

Service outcomes in telecare are based on individual cases and particularly user experience from both clinical and a social point of view.

For each case there needs to be agreed service objectives that are understood and agreed by all stakeholders involved. Introducing technology in socially dominated environments introduces typical services errors in the home and at the same time introduces unfamiliar errors, which are related to the systems and technology applied. In the majority of cases stakeholders are acquiring new knowledge be it on the expectations of the user, the capabilities of the service provider or the functional boundaries of the devices. The increase in the application of telecare solutions has seen design methods that are inconsistent and different from provider to provider. In current applications the role of the user is trivialised and telecare solution design becomes a mechanical process driven by the technology push. Best practice and benchmarking becomes difficult because of the disparate methods of design. This calls for a new approach in the provision of telecare hence the guideline proposed.

The proposed Normative Home Telecare Framework offers a guide on which telecare solution design can be based and therefore provides a means of identifying similar quality and patient safety metrics. A user centred approach is proposed. Solutions can only be made richer by a cooperative approach that helps to understand user and provider related aspects of the service. Social constructivism is applied to manage the expectations from the user and from the provider side. Improved commitment to the success of the service is achieved willingly from the user by abandoning the prescriptive approach to system design. This sharing of knowledge improves understanding by the user, which improves user experience and raises satisfaction. This improved user experience raises the quality of service.

There is evidence that contextual factors can be linked to positive outcomes of patient safety, reduction of medication errors, reduction of hospital admission rates, reduction of falls and health care associated infections (RCN 2009). Defining safety aspects in the home will always include a contextual element and the best way to agree on the meaning to adopt is by cooperative design approach. Quality has to be related to user experience and user experience is related to user expectation. The public interest in care quality and the desire by professionals to demonstrate quality lead to an interest in identifying the aspects to monitor and measure. To have consistency in the monitoring and measuring of quality metrics there is need to have a shared understanding of the issues and the terms applied to them. Terms like benchmarking need to have an agreed standard in order to compare performance between similar systems, which is the reason a guideline to designing telecare solutions is proposed in the form of a normative framework.

Social aspects are by nature ambiguous and dynamic. They are influenced by the culture, community and individual values and therefore differ between communities and individuals. The framework provides method of structuring the captured social aspects and applying them to the solutions. An improved understanding of the objectives and provider capabilities will reduce service errors. Norm analysis provides a much-needed link between the technical objectives and the social objectives. Furthermore the framework provides a means by which those structured norms can be configured on the selected devices so that the solution behaviour mirrors the user expectations.

REFERENCES

Baek, E.-O., & Cagiltay, K. et al. (2008). User centred design and development. In *Handbook of research on educational communication and technology* (3rd ed.). New York: Taylor & Francis Group, LLC.

Bandura, A. (1982). Self efficacy mechanism in human agency. *The American Psychologist, 37*(2), 122–147. doi:10.1037/0003-066X.37.2.122

Barlow, J., & Bayer, S. et al. (2006). Implementing complex innovations in fluid multi-stakeholder environments: Experiences of telecare. *Technovation, 26*(3), 396–406. doi:10.1016/j.technovation.2005.06.010

Baxter, G., & Monk, A. (2006). A technique for client-centred evaluation of electronic assistive technology. *Contemporary Ergonomics*, 236-240.

BC-Government. (2004). *Prevention of falls and injuries among the elderly. M. O. Health. B C Canada.* B C Government.

Brook, R. H., McGlynn, et al. (2000). Defining and measuring quality of care: A perspective from US researchers. *International Journal for Quality in Health Care, 12*(4), 281–295. doi:10.1093/intqhc/12.4.281 PMID:10985266

Campbell, S., Roland, et al. (2000). Defining quality of care. *Social Science & Medicine, 51*(11). doi:10.1016/S0277-9536(00)00057-5 PMID:11072882

Chan, M., Esteve, et al. (2008). A review of smart homes - Present state and future challenges. *Computer Methods and Programs in Biomedicine, 91*(1), 55–81. doi:10.1016/j.cmpb.2008.02.001 PMID:18367286

Chaplin, M., & Bucke. (1990). *What are biosensors: Enzyme technology.* Cambridge, UK: Cambridge University Press.

Chidzambwa, L. (2013). The social considerations for moving health services into the home: A telecare perspective. *Health Policy and Technology, 2*(1), 10–25. doi:10.1016/j.hlpt.2012.12.003

Clark, M., & Goodwin, N. (2010). *Sustaining innovation in telehealth and telecare.* WSD Action Network.

Crabtree, A. (2003). *Designing collaborative systems: A practical guide to ethnography.* Berlin: Springer.

Dewsbury, G. (2001). The social psychological aspects of smart home technology within the care sector. *New Technology in Human Services, 14*(1), 9–17.

DoH, U. G. (2011). *Whole system demonstrator programme: Headline findings.* London: D. o. Health.

Donabedian, A. (1997). The quality of care How can it be assessed. *Archives of Pathology & Laboratory Medicine, 121*(11), 1145. PMID:9372740

Edge, M., Taylor, et al. (2000). The potential for 'smart home' systems in meeting the care needs of older persons and people with diabilities. *Seniors Housing Updates, 2.*

Golafshani, H. (2003). Understanding reliability and validity in qualitative research. *Qualitative Report, 8*(4), 597–607.

Hanson, J. Percival, et al. (2007). Attitudes to telecare among older people, professional care workers and onformal carers: A preventive strategy or crisis management. Universal Access in the Information Society, 6(2).

Jackson, P., & Klobas, J. (2001). Assessing your organisation's knowledge management health. In *Proceedings of 9th Specials, Health and Law Libraries Conference.* Australian Library and Information Association.

Kane, R. (2001). Long term care and a good quality of life: Bringing them together. *The Gerontologist, 41*(3), 293–304. doi:10.1093/geront/41.3.293 PMID:11405425

Klockner, C. A., & Matthies, E. (2004). How habits interfere with norm-directed behaviour: A normative decision-making model for travel mode choice. *Journal of Environmental Psychology, 24,* 319–327. doi:10.1016/j.jenvp.2004.08.004

Koch, S. (2006). Home telehealth - Current state and future trends. *International Journal of Medical Informatics, 7*(8), 565–576. doi:10.1016/j.ijmedinf.2005.09.002 PMID:16298545

Lang, A., Edwards, et al. (2007). Safety in home care: A broadened perspective of patient safety. *International Journal for Quality in Health Care, 20*(2), 130–135. doi:10.1093/intqhc/mzm068 PMID:18158294

Lawson, S., & Nutter, D. (2008). *Technology to support ageing in place: Meeting the challenges of an ageing society.* SPARC.

Liu, K. (2000). *Semiotics in information systems engineering.* Cambridge, UK: Cambridge University Press. doi:10.1017/CBO9780511543364

Lords, H. o. S. C. o. S. a. T. (2005). *The environmental challenge and assistive technology.* London: H. o. Lords.

Mattke, S. Klautzer, et al. (2010). Health and wellbeing in the home. The RAND Corporation.

Max-Neef, M. (1992). *Development and human needs.* Retrieved 16/09/2011, 2011, from http://208.106.164.92/general/resources/2007-Manfred-Max-Neef-Fundamental-Human-Needs.pdf

McGee-Lennon, M. R., & Gray, P. D. (2007). Including stakeholders in the design of home care systems: Identification and categorisation of complex user requirements. Paper presented atINCLUDE 2007 - Designing with People. London, UK.

Percival, J., & Hanson, J. (2006). Big brother or brave new world? Telecare and its implications for older people's independence and social inclusion. *Critical Social Policy, 26*(24), 888–909. doi:10.1177/0261018306068480

Perry, J. Beyer, et al. (2010). Ethical issues in the use of telecare: Adult services report. London: Social Care Institute for Excellence.

Perry, J., & Beyer, S. (2010). *Ethical issues in the use of telecare*. London: Social Care Institute for Excellence.

Porteous, J., & Brownsell, S. J. (2000). *Using telecare: Exploring technologies for independent living for older people*. London: Anchor Trust.

RCN. (2009). *Measuring for quality in health and social care: An RCN position statement*. London: Royal College of Nursing.

Salter, A., & Liu, K. (2002). *Using semantic analysis and norm analysis to model organisations*. ICEIS.

Schwartz, S. H., & Fleishman, J. A. (1978). Personal norms and the mediation of legitimacy effects on helping. *Social Psychology*, *41*(4), 306–315. doi:10.2307/3033583

Sethi, R. Azzi, et al. (2011). *Trend and issues in community telecare in the United Kingdom*. Paper presented at the IET Conference on Assisted Living. London, UK.

Sethi, R., & Khusainov, R. (2012). *Trends and issues in community telecare in the United Kingdom*. Academic Press.

Stockdale, R., & Standing, C. (2006). An interpretive approach to evaluating information systems: A content, context, process framework. *European Journal of Operational Research*, *173*(3), 1090–1102. doi:10.1016/j.ejor.2005.07.006

Tolmie, P. Pycock, et al. (2002). Unremarkable computing. In *Proceedings of the 2002 CHI Conference on Human Factors in Computing Systems*. ACM.

UN. D. o. E. a. S. A. P. D. (2009). World population ageing. New York: United Nations.

von Niman, B. Rodriguez-Ascaso, et al. (2006). User experience design guidelines for telecare services. In *Proceedings of the 8th Conference on Human-Computer Interaction with Mobile Devices and Services*. Helsinki, Finland: ACM.

Walshman, G. (1995). Interpretive case studies in IS research: Nature and method. *European Journal of Information Systems*, *4*(2), 74–81. doi:10.1057/ejis.1995.9

Wenzel, M. (2002). *The social side of sanctions - Personal and social norms as moderators of deterrence* (Working Paper 34). Australian National University.

Whitworth, B., & de Moor, A. (2003). Legitimate by design: Towards trusted socio-technical systems. *Behaviour & Information Technology*, *22*(1), 31–51. doi:10.1080/01449290301783

Chapter 54

A Case for Enterprise Interoperability in Healthcare IT:
Personal Health Record Systems

Mustafa Yuksel
Software Research Development and Consultancy Ltd. (SRDC), Turkey & Middle East Technical University (METU), Turkey

Asuman Dogac
Software Research Development and Consultancy Ltd. (SRDC), Turkey

Cebrail Taskin
Argela Software and Informatics Technologies, Turkey

Anil Yalcinkaya
Argela Software and Informatics Technologies, Turkey

ABSTRACT

The PHR systems need to be integrated with a wide variety of healthcare IT systems including EHRs, electronic medical devices, and clinical decision support services to get their full benefit. It is not possible to sustain the integration of PHRs with other healthcare IT systems in a proprietary way; this integration has to be achieved by exploiting the promising interoperability standards and profiles. This chapter provides a survey and analysis of the interoperability standards and profiles that can be used to integrate PHRs with a variety of healthcare applications and medical data resources, including EHR systems to enable access of a patient to his own medical data generated by healthcare professionals; personal medical devices to obtain the patient's instant physiological status; and the clinical decision support services for patient-physician shared decision making.

INTRODUCTION

The Personal Health Record (PHR) systems have evolved from Web pages where patients entered their own data manually to the systems giving patients access to their electronic health records (EHRs) from a healthcare provider. The latter is called a provider-tethered PHR system, and the data from a healthcare provider's information system such as an EHR or a laboratory system is entered into the PHRs automatically via the data exchange interfaces established among these systems. There are also employer/payer portals providing patients access to claims data and more

DOI: 10.4018/978-1-4666-8756-1.ch054

recently third party PHR systems such as Microsoft HealthVault (http://www.healthvault.com) that provides a secure storage for PHR data together with data exchange interfaces so that third parties can develop applications to upload patient data from a specific system or source, for example, home health devices.

The intent of all of these systems is to give patients better access to their own healthcare data (Halamka et al., 2008). The PHR is defined as "a tool for collecting, tracking and sharing important, up-to-date information about an individual's health or the health of someone in their care" (American Health Information Management Association et al., 2007, p. 1). It typically contains information about an individual's diagnoses, medications, allergies, procedures, lab test results, immunization records and other personal health information. Many PHR systems also provide linkages to convenience tools such as requesting appointments, requesting prescription renewals, asking billing questions and communication tools to assist the patient in connecting with various healthcare professionals.

However, currently all this integration is achieved mostly in a proprietary way and in a fragmented fashion rather than using the standard interfaces. A recent survey investigating the major 48 PHR systems on the market discovered that almost none of the PHRs use existing medical standards for the storage and communication of their data (Helmer et al., 2011). Given the existing semantic and technical diversity of eHealth platforms, each integration effort with a new system will be an expensive process unless standard interfaces are used for data exchange.

In this chapter, we present a survey and analysis of interoperability standards to connect the PHR systems to healthcare applications and medical data resources including EHR systems, personal medical devices and clinical decision support services. Some of these standards are specifically developed for the PHR systems; some are general

standards that can also be used in the PHR systems. Additionally, because PHR systems contain a summary of EHR data, some EHR standards directly apply. For the sake of completeness, we present an analysis of all these standards as they apply to the PHR systems.

The chapter is organized as follows: A motivating example based on a visionary scenario is presented in the next section. Then, a classification of the PHR interoperability standards is provided, which is followed by a section on the EHR-PHR interoperability content standards and profiles. The succeeding section classifies the terminology systems based on the underlying structure and the knowledge representation formalism which determine the way they express the semantics and hence help with the interoperability. After that, the medical device interoperability standards and profiles for importing medical device data to patient's PHR are introduced. The standards relevant for clinical decision support services are covered in another section. Finally, the last section concludes the chapter.

A MOTIVATING EXAMPLE

Mr. Smith visits his general practitioner (GP) with the symptoms of pain in his joints. The results of laboratory tests as well as radiographs indicate rheumatoid arthritis with high risk of damage in the joints. The GP refers the patient to a rheumatologist in the local hospital.

The local hospital that Mr. Smith is referred to has a care management system for rheumatoid arthritis, which provides a care plan for shared decision making between the physician and the patient to help them monitor the progress jointly. The care plan is a workflow based on "National clinical guideline for management and treatment of rheumatoid arthritis in adults," and it is processed and visualized through a clinical decision support service.

Mr. Smith decides to enroll in this program, and a care plan is created for him using this guideline, which specifies all the decision, action, branch and synchronization steps including medical tests, medications, home monitoring and follow-up appointments recommended for the care of his condition. To execute these steps, the care management workflow needs to retrieve data from the Electronic Medical Record (EMR) system at the GP's office; the Electronic Health Record (EHR) system at the hospital; the Laboratory Information System (LIS) at the local lab, and from the PHR of the patient. Fortunately for Mr. Smith, his PHR system provides a single point of access and control to all this information because it is interoperable with all the mentioned systems based on relevant standards. Additionally, the consent management mechanism of the PHR controls access to this data according to his privacy consent.

The rheumatologist goes over the steps of the care plan and describes them to Mr. Smith. He also wants Mr. Smith to record the symptoms and signs of the disease, his emotional state and side effects of the medications to his PHR.

At his next appointment with the GP, standard physical exam reveals that Mr. Smith suffers from hypertension, which is the side effect of his arthritis medication. For hypertension control, the GP recommends him benazepril. The PHR system of Mr. Smith has standard interfaces to external decision support services, one of which checks drug-to-drug interactions. When this medication record appears in his PHR, the drug-to-drug interaction checker recommends medication replacement because his current drug for rheumatoid arthritis, namely ibuprofen, might decrease the antihypertensive efficacy of benazepril. The rheumatologist replaces the drug and recommends blood pressure measurements to Mr. Smith four times daily. The PHR system uses standard interfaces for importing medical device data and therefore the off-the-shelf blood pressure device he purchases is capable of automatically uploading his measurements to his PHR so that both the patient himself and the GP can follow the results.

The GP monitors remotely both the progress of the care plan, the measurements provided by the medical device and status updates provided by Mr. Smith, and confirms that everything is under control. He motivates Mr. Smith through the instant messaging service of the PHR for his continuous dedication to the care plan, and notifies him for his next regular appointment.

CLASSIFICATION OF THE INTEROPERABILITY STANDARDS FOR THE PHR SYSTEMS

PHRs are not only electronic repositories of health information controlled or accessed by patients. They are also integrated with a wide variety of healthcare information technology systems. Therefore, the interoperability standards for the PHR systems can be categorized according to the systems they are communicating with:

- Electronic Health Record standards,
- Personal Medical Device standards, and
- Clinical Decision Support Service (CDSS) standards.

It should be noted that the interoperability of IT systems can be assessed on different layers, from the lowest physical layer in the ISO/OSI model to the behavior of the system as perceived by the end users. It is feasible to organize these into three major layers in the case of interoperability of healthcare IT systems: the communication layer, the content layer and the business process layer. The communication layer covers the messaging specifications that are built on top of the application layer of the ISO/OSI model or the TCP/IP model, such as HL7 SOAP Web Services Profile; or rarely some lower layers such as the OSI session layer in the case of HL7 Minimal Lower Layer Protocol (MLLP). The content layer involves the format of the exchanged clinical messages and documents as well as their semantics expressed through the clinical terminology systems used. The business process layer involves the choreography of the interactions among the healthcare IT systems, by defining high-level transactions and then binding them to specific standards from the communication layer and content models from the content layer.

This article focuses mainly on the standards in the content layer. It also covers the profiling approach that corresponds to the business process layer as described above. The communication layer is not directly within the scope of the article, as it is built on top of very well known standards such as Web services and used similarly in other domains. However, relevant healthcare communication standards are referred within interoperability profiles.

Enterprise Interoperability Perspective

Building on the well-established state of the art, the interoperability layers are specified as legal, organizational, semantic and technical interoperability within the European Interoperability Framework (EIF) (European Commission, 2004). This classification is adopted by several initiatives including the European Interoperability Architecture (EIA), which explores the need for a European interoperability architecture facilitating the establishment of European public services (Van Langenhove et al., 2011). Although interoperability in PHR systems covers all four layers of enterprise interoperability, this chapter focuses specifically on two layers: technical and semantic interoperability.

In parallel with this layered approach, in order to identify a proper structure dedicated to enterprise interoperability, the ENSEMBLE project (Envisioning, Supporting and Promoting Future Internet Enterprise Systems Research through Scientific Collaboration) has formulated 12 scientific areas of enterprise interoperability in 4 granularity levels by analyzing the technological trends and the background knowledge (Pop-

plewell et al., 2012). Among the 6 fundamental scientific areas that constitute the 1st granularity level, the interoperability standards and profiles presented in this chapter address directly all but one; i.e. data, process, rules, objects and software interoperability are covered, but cultural interoperability is not. Most of the remaining areas in other granularity levels (e.g. eID interoperability at 2nd level or cloud interoperability at 3rd level) are not addressed directly but since these levels are derived by iterative combination of core scientific areas at the 1st level, they are addressed indirectly.

As a highly interdisciplinary domain, interoperability in PHR systems affects and is affected by a number of neighboring scientific domains. Inspired by the needs of enterprise interoperability and several state of the art classification structures, the ENSEMBLE project provides a reusable classification of the scientific domains, which is termed as Enterprise Interoperability Science Base - Scientific Domain Reference Taxonomy (EISB-SDRT). Social sciences, applied sciences and formal sciences are recognized in the three-level general classification of this taxonomy. Within the social sciences category, we have identified sociology, economics and political science as the neighboring scientific domains since management of healthcare data by the patients themselves as the true owners of their data has social and legal aspects, as well as financial implications such as reducing costs by reducing the number of unnecessary physical patient visits through remote monitoring and communication. Among the main scientific domains within the applied sciences, medicine and engineering are directly involved in establishing interoperability in PHR systems. Finally, a majority of the scientific areas within the formal sciences category as the fundamentals of enterprise interoperability are again neighboring domains of interoperability in PHR systems. These can be listed as mathematics (logic especially for semantic interoperability), computer science (almost all sub-domains like data structures, software engineering, information theory) and other interdisciplinary sciences (systems, network, Web,...). Since our work in this chapter focuses on technical and semantic interoperability layers, following sections detail the interoperability problems by considering the neighboring scientific domains within applied and formal sciences categories.

In order to address the semantic and technical interoperability problems in establishing interoperability among PHR systems and several other healthcare information technology systems by making use of reusable patterns, we prioritize the work done by following the profiling approach. Profiling starts with analyzing the required use cases in a specific domain. As the next step, the actors, transactions among them and the requirements of these transactions are identified in detail. Finally, instead of developing technical data exchange specifications from scratch, the identified technology independent transactions are bound to the most appropriate state of the art interoperability standards, which are further refined or extended when necessary. It is also possible to switch technology bindings of or provide several technology bindings to these technology independent transactions. The profiling approach is widely used by Integrating the Healthcare Enterprise (IHE) initiative (http://www.ihe.net/), several interoperability profiles of which are presented in the following sections. The profiling approach is also totally in line with the European Interoperability Architecture guidelines of the European Commission.

PHR-EHR INTEROPERABILITY STANDARDS

PHR/EHR Content Standards

Electronic Health Record (EHR) is defined as "digitally stored health care information about an individual's lifetime with the purpose of supporting continuity of care, education and research,

and ensuring confidentiality at all times" (Iakovidis, 1998). EHR data is stored in a multitude of medical information systems, which are used by health professionals but not directly accessible by the patients. A PHR contains the summary of the patient's EHR data. Therefore PHR content standards, just like EHR content standards (Eichelberg et al., 2005), define document structures consisting of document components such as sections, entries and data elements and are in fact based on the EHR content standards most of the time.

One of the most widely used standards that define PHR summary data is the E2369-05 Standard Specification for Continuity of Care Record (CCR) (ASTM International, 2005) by the American Society for Testing and Materials (ASTM) International. CCR defines a core data set for the most relevant administrative, demographic, and clinical information facts about a patient's healthcare, covering one or more healthcare encounters. It contains various sections such as patient demographics, insurance information, diagnosis and problem list, medications, allergies and care plan. CCR specification has its own XML schema definition; but it is also used in constraining other EHR content standards to obtain PHR/EHR content templates.

Generic EHR content standards that can also be used for EHR-PHR interoperability include HL7 Clinical Document Architecture, Release 2 (CDA) (Health Level Seven, 2005), ISO/CEN 13606-1: Reference Model (International Organization for Standardization et al., 2008) and openEHR (The openEHR Foundation, 2006). Unlike CCR, all these standards define quite generic structures such as folder, section, entry, observation and substance administration that can be used to represent any kind of clinical statement. The specialization of these generic structures is done by refining their semantics through the use of coded terms and/or free text explanations. For example, a 13606-1 section can be declared to be an allergies section by setting its name (free text) and meaning (coded value) attributes accordingly.

Formal expressions of such specializations result in content templates as explained in *PHR/EHR Content Templates* Section.

Another PHR content standard is the HealthVault Thing Types that are defined by Microsoft. Instead of using the existing content standards, Microsoft preferred defining a simple proprietary XML syntax for each possible clinical statement (e.g. blood glucose measurement, body dimension, insulin injection, etc.). Yet, the underlying information model of these Thing Types is compatible with the data types and structures of the well-known standards such as CCR and CDA which facilitates the interchange of clinical data complying with these standards in HealthVault.

Analysis of PHR/EHR Content Standards

All PHR/EHR content standards serve similar purposes, that is, consistent and machine processable representation of healthcare information. The main distinguishing property among various content standards is the specificity (expressivity) of the underlying information model; that is, how generic or specific their schemas are (Table 1).

ISO/CEN 13606 and openEHR provide the most generic schema. It is possible to represent any kind of clinical statement with the combination of just three classes, namely Entry, Cluster and Element. HL7 CDA R2, on the other hand, has multiple structures each specialized for a group of medical activities; hence it has a more specialized schema. It has nine entry classes derived from the HL7 v3 Reference Information

Model (RIM) (Health Level Seven, 2010c), such as Act, Observation, SubstanceAdministration and Encounter. It is possible to classify ASTM CCR schema similarly with CDA. Some CCR classes like Immunization, Plan and Alert are more specific than CDA classes but still, there are no dedicated structures for representing individual medical events such as blood pressure or insulin injection, which are provided by HealthVault.

The advantage of a specialized schema such as HealthVault is that it is self-explanatory and easy to implement at first. However, in the long run, they might create maintenance issues for the implementers because each time the information model of a dedicated clinical event is modified or a new one is created, the syntax completely changes as well. Consider for instance, a Web service endpoint that accepts HL7 CDA R2 documents; this single endpoint can accept any CDA document, perform XSD validation on it, and then invoke the corresponding validation procedure according to the content, actually according to the content template (*PHR/EHR Content Templates* Section). When there is a change in the content template, the endpoint stays the same and the validation rules are modified. This is not easily achievable with specialized schemas.

The disadvantage of the generic and semi-generic schemas is that the footprint of clinical documents can become quite large. There can be many repeating constructs and attributes for representing a very simple medical event, especially with fully generic schemas. Therefore, it is better to have at least some common structures for modeling a group of medical activities, as in the case of CDA. Even with CDA, the experience shows that it is not easy to deal with tens of attributes just for modeling a diagnosis with an ICD-10 code for instance. In order to overcome these issues, recently greenCDA (Health Level Seven, 2011a) has been proposed by the HL7 CDA community. greenCDA is the strategy of hiding certain CDA complexities such as fixed attributes (e.g. classCode, moodCode) and generic XML tags

Table 1. Comparison of PHR/EHR content schema expressivities

Totally Generic Schema	Semi-Generic Schema	Specialized Schema
ISO/CEN 13606, openEHR	HL7 CDA R2, ASTM CCR	HealthVault Thing Types

by introducing an intermediary XML schema with clinically meaningful XML element and attribute names, such as resultId, procedureType and problemCode. This intermediary schema is supported with transformation rules expressed in XSLT to automatically convert greenCDA instances to valid CDA instances. It is more meaningful to implement greenCDA together with content templates such as Continuity of Care Document (CCD) and Patient Care Coordination (PCC) templates (*PHR/EHR Content Templates* Section). The first release of greenCDA implementation guide by HL7 provides an intermediary greenCDA schema conforming to Health Information Technology Standards Panel (HITSP) C32/C83 content modules (Healthcare Information Technology Standards Panel, 2009) and generating CDA instances through transformation that comply with the corresponding CCD templates.

Finally regarding the analysis of existing PHR/EHR content standards, in order to foster unique representation and hence interoperability, there has to be a normative computer processable schema of a content standard. To remain technology independent, ISO/CEN states that compliance to 13606 standard is achieved by implementing the 13606 UML model. However, because XML is the de facto data exchange standard, it would be good to have a normative XML Implementation Technology Specification of the 13606 UML model. In this way, when two 13606 implementing systems need to interoperate, the implementers can directly skip interoperability at the syntactic level and concentrate on the actual clinical content. It should be noted that, although it is not official, there is an XML schema of ISO/CEN 13606 for the last three years, maintained by the EN 13606 Association (2010).

PHR/EHR Content Templates

The content templates are built on top of the well-accepted content standards to further refine these standards by:

- Restricting the alternative hierarchical structures to be used within the instances,
- Constraining optionality and cardinality of some elements,
- Defining the code systems and codes used to classify parts of the content, and also
- Describing the specific data elements that are included.

One of the most prominent PHR content templates, namely Continuity of Care Document (CCD) (Health Level Seven, 2008) is defined by constraining an EHR content markup standard, namely, HL7 Clinical Document Architecture, Release 2 (CDA) with requirements set forward in ASTM CCR. CCD defines a single document template, but there are several section templates and clinical statement templates to be used within this main document template. IHE Patient Care Coordination (PCC) Technical Framework further details and multiplies the CCD templates at the document, section and clinical statement levels according to the content module requirements of its integration profiles such as Exchange of Personal Health Record Content (XPHR) (Integrating the Healthcare Enterprise, 2010d) and Query for Existing Data (QED) (Integrating the Healthcare Enterprise, 2008b). For example, currently PCC has six main document templates (Discharge Summary, Medical Document, Medical Summary, PHR Extract, PHR Update, Scanned Document) in comparison to the single CCD document template. Similarly, HITSP has defined CDA content modules that reuse and further restrict the IHE PCC templates and the underlying CCD templates according to the requirements in the US (Healthcare Information Technology Standards Panel, 2010). In December 2011, within the US Office of the National Coordinator's (ONC) Standards and Interoperability (S&I) Framework, through the joint efforts of HL7, IHE, ONC and the Health Story Project (2011), the Consolidated CDA Templates guide was released as the single source incorporating and harmonizing CDA templates from CCD,

PCC, HITSP C32, HL7 Health Story guides and Stage 1 Meaningful Use. Consolidated CDA is by far the most comprehensive and complete single source library of CDA templates, which makes it very valuable for CDA implementers all over the world.

As a result, although the CCR specification itself defines an XML schema as a content template for the exchange purposes, the HL7 CDA implementation of CCR, that is the HL7/ASTM CCD, and the other templates building on top of the CCD, are more widely-accepted than CCR's own XML schema.

In all CDA based templates, the most common way of formally expressing the constraints defined in templates and checking these constraints on clinical document instances is to create machine processable versions of templates as schematron rules, which then can be executed on the instances and present validation results automatically. Recently, model based validators that are implemented with Model Driven Health Tools (MDHT) (https://mdht.projects.openhealthtools. org/) have become popular as well. In MDHT, the validation rules are executed as Java and Object Constraint Language (OCL) code generated from the UML models.

ISO/CEN 13606 and openEHR adopt the concept of archetype, which is a computable expression of a domain level concept (e.g. blood pressure, physical examination or laboratory result) in the form of structured constraint statements, based on a reference information model (Beale et al., 2007). Hence, openEHR archetypes are based on the openEHR reference model, and 13606 archetypes are based on the 13606 reference model (i.e. 13606-1). It should be noted that the term "template" in openEHR has a more specific meaning than its generic usage in the HL7 and IHE domains; it corresponds to a directly usable definition that composes archetypes into larger structures such as a screen form, document or report. It can be said that clinical statement templates and section templates of ASTM/HL7, IHE and HITSP correspond to archetypes of ISO/CEN and openEHR; while document templates in the former correspond to templates in the latter. Both 13606 and openEHR use the ISO/CEN standardised Archetype Definition Language (expressed in ADL syntax or its XML equivalent) to formally define archetypes. openEHR also maintains the openEHR Clinical Knowledge Manager (CKM) (http://www. openehr.org/knowledge/) as a collaborative environment to build and host archetypes, templates and termsets. CKM is a valuable repository not only for openEHR and 13606 implementers, but for all; since it serves hundreds of archetypes in various representations (tabular, mindmap, ADL and XML) and languages, and all these archetypes are a result of harmonization of contributions from healthcare professionals all around the world.

Finally, HealthVault Thing Types can be considered as content templates as well, since they are specific to domain level concepts as in the case of CDA based templates and openEHR archetypes.

Analysis of PHR/EHR Content Templates

Content standards are not enough for interoperability because there can be many different ways of organizing the same clinical information even when the same PHR/EHR content standard is used: the same information can be expressed through different components and these components can be nested differently. Therefore, the templates/ archetypes are necessary to constrain the structure and format of generic PHR/EHR content standards. There is already much effort in defining content templates on top of content standards as explained in the previous section.

However, overlapping terminology systems as well as the structural differences in document templates create semantic interoperability problems in content templates which can be categorized as follows:

- Different terminology systems used by different healthcare applications in the same compositional structure within the same document template; and
- Different compositional structures within the same document template that express the same meaning differently.

As an example, consider the glucose measurement representations in HL7/ASTM CCD given in Figure 1. In this figure, there are two instances of the "CCD result organizer" template for reporting 104 mg/dL glucose in the plasma of a patient, which is measured in a laboratory setting. Both instances present the same information, are valid CCD result organizer extracts and can be used in various integration profiles of IHE, such as XPHR (Exchange of Personal Health Record Content), XDS-MS (Cross Enterprise Sharing of Medical Summaries) or XD-LAB (Sharing Laboratory Reports).

In the following subsections, we investigate these types of interoperability problems and address possible solutions.

Different Terminology Systems in the Same Compositional Structure

Consider the third shaded block of the first instance in Figure 1, which states that the observed value is within the normal ranges by using SNOMED CT code for "within reference range" (281301001) as the interpretation code of the observation class. Because, there is no CCD constraint on the value of interpretation code, in the second instance, this time the HL7 ObservationInterpretation code for "normal" (N) is used for the same purpose. Semantically, this code is an exact match with the SNOMED CT code used in the first instance.

Possible Solutions for Addressing Different Terminology Systems in the Same Compositional Structure

When different terminology systems are used in the same compositional structure, it is necessary to semantically mediate them for interoperation. There are some repositories of biomedical vo-

Figure 1. An example on some of the semantic interoperability problems in content templates

CCD Result Entry 1

```
<organizer classCode="BATTERY" moodCode="EVN">
  <!-- Result organizer template -->
  <templateId root="2.16.840.1.113883.10.20.1.32"/>
  <id root="7d5a02b0-67a4-11db-bd13-0800200c9a66"/>
  <!-- SNOMED CT code for Plasma glucose measurement procedure -->
  <code code="119958019" codeSystem="2.16.840.1.113883.6.96"
    displayName="Glucose measurement, plasma"/>
  <statusCode code="completed"/>
  <effectiveTime value="200003231430"/>
  <component>
    <observation classCode="OBS" moodCode="EVN">
      <!-- Result observation template -->
      <templateId root="2.16.840.1.113883.10.20.1.31"/>
      <id root="107c2dc0-67a5-11db-bd13-0800200c9a66"/>
      <!-- SNOMED CT code for Blood glucose status -->
      <code code="405176005" codeSystem="2.16.840.1.113883.6.96"
        displayName="Blood glucose status"/>
      <statusCode code="completed"/>
      <effectiveTime value="200003231430"/>
      <value xsi:type="PQ" value="104" unit="mg/dL"/>
      <!-- SNOMED CT Code for Within Reference Range (Qualifier)-->
      <interpretationCode code="281301001"
        codeSystem="2.16.840.1.113883.6.96"/>
    </observation>
  </component>
</organizer>
```

CCD Result Entry 2

```
<organizer classCode="BATTERY" moodCode="EVN">
  <!-- Result organizer template -->
  <templateId root="2.16.840.1.113883.10.20.1.32"/>
  <id root="7d5a02b0-67a4-11db-bd13-0800200c9a67"/>
  <!-- SNOMED CT code for Laboratory test procedure (generic) -->
  <code code="15220000" codeSystem="2.16.840.1.113883.6.96"
    displayName="Laboratory Test"/>
  <statusCode code="completed"/>
  <effectiveTime value="200003231430"/>
  <component>
    <observation classCode="OBS" moodCode="EVN">
      <!-- Result observation template -->
      <templateId root="2.16.840.1.113883.10.20.1.31"/>
      <id root="107c2dc0-67a5-11db-bd13-0800200c9a67"/>
      <!-- LOINC Code for Glucose in serum or plasma -->
      <code code="2345-7" codeSystem="2.16.840.1.113883.6.1"
        displayName="Glucose in serum or plasma"/>
      <statusCode code="completed"/>
      <effectiveTime value="200003231430"/>
      <value xsi:type="PQ" value="104" unit="mg/dL"/>
      <!-- HL7 ObservationInterpretation code for Normal -->
      <interpretationCode code="N"
        codeSystem="2.16.840.1.113883.5.83"/>
    </observation>
  </component>
</organizer>
```

cabularies that also provide mapping information among the terms of these vocabularies, such as the Unified Medical Language System (UMLS) (http://www.nlm.nih.gov/research/umls/) Metathesaurus that integrates over 2 million names for some 900,000 concepts from more than 60 families of biomedical vocabularies, as well as 12 million relations among these concepts. Similarly, BioPortal initiative (http://bioportal. bioontology.org/) serves more than 290 biomedical ontologies including ontological representations of major terminology systems like SNOMED CT, LOINC, ICD-10 and MedDRA, as well as mapping information between the coded terms of these terminology systems through ontological constructs. Such repositories can be exploited for automated or semi-automated mapping of coded terms from different terminology systems.

Yet, neither UMLS, nor BioPortal is perfect regarding the quality of the terminology mappings they provide. There are some mappings between the terms that are not at the same hierarchical level. For example, in one BioPortal mapping, "bronchitis" in one terminology system is matched with "respiratory diseases" in another terminology system. Furthermore, some of the mappings provided by these repositories are automatically generated with the help of NLP based methods, and they need to be validated.

Therefore, it is necessary to involve clinical terminology experts to increase the quality of the mappings, during both the mapping creation phase and the clinical statement translation phase. Creation of mapping definitions among entire terminology systems is an ambitious task. Instead, focusing on particular sub-topics such as cardiovascular diseases with the involvement of related experts is more achievable. When the quality of the mappings is not assured, semi-automatic translation of clinical statements should be preferred over fully automatic translation. In this case, the translation mechanism can be a living system that can be improved with the integration of feedback received from terminology experts.

Different Compositional Structures

Another type of semantic interoperability challenge comes from different compositional structures for encoding the same medical information.

Consider the first shaded block of the first instance in Figure 1. The result organizer code is the SNOMED CT code for plasma glucose measurement procedure (119958019). In the second instance, the code of the result organizer template is again from SNOMED CT; however, this time the code refers to a more generic meaning, i.e. laboratory test procedure (15220000). Because the CCD constraint for the result organizer code is to use an appropriate code from SNOMED CT or LOINC or optionally CPT-4, by using the codes from SNOMED CT, both of these documents satisfy this constraint.

In the first instance, the second coded attribute presents the topic of the observable entity of the result organizer, and the SNOMED CT code for blood glucose status (405176005) is used for this purpose. This code encodes the meaning for the actual observed value, which is 104 mg/dL glucose.

In the second instance, the code system preferred in the code attribute of observation class is different. Here, the LOINC code for glucose in serum or plasma (2345-7) is used for encoding the meaning of the actual observed value.

As a result, the result organizer codes and the observation codes of the first and second instances do not directly correspond to each other; the first result organizer code is restricted to glucose measurement domain while the second one is generic, and the observation codes are quite similar but not identical. However, when we consider the medical information represented in these instances, the combined meaning of organizer and observation codes are almost identical.

Possible Solutions for Addressing Different Compositional Structures

This problem is well-known and to address it, terminology bindings (Browne, 2008) have been proposed which specify the association between a data point (node) of an information or data model and the set of terms that can be used to populate that data point's value. The set of permissible values for a data point can be expressed by a query or a rule. As an example, the HL7 TermInfo (Health Level Seven, 2006) guidelines specify how SNOMED CT can be used in HL7 v3 standards, in order to communicate healthcare information in an agreed, consistent and adequately expressive form. In SNOMED CT, concepts are defined by relationships (e.g. method, procedure site, etc.) among them, and they can also be qualified (combined) to represent more precise meanings. Hence, even a single SNOMED CT concept may represent a meaning that the HL7 v3 RIM is able to represent using a combination of classes and attributes. TermInfo identifies options for use of SNOMED CT concepts in various attributes of HL7 RIM classes, and also provides an evaluation of such options. Unfortunately, although TermInfo is a very important project to contribute to consistent usage of terminology systems within content templates, its activities have been suspended for the last few years.

Another practical approach to this type of semantic interoperability has been developed in epSOS (http://www.epsos.eu), which is a pan-European project for piloting cross-border interoperability among national and regional EHR systems in Europe. For this purpose, first, the content templates of the three document types (i.e. patient summary, ePrescription and eDispensation) to be exchanged are defined as pivot documents by using and further restricting IHE PCC templates. Each country defines its own mapping from its national data structures onto these pivot document schemas. For the coded and unique representation of clinical content within these schemas, subsets from existing terminology systems such as SNOMED CT, ICD-10, LOINC and ATC have been selected to create the epSOS Master Value Sets Catalogue (MVC). The latest version of MVC contains 46 value sets. For example, the procedures value set contains 102 terms from SNOMED CT and illnesses and disorders value set contains 1685 terms from ICD-10. Each epSOS participating nation provides mapping of any locally used terminology system to MVC content and also translation of the MVC content into its own language, resulting in the epSOS Master Translation/Transcoding Catalogue. There are plans to provide MVC as an ontology (coded in OWL) to foster semantic interoperability.

As in the case of epSOS, the Clinical Info Model & Vocabulary Work Group of Transitions of Care (ToC) Initiative in the US has defined "Meaningful Use Subsets" of SNOMED CT, ICD-10, LOINC and RxNorm.

EHR-PHR INTEROPERABILITY PROFILES

IHE Exchange of Personal Health Record Content (XPHR) Integration Profile

The XPHR profile (Integrating the Healthcare Enterprise, 2010d) provides an interoperability mechanism to exchange data between PHR systems and the healthcare providers' information systems. Two actors have been defined: the "Content Creator" that creates the content to be exchanged and the "Content Consumer" that consumes this content. The data exchange is in both directions: a PHR system can get data from the healthcare information systems and can also feed data to these systems. A PHR system in the "Content Creator" role provides a summary of patient PHR information to providers' information systems, and the providers' systems in the "Content

Creator" role can suggest updates to the patient's PHR upon completion of a healthcare encounter.

The content to be exchanged is specified through two content templates, namely PHR Extract Module and the PHR Update Module. The PHR Extract Module describes the document content that summarizes information contained within a Personal Health Record. The purpose of the PHR Update Module is to provide a mechanism to update an existing PHR Extract content to reflect the changes in patient information in other healthcare information systems. Both PHR Extract and Update modules are defined as IHE PCC templates based on HL7/ASTM CCD.

XPHR relies on the previously defined document exchange profiles such as Cross-Enterprise Document Sharing (XDS) (Integrating the Healthcare Enterprise, 2010c), Cross-Enterprise Document Media Interchange (XDM) (Integrating the Healthcare Enterprise, 2010a) or Cross-Enterprise Document Reliable Interchange (XDR) (Integrating the Healthcare Enterprise, 2010b).

As an example, in Figure 2 we describe how IHE XPHR profile can be implemented based on IHE XDS Profile. A PHR system in the "Content Creator" role stores patient information to a Content Repository using XDS "Provide & Register Document Set" transaction whose content complies with the "PHR Extract Module" content template (Optionally, the Content Creator and Content Repository actors can be grouped as a single actor as shown by the dotted lines in Figure 2, in which case the "Provide & Register Document Set" transaction becomes irrelevant). Then the metadata of the stored content is sent to the Content Registry by using "Register Document Set" transaction of XDS to facilitate its discovery. Similarly, an EHR system can take the role of a "Content Creator" and store patient information again complying with the "PHR Extract Module" content template. Additionally, an EHR system may provide patient data through "PHR Update Module" to update the PHR Extract.

IHE Query for Existing Data (QED) Integration Profile

Using the Query for Existing Data (QED) Profile (Integrating the Healthcare Enterprise, 2008b), it is possible to access clinical data sources with predefined queries and hence this profile is quite relevant for PHR-EHR data exchange. There are two actors in this profile, namely the "Clinical Data

Figure 2. IHE XPHR profile based on IHE XDS

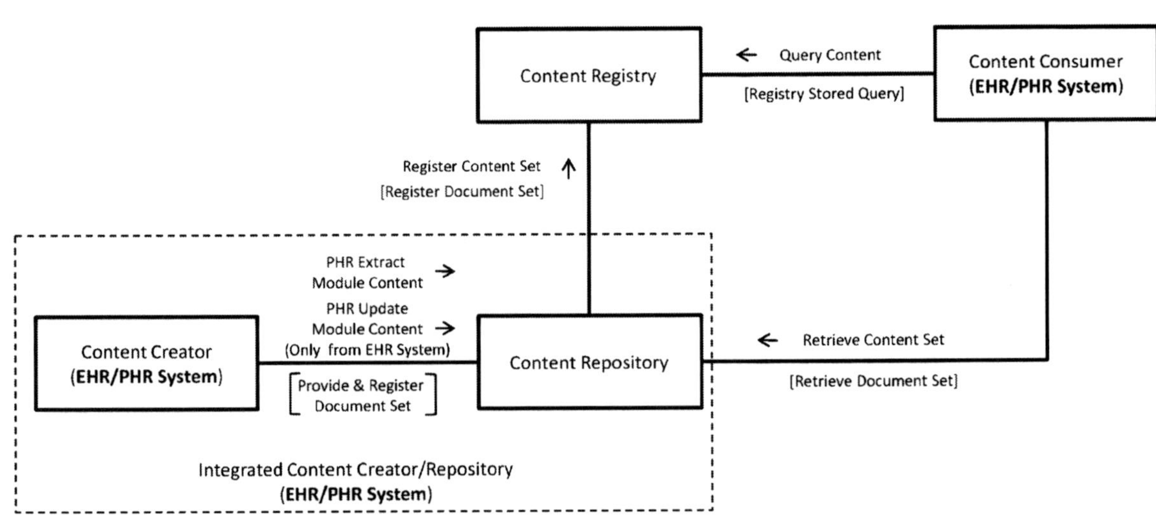

Consumer" and the "Clinical Data Source," and the business process layer involves one transaction, namely, "Query Existing Data" that is used by the consumer to query the source. This transaction gets a number of query parameters such as "patientId," "patientName," "careProvisionCode" and "careRecordTimePeriod." Six different types of queries are defined and each of them is indicated as an option of the "Query Existing Data" transaction. The actor implementing this transaction must support at least one of them:

- Vital Signs Option;
- Problems and Allergies Option;
- Diagnostic Results Option;
- Medications Option;
- Immunizations Option;
- Professional Services Option.

A content template is specified for each result to be returned by the query. Each content template inherits constraints from the CCD and PCC entry level templates, and defines further constraints such as by setting the units to be used and a specific vocabulary.

For example, a "Clinical Data Consumer" that implements the "Problems and Allergies Option" can retrieve all problem entries by specifying the code "MEDCCAT" and the result will conform to the PCC Problem Entry template, or can specify the code "INTOLIST" that will return the results conforming to the PCC Allergy and Intolerance Concern template.

A "Clinical Data Source" that implements the "Problems and Allergies Option" on the other hand, must be able to respond to all vocabulary specified for problems and allergies including "MEDCCAT" and "INTOLIST." An example QED usage scenario is depicted in Figure 3.

For the communication layer, the IHE ITI Web services (Integrating the Healthcare Enterprise, 2010f) and HL7 Web services guidelines (Health Level Seven, 2010b) are used. The "Query Existing Data" transaction is mapped to the Query Care Record Event Profile Query of HL7 v3 Care Record Query topic. It is important to note that in these transactions that are defined by the HL7 v3 Care Provision domain (used by IHE RCG and CM profiles as well), it is not possible to exchange a complete CDA document instance. The payload of a Care Provision Event instance as used in these transactions can contain only Care Statement instances, which are almost identical with CDA entry classes. Hence, IHE QED (also RCG and CM) profile refers to only entry level PCC templates.

Figure 3. The use of IHE QED Profile for data exchange

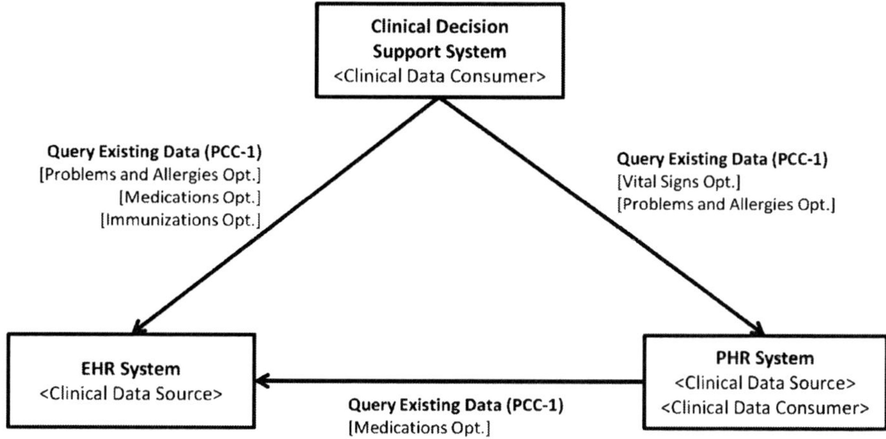

Analysis of PHR Interoperability Profiles

Being interoperability profiles, both XPHR and QED address all the layers in the interoperability stack. Their difference is that with QED, it is possible to get parts of a patient's EHR as specified through the options such as "vital signs" or "medications." Indeed, such partial queries are important because exchange of a complete patient history is not necessary all the time; it might be necessary to get only the active medications of a patient for example. QED is relevant for decision support services as well; it can be used to retrieve only relevant portions of patient data according to the requirements of the specific decision support service. However, in the future, it might be necessary to extend the existing set of options.

A disadvantage of QED is that it lacks support for asynchronous communication. XPHR on the other hand, when implemented with XDS for instance, can support asynchronous Web services exchange. This issue is further detailed in *Clinical Decision Support Service Standards* Section while describing the Clinical Decision Support Service standards.

TERMINOLOGY SYSTEMS

In medicine, the clinical data structures such as EHR and PHR content templates refer to "controlled vocabularies" or "terminologies" to express semantics, i.e., the meaning of the terms used. For example, the observation for a patient can be expressed as a "heart attack" or a "myocardial infarction," and these mean the same thing to medical professionals. But unless the term is associated with a unique code from a terminology system, automated processing of the exchanged term is very difficult because an application, programmed to use "heart attack," would not understand "myocardial infarction." When the observation refers to a medical terminology system such as SNOMED CT and the code 22298006 for "Myocardial infarction" is used to represent the observation, the meaning exchanged can be shared in a consistent and automated way as long as both of the applications use this code.

In this section, we will briefly mention some of the well-known terminology systems and provide an analysis especially for terminology systems' mapping.

Analysis of Terminology Systems

The terminology systems can be classified based on the underlying structure and related knowledge representation formalism that determine the way they express the semantics of the relationships between the coded terms: Some are plain lists, for example the Standard Terms of the European Directorate for the Quality of Medicines and Healthcare (EDQM); some are terminology systems organized into a hierarchy, for example ICD-10 and hence give the parent-child information among the terms; and some express the relationships between the coded terms through ontological constructs, for example SNOMED CT or semantic networks like Unified Medical Language System (UMLS). This classification together with some example terminology systems and resources is provided in Table 2.

Currently, SNOMED CT is the most comprehensive clinical vocabulary available, in terms of coverage and the relationships among concepts. It contains approximately 350,000 active concepts, more than 1 million terms including synonyms and about 1.5 million relations between the concepts. On the other hand, SNOMED CT has both logical and ontological problems as has been discussed in the literature (Heja et al., 2008; Bodenreider et al., 2007; Schulz et al., 2009). The identified problems include mixing the subsumption relation with other relations such as "part of;" redundant concepts; omission of obvious relationships and contracting disjoint entities into one concept. A number of recommendations have been proposed

Table 2. Classification of some medical terminology systems and resources

Simple Lists (No Relationship Among the Terms)	Classification Systems (Hierarchical Relationship Among the Coded Terms)	Semantic Relationship Among the Concepts	Mapping Information Among Different Terminology Systems
EDQM Standard Terms	ICD-9, ICD-10, MedDRA	SNOMED CT, UMLS Metathesaurus and Semantic Network	UMLS Metathesaurus, BioPortal

to overcome these problems such as arranging SNOMED CT upper ontology according to a standard upper ontology (Heja et al., 2008; Schulz et al., 2009); assigning SNOMED CT concepts to four disjoint groups such as classes, instances, relations and meta-classes (Schulz et al., 2009) and a high level core reference ontology of shared medical knowledge (Heja et al., 2008). However, the use of SNOMED CT as a terminology service as a plain or loosely structured list does not need substantial restructuring.

To achieve interoperability among terminology systems, not only the mapping information between them but also the semantic relationships among the terms (or, concepts) are necessary because this helps discovering the implicit equivalences between two terms from different terminology systems by using reasoning. As an example, assume a patient's acute heart failure condition is expressed with SNOMED CT code 56675007 in a clinical document and the receiving application understands only the MedDRA terminology system. Through reasoning, it is possible to discover that the equivalent MedDRA code is 10019279 for "heart failure," because the SNOMED CT class for "acute heart failure" (56675007) is a subclass of the class for "heart failure" (84114007) and given that MedDRA code for "heart failure" (10019279) maps to 84114007 in SNOMED CT; a reasoner can deduce this result by using subsumption reasoning.

Currently, several sources provide terminology system mappings. More than 60 families of biomedical vocabularies together with context and inter-context relationships among these various vocabularies are available within the UMLS.

Also, ontological representations of more than 290 terminology systems and their mappings are accessible through BioPortal, which is maintained by the US National Center for Biomedical Ontology. However, not all the mappings are fully reliable. Therefore, as discussed in *Possible solutions for addressing different terminology systems in the same compositional structure* Section, although there is a need to develop tools to map terms from different terminology systems, continuous involvement of terminology experts and healthcare professionals in this process is necessary to guarantee reliable translation of clinical statements/documents.

STANDARDS FOR EHR-PHR-MEDICAL DEVICE INTEROPERABILITY

Personal medical devices are essential to the practice of modern healthcare services, including the PHR systems. A number of applications have been developed to store personal medical device data to PHR systems.

The prominent standards for the integration of medical device data into electronic and personal health records (EHR/PHR) include the IHE Patient Care Device (PCD) integration profiles (Integrating the Healthcare Enterprise, 2010e) and Electronic/Personal Health Record Network Interface (xHRN-IF) (Carroll et al., 2007) by the Continua Health Alliance.

Both of these standards address how to map the device data obtained through the ISO/IEEE 11073 standard (International Organization for

Standardization et al., 2004a) to the healthcare application interfaces. This is because the most widely used standard to obtain data from the medical devices is ISO/IEEE 11073 set of standards. 11073 standards define an object-oriented Domain Information Model (DIM) (International Organization for Standardization, 2004b) to model medical device domain. It is possible to represent a medical device and its measurements with objects using the DIM. However, in order to define interoperable medical devices, the attributes of these objects must consist of codes that are specified in a data dictionary. ISO/IEEE 11073 - 10101: Nomenclature (International Organization for Standardization, 2004c) is a data dictionary of vital signs domain which is used to represent the DIM objects with common codes.

IHE Device Enterprise Communication (DEC) Profile is used for transmitting information from medical devices at the point of care to the enterprise applications. For this purpose, ISO/IEEE 11073 Domain Information Model is mapped to HL7 v2.5 Observation Report and the ISO/IEEE 11073 Data Types are mapped to HL7 v2.5 Data Types. For semantic interoperability, IHE has developed the Rosetta Terminology Mapping (RTM) Profile to provide the mapping between the proprietary device parameters to ISO/IEEE 11073 Nomenclature. Each row of the Rosetta table, which is under development, gives the vendors' displayed name and units of measure together with the equivalent ISO/IEEE 11073 identifier and the unit from the Unified Code for Units of Measure (UCUM) code system (http://www.unitsofmeasure.org/).

The Continua Health Alliance Electronic/Personal Health Record Network Interface (xHRN-IF) is based on the HL7 Personal Health Monitoring Report (PHMR) (Health Level Seven, 2008) document format. The PHMR carries personal healthcare monitoring information including the representation of the measurements captured by devices, notes, summaries and graphs. In order to represent such varying data, templates are defined by reusing HL7 Continuity of Care Document. The health record systems like PHRs need to implement xHRN-IF to be able to exchange personal health information with healthcare entities conforming to this standard.

Analysis of the Standards for EHR-PHR-Medical Device Interoperability

As already mentioned, the EHR-PHR-Medical Device Interoperability standards address how to map the device data obtained through the ISO/IEEE 11073 standards to the healthcare application interfaces. Considering that there are different EHR/PHR content standards and templates, generating a mapping from ISO/IEEE 11073 Domain Information Model to each of them is not very practical.

A recent work (Yuksel et al., 2011) addresses this challenge by specializing the HL7 v3 Reference Information Model (RIM) to the medical device domain using the ISO/IEEE 11073 Domain Information Model (DIM) to obtain its Refined Message Information Model (RMIM). The novelty of this approach is that it provides a common denominator for different HL7 v3 RIM based interfaces of various EHR/PHR content models rather than using the bilateral mappings between the device models and different application standards. This facilitates EHR/PHR and personal medical device data interoperability because the concepts are derived from a common RIM through a well-defined refinement process and hence the building blocks of the interfaces are similar, and they can be traceable back to the RIM.

CLINICAL DECISION SUPPORT SERVICE STANDARDS

Clinical Decision Support Services (CDSSs) are used in care management to provide clinicians, staff and patients with knowledge, intelligently filtered or presented at appropriate times, to enhance health and healthcare (Kawamoto et al., 2007). Common uses of CDSSs include computerized provider order entry systems that give patient-specific recommendations as part of the order entry process; listing health maintenance procedures due when patient age, gender, past health maintenance procedures are provided; or laboratory alerting systems that page physicians when critical lab values are detected.

Although the CDSSs are designed primarily to assist patient-specific decision making by clinicians, it is anticipated that CDSSs will be adapted to provide patient guidance services from the PHR systems to be used by patients themselves (European Commission, 2010). In this respect, a relevant topic that is indirectly linked with the CDSS concept is enabling patients' access to evidence-based health information available as text or multimedia resources presented in layman terms, to foster their engagement in the management of their care. Some PHR systems automatically link the key terms or phrases in the patient's records with relevant evidence-based health information on the Web. A further improvement in this direction is provided by the HL7 International Context-Aware Knowledge Retrieval Standard, known as Infobutton (Health Level Seven, 2010a), which rather than providing a direct link, helps a user (not necessarily a patient; can be a health professional as well) to refine his query based on automatically collected contextual information (e.g. user type, patient age and gender, the term of interest) and user feedback. Then it allows the user to easily access the preferred evidence-based resource through World Wide Web links.

CDSSs generally include a knowledge base containing information such as compiled clinical information on diagnoses, drug interactions and guidelines; a program for combining that knowledge with patient-specific information to draw machine interpretable conclusions regarding patients; and a mechanism to enter or import patient data from the EHR/PHR systems into the CDSS so that the relevant information, such as

lists of possible diagnoses, drug interaction alerts, or preventive care reminders can be provided (Berner et al., 2009).

The main challenge to wider use of CDSSs is the need to implement different interfaces when dealing with different CDSSs. There are three major initiatives to address this challenge: the service oriented model by the Healthcare Services Specification Project (HSSP) to expose clinical decision support services in a uniform way, the IHE Request for Clinical Guidance (RCG) Profile and the IHE Care Management (CM) Profile that provides a mechanism for EHR/PHR and other health IT systems to communicate information to care management systems.

HSSP developed first a service functional model (SFM) (Kawamoto et al., 2006) and then a technical specification built upon this SFM for exposing CDSS modules as decision support services. The aim is to let the CDSS client applications have uniform access to different knowledge modules. By using the specified service interfaces, a service client is able to determine which knowledge module to use, what data are needed for requesting a patient evaluation, as well as what will be returned by the CDSS as a result of the patient evaluation request.

IHE has published the Request for Clinical Guidance profile (Integrating the Healthcare Enterprise, 2009b) that describes how to exchange patient data as the payload needed to drive the clinical decision support service for certain decision support modules such as drug and allergy interaction detection, forecasting a vaccine schedule, identifying eligible patients for research or other programs, and cost effective selection of antibiotics based on recent institutional data.

Another related IHE profile is the Care Management profile (Integrating the Healthcare Enterprise, 2008a). This profile is more generic than the RCG profile in that it provides a mechanism for EHR/PHR and other health IT systems to communicate information to care management systems through the use of evidence based guidelines.

HSSP Clinical Decision Support Service Specification

In 2006, Healthcare Services Specification Project (HSSP), which is a joint effort by Health Level Seven (HL7) and the Object Management Group (OMG), developed a service functional model for exposing CDSS modules as decision support services. The aim is to facilitate CDSS client applications to:

- Identify the knowledge modules that could be used to meet their needs;
- Know what patient data must be submitted to the CDSS in order to obtain an accurate evaluation; and
- Know the meaning and format of any results that will be returned by the CDSS following a patient evaluation (Kawamoto et al., 2006).

In order to realize this functionality, three interface specifications are developed:

- The Meta-data Discovery interface provides operations for discovering and examining meta-data associated with a CDSS or its knowledge modules.
- The Query interface provides operations for discovering and examining knowledge modules of interest. This interface includes operations for identifying the data required for evaluating a patient using a knowledge module.
- The Evaluation interface provides operations for obtaining evaluation results using specified knowledge modules. A CDSS is permitted to return evaluation results using a variety of information constructs including the RIM acts (e.g., an HL7 medication entity with a mood code indicating that the medication should be ordered), dates (e.g., the date that a test was last performed, or the date at which a test will be due), and boolean values (e.g., whether a patient is in need of a pneumococcal vaccine).

Building on this functional model, OMG developed a fully implementable Clinical Decision Support Service (CDSS) specification as a normative standard in 2010 (the latest version is from 2011) (Object Management Group, 2011), which is then proceeded by the HL7 Decision Support Service (DSS) specification (Health Level Seven, 2011b). HL7 DSS and OMG CDSS technical specifications are almost identical; minor differences will be resolved in future releases. They include both a platform-independent model (PIM) for the DSSs as well as a platform-specific model (PSM) for SOAP XML Web services. The PIM represents the platform-independent definitions of the DSS interfaces and the elements used within these interfaces as a UML model. The PSM describes technical details for implementation including WSDLs and XSDs that are generated according to the PIM. The XML syntax of these schemas are mostly custom defined by OMG, but some data elements are built upon the HL7 v3 RIM XSD representation as well. The HL7/OMG Decision Support Service technical specifications also define several profiles and semantic requirements to ensure a minimum level of interoperability among DSSs.

OpenCDS (http://www.opencds.org/) is a multi-institutional, collaborative effort to develop an open-source reference implementation of the HL7/OMG DSS technical specifications, and 1.1 release of the implementation is already available.

IHE Request for Clinical Guidance (RCG) Profile

The IHE Request for Clinical Guidance (RCG) profile supports integration of clinical decision support into healthcare IT systems by describing how to exchange patient data as the payload needed to drive the clinical decision support service.

There are two actors in this profile, namely, the "Care Manager" and the "Decision Support Service" actors. "Request for Clinical Guidance" transaction requests and returns information between these actors. At the communication layer HL7 v3 Web Services Profile is used, and the Report Care Provision transaction that is defined by the HL7 v3 Care Provision domain is utilized. In general, RCG profile suggests leveraging the existing PCC content modules to deliver information to a CDSS. The CDSS then responds with a suggested care plan or additional clinical information. As an example, consider an immunization forecasting scenario (Integrating the Healthcare Enterprise, 2009b). The "Care Manager" actor obtains patient age, gender, and current immunization status, allergies and problem information from the EHR/PHR system. The "Care Manager" actor submits the relevant portions of this information to the decision support service using "Request for Clinical Guidance" transaction. The "Decision Support Service" actor, which in this case is an immunization forecasting service, processes this information and returns a response to the "Care Manager" actor in the same transaction. The response includes the evaluations of the immunizations and one or more immunization schedules.

It is clear that content templates are needed for describing the payloads used in the request and response messages of the request for clinical guidance transaction. Currently, only immunization content template is available through the Immunization Content Profile (Integrating the Healthcare Enterprise, 2009a). It is anticipated that additional content profiles that work with these actors will be created in the future.

IHE Care Management (CM) Profile

The Care Management (CM) profile supports the exchange of information between health IT systems and applications used to manage care for specific conditions. The Care Management profile describes a publish/subscribe mechanism between source and the consumer systems. It is almost the same with the QED profile (*IHE Query for Existing Data (QED) Integration Profile* Section), but rather than getting an immediate response only for once; the source system keeps sending back the new results that matches the criteria as they become available. This query is maintained indefinitely until the requesting system cancels it.

As in the case of QED and RCG profiles, Care Management profile uses transactions and messages that are defined by the HL7 v3 Care Provision domain. For this reason, it is not possible to use document level content templates directly within the CM profile, as Care Provision Event messages allow only entry level instances as the payload.

Unlike QED and RCG, CM profile supports HL7 v2 messaging in addition to HL7 v3 Web services implementation.

Analysis of the Clinical Decision Support Service Standards

Among the three major initiatives explained above, the HL7/OMG DSS technical specifications, which are defined on top of the HSSP service functional model, cover the widest range of accessible interfaces for the CDSSs. For example, meta-data discovery and query interfaces together provide several methods to find knowledge modules of interest. IHE RCG and CM profiles on the other hand do not provide discovery functionalities. OpenCDS, that is, the collaborative and open-source reference implementation effort for HL7/OMG DSS technical specifications is another advantage of HSSP functional model.

The main advantage of the Care Management profile over the rest, and also over the IHE QED profile, is that, it enables asynchronous stateful clinical decision support.

The major drawback of all three efforts is their low-profile support for the structured content modules to exchange patient and decision support data. HL7/OMG DSS technical specifications state that ASTM CCR, HL7/ASTM CCD or any other HL7 v3 RIM based syntax can be used to exchange patient data with CDSSs, which in fact is quite a loose restriction. IHE CM and RCG profiles on the other hand, necessitate the usage of messages that are defined by the HL7 v3 Care Provision domain; but the profiles are always explained with IHE PCC content modules that are defined on top of CCD. As explained previously, it is not possible to use PCC document and section level templates in the Care Provision Event messages, and entry level templates are subject to some changes while transforming them to Care Statement instances used within Care Provision Event messages. However, transformation of complete CDA documents to valid Care Provision messages is presented very briefly in the profiles. Such issues impede the use of the CDSS standards and profiles.

CONCLUSION

Personal Health Records (PHRs) have the potential to dramatically change healthcare over the coming years (Kaelber et al., 2008). It is anticipated that empowering patients with PHRs and thus making their active participation possible in their own healthcare management will produce better health outcomes at lower costs.

A notable report by some of the leading industry organizations including Google, HIMSS, Kaiser Permanente and Microsoft investigates the value of PHR systems in the context of four PHR system architectures: provider-tethered, payer-tethered, third-party, and interoperable PHRs (Kaelber et al., 2008). Provider tethered, payer-tethered, and third-party PHRs all have related examples in the current marketplace. These systems mostly use ad hoc interfaces to pass information from each healthcare application to the PHR system. Given the large number of applications involved, it is not practical or cost effective to design one-off interfaces.

Interoperable PHRs, on the other hand, represent a future type of PHR in which all entities have access to data due to health data communication standards and interoperability. The report concludes that from the perspective of the healthcare system, interoperable PHRs provide the greatest value.

This chapter surveys the interoperability standards that can be used to import/export data to and from the PHR systems to a large number of healthcare applications and medical data resources. It is an analysis harmonizing the state-of-the-art and the authors' experiences in developing systems using these standards which are presented through clear examples rather than a compilation of descriptions from the standards' specifications. The study also aims to provide an entry point for the researchers in this domain.

The interoperable PHRs, when realized, will reinforce patient participation in care processes and health management, improve health outcomes by improved decision support, enhance adherence to treatment by making it possible to measure patients' compliance and to demonstrate their progress and have positive impact on lifestyle diseases by empowering patients with better information, communication and means for shared decision making.

REFERENCES

American Health Information Management Association (AHIMA) & American Medical Informatics Association. (AMIA). (2007). *The value of personal health records: A joint position statement for consumers of health care*. Retrieved from http://www.amia.org/sites/amia.org/files/ahima-amia-phr-statement.pdf

ASTM International. (2005). *E2369 - 05e1 standard specification for continuity of care record (CCR)*. Retrieved from http://www.astm.org/Standards/E2369.htm

Beale, T., & Heard, S. (2007). *Archetype definitions and principles.* Retrieved from http://www.openehr.org/svn/specification/TRUNK/publishing/architecture/am/archetype_principles.pdf

Berner, E. S. (2009). *Clinical decision support systems: State of the art.* Retrieved from http://healthit.portaldev.ahrq.gov/portal/server.pt/gateway/PTARGS_0_1248_874024_0_0_18/09-0069-EF.pdf

Bodenreider, O., Smith, B., Kumar, A., & Burgun, A. (2007). Investigating subsumption in SNOMED CT: An exploration into large description logic-based biomedical terminologies. *Artificial Intelligence in Medicine, 39*(3), 183–195. doi:10.1016/j.artmed.2006.12.003 PMID:17241777

Browne, E. (2008). *openEHR archetypes and terminology.* Retrieved from http://www.openehr.org/wiki/display/healthmod/Archetypes+and+Terminology

Carroll, R., Cnossen, R., Schnell, M., & Simons, D. (2007). Continua: An interoperable personal healthcare ecosystem. *IEEE Pervasive Computing / IEEE Computer Society [and] IEEE Communications Society, 6*(4), 90–94. doi:10.1109/MPRV.2007.72

Eichelberg, M., Aden, T., Riesmeier, J., Dogac, A., & Laleci, G. B. (2005). A survey and analysis of electronic healthcare record standards. *ACM Computing Surveys, 37*, 277–315. doi:10.1145/1118890.1118891

EN 13606 Association. (2010). *Unofficial ISO/CEN 13606 XML schema.* Retrieved from http://www.en13606.org/resources/files/cat_view/53-xml-schemas

European Commission. (2004). *European interoperability framework for pan-European egovernment services.* Retrieved from http://ec.europa.eu/idabc/servlets/Docd552.pdf?id=19529

European Commission. (2010). *FP7 ICT work programme 2011 - Objective ICT-2011.5.3 patient guidance services (PGS).* Retrieved from ftp://ftp.cordis.europa.eu/pub/fp7/docs/wp/cooperation/ict/c-wp-201101_en.pdf

Halamka, J. D., Mandl, K. D., & Tang, P. C. (2008). Early experiences with personal health records. *Journal of the American Medical Informatics Association, 15*(1), 1–7. doi:10.1197/jamia.M2562 PMID:17947615

Health Level Seven. (2005). *Clinical document architecture (CDA), release 2.* Retrieved from http://www.hl7.org/implement/standards/cda.cfm

Health Level Seven. (2006). *TermInfo: Using SNOMED CT in HL7 version 3.* Retrieved from http://www.hl7.org/library/committees/terminfo/TermInfo_Ballot_DRAFT.30Jan2006.doc

Health Level Seven. (2008). *Personal healthcare monitoring report (PHMR).* Retrieved from http://www.hl7.org/documentcenter/ballots/2008SEP/support/CDAR2_PHMRPTS_R1_DSTU_2008NOV.zip

Health Level Seven. (2010a). *Context-aware retrieval application (infobutton), knowledge request, release 1.* Retrieved from http://www.hl7.org/v3ballot/html/domains/uvds/uvds_Context-awareKnowledgeRetrieval(Infobutton).html

Health Level Seven. (2010b). *HL7 version 3 standard: Transport specification - Web services profile, release 2.* Retrieved from http://www.hl7.org/v3ballot/html/infrastructure/transport/transport-wsprofiles.html

Health Level Seven. (2010c). *Reference information model (RIM) release 3.* Retrieved from http://www.hl7.org/v3ballot/html/infrastructure/rim/rim.html

Health Level Seven. (2011a). *greenCDA project.* Retrieved from http://wiki.hl7.org/index.php?title=GreenCDA_Project

Health Level Seven. (2011b). *HL7 version 3 standard: Decision support service, release 1*. Retrieved from http://www.hl7.org/v3ballot/html/infrastructure/dss/HL7_Decision_Support_Service_%20Normative_Specification_Release_1.pdf

Health Level Seven & ASTM International. (2008). *Continuity of care document (CCD) release 1*. Retrieved from http://wiki.hl7.org/index.php?title=Product_CCD

Healthcare Information Technology Standards Panel. (2009). *HITSP C32 - Summary documents using HL7 continuity of care document (CCD) component*. Retrieved from http://www.hitsp.org/ConstructSet_Details.aspx?&PrefixAlpha=4&PrefixNumeric=32

Healthcare Information Technology Standards Panel. (2010). *HITSP C83 - CDA content modules component*. Retrieved from http://www.hitsp.org/Handlers/HitspFileServer.aspx?FileGuid=717d69a5-6bc4-4f8b-a22c-197130b50567

Heja, G., Surjan, G., & Varga, P. (2008). Ontological analysis of SNOMED CT. *BMC Medical Informatics and Decision Making, 8*(S1), S8. doi:10.1186/1472-6947-8-S1-S8 PMID:19007445

Helmer, A., Lipprandt, M., Frenken, T., Eichelberg, M., & Hein, A. (2011). Empowering patients through personal health records: A survey of existing third-party web-based PHR products. *Electronic Journal of Health Informatics, 6*(3), 1–19.

Iakovidis, I. (1998). Towards personal health records: Current situation, obstacles and trends in implementation of electronic healthcare. *International Journal of Medical Informatics, 52*(1-3), 105–115. doi:10.1016/S1386-5056(98)00129-4 PMID:9848407

Integrating the Healthcare Enterprise. (2008a). *Care management (CM) integration profile*. Retrieved from http://www.ihe.net/Technical_Framework/upload/IHE_PCC_Care_Management_CM_Supplement_TI_2008-08-22.pdf

Integrating the Healthcare Enterprise. (2008b). *Query for existing data (QED) integration profile*. Retrieved from http://www.ihe.net/Technical_Framework/upload/IHE_PCC_Query_for_Existing_Data_QED_SupplSuppl_TI_2008-08-22.pdf

Integrating the Healthcare Enterprise. (2009a). *Immunization content (IC) integration profile*. Retrieved from http://www.ihe.net/Technical_Framework/upload/IHE_PCC_Immunization_Content_IC_Supplement_TI_-2009-08-10.pdf

Integrating the Healthcare Enterprise. (2009b). *Request for clinical guidance (RCG) integration profile*. Retrieved from http://www.ihe.net/Technical_Framework/upload/IHE_PCC_Request_for_Clinical_Guidance_RCG_TI_-2009-08-10.pdf

Integrating the Healthcare Enterprise. (2010a). *Cross-enterprise document media interchange (XDM) integration profile*. Retrieved from http://www.ihe.net/Technical_Framework/upload/IHE_ITI_TF_Rev7-0_Vol1_FT_2010-08-10.pdf

Integrating the Healthcare Enterprise. (2010b). *Cross-enterprise document reliable interchange (XDR) integration profile*. Retrieved from http://www.ihe.net/Technical_Framework/upload/IHE_ITI_TF_Rev7-0_Vol1_FT_2010-08-10.pdf

Integrating the Healthcare Enterprise. (2010c). *Cross-enterprise document sharing (XDS) integration profile*. Retrieved from http://www.ihe.net/Technical_Framework/upload/IHE_ITI_TF_Rev7-0_Vol1_FT_2010-08-10.pdf

Integrating the Healthcare Enterprise. (2010d). *Exchange of personal health record content (XPHR) integration profile*. Retrieved from http://www.ihe.net/Technical_Framework/upload/IHE_PCC_TF_Rev6-0_Vol_1_2010-08-30.pdf

Integrating the Healthcare Enterprise. (2010e). *Patient care device (PCD) technical framework, volume 1, revision 1.2*. Retrieved from http://www.ihe.net/Technical_Framework/upload/IHE_PCD_TF_Rev1-2_Vol1_TI_2010-09-30.pdf

Integrating the Healthcare Enterprise. (2010f). *Web services for IHE transactions*. Retrieved from http://www.ihe.net/Technical_Framework/upload/IHE_ITI_TF_Rev7-0_Vol2x_FT_2010-08-10.pdf

International Organization for Standardization & Comité Européen de Normalisation. (2008). *EN 13606-1, health informatics – Electronic health record communication – Part 1: Reference model*.

International Organization for Standardization & The Institute of Electrical and Electronics Engineers. (2004a). *ISO/IEEE 11073 family of standards*.

International Organization for Standardization & The Institute of Electrical and Electronics Engineers. (2004b). *ISO/IEEE 11073-10201:2004(E) health informatics – Point-of-care medical device communication – Part 10201: Domain information model*.

International Organization for Standardization & The Institute of Electrical and Electronics Engineers. (2004c). *ISO/IEEE 11073-10101:2004(E) health informatics – Point-of-care medical device communication – Part 10101: Nomenclature*.

Kaelber, D. C., Shah, S., Vincent, A., Pan, E., Hook, J. M., Johnston, D., et al. (2008). *The value of personal health records*. Retrieved from http://www.citl.org/publications/_pdf/CITL_PHR_Report.pdf

Kawamoto, K., & Esler, B. (2006). *Service functional model specification - Decision support service (DSS)*. Retrieved from http://archive.hl7.org/v3ballotarchive/v3ballot2009jan/html/infrastructure/dss/Decision%20Support%20Service%20v1_0.pdf

Kawamoto, K., & Lobach, D. (2007). Proposal for fulfilling strategic objectives of the U.S. roadmap for national action on clinical decision support through a service-oriented architecture leveraging HL7 services. *Journal of the American Medical Informatics Association, 14*(2), 146–155. doi:10.1197/jamia.M2298 PMID:17213489

Object Management Group. (2011). *OMG clinical decision support service (CDSS), version 1.0*. Retrieved from http://www.omg.org/spec/CDSS/1.0/PDF

Popplewell, K., Lampathaki, F., Koussouris, S., Mouzakitis, S., Charalabidis, Y., Goncalves, R., & Agostinho, C. (2012). *ENSEMBLE deliverable D2.1 - EISB state of play report*. Retrieved from http://www.fines-cluster.eu/fines/jm/Publications/Download-document/339-ENSEMBLE_D2.1_EISB_State_of_Play_Report-v2.00.html

Schulz, S., Suntisrivaraporn, B., Baader, F., & Boeker, M. (2009). SNOMED reaching its adolescence: Ontologists' and logicians' health check. *International Journal of Medical Informatics, 78*(S1), 86–94. doi:10.1016/j.ijmedinf.2008.06.004 PMID:18789754

Seven, H. L. Integrating the Healthcare Enterprise, The Office of the National Coordinator for Health Information Technology & Health Story Project. (2011). *Implementation guide for CDA release 2.0 - Consolidated CDA templates (US realm)*. Retrieved from http://wiki.hl7.org/images/b/be/CDAConsolidationR12011.zip

The openEHR Foundation. (2006). *Introducing openEHR*. Retrieved from http://www.openehr.org/releases/1.0.2/openEHR/introducing_openEHR.pdf

Van Langenhove, P., Dirkx, M., & Decreus, K. (2011). *European interoperability architecture (EIA), phase 2 - Final report: Common vision for an EIA*. Retrieved from http://ec.europa.eu/isa/documents/isa_2.1_eia-finalreport-common-visionforaneia.pdf

Yuksel, M., & Dogac, A. (2011). Interoperability of medical device information and the clinical applications: An HL7 RMIM based on the ISO/IEEE 11073 DIM. *IEEE Transactions on Information Technology in Biomedicine, 15*(4), 557–566. doi:10.1109/TITB.2011.2151868 PMID:21558061

KEY TERMS AND DEFINITIONS

Clinical Decision Support Service: An interactive information system to assist health professionals, ideally with the involvement of patients, in their decision making tasks by reusing existing healthcare knowledge.

Electronic Health Record (EHR): Digitally stored healthcare information by the care givers about an individual's lifetime with the purpose of supporting care.

Personal Health Record (PHR): A tool for collecting, tracking and sharing important, up-to-date information about an individual's health or the health of someone in their care.

Personal Medical Device: Portable, wearable or implantable devices that can monitor vital signs and manage chronic diseases of an individual. These devices are able to communicate with other computer systems through electronic means.

Semantic Interoperability: The ability of two or more information systems to actually interpret and understand the exchanged data.

Technical Interoperability: The ability of two or more information systems to communicate and exchange data.

Chapter 55
Knowledge Discovery and Data Mining Applications in the Healthcare Industry:
A Comprehensive Study

Iman Barazandeh
Iran University of Science and Technology, Iran & Islamic Azad University, Mahshahr Branch, Iran

Mohammad Reza Gholamian
Iran University of Science and Technology, Iran

ABSTRACT

The healthcare industry is one of the most attractive domains to realize the actionable knowledge discovery objectives. This chapter studies recent researches on knowledge discovery and data mining applications in the healthcare industry and proposes a new classification of these applications. Studies show that knowledge discovery and data mining applications in the healthcare industry can be classified to three major classes, namely patient view, market view, and system view. Patient view includes papers that performed pure data mining on healthcare industry data. Market view includes papers that saw the patients as customers. System view includes papers that developed a decision support system. The goal of this classification is identifying research opportunities and gaps for researchers interested in this context.

INTRODUCTION

Since human learned to inscribe his thinks in the world out of his/her mind, Data has been created and started to growing and its growing accelerates through continuous advances in storing technology during the years and recent years are explosion age of data. Large and valuable volume of data is accumulated in databases and data warehouses in all domains. Online stores store sale details and customer information and interests in their databases. In banking industry account information and transactions are stored. In healthcare industry general patient information and his/her point of care information are stored in databases. These days information is stored either digital or manual because it is proved that information and knowledge are the main success driver in every domain and industry.

DOI: 10.4018/978-1-4666-8756-1.ch055

However, what we can do with this large volume of data and how we can extract high level knowledge from low level and raw data. It is obvious that we can mine the data to find new and valuable relations and patterns. Pattern is an expression in some language describing a subset of the data or a model applicable to the subset and we can consider a pattern to be knowledge if it exceeds some interestingness threshold that is depends on domain and user definition (Fayyad, Piatetsky-Shapiro & Smyth, 1996). Extracted knowledge can be used to make more effective decisions.

For long years, statisticians used classical statistic methods for pattern identification. Statistics, especially as taught in most statistics texts, might be described as being characterized by data sets which are small and clean, which permit straightforward answers via intensive analysis of single data sets, which are static, which were sampled in an iid manner, which were often collected to answer the particular problem being addressed, and which are solely numeric. None of these apply in the data mining context (Hand, 1998). Data mining technology is presented to pass the constraints of statistic methods. Data mining is a technology that blends traditional data analysis methods with sophisticated algorithms for processing large volumes of data. It has also opened up exciting opportunities for exploring and analyzing new types of data (Tan, Steinbach & Kumar, 2005). Brossette and Hymel (2008) believe that the main tenet of data mining is that the models and patterns contain insights that were previously unsuspected. For that reason alone, data mining is not an exercise in hypothesis-driven exploratory statistics, or hypothesis-driven statistical model building, because "hypothesis-driven" implies previously suspected. Data mining is a new discipline lying at the interface of statistics, database technology, pattern recognition, machine learning, and other areas (Hand, 1998).

There are several definitions for data mining, but all of these definitions have a same understating of underlying concept and there are keywords that are common in all of them. Tan et al. (2005) define data mining as the process of automatically discovering useful information in large data repositories. From Fayyad et al. (1996) point of view knowledge discovery in databases (KDD) is the overall process of discovering useful knowledge from data, and data mining refers to a particular step in this process that is the application of specific algorithms for extracting patterns from data. Usefulness is depends to domain of problem and user definition. Data mining is always associated with analysis. Everywhere that analysis of a small or large data set is needed, data mining can be useful.

Healthcare industry is one of the most interesting areas in which data mining may have an important practical impact. In healthcare, data mining is becoming increasingly popular for several reasons: the extremely large amounts of data; the need for organizations to make decisions based on the analysis of clinical and financial data; and the power to generate information that is fundamentally useful to all parties involved in the healthcare industry (Santos, Malheiros, Cavalheiro & Parente de Oliveira, 2013). Databases are growing in hospitals, clinics, medical research centers, pharmaceutical companies and other related businesses. Researchers and practitioners of this industry seek for solutions to enable them using hidden patterns of data, to extract valid knowledge for more accurate and timely diagnosis, effective genetic data analysis, more effective care, drug discovery, drug repositioning, more effective monitoring and evaluating system, outlier detection, reducing errors, improving decision making for physicians and personnel performance, improving customer relationship management in hospitals and clinics, healthcare tourism and also better understanding of characteristics of care processes. To the best of our knowledge there is not a survey that investigates general applications of knowledge discovery and data mining in healthcare industry. Thus, this chapter proposes a new classification of applications of knowledge discovery and data mining in healthcare industry through studying of recent five years researches. Studies show that knowledge discovery and data mining applications in healthcare industry can be classified to three major classes named patient view, market view and system view. Patient view includes papers that performed pure data mining on healthcare industry data. Market view includes papers that saw the patients as customers. System view includes papers that developed a decision support system.

The rest of chapter organized in two main sections. First section introduces knowledge discovery in databases, data mining and its main techniques, and also domain driving data mining (D^{3}M) methodology in short. Second section discusses data mining in healthcare industry, healthcare data set characteristics and challenges of applying domain driving data mining in this industry. Proposed classification is presented and chapter is concluded finally.

KNOWLEDGE DISCOVERY AND DATA MINING

Data Mining Tasks

Data mining tasks can be generally classified into two tasks of predictive and descriptive tasks (Tan et al, 2005). Predictive tasks predict the value of a particular attribute based on the values of other attributes. Classification, regression and anomaly detection are three types of predictive tasks. Descriptive tasks find human-interpretable patterns and relations that describe particular characteristics in data. Clustering, association rule mining and sequential pattern discovery are three types of descriptive tasks. These tasks are briefly explained in following.

- **Classification:** It is used for building predictive models for discrete target variables. In classification objects are assigned to one of several predefined categories. Decision tree classifiers, rule-based classifiers, neural networks, support vector machines and naïve Bayes classifiers are of this type. Each technique employs learning algorithm to identify a model that best fits the relationship between the attribute set and class label of input data. Obviously these techniques use supervised learning algorithm.

- **Regression:** It is used for building predictive models for continuous target variables assuming a linear or nonlinear model of dependency. Regression is greatly studied and discussed in statistics and neural networks. Regression uses supervised learning algorithm like classification.

- **Anomaly Detection:** It is the task of identifying observation known as anomalies or outliers whose characteristics are significantly different from the rest of the data. Applications like detection of fraud and unusual patterns of disease are of this type.

- **Clustering:** It seeks to find groups of closely related observation so that observations that belong to the same cluster are more similar to each other than observations that belong to other clusters. The greater the similarity (or homogeneity) within a group and the greater the difference between groups, the better or more distinct the clustering. There are not predefined class labels in clustering problems.

- **Association Rule Mining:** It is used to discover patterns in the form of implication rules or feature subsets that describe strongly associated features in the data. Association analysis includes two main parts. First part is discovering patterns from a large data set and second is selecting interesting patterns from the set of all possible patterns.

- **Sequential Pattern Discovery:** It is used to find rules that predict strong sequential dependencies among different events. It is applicable on databases that consist of sequences of ordered elements or events, recorded with or without a concrete notion of time.

DOMAIN DRIVEN DATA MINING (D³M)

Cao and his colleagues (Cao, Yu, Zhang & Zhao, 2010; Cao, 2010) has presented a methodology that emphasis on the importance of actionability of the knowledge presented in academic researches. They try to warn the existing big gap between academic objectives and what business managers needs for decision making in real world problems and situations. Actionable knowledge discovery aims to deliver knowledge that is business friendly, and which can be taken over by business people for seamless decision making. They believe that the process of data mining should not stop at pattern identification and building a model and satisfying technical significances, but also it should be able to solve real world problems.

Domain driven data mining has been proposed to engage the relevant aspects in actionable knowledge discovery. On top of the data-driven framework, domain driven data mining aims to develop proper methodologies and techniques for integrating domain knowledge, human roles and interaction, as well as actionability measures into the KDD process to discover and deliver actionable knowledge in the constrained environment. Furthermore, it aims to ensure the delivery of actionable and dependable knowledge that can be taken over by business people for direct decision-making and business operation purposes. Table 1 compares major dimensions of the traditional data-centered data mining and domain driven data mining (Cao, Yu, Zhang & Zhao, 2010).

KNOWLEDGE DISCOVERY IN HEALTHCARE INDUSTRY

Data Analysis in Healthcare Industry

Data mining is effectively nowadays employed in various industries like insurance, marketing,

Figure 1. The gap between academic and business objectives

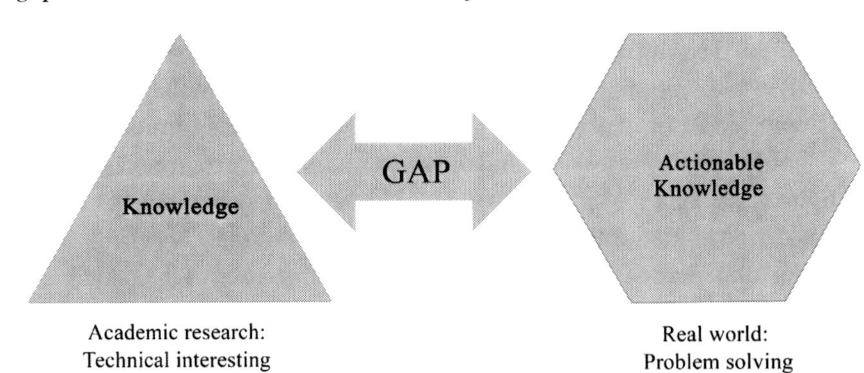

Table 1. Data-centered vs. domain driven data mining

Domain Driven	Traditional Data-Centered	Dimensions
Solving business problems	Developing innovative approaches	Aims
Let data and domain knowledge Tell hidden story in business; discovering actionable knowledge to satisfy real user needs	Let data create/verify research innovation; Demonstrate and push the use of novel algorithms discovering knowledge of interest technically	Goals
Problem-solving is the target	Algorithms are the focus	Objectives
Data and domain-oriented factors tell the story	Data tells the story	Object mined
Mining constrained real-life data	Mining abstract and refined datasets	Datasets
Ad-hoc, running-time and personalized model customization	Predefined	Models and methods
Human is in the circle of data mining process	Data mining is an automated process	Process
Technical and business aspects such as actionability	Technical sides such as accuracy and computational aspects	Performance
Business says "yes" or "no"	Evaluation based on technical metrics	Evaluation
Operationalizable business rules	Hidden patterns	Deliverables

banking, agriculture, customer relationship management, genetic, human right and other sciences. The World Health Organization (WHO) identified the potential of data mining for improving the problems in the medical domain as early as 1997. In the WHO research, emphasis was placed on the usefulness of knowledge detection from medical data repositories that could benefit medical diagnosis and prediction, patient health planning and progress, healthcare system monitoring and assessment, hospital and health services management, and disease prevention (Nahar, Imam, Tickle, & Chen, 2013). Researchers believe that data analysis in healthcare industry is different from other industries because of its heavy relying to background knowledge (Fig. 2). Bellazzi et al. (2011) reports the reasons as safety critical aspect of medical decision making, hardly reproducibility of data, affection of data by several sources of uncertainty and etc. Yeh, Wu and Tsao (2011) explain that Medical data analysis includes data gathering, preprocessing, result evaluation, favorable interaction, and discussions with clinicians for correct analytic results. Lavrac et al. (2007) believe that Healthcare are a knowledge-intensive

domain, in which neither data gathering nor data analysis can be successful without using knowledge about both the problem domain and the data analysis process.

HEALTHCARE DATA SETS CHARACTERISTICS

Data sets in healthcare industry have unique characteristics. Harrison (2008) and Cios and Moore (2002) comprehensively investigate these characteristics and some of them are explained at following. Raw medical data are voluminous and heterogeneous. Medical data may be collected from various images, interviews with the patient, laboratory data, and the physician's observations and interpretations. All these components may bear upon the diagnosis, prognosis, and treatment of the patient, and cannot be ignored. Each record may includes many different data elements, each representing a dimension that can vary in type and value, characterize an item of interest, such as a patient, disease, or specimen. Thus, high dimensionality is one the main characteristics of

Figure 2. All of the KDD steps need domain knowledge to be effective

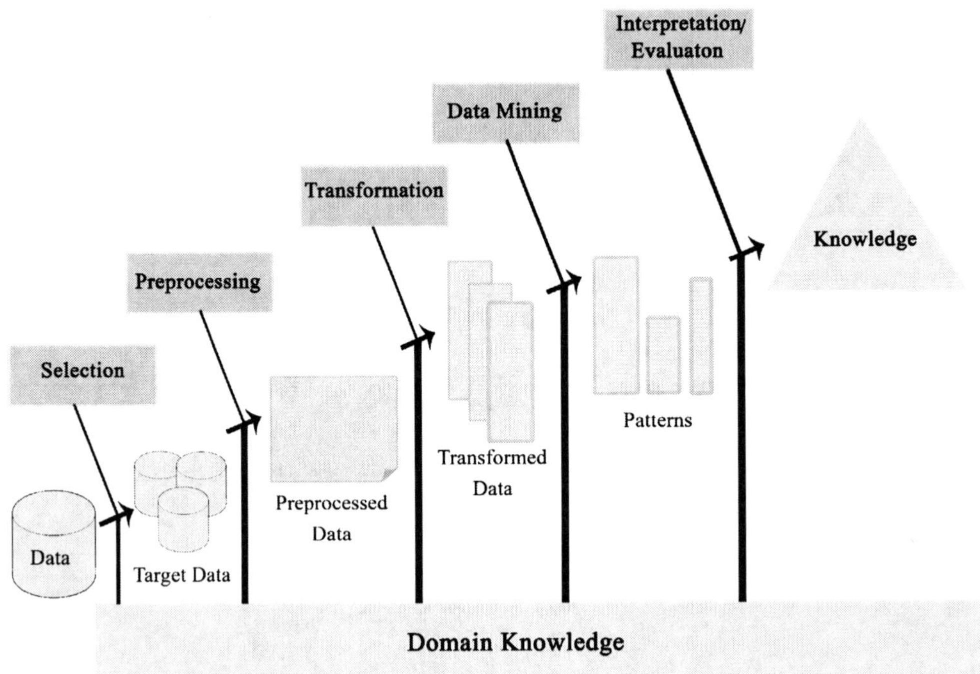

healthcare data. Diagnoses and other summary data in medical records are generally human interpretations of aggregates of observations and objective data values. Interpretations by different individuals may differ or even conflict.

Data elements in clinical records may not be meaningful outside of a particular temporal context. This phenomenon is particularly true for laboratory databases, which are largely composed of time sequences. So, temporal structure of data should be considered in analysis. Another issue is that data mining methods themselves, especially statistics, and the basic assumptions underlying these methods, may be fundamentally different for medical data and these differences should be considered before analysis. Finally, because medical data are collected on human subjects, there is an enormous ethical and legal tradition designed to prevent the abuse of patients and misuse of their data. Thus for working on such a data all of these constraints should be considered.

Many of data analysis constraint are resolved if data stored in an integrated and standard manner. This is caused data analysis gets more and more simple and precise and extracted knowledge will be more useful in practice. From a research perspective, integrated patient data constitute a computable collection of fine-grained longitudinal phenotypic profiles, facilitating cohort-wide investigations and knowledge discovery on an unprecedented scale (Jensen, Jensen & Brunak, 2012). The Electronic Health Records (EHR) offers the hope for such improved access to patient-specific information and should provide a major benefit both for the quality of care and for the quality of life for clinicians in practice (Shortliffe & Cimino, 2006). Jensen et al. (2012) believe that EHRs capture and integrate data on all aspects of care over time, with the data being represented according to relevant controlled vocabularies. EHR data comprise various data types, from structured information such as drug prescription data consisting of dates and dosages that are captured through a standardized ePrescription system, to unstructured data such as clinical narratives that describe the medical reasoning behind the prescription. This range of different data types highlights the challenge in EHR integration. However, knowledge discovery and data mining in EHRs make delivering personalized and stratified medicine, discovering disease comorbidities and adverse drug events, predicting future patient outcomes, genotype– phenotype association studies and other important applications of data mining in healthcare industry more simple and precise.

CLASSIFICATION OF KNOWLEDGE DISCOVERY AND DATA MINING APPLICATIONS IN HEALTHCARE INDUSTRY

Method

Figure 3 describes the analysis process of conducted survey. The main objective is to create a road map that clearly represents current research trends in this domain. Reviewed papers are mostly of recent five years, from 2008 to mid-2013 and are results of searching "data mining" keyword next to other keywords like "health", "clinic", "patient", "medicine" or "decision support systems" in several online databases include Elsevier, IEEE, ACM, Wiley and Springer. These keywords are generally key components of healthcare industry and can be found in title, keyword indices or abstract of papers in surveyed domain. Selected papers add some knowledge to healthcare industry and those that solely use health data sets for evaluating their algorithms were not considered. Also text mining papers were not considered. This filtering reduced the number of search results to 60 papers, from 24 journals and one proceeding, which were closely related to the survey objectives. The number of papers published in this domain is enormous and it is impossible to consider all of them. So, these papers are not covered all papers in this domain but in researchers belief other existing papers certainly lie in one of the classes of the proposed classification.

Classification

This section classifies knowledge discovery and data mining applications in healthcare industry. The proposed classification is based on main healthcare industry pillars. These pillars can be

Figure 3. Analysis process

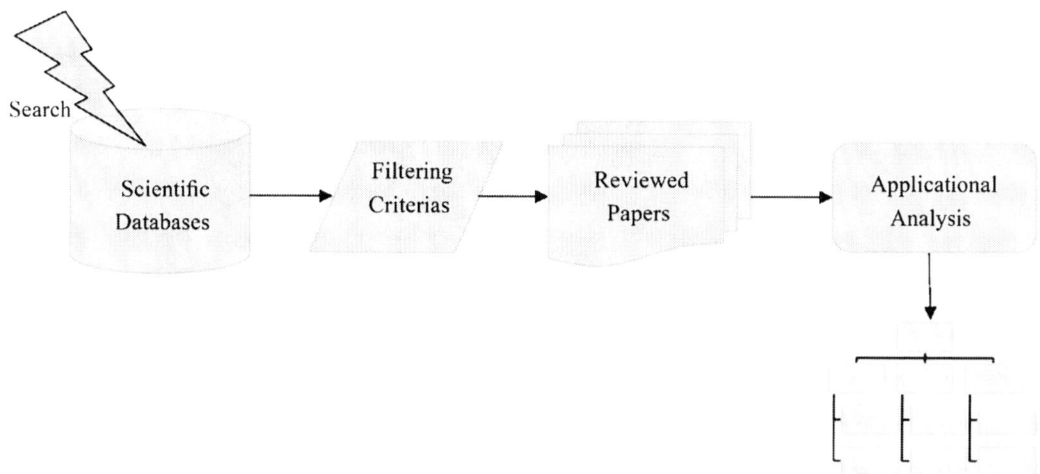

patient as most important pillar, information and knowledge of healthcare activities, practitioners include managers, physicians, nurses and other personnel, and business issues that cause the industry survive and establish the relationship between all pillars. Patients need high quality services and these services are based on high quality knowledge. Practitioners that deliver these services need high quality and available information and knowledge that enable them to make best decisions. Thus, they need systems and tools that at proper time and intelligently provide them latest and up-to-date knowledge. Healthcare businesses need customer acquisition and retention to increase their revenue and profit and automatically it cases businesses to improve their service quality. Thus, as it is shown in Figure 4 and Table 2, based on these pillars and reviewed papers, knowledge discovery and data mining applications in healthcare industry can be classified to three major classes named patient view, market view and system view. Patient view includes papers that their goal is discovering knowledge for improving patient care and treatment. Market view includes papers that their goal is discovering knowledge for improving healthcare businesses revenue.

System view includes papers that their goals is discovering knowledge and make it available to healthcare practitioners in an intelligent manner.

Patient View

Patient view includes papers that purely mined clinical data sets to derive models and discovered patterns. Patient view is divided to predictive models and pattern mining groups. Predictive models include papers that mine records of patients with specific diseases or characteristics to derive a predictive model for in time diagnosis, therapy and trial outcome prediction, determining risk factors of a disease and improving monitoring tasks. Some papers worked on administrative data of hospitals and clinics to improve services and reduce errors. As it can be seen in Table 3 almost 42 percent of the reviewed papers are in this group. Apparently predictive models group are most investigated field in this context. Building predictive models can be simple or complicated based on adopted data sets and techniques. Decision tree is one of the simplest techniques for implementation from technical perspective and for interpreting from a domain expert perspective. Moon, Kang, Jitpita-

Figure 4. The proposed classification

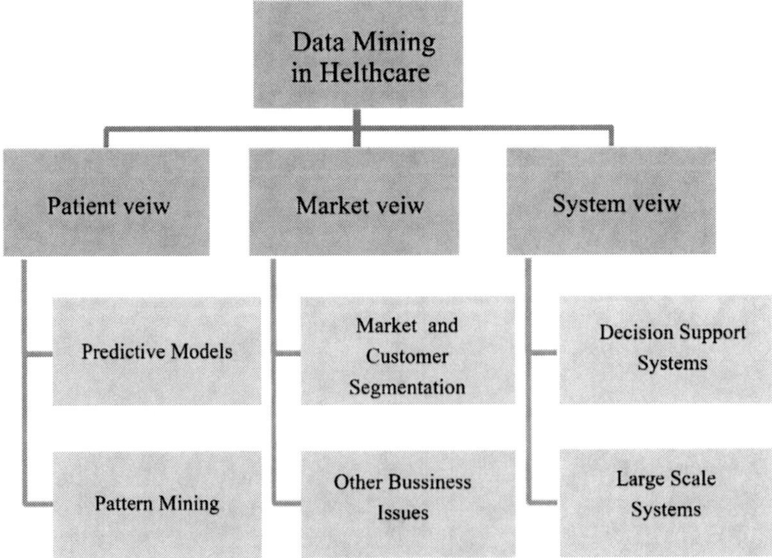

Table 2. The proposed classification including reviewed papers

Percent	Number	References	Group	Class
42%	25	(Bellazzi et al, 2008), (Moon et al, 2012), (Rahman et al, 2011), (Gregori et al, 2011), (Meng et al, 2013), (Marcano-Cedeno et al, 2013), (Yang et al, 2009), (Ghazavi et al, 2008), (Parhizi et al, 2013), (Alizadehsani et al, 2013), (Lehman et al, 2005), (Gil & Johnsson, 2010), (Chi et al, 2010), (Yan et al, 2009), (Zayed et al, 2013), (Roham et al, 2012), (Delen et al, 2009), (Kandula et al, 2011), (Zhao & Weng, 2011), (Bennett et al, 2012), (Hauskrecht et al, 2013), (Lee et al, 2011), (Bellazzi et al, 2011), (Chen et al, 2011), (Shimada et al, 2008)	**Predictive Models**	**Patient view**
18%	11	(Nahar et al, 2013), (Guerrero et al, 2012), (Lazarou et al, 2012), (Kakilehto et al, 2009), (Tai & Chiu, 2009), (Ou-Yang et al, 2013), (Cruz, 2013), (Semenova, 2004), (Yao et al, 2011), (Lee & Giraud-Carrier, 2013), (Lavrac et al,2007)	**Pattern Mining**	
8%	5	(Chen et al, 2012), (Lee & Shih, 2009), (Wei et al, 2012), (Jo et al, 2010), (Hung et al, 2010)	**Market and Customer Segmentation**	**Market view**
5%	3	(Lee et al, 2008), (Orentlicher, 2010), (Shanmugam, 2012)	**Other Business Issues**	
20%	12	(Chae et al, 2003), (Chi et al, 2008), (Yeh et al, 2011), (Alonso et al, 2002), (Kumar et al, 2010), (Da Silva et al, 2011), (Aral et al, 2012), (Ting et al, 2011), (Tenorio et al, 2011), (Cho et al, 2013), (Brossette& Hymel, 2008), (Tartarisco et al, 2012)	**Decision Support Systems**	**System view**
7%	4	(Santos et al, 2013), (El-Sappagh & El-Masri, 2013), (Yan et al, 2004), (Vicente et al, 2004)	**Large Scale Systems**	
	60			

klert & Kim (2012) have used Classification and regression trees (CART) to characterize smoking behavior among older adults by assessing the psychological distress, physical health status, alcohol use, and demographic variables in relations to the current smoking. Parhizi, Steege and Pasupathy (2013) have used a tree-based Chi-Square Automatic Interaction Detection (CHAID) to identify relationships between multiple psychosocial factors and dimensions of fatigue using data mining classification methods. Kumar et al. (2010) believe that people typically use decision trees because they are easy to explain the classification to domain experts. Often, this comprehensibility comes at the expense of accuracy. Artificial Neural Networks (ANNs) are black box artificial intelligence-based algorithms that have been until recently quite popular in clinical medicine, although they are prone to overfitting (Bellazzi et al, 2011). Accuracy and performance of ANN based models are mostly depends on domain, selected features, data set and mining software. In Marcano-Cedeno et al. (2013) in contrast to most of studies that are focused in determining survival, predicting disability or the recovery of patients, and looking for the factors that are better at predicting the patient's condition after suffering an acquired brain injury (ABI), the purpose was the novel application of data mining to predict the outcomes of the cognitive rehabilitation of patients with ABI. They used decision tree, multilayer perceptron and general regression neural network to construct the prediction models. In Delen, Fuller, McCann & Ray (2009) the healthcare coverage of individuals has been examined by applying artificial neural network and decision tree on a wide-variety of predictive factors and they claimed that experimental results indicated that the most accurate classifier for this phenomenon was the multi-layer perceptron type artificial neural network model. A more robust approach, grounded in statistical learning theory, is provided by support vector machine (SVM), which may handle both linear and nonlinear decision boundaries. Although the learned classifiers may be difficult to interpret, the classification performance can be quite high (Bellazzi et al, 2011). In Kandula, Zeng-Treitler, Chen, Salomon & Bray (2011) proposed a bootstrapping method that supplements ICD-9 codes with lab results, medications, etc. to build classification models that can be used to identify cohorts more accurately. The proposed method does not require prior information about the true class of the patients. They used SVM to build the models. Probabilistic classifiers, such as Naive Bayes classifiers and Bayesian networks are also exploited in the medical literature, although less frequently (Bellazzi et al, 2011). In Zhao & Weng (2011) a novel method have been proposed that combines PubMed knowledge and Electronic Health Records to develop a weighted Bayesian Network Inference (BNI) model for pancreatic cancer prediction. They claimed that in an evaluation using a case-control dataset, the weighted BNI model significantly outperformed the conventional BNI and k-Nearest Neighbor (KNN) and SVM. Anomaly or outlier detection is another predictive data mining task that is exploited in the literature, although less frequently. Hauskrecht et al. (2013) have developed and evaluated a data-driven approach for detecting unusual (anomalous) patient-management decisions using past patient cases stored in electronic health records (EHRs). Their hypothesis was that a patient-management decision that is unusual with respect to past patient care may be due to an error and that it is worthwhile to generate an alert if such a decision is encountered. They used SVM to build their model. Bennett, Doub and Selove (2012) believe that next version of predictive models in future are the patient personalized ones and it is possible through combining mixing

genetic and clinical indicators, rather than using one or the other.

Second group of patient view is pattern mining. Papers in this group investigates mining hidden relations, dependencies and interesting patterns, finding useful and meaningful groups, determining effective and key factors in patients data with a specific disease and also in administrative data sets. Patterns embedded in large volumes of clinical data may provide important insights into the characteristics of patients or care delivery processes, but may be difficult to identify by traditional means (Rahman & Hasan, 2011). Almost 18 percent of the reviewed papers are in this group. In this context, association rule discovery is the most popular descriptive technique. In contrast to other data mining techniques, association rule is not driven from statistics. In Healthcare, association rules are considered to be quite useful as they offer the possibility to conduct intelligent diagnosis and extract invaluable information and build important knowledge bases quickly and automatically (Rahman & Hasan, 2011). Nahar, Imam, Tickle and Chen (2013) investigate the sick and healthy factors which contribute to heart disease for males and females. Association rule mining, a computational intelligence approach, is used to identify these factors. In Tai & Chiu (2009) association rule mining has been applied to explore the labyrinthian network of Attention Deficit/Hyperactivity Disorder (ADHD) comorbidity, and to examine the practicality of association rule mining in comorbidity studies using clinic databases. Clustering is also used frequently in this context especially in business related issues. Self organizing map (SOM) is a type of artificial neural network that because it produces a low-dimensional (typically two-dimensional), discretized representation of the high dimensional input space that is one of the main characteristics of clinical data sets, called a map, is one of the most popular clustering techniques in this context. SOMs are different from other artificial neural networks in the sense that they use a neighborhood function to preserve the topological properties of the input space (Wikipedia, Self-organizing map, n. d.). Guerrero et al. (2012) have used SOM to detect a residual area of low satisfaction in dialysis patients. Lee and Giraud-Carrier (2013) have adapted and extended association rule mining and clustering algorithms to extract useful knowledge regarding diabetes and high blood pressure from mined data set and to demonstrate how data mining techniques may be used to support evidence-based medicine.

Market View

One of the interesting issues for businesses in every industry is customer relationship management (CRM) for better customer acquisition and retention. Improving quality of care and customer satisfaction are the key business drivers in healthcare industry (Hung, Hung, Tsai & Jiang, 2010). The effective and efficient utilization of IT is a method for implementing a successful CRM strategy to understand customer needs, satisfy customer demands, mine for valuable customer information, identify target and potential customers, realize the maximum customer value, increase customer loyalty, and finally maximize profits (Chen, Cheng, Lai, Hsu & Syu, 2012). Market view includes papers that look at the patient as a potential customer. These papers are 13 percent of all the reviewed papers and divide to market and customer segmentation, and other business related issues groups. Market and customer segmentation through data mining are one of the most popular research fields in CRM context. The health care industry is one of the world's largest and fastest-growing industries (Wikipedia, Healthcare industry, n. d.). As the competition increased in this industry, related businesses like hospitals, clinics, pharmaceutical companies and others needed to identify their core competencies and increase their competitive advantages. CRM can be the most valuable core competency that a business can have especially in health related

business as people care about their health more than anything else. However, apparently market view is the smallest research area in this context and it can be because of difficulties of accessing to financial data for researches and also constraints that exist because of ethical and legal issues. But definitely like other industries, businesses in healthcare industry can use data mining for market analysis, discovering customer behavior patterns and designing effective marketing strategies. Papers in market and customer segmentation group mostly mine customer and market data to find the profitable segments of customers and maximize the profit through developing targeted effective marketing strategies. Chen et al. (2012) propose a two-stage clustering-classification model through initially integrating the RFM attribute and K-means algorithm for clustering the target customer segment (TCS) patients and then integrating the global discretization method and the rough set theory for classifying hospitalized departments and optimizing healthcare services. Wei, Lin, Weng and Wu (2012) develop an extended RFM (recency, frequency, and monetary) model, namely LRFM (length, recency, frequency, and monetary) model, by adopting SOM technique for a children's dental clinic to segment its dental patients. Second group in market view include papers in others business related issues like hospital selection, health tourism and pharmaceutical marketing. Shanmugam, (2012) explains that mainly for the sake of affordability, many patients in much advanced nations, often voluntarily, seek medical services in far less underdeveloped nations. He applies a data mining approach to compute and interpret economic indices and portray the economic booming in the hosting nations which render the medical treatments to the patients who emanate from the guest nations.

System View

Clinical decision support systems (CDSS) are systems that support clinician to make effective decisions in diagnosis, prognosis, therapy and prescription and also used for preventing medical errors, especially diagnostic errors, reducing cost, and improving patient safety (Mitchell et al, 2011). System view is divided into two groups of decision support systems and large scale systems. Former includes papers that explicitly propose an algorithm, information flow diagram, application or architecture for decision support systems. Yeh et al. (2011) have combined temporal abstraction with data mining techniques for analyzing dialysis patients' biochemical data to develop a decision support system. The mined temporal patterns are helpful for clinicians to predict hospitalization of hemodialysis patients and to suggest immediate treatments to avoid hospitalization. Chi, Street and Katz (2010) have proposed a machine learning based expert system approach, called optimal decision path finder (ODPF), to dynamically determine the test that is most likely to be informative in terms of diagnostic accuracy while minimizing the time and money spent on diagnostic testing. Tartarisco et al. (2012) have proposed an automatic simple, compact, wireless, personalized and cost efficient pervasive architecture for the evaluation of the stress state of individual subjects suitable for prolonged stress monitoring during normal activity. It used SOM to cluster the received bio-signals from a wearable device. Papers propose architecture or systems that can perform or have potential to perform knowledge discovery and data mining in a large scale manner are in the large scale system group. Santos et al. (2013) have described that the large-scale adoption of data mining has been limited thus far because it is difficult to use, especially for non-expert users and one way to facilitate data mining by non-expert users is to automate the process. They presented an automated data mining system that allows public health decision makers that probably do not have any knowledge about data mining techniques and tools, to access analytical information regarding brain tumors. The difference between previous data mining approaches and the approach proposed in

their study is that the proposed approach is concept-centric; the reports stem from concepts selected by users from the domain ontology. In addition, the approach does not require users to select input parameters; instead, they only select the concepts to be analyzed. System view includes the considerable number of reviewed papers, about 20 percent. It is considerable because developing a decision support system in small or large scale, have their own complexity and challenges in addition of all of common challenges of applying knowledge discovery and data mining in healthcare industry. Mitchell et al. (2011) believe that these challenges are of three major types. The first is domain challenges that related to large number of interacting and complicating conditions or factors that is usually involved in clinical decisions; relevant information and available options are incomplete, uncertain, and often changing with the progression of the disease(s), the genetic makeup of the patients, and the outcome of the actions. Second challenge is system challenges that related to the constantly varying clinical workflows, rapidly changing information technology platforms, and exponentially accumulating information and data of various forms that render many subsystems or processes incompatible or obsolete very quickly. These in turn complicate the proper encoding, maintenance, and integration of the information and knowledge needed to support cost-effective decision making; and the third challenge is usage challenges that related to existing of different users with vastly different backgrounds, different objectives, and even different preferences in their decision making approaches for the same system and difficulty of fulfilling their needs.

DISCUSSION

According to the united nation International Standard Industrial Classification (ISIC) definition, the healthcare industry generally consist of three major activities include hospital activities, medical and dental practice activities, and other human health activities (Wikipedia, Healthcare industry, n. d.). Knowledge discovery and data mining have powerful capability to discover hidden patterns in data related to all of these activities. Wherever significant volume of stored data are accessible, knowledge discovery and data mining can effectively improve system performance or enhance the knowledge related to mined data. Discovered patterns and derived models help practitioners to make the right, effective and timely decisions and lead to better services.

Knowledge discovery and data mining in healthcare industry is much more knowledge intensive in compared to other industries and this should be considered in all of KDD steps from feature selection to choosing the data mining techniques and evaluation and interpretation of results. Problem and data set characteristics and analyzing goals should be considered in choosing every techniques used in KDD steps. Because for example selecting an unrelated feature or ignoring an important feature can heavily affect final results or can lead to incorrect results. Also an analysis that does not solve the healthcare practitioner problems is not useful even if it satisfies technical measures. That is why the synergy between technical and healthcare domain experts to recognize data characteristics, to determine significance and effectivity of every feature and to choose the most effective techniques for all steps of data analysis is the key success factor in KDD. If we determine the criteria of success assessment rigidly the ability of extracted knowledge to solve real world problems, the necessity and importance of existence of this synergy will be much more. Lack or incompleteness of both sides leads to poor problem definition and analysis and therefore results to less valuable or worthless knowledge.

Each data mining techniques include classification or clustering or association rules mining has specific characteristics and analyze the data in a different manner. If these characteristics and extracted knowledge of these techniques used to complete each other rather than using them in a divergence manner, final results will be more valuable. However, data mining techniques are not without imperfections. Being imperfect for any reason, intrinsic or data set, other techniques such as statistical techniques and algorithms, case based reasoning, rule-based methods, evolutionary algorithms and machine learning techniques can help to improve data analysis.

One of the advantages of research in patient view class is its variety of research areas. Literature review shows that available data sets of large number of diseases including mortal ones such as heart disease and cancer to less mortal ones like children's obesity or urological dysfunctions are investigated. Each data set can be inspiration for new models and patterns. Wherever patients data set with a specific disease are available, it can be used to build predictive models and discovered valuable patterns. These models and patterns can be related to final state or trial and rehabilitation activities results of patients.

Wherever the aim of data miner is discovering hidden relationships between data elements, there is no technique more applicable than association rule mining. Healthcare industry is not an exception too. These elements in the healthcare are disease symptoms, trials, medications, prescription and reaction. These elements along with demographic and psychographic data are almost fixed in most data sets. Mining association rules elegantly discover hidden relationships between these elements and lead to producing new knowledge, improving care processes and reducing care and service errors. Clustering in this domain in most cases is used as a supplement for mining association rules.

Competition among businesses in healthcare industry has grown like other industries. Knowledge about customers and market to create competitive advantage and implement powerful CRM is the most important assets of a business. In order to manage customers better, organizations need to classify their customers. Among the customers that organizations deal with them, few ones are most profitable. These are customers that an organization try to continue its relationship with them. Additionally, segmenting customers to separate groups in which all members are similar in many characteristics, allowing the organization to design marketing strategies tailored to the needs and desires of each group. Most of researches on market view area were somehow related to CRM and it reflects the importance of this issue in healthcare industry businesses.

The development of decision support systems is a step forward to solve real world problems, where uncertainty and high dimensionality cause decision making be a difficult task. It causes extracted knowledge be applicable for managers, physicians in care environment, and individuals outside of care environment through personal health systems. Heart of a decision support system is the knowledge that it uses to make decision. The challenges facing researchers interested in developing decision support systems are getting the data and processing them automatically or semi-automatically and efficiently, optimal knowledge updatability and dynamic learning of system, efficient result evaluation and presentation. It seems that one of the limitations in developing of decision support systems is automating preprocessing step. However, research shows that the role of the user in this step should still remain strong. Technically it is not simply possible, but the standard and structured data storages like electronic health records is a step towards improving data sets structure and optimizing preprocessing step. Also, systems must be able to be compatible with multi-class decision making problems, because most of real world problems in this industry deal with several complicated conditions that are even unknown in worst case. For this reason the main criticism that can make on several number researches is oversimplification of problems. Ongoing advances in computer networks and distributed systems as well as powerful software architectures provide interesting research areas in designing and implementing large-scale systems to improve collaboration and resource sharing.

Several numbers of papers explicitly or implicitly considered D^3M methodology and could get close to real world problem solving without exorbitance problem simplification. However, there is a long way to realize all the specifications of D^3M methodology in healthcare industry as it is described in Cao et al. (2010). Wide research areas, different approaches in diagnosis, prognosis, therapy and other car processes, continuous developments in information technology and medicine cause that presenting comprehensive solutions harder. However, there are researches (Sebastian and Then, 2011; Kuo, Lonie, Sonenberg and Paizis, 2007; Santos et al, 2013) that make well considerable progression toward realizing D^3M visions.

The main limitations of our research were dependency of knowledge discovery and data mining in healthcare industry to background knowledge and also its variety of applications. Analyzing models and parameters used to build the models, evaluating discovered pattern and derived models and generally presented results are affected by mentioned limitations. On the other hand, dependency of data mining in healthcare industry to context and data makes accurate comparing of data mining techniques difficult.

According to our research's applicational perspective, the ideas at macro level to improve using knowledge discovery in healthcare industry can be as following:

- Using domain driven data mining in healthcare industry to enhance the actionability of extracting knowledge.
- Defining the problem, designing and conducting knowledge discovery toward solving real world problems in healthcare industry.
- Designing a healthcare driven data mining (HD^2M) framework in all dimensions.

- Proposing customized KDD techniques according to general characteristics of healthcare data.

These four ideas stress on D³M primary objective that is reducing the gap exists between research and real world problem solving. Here the domain is healthcare, so we seek for healthcare specific data mining problem definition and design, techniques and frameworks, or in other words, healthcare driven data mining (HD²M). The aim is making extracted knowledge or models and pattern more useful and executable and somehow easier to understand and to use for healthcare industry practitioners.

- Making discovered patterns and derived models usable for healthcare industry practitioners through developing decision support systems to help them for making better decisions.
- Proposing large scale and distributed architectures for decision support systems using novel technologies to enhance system availability.

As discussed before, one of the main ways of making extracted knowledge from knowledge discovery and data mining easier to use and also executable for practitioners is providing it in small and large scale decision support systems. Developing intelligent decision support systems that their knowledge is provided through knowledge discovery and data mining engine is another major research area.

- Proposing large scale and distributed architectures for decision support systems that consider knowledge integration after KDD.

The world contains a vast array of complex and diverse data, but locating and connecting the information are difficult (Cases et al, 2013). One of the ways to overcome these problems is developing a framework to connect and integrate different data mining processes and extracted knowledge without completely integrating original data sets.

- Proposing real time data analysis frameworks to use KDD in real time healthcare applications.

Another research idea can be developing decision support systems that use data mining for analyzing instant patient data in real time situations that timely decision making is very crucial such as operating room, intensive care unit (ICU) or emergency department to help practitioners make vital decisions better and quicker.

- Proposing methods and approaches for mining EHRs more efficient.
- Discovering analysis opportunities to improve CRM in healthcare industry businesses with respect to the ethical and legal constraints.

CONCLUSION

This chapter has reviewed recent studies on knowledge discovery applications in healthcare industry and proposes a new classification of these applications. Studies has shown that knowledge discovery and data mining applications in healthcare industry can be classified to three major classes named patient view, market view and system view. Patient view includes papers that performed pure data mining on healthcare industry data. Market view includes papers that saw the patients as customers. System view includes papers that developed a decision support system. The goal of this classification was identifying research opportunities and gaps for researchers are interested to this context.

ACKNOWLEDGMENT

The authors would like to thank the anonymous reviewers and the editor for their insightful comments and suggestions.

REFERENCES

Alizadehsani, et al. (2013). A data mining approach for diagnosis of coronary artery disease. *Computer Methods and Programs in Biomedicine, 111*(1), 52–61. doi:10.1016/j.cmpb.2013.03.004 PMID:23537611

Alonso, F., Caraca-Valente, P. J., Gonzalez, A. L., & Montes, C. (2002). Combining expert knowledge and data mining in a medical diagnosis domain. *Expert Systems with Applications, 23*(4), 367–375. doi:10.1016/S0957-4174(02)00072-6

Aral, K. D., Guvenir, H. A., Sabuncuoglu, I., & Akar, A. R. (2012). A prescription fraud detection model. *Computer Methods and Programs in Biomedicine, 106*(1), 37–46. doi:10.1016/j.cmpb.2011.09.003 PMID:22088866

Bellazzi, R., Ferrazzi, F., & Sacchi, L. (2011). Predictive data mining in clinical medicine: a focus on selected methods and applications. *WIREs Data Mining and Knowledge Discovery, 1*(5), 416–430. doi:10.1002/widm.23

Bellazzi, R., & Zupan, B. (2008). Predictive data mining in clinical medicine: Current issues and guidelines. *International Journal of Medical Informatics, 77*(2), 81–97. doi:10.1016/j.ijmedinf.2006.11.006 PMID:17188928

Bennett, C. C., Doub, T. W., & Selove, R. (2012). EHRs connect research and practice: Where predictive modeling, artificial intelligence, and clinical decision support intersect. *Health Policy and Technology, 1*(2), 105–114. doi:10.1016/j.hlpt.2012.03.001

Brossette, S. E., Hymel P. A. (2008). Data mining and infection control. *Clinics in Laboratory Medicine, 28*(1), 119–126.

Cao, L. (2010). Domain-driven data mining: challenges and prospects. *IEEE Transactions on Knowledge and Data Engineering, 22*(6), 755–769. doi:10.1109/TKDE.2010.32

Cao, L., Yu, S. P., Zhang, C., & Zhao, Y. (2010). *Domain driven data mining.* Springer. doi:10.1007/978-1-4419-5737-5

Cases, et al. (2013). Improving data and knowledge management to better integrate health care and research. *Journal of Internal Medicine, 274*(4), 321–328. doi:10.1111/joim.12105 PMID:23808970

Chae, Y., Kim, H., Tark, H., Park, H., & Ho, S. (2003). Analysis of healthcare quality indicator using data mining and decision support system. *Expert Systems with Applications, 24*(2), 167–172. doi:10.1016/S0957-4174(02)00139-2

Chen, H. Y., Chuang, C. H., Yang, Y. J., & Wu, T. P. (2011). Exploring the risk factors of preterm birth using data mining. *Expert Systems with Applications, 38*(5), 5384–5387. doi:10.1016/j.eswa.2010.10.017

Chen, Y. S., Cheng, C. H., Lai, C. J., Hsu, C. Y., & Syu, H. J. (2012). Identifying patients in target customer segments using a two-stage clustering-classification approach: A hospital-based assessment. *Computers in Biology and Medicine, 42*(2), 213–221. doi:10.1016/j.compbiomed.2011.11.010 PMID:22177941

Chi, C. L., Street, W. N., & Katz, D. A. (2010). A decision support system for cost-effective diagnosis. *Artificial Intelligence in Medicine, 50*(3), 149–161. doi:10.1016/j.artmed.2010.08.001 PMID:20933375

Chi, C. L., Street, W. N., & Ward, M. M. (2008). Building a hospital referral expert system with a prediction and optimization-based decision support system algorithm. *Journal of Biomedical Informatics*, *41*(2), 371–386. doi:10.1016/j.jbi.2007.10.002 PMID:18054523

Cho, I., Park, I., Kim, E., Lee, E., & Bates, D. W. (2013). Using EHR data to predict hospital-acquired pressure ulcers: A prospective study of a bayesian network model. *International Journal of Medical Informatics*, *82*(11), 1059–1067. doi:10.1016/j.ijmedinf.2013.06.012 PMID:23891086

Cios, K., & Moore, G. W. (2002). Uniqueness of medical data mining. *Artificial Intelligence in Medicine*, *26*(1-2), 1–24. doi:10.1016/S0933-3657(02)00049-0 PMID:12234714

Cruz, A. M. (2013). Evaluating record history of medical devices using association discovery and clustering techniques. *Expert Systems with Applications*, *40*(13), 5292–5305. doi:10.1016/j.eswa.2013.03.034

Da Silva, S. F., Ribeiro, M. X., Batista Neto, J. D. E. S., Traina-Jr, C., & Traina, A. J. M. (2011). Improving the ranking quality of medical image retrieval using a genetic feature selection method. *Decision Support Systems*, *51*(4), 810–820. doi:10.1016/j.dss.2011.01.015

Delen, D., Fuller, C., McCann, C., & Ray, D. (2009). Analysis of healthcare coverage: A data mining approach. *Expert Systems with Applications*, *36*(2), 995–1003. doi:10.1016/j.eswa.2007.10.041

El-Sappagh, S. H., & El-Masri, S. (2013). A distributed clinical decision support system architecture. *Journal of King Saud University-Computer and Information Sciences*, *26*(1), 69–78. doi:10.1016/j.jksuci.2013.03.005

Fayyad, U., Piatetsky-Shapiro, G., & Smyth, P. (1996). From Data Mining to Knowledge Discovery in Databases. *AI Magazine*, *17*(3), 37–54.

Garrett, P., & Seidman, P. (2011). *EMR vs EHR – What is the Difference?*. Retrieved August 10, 2013, from http://www.healthit.gov/buzz-blog/electronic-health-and-medical-records/emr-vs-ehr-difference/

Ghazavi, S. N., & Liao, T. W. (2008). Medical data mining by fuzzy modeling with selected features. *Artificial Intelligence in Medicine*, *43*(3), 195–206. doi:10.1016/j.artmed.2008.04.004 PMID:18534831

Gil, D., & Johnsson, M. (2010). Using support vector machines in diagnoses of urological dysfunctions. *Expert Systems with Applications*, *37*(6), 4713–4718. doi:10.1016/j.eswa.2009.12.055

Gregori, D., Petrinco, M., Bo, S., Rosato, R., Pagano, E., Berchialla, P., & Merletti, F. (2011). Using data mining techniques in monitoring diabetes care. The simpler the better? *Journal of Medical Systems*, *35*(2), 277–281. doi:10.1007/s10916-009-9363-9 PMID:20703563

Guerrero, et al. (2012). Self-Organising Maps: A new way to screen the level of satisfaction of dialysis patients. *Expert Systems with Applications*, *39*(10), 8793–8798. doi:10.1016/j.eswa.2012.02.001

Hand, D. J. (1998). Data mining: statistics and more? *American Statistical Association*, *52*, 112–118.

Harrison, J. H. (2008). Introduction to the mining of clinical data. *Clinics in Laboratory Medicine*, *28*(1), 1–7. doi:10.1016/j.cll.2007.10.001 PMID:18194715

Hauskrecht, M., Batal, I., Valko, M., Visweswaran, S., Cooper, G. F., & Clermont, G. (2013). Outlier detection for patient monitoring and alerting. *Journal of Biomedical Informatics*, *46*(1), 47–55. doi:10.1016/j.jbi.2012.08.004 PMID:22944172

Healthcare Industry. (n.d.). In *Wikipedia*. Retrieved Sep 17, 2013, from http://en.wikipedia.org/wiki/Health_care_industry

Hung, S. Y., Hung, W. H., Tsai, C. A., & Jiang, S. C. (2010). Critical factors of hospital adoption on CRM system: Organizational and information system perspectives. *Decision Support Systems*, *48*(4), 592–603. doi:10.1016/j.dss.2009.11.009

Jensen, P. B., & Jensen, L, J, Brunak, S. (2012). Mining electronic health records: towards better research applications and clinical care. *Nature Reviews. Transactional Genetics*, *13*(6), 395–405.

Jo, H. S., Hwang, M. S., & Lee, H. (2010). Market segmentation of health information use on the Internet in Korea. *International Journal of Medical Informatics*, *79*(10), 707–715. doi:10.1016/j.ijmedinf.2010.07.006 PMID:20810307

Kakilehto, T., Salo, S., & Larmas, M. (2009). Data mining of clinical oral health documents for analysis of the longevity of different restorative materials in Finland. *International Journal of Medical Informatics*, *78*(12), e68–e74. doi:10.1016/j.ijmedinf.2009.04.004 PMID:19428290

Kandula, S., Zeng-Treitler, Q., Chen, L., Salomon, W. L., & Bray, B. E. (2011). A bootstrapping algorithm to improve cohort identification using structured data. *Journal of Biomedical Informatics*, *44*(1), S63–S68. doi:10.1016/j.jbi.2011.10.013 PMID:22079803

Kumar, M., Ghani, R., & Mei, Z. S. (2010). Data mining to predict and prevent errors in health insurance claims processing. In *Proceedings of the 16th ACM SIGKDD International Conference on Knowledge Discovery and Data Mining* (pp. 65-74). ACM.

Kuo, Y. T., Lonie, A., Sonenberg, L., & Paizis, K. (2007). Domain Ontology Driven Data Mining. In *Proceedings of the 2007 international Workshop on Domain Driven Data Mining* (pp 11-17). Academic Press.

Lavrac, N., Bohanec, M., Pur, A., Cestnik, B., Debeljak, M., & Kobler, A. (2007). Data mining and visualization for decision support and modeling of public health-care resources. *Journal of Biomedical Informatics*, *40*(4), 438–447. doi:10.1016/j.jbi.2006.10.003 PMID:17157076

Lazarou, C., Karaolis, M., Matalas, A. L., & Panagiotakos, D. B. (2012). Dietary patterns analysis using data mining method. An application to data from the CYKIDS study. *Computer Methods and Programs in Biomedicine*, *108*(2), 706–714. doi:10.1016/j.cmpb.2011.12.011 PMID:22296977

Lee, J. W., & Giraud-Carrier, C. (2013). Results on mining NHANES data: A case study in evidence-based medicine. *Computers in Biology and Medicine*, *43*(5), 493–503. doi:10.1016/j.compbiomed.2013.02.018 PMID:23566395

Lee, T. T., Liu, C. Y., Kuo, Y. H., Mills, M. E., Fong, J. G., & Hung, C. (2011). Application of data mining to the identification of critical factors in patient falls using a web-based reporting system. *International Journal of Medical Informatics*, *80*(2), 141–150. doi:10.1016/j.ijmedinf.2010.10.009 PMID:21115393

Lee, W., & Shih, B. (2009). Application of neural networks to recognize profitable customers for dental services marketing-a case of dental clinics in Taiwan. *Expert Systems with Applications*, *36*(1), 199–208. doi:10.1016/j.eswa.2007.09.028

Lee, W., Shih, B., & Chung, Y. S. (2008). The exploration of consumers' behavior in choosing hospital by the application of neural network. *Expert Systems with Applications*, *34*(2), 806–816. doi:10.1016/j.eswa.2006.10.020

Lehman, T. M., Guld, M. O., Deselaers, T., Keysers, D., Schubert, H., & Spitzer, K. et al. (2005). Automatic categorization of medical images for content-based retrieval and data mining. *Computerized Medical Imaging and Graphics*, *29*(2-3), 143–155. doi:10.1016/j.compmedimag.2004.09.010 PMID:15755534

Liao, S. H., Chu, P. H., & Hsiao, P. Y. (2012). Data mining techniques and applications – A decade review from 2000 to 2011. *Expert Systems with Applications*, *39*(12), 11303–11311. doi:10.1016/j.eswa.2012.02.063

Marcano-Cedeno, A., Chausa, P., Garcia, A., Caceres, C., Tormos, J. M., & Gomez, E. J. (2013). Data mining applied to the cognitive rehabilitation of patients with acquired brain injury. *Expert Systems with Applications*, *40*(4), 1054–1060. doi:10.1016/j.eswa.2012.08.034

Meng, X. H., Huang, Y. X., Rao, D. P., Zhang, Q., & Liu, Q. (2013). Comparison of three data mining models for predicting diabetes or prediabetes by risk factors. *The Kaohsiung Journal of Medical Sciences*, *29*(2), 93–99. doi:10.1016/j.kjms.2012.08.016 PMID:23347811

Mitchell, et al. (2011). 50 Years of Informatics Research on Decision Support: What's Next. *Methods of Information in Medicine*, *50*, 525–535. doi:10.3414/ME11-06-0004 PMID:22146915

Moon, S. S., Kang, S. Y., Jitpitaklert, W., & Kim, S. B. (2012). Decision tree models for characterizing smoking patterns of older adults. *Expert Systems with Applications*, *39*(1), 445–451. doi:10.1016/j.eswa.2011.07.035

Nahar, J., Imam, T., Tickle, K. S., & Chen, Y. P. (2013). Association rule mining to detect factors which contribute to heart disease in males and females. *Expert Systems with Applications*, *40*(4), 1086–1093. doi:10.1016/j.eswa.2012.08.028

Orentlicher, D. (2010). Prescription data mining and the protection of patients' interests. *The Journal of Law, Medicine & Ethics*, *38*(1), 74–84. doi:10.1111/j.1748-720X.2010.00468.x PMID:20446986

Ou-Yang, C., Agustianty, S., & Wang, H. C. (2013). Developing a data mining approach to investigate association between physician prescription and patient outcome – A study on re-hospitalization in Stevens–Johnson Syndrome. *Computer Methods and Programs in Biomedicine*, *112*(1), 84–91. doi:10.1016/j.cmpb.2013.07.004 PMID:23910224

Parhizi, S., Steege, L. S., & Pasupathy, K. S. (2013). Mining the relationships between psychosocial factors and fatigue dimensions among registered nurses. *International Journal of Industrial Ergonomics*, *43*(1), 82–90. doi:10.1016/j.ergon.2012.11.010

Patel, et al. (2009). The coming of age of artificial intelligence in medicine. *Artificial Intelligence in Medicine*, *46*(1), 5–17. doi:10.1016/j.artmed.2008.07.017 PMID:18790621

Rahman, R. M., & Hasan, F. R. M. (2011). Using and comparing different decision tree classification techniques for mining ICDDR,B Hospital Surveillance data. *Expert Systems with Applications*, *38*(9), 11421–11436. doi:10.1016/j.eswa.2011.03.015

Roham, M., & Gabrielyan, A, R., Archer, N. P. (2012). Predicting the impact of hospital health information technology adoption on patient satisfaction. *Artificial Intelligence in Medicine*, *56*(2), 123–135. doi:10.1016/j.artmed.2012.08.001 PMID:22964161

Santos, R. S., Malheiros, S. M. F., Cavalheiro, S., & Parente de Oliveira, J. M. (2013). A data mining system for providing analytical information on brain tumors to public health decision makers. *Computer Methods and Programs in Biomedicine*, *109*(3), 269–282. doi:10.1016/j.cmpb.2012.10.010 PMID:23122302

Sebastian, Y., & Then, P. H. H. (2011). Domain-driven KDD for mining functionally novel rules and linking disjoint medical hypotheses. *Knowledge-Based Systems*, *24*(5), 609–620. doi:10.1016/j.knosys.2011.01.008

Self-Organizing Map. (n.d.). In *Wikipedia*. Retrieved Sep 10, 2013, from http://en.wikipedia.org/wiki/Self-organizing_map

Semenova, T. (2004). Discovering patterns of medical practice in large administrative health databases. *Data & Knowledge Engineering*, *51*(2), 149–160. doi:10.1016/j.datak.2004.02.001

Shanmugam, R. (2012). Booming medical tourism and economic indices. *International Journal of Research in Nursing*, *3*(2), 38–47. doi:10.3844/ijrnsp.2012.38.47

Shimada, K., Wang, R., Hirasawa, K., & Furuzuki, T. (2008). Medical association rule mining using genetic network programming. *Electronics and Communications in Japan*, *91*(2), 46–54. doi:10.1002/ecj.10022

Shortlife, E. H., & Cimino, J. J. (2006). Biomedical informatics: Computer applications in health care and biomedicine (3rd ed.). New York: Springer.

Shortliffe, E. H. (1993). The adolescence of AI in medicine: will the field come of age in the 90s? *Artificial Intelligence in Medicine*, *5*(2), 93–106. doi:10.1016/0933-3657(93)90011-Q PMID:8358494

Tai, Y. M., & Chiu, H. W. (2009). Comorbidity study of ADHD: Applying association rule mining (ARM) to National Health Insurance Database of Taiwan. *International Journal of Medical Informatics*, *78*(12), e75–e83. doi:10.1016/j.ijmedinf.2009.09.005 PMID:19853501

Tan, P. N., Steinbach, M., & Kumar, V. (2005). *Introduction to data mining*. Pearson Addison-Wesley.

Tartarisco, G., Baldus, G., Corda, D., Raso, R., Arnao, A., & Ferro, M. et al. (2012). Personal Health System architecture for stress monitoring and support to clinical decisions. *Computer Communications*, *35*(11), 1296–1305. doi:10.1016/j.comcom.2011.11.015

Tenorio, J. M., Hummel, A. D., Cohrs, F. M., Sdepanian, V. L., Pisa, I. T., & Marin, H. D. F. (2011). Artificial intelligence techniques applied to the development of a decision–support system for diagnosing celiac disease. *International Journal of Medical Informatics*, *80*(11), 793–802. doi:10.1016/j.ijmedinf.2011.08.001 PMID:21917512

Ting, S. L., Kwok, S. K., Tsang, A. H. C., & Lee, W. B. (2011). A hybrid knowledge-based approach to supporting the medical prescription for general practitioners: Real case in a Hong Kong medical center. *Knowledge-Based Systems*, *24*(3), 444–456. doi:10.1016/j.knosys.2010.12.011

Vicente, J., Garcia-Gomez, J. M., Vidal, C., Marti-Bonmati, L., Arco, A. D., & Robles, M. (2004). SOC: A Distributed Decision Support Architecture for Clinical Diagnosis. *Biological and Medical Data Analysis. Lecture Notes in Computer Science*, *3337*, 96–104. doi:10.1007/978-3-540-30547-7_11

Wei, J., Lin, S., Weng, C., & Wu, H. (2012). A case study of applying LRFM model in market segmentation of a children's dental clinic. *Expert Systems with Applications*, *39*(5), 5529–5533. doi:10.1016/j.eswa.2011.11.066

Yan, H., Jiang, Y., & Zheng, J., Fu, B., Xiao, S., & Peng, C. (2004). The internet-based knowledge acquisition and management method to construct large-scale distributed medical expert systems. *Computer Methods and Programs in Biomedicine*, *74*(1), 1–10. doi:10.1016/S0169-2607(03)00076-2 PMID:14992822

Yan, Q., Yan, H., Han, F., Wei, X., & Zhu, T. (2009). SVM-based decision support system for clinic aided tracheal intubation predication with multiple features. *Expert Systems with Applications*, *36*(3), 6588–6592. doi:10.1016/j.eswa.2008.07.076

Yang, C. C., Lin, W. T., Chen, H. M., & Shi, Y. H. (2009). Improving scheduling of emergency physicians using data mining analysis. *Expert Systems with Applications*, *36*(2), 3378–3387. doi:10.1016/j.eswa.2008.02.069

Yao, L., Zhang, Y., Li, Y., Sanseau, P., & Agarwal, P. (2011). Electronic health records: Implications for drug discovery. *Drug Discovery Today*, *16*(13/14), 594–599. doi:10.1016/j.drudis.2011.05.009 PMID:21624499

Yeh, J. Y., Wu, T. H., & Tsao, C. W. (2011). Using data mining techniques to predict hospitalization of hemodialysis patients. *Decision Support Systems*, *50*(2), 439–448. doi:10.1016/j.dss.2010.11.001

Zayed, N., Awad, A. B., El-Akel, W., Doss, W., Awad, T., Radwan, A., & Mabrouk, M. (2013). The assessment of data mining for the prediction of therapeutic outcome in 3719 Egyptian patients with chronic hepatitis C. *Clinics and Research in Hepatology and Gastroenterology*, *37*(3), 254–261. doi:10.1016/j.clinre.2012.09.005 PMID:23141214

Zhao, D., & Weng, C. (2011). Combining PubMed knowledge and EHR data to develop a weighted Bayesian network for pancreatic cancer prediction. *Journal of Biomedical Informatics*, *44*(5), 859–868. doi:10.1016/j.jbi.2011.05.004 PMID:21642013

KEY TERMS AND DEFINITIONS

Actionable Knowledge Discovery: Actionable knowledge discovery aims to deliver knowledge that is business friendly, and which can be taken over by business people for seamless decision making.

Data Mining: Tan et al. (2005) define data mining as the process of automatically discovering useful information in large data repositories.

Healthcare Industry: According to the united nation International Standard Industrial Classification (ISIC) definition, the healthcare industry generally consist of three major activities include hospital activities, medical and dental practice activities, and other human health activities (Wikipedia, Healthcare industry, n. d.).

Knowledge Discovery: From Fayyad et al. (1996) point of view knowledge discovery in databases (KDD) is the overall process of discovering useful knowledge from data, and data mining refers to a particular step in this process that is the application of specific algorithms for extracting patterns from data.

Market View: Market view is one of the proposed classification groups. Market view includes papers that look at the patient as a potential customer. Most of researches on market view area were somehow related to CRM and it reflects the importance of this issue in healthcare industry businesses.

Patient View: Patient view is one of the proposed classification groups. It includes papers that purely mined clinical data sets to derive models and discovered patterns. Patient view is divided to predictive models and pattern mining groups.

System View: System view is one of the proposed classification groups. It includes papers that explicitly propose an algorithm, information flow diagram, application or architecture for decision support systems and also papers that propose architecture or systems that can perform or have potential to perform knowledge discovery and data mining in a large scale manner.

This work was previously published in Healthcare Informatics and Analytics edited by Madjid Tavana, Amir Hossein Ghapanchi, and Amir Talaei-Khoei, pages 241-262 copyright year 2015 by Medical Information Science Reference (an imprint of IGI Global).

Chapter 56
A Balanced Perspective to Perioperative Process Management Aligned to Hospital Strategy

Jim Ryan
Troy University, USA

Sandra Daily
University of Alabama at Birmingham Hospital, USA

Barbara Doster
University of Alabama at Birmingham Hospital, Birmingham, AL, USA

Carmen Lewis
Troy University, USA

ABSTRACT

Dynamic technological activities of analysis, evaluation, and synthesis can highlight complex relationships within integrated processes to target improvement and ultimately yield improved processes. Likewise, the identification of existing process limitations, potential capabilities, and subsequent contextual understanding are contributing factors that yield measured improvement. Based on a 120-month longitudinal study of an academic medical center, this study investigates how integrated information systems and business analytics can improve perioperative efficiency and effectiveness across patient quality of care, stakeholder satisfaction, clinical operations, and financial cost effectiveness. This case study examines process management practices of balanced scorecard and dashboards to monitor and improve the perioperative process, aligned to overall hospital goals at strategic, tactical, and operational levels. The conclusion includes discussion of study implications and limitations.

1. INTRODUCTION

A hospital's perioperative process provides surgical care for inpatients and outpatients during preoperative, intra-operative, and immediate post-operative periods. Accordingly, the perioperative sub-processes (e.g. preoperative, intra-operative, and post-operative activities) are sequential where each activity sequence paces the efficiency and effectiveness of subsequent activities. As a result, a hospital's perioperative process is tightly coupled to patient flow, patient safety, patient quality of

DOI: 10.4018/978-1-4666-8756-1.ch056

care, and stakeholders' satisfaction (i.e. patient, physician/surgeon, nurse, perioperative staff, and hospital administration).

Implementing improvements that will result in timely patient flow through the perioperative process is both a challenge and an opportunity for hospital stakeholders, who often have a variety of opinions and perceptions as to where improvement is needed. The challenge of delivering quality, efficient, and cost-effective services affects all healthcare stakeholders. Perioperative improvements ultimately affect not only patient quality of care, but also the operational and financial performance of the hospital itself. From an operational perspective, a hospital's perioperative process requires multidisciplinary, cross-functional teams to maneuver within complex, fast-paced, and critical situations–the hospital environment (McClusker et al., 2005).

Similarly from a hospital's financial perspective, the perioperative process is typically the primary source of hospital admissions, averaging between 55 to 65 percent of overall hospital margins (Peters & Blasco, 2004). Macario et al. (1995) identified 49 percent of total hospital costs as variable with the largest cost category being the perioperative process (e.g. 33 percent). Given the rising cost of healthcare, the public demand for healthcare transparency and accountability, and the current economic environment–managing and optimizing a quality, efficient, flexible, and cost-effective perioperative process are critical success factors (CSFs), both operationally and financially, for any hospital.

Recently, the focus of healthcare in the United States has shifted toward monitoring and improving clinical outcomes to meet new regulatory and reimbursement requirements. Likewise, hospitals in the United States must report and improve clinical outcomes more now due to the American Recovery and Reinvestment Act of 2009 and the Joint Commission on Accreditation of Healthcare Organizations (TJC) / Centers for Medicare & Medicaid Services (CMS) core measures. These

performance and reporting challenges require leveraging information systems (IS) and technologies (IT) to meet these demands. Furthermore, hospital administration could benefit by considering the strategic IS and business alignment challenges experienced in other industries over the past decades (Luftman & Ben-Zvi, 2010) as well as within the healthcare industry (Bush, 2009). With respect to hospital IS/IT alignment, this study investigates the research question of how business process management (BPM) is an applicable approach for perioperative process management as well as overall hospital's strategic vision execution with monitored clinical outcomes.

This study highlights BPM practices of balanced scorecards (BSC) and dashboards within a hospital's perioperative process. Empowered individuals driven by integrated internal and external organizational data facilitate the case results. The investigation method covers a longitudinal study of an integrated clinical scheduling information system (CSIS) within the perioperative process of a large, teaching hospital (e.g. academic medical center). The implementation of an agile CSIS and subsequent contextual understanding of the perioperative process and its sub-processes prescribed opportunity for measured improvements. Specifically, the extension of business analytics into BSCs and dashboards at different levels (e.g. strategic, tactical, and day-to-day operations), coupled with internal and external best-practice benchmarks, provide the framework for targeting improvement opportunities and evoking improvement changes to the perioperative process. The planning and development of the BSCs and dashboards also provide change dynamics for evaluation and improvement to the overall perioperative process. This case study also identifies complex dynamics within the perioperative process nested in the hospital environment.

The following sections review previous literature on BPM and BPM efforts in healthcare, as well as healthcare performance indicators and quality measures. Following the literature review, we present our methodology, case study background, and a discussion of the observed results from the BSCs and dashboard efforts. By identifying a holistic framework for analysis, evaluation, and synthesis of end-to-end process measures with established benchmarks, this paper prescribes an a priori environment to support perioperative process measurement, control, and improvement aligned to hospital strategy. The conclusion also addresses study implications and limitations.

2. LITERATURE REVIEW

Industry competition, first mover advantage on innovations, adaptation of better management practices, and/or government regulations are examples of the many factors that drive process improvements. Traditionally, the hospital environment lacked similar industrial pressures beyond government regulations. However, hospital administration currently face increasing pressure to provide objective evidence of patient outcomes in respect to organizational quality, efficiency, and effectiveness (CMS, 2005; CMS, 2010; PwC, 2012), all while preserving clinical quality standards.

Hospital administrators and medical professionals must focus on both the patient quality of care as well as management practices that yield efficiency and cost effectiveness (PwC, 2012). To this end, industrial and operations management practices of BSC, business analytics, and dashboards borrowed from BPM provide a framework to target and measure process improvement (Jeston & Nelis, 2008; Kaplan & Norton 1996; Tenner & DeToro, 1997). Measured utilization of these practices is not a result from lack of research as a body of knowledge exists concerning their application in healthcare (Albanese et al., 2010; Fairbanks, 2007; Herzer et al., 2008; Kruskal et al., 2012; Kujala et al., 2006; Zbinden, 2002). Moreover, the literature suggests that such approaches and interventions can yield positive results with significant variations in implementation success.

2.1. Business Process Management (BPM)

Specifically, this study examines BPM applications of BSCs and dashboards to monitor and measure improvement within the perioperative process, aligned to hospital strategy. This study uses the BPM definition provided by Jensen and Nelis (2008, p. 10) as "the achievement of an organization's objectives through the improvement, management, and control of essential business processes." The authors further elaborate that process management and analysis is integral to BPM, where there is no finish line for improvement. Hence, this study views BPM as an organizational commitment to consistent and iterative process performance improvement that meets organizational objectives. To this end, BPM embraces the concept of continuous process improvement (CPI) aligned with business strategy.

CPI is a systematic approach toward understanding the process capability, the customer's needs, and the source of observed variation. Tenner and DeToro (1997) views CPI as an organizational response to an acute crisis, a chronic problem, and/or an internal driver. The incremental realization of improvement gains occurs through an iterative cycle of analysis, evaluation, and synthesis or plan-do-study-act (Walton, 1986) to minimize observed variation. CPI encourages bottom-up communication at the day-to-day operations level and requires process data comparisons to control metrics. Doubt can exist as to: whether the incremental improvement addresses symptoms versus causes; whether the improvement effort is sustainable year after year; and/or whether management is in control of the process (Jensen & Nelis, 2008).

As BPM requires alignment to strategic objectives, a BSC approach (Kaplan & Norton, 1996) embraces the ability to quantify organizational control metrics aligned with strategy across perspectives of: (1) financial; (2) customer; (3) process; and (4) learning/growth. Business analytics is the body of knowledge identified with the deployment and use of technology solutions that incorporate BSCs, dashboards, performance management, definition and delivery of business metrics, as well as data visualization and data mining. Business analytics within BPM focus on the effective use of organizational data and information to drive positive business action (Turban et al., 2008). The effective use of business analytics demands knowledge and skills from subject matter experts and knowledge workers. Similarly, Wears and Berg (2005) concur that IS/IT only yield high-quality healthcare when the use patterns are tailored to knowledge workers and their environment. Therefore, BPM success through BSCs and dashboards has a strong dependence on contextual understanding of end-to-end core business processes (Jensen & Nelis, 2008).

2.2. Key Performance Indicators (KPIs)

An integral part of CPI is information about performance before and after the intervention. Thus, performance measurement is an essential requirement for purposeful BPM. Early in the IT literature, Ackoff (1967) proposed IS design should embed feedback as a control to avoid management misinformation. Other authors (Zani, 1970; Rockart, 1979; Munroe & Wheeler, 1980) proposed the selection and supervision of defined data as KPIs to assist management in qualifying measurement of CSFs and subsequently managing organizational action (i.e. business processes) through IS feedback. Similarly, hospital processes are becoming increasingly information intensive and doubt exists as to whether process management understanding can meet the increasing hospital environmental demands for value and cost efficiency (Catalano & Fickenscher, 2007).

The following scenario of operational, tactical, and strategic KPIs illustrate the complexity, dynamic nature, and nested relationships among hospital processes. Operational and tactical KPIs in managing and optimizing a hospital's

perioperative process include monitoring the percentage of surgical cases that start on-time (OTS) and the number of first-of-the-day surgical cases (FCOD_OTS) that start on-time, as well as operating room (OR) turn times (TURNS) and utilization (UTIL) (Barnes, 2010; Herzer et al., 2008). The Thomson Group (2010) noted how OR suite TURNS between cases, along with a flexible and efficient perioperative work environment, are CSFs for physician/surgeon satisfaction, which in turn is a CSF for hospital margin. Poor KPIs on operational and tactical metrics (i.e. OTS, FCOD_OTS, TURNS or UTIL) affect strategic CSFs of patient safety, patient quality of care, surgeon/staff/patient satisfaction, and hospital margin (Marjamaa et al., 2008; Peters & Blasco, 2004).

2.3. Healthcare Quality Benchmark Standards

Healthcare industry benchmark standards focus on patient quality of care via self-reported outcome measures or patient satisfaction survey results. The CMS and the Hospital Quality Alliance (HQA) began publicly reporting inpatient quality reporting (IQR) outcomes on 30-day mortality measures for acute myocardial infarction (AMI) and heart failure (HF) in 2007 and for pneumonia (PN) in 2008 (CMS, 2010).

Patient satisfaction measures began development as the Hospital Consumer Assessment of Healthcare Providers and Systems (HCAHPS) survey in 2002. The collaboration effort was between CMS and the Agency for Healthcare Research and Quality (AHRQ), another federal agency under the Department of Health and Human Services. The evolved HCAHPS survey measures report patient perspectives on care received across items that encompass ten key topics: (1) communication with doctors, (2) communication with nurses, (3) responsiveness of hospital staff, (4) pain management, (5) communication about medicines, (6) discharge information, (7) cleanliness of the hospital environment, (8) quietness of the hospital environment, (9) overall rating of the hospital, and (10) whether the patient would recommend the hospital to family and friends (HCAHPS, 2012).

In 2005, CMS began a major priority to encourage improvements in the quality of care provided to Medicare beneficiaries (CMS, 2005). The result was pay-for-performance (P4P) or value-based purchasing (VBP) as a CMS payment model that rewards healthcare providers for meeting certain performance measures in quality and efficiency. In a 2007 study, hospitals reporting both public and P4P achieved modestly greater quality improvements than hospitals engaged only in public reporting (Lindenauer et al., 2007). In 2008 as an additional rule to P4P, CMS included disincentives of reducing payments for negative consequences of care that should never occur, as defined by the National Quality Forum, including hospital infections under the surgical care improvement project (SCIP) (NQF, 2008).

3. RESEARCH METHOD

The objective of this study is to examine BPM practices of BSCs and dashboards within a hospital's perioperative process that target opportunities and measure improvement, aligned to hospital strategy. To this end, case research is particularly appropriate (Eisenhardt, 1989; Yin, 2003). An advantage of the positivist approach (Weber, 2004) to case research allows concentrating on specific hospital processes in a natural setting to analyze the associated qualitative problems and environmental complexity. Hence, our study took an in-depth case research approach.

Our research site is an academic medical center (e.g. University Hospital), licensed for 1,044 beds and located in the southeastern region of the United States. University Hospital is one of two magnet hospitals in the state and the U.S. News and World Report has repeatedly recognized University Hospital as a Best Hospital over the past

two decades. Concentrating on one research site facilitated the research investigation and allowed the continued collection of longitudinal data. This study spans activities from 2003 to 2013. During the 120-month study, we conducted field research and gathered data from multiple sources including interviews, field surveys, site observations, field notes, archival records, and document reviews.

The initial perspective of this research focused on University Hospital's perioperative process for its 32 general operating room (OR) suites. Perioperative Services is the University Hospital department that coordinates the hospital's perioperative process across Admissions, PREP having 42 beds, Post Anesthesia Care Unit (PACU) having 45 beds, and Central Sterile Supply (CSS).

4. CASE BACKGROUND

Perioperative Services implemented a new CSIS in 2003, after using its prior CSIS for 10 years. The old CSIS and its vendor were not flexible in adapting to new data collection needs of Perioperative Services. Figure 1 depicts University Hospital's CSIS architecture as of October 2004. University Hospital had six main IS: (1) a large-scale hospital materials management IS, which included pharmacy, material and medical device management (Vendor L); (2) a large scale enterprise resource planning IS (Vendor O); (3) a patient record Admit/Discharge IS (Vendor Q); (4) a cost accounting IS (Vendor T); (5) a financial budgeting IS (Vendor H); and (6) a CSIS (Vendor C) that included three modules for clinical scheduling, routing sheets, and cost data.

All IS were integrated with uni-directional constraints placed on sensitive information. The institutional intranet served as portal access to extend each of the six IS. User authentication via the intranet was single entry with particular user-IS rights and privileges negotiated upon authentication.

Figure 1. IS architecture (October 2004)

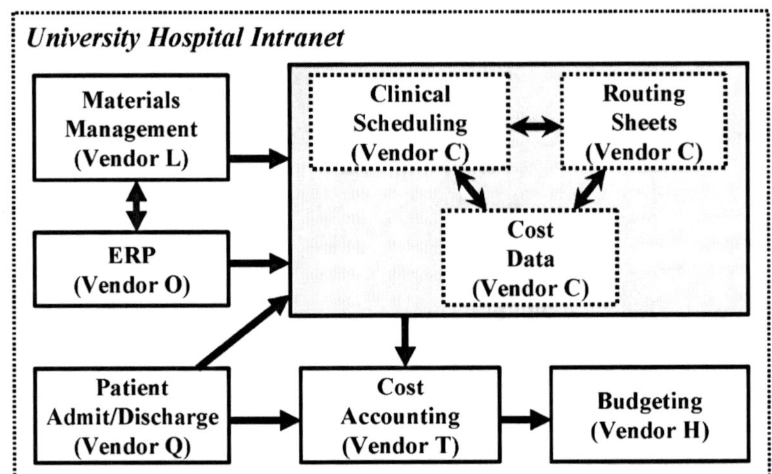

4.1. November 2004

University Hospital opened a new diagnostic and surgical facility in November 2004, which covers three-fourths of a city block rising 12 stories. Perioperative Services were relocated into three floors, with ORs located over two floors and CSS located separately on the third. The move expanded Perioperative Services to cover an additional floor and nine additional ORs. The new facility housed 40 state-of-the-art OR suites (32 general OR), each equipped with new standardized equipment as well as equipment by surgical specialty. Within six weeks of occupying the new perioperative facility, scheduling KPIs reflected chaos. On-time surgical case starts plunged to 18% during December 2004. Within a highly competitive hospital industry, having only 18% OTS was unacceptable as 82% of scheduled surgeries experienced delays and risked patient care and safety. University Hospital had failed to adjust its perioperative process to compensate for the introduction of radical innovations–existing perioperative processes were disparate within the new environment.

4.2. Perioperative Continuous Process Improvement (CPI)

In January 2005, perioperative concerns were laid out before a quickly convened executive council. The meeting included the chief executive officer, the chief financial officer, the chief information officer, the chief nursing officer, and top representatives of surgeons, anesthesia, and Perioperative Services. The end-result of this meeting was changed governance for Perioperative Services in the formation of a cross-functional, multidisciplinary executive team, similar to matrix-style management. The executive team consisted of a cross-section of perioperative stakeholders (i.e. surgeons, nurses, anesthesiologists, and perioperative management), chartered and empowered to evoke change.

University Hospital's executive team launched a CPI effort to address the perioperative crisis through soft innovations (Ryan et al., 2008). The executive team and numerous task forces, formed to address specific problems and/or opportunities, were chartered to systematically identify issues and enlist working managers for solutions that focus on patient care and safety, attack difficult questions, and no issue was "off-limits."

Given the slow learning curve associated with the OR relocation and radical innovation disruption, a new KPI was established to track surgical case OTS within 10 minutes. This particular KPI provided motivation for CPI and was retired in 2008. Figure 2 represents the perioperative process improvement in the surgical case OTS through May 2007.

Since the OR relocation in 2004, University Hospital has sustained an annual 10% growth in surgical case procedures in its original 32 general OR suites (GENOR). Perioperative Services has also assumed the management and scheduling of an additional 36 ORs that include 8 cardio-vascular OR suites (CVOR), 19 OR suites at the Hygh Hospital campus (HHOR), and 9 OR suites at the Eye Foundation Hospital (CEFH). University Hospital has continued a systematic approach to perioperative CPI across all of its surgical locations and services, achieving improvement success that targeted perioperative process analysis and redesign (Ryan et al., 2010), heuristic OR scheduling (Ryan et al., 2011a), hospital-wide patient flow (Ryan et al., 2011b), preoperative clinic benchmarking and re-engineering (Ryan et al., 2012), and radio-frequency identification implementation (Ryan et al., 2013). Figure 3 depicts the improved patient flow through the University Hospital Health System (UHHS) resulting from these CPI efforts.

5. RESULTS AND DISCUSSION

The executive team and perioperative management consistently focus on data-driven, end-to-end CPI efforts. Initially as needed to facilitate perioperative process management and improvement, the executive team and subsequent task groups defined process control measures based on internal process data collected through the CSIS and external industry standards. Initially, these control measures benchmarked previous months' metrics to establish trends for tracking improvement and/or targeting areas for improvement. When reviewing what could have been done better during the initial CPI efforts, the executive team and Perioperative Services management

Figure 2. OTS KPIs December 2004 to May 2007

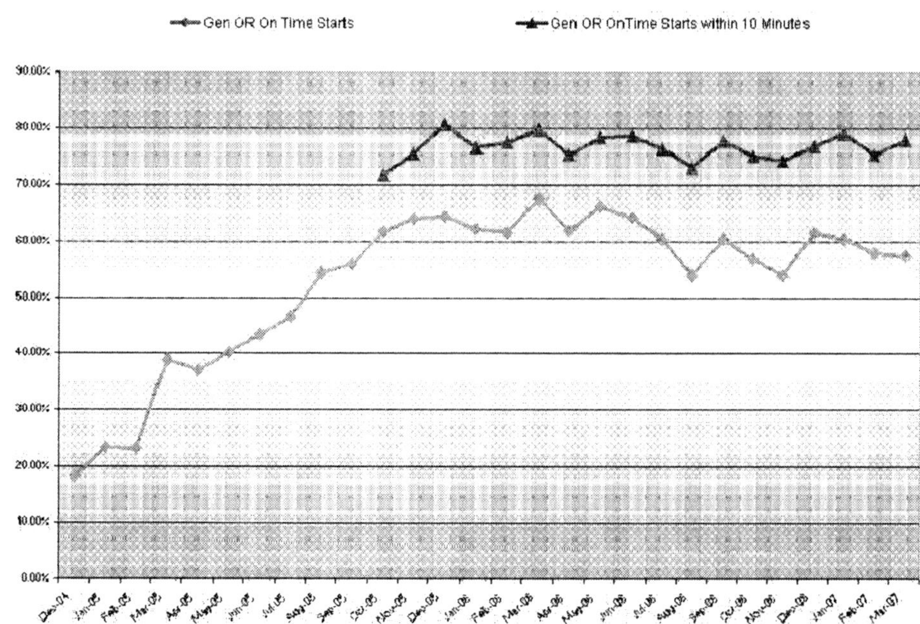

Figure 3. UHHS improved patient flow

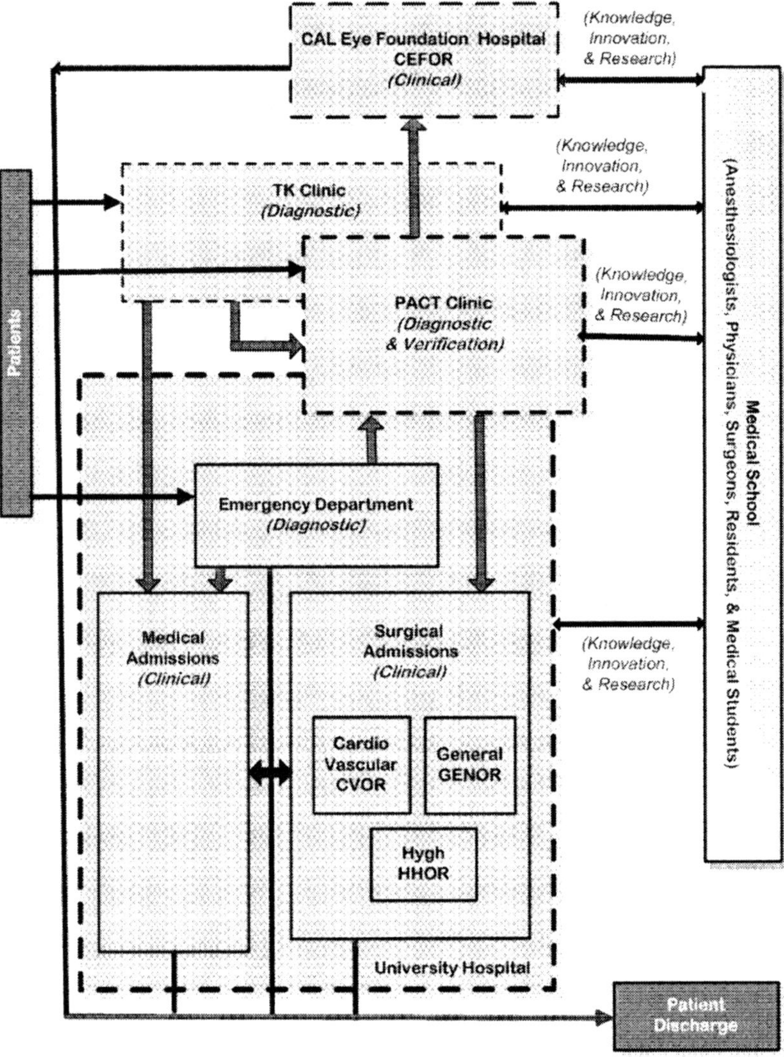

recognized the need to involve perioperative stakeholders in the entire improvement process and not just end-result to-do lists. As a result in 2008, the executive team launched an initiative to categorize, qualify, and quantify perioperative performance measures for process management and control feedback as well as meet regulatory requirements for CMS and TJC. The initiative set out to identify and define measures associated with core perioperative processes, establish a BSC of measures, and develop a means to disseminate the process feedback to perioperative stakeholders.

The following sections elaborate on the initiative's results through May 2013.

5.1. Core and Operational Measures

The identification and definition of perioperative operational control measures has been an iterative evolution for University Hospital since 2005, similar to the core healthcare industry quality standards coordinated and adopted by CMS and TJC. University Hospital currently has 53 core and operational measures identified and defined

Table 1. Sample strategic measure

Outcome Category	Measure	Source	Operational Definition	Sch	Rpt	Target
Patient Safety	Time Outs Documented	CSIS	OR/Bedside procedures	Mth	Avg	TJC

at the strategic level that measure perioperative performance on a monthly or quarterly basis. Each measure maps to a process, definition, outcome, data source, data type, personnel responsible, reporting frequency, and control target. Table 1 represents a sample of the 53 strategic core and operational measures.

Table 2 lists the specific strategic outcome categories and number of associated core and operational measures. The 53 strategic measures are spread over outcome categories that cover patient safety, patient satisfaction, patient satisfaction–HCAPHS, employee satisfaction, patient throughput, mortality/readmissions, financial, and IQR quality measures over AMI, HF, PN, and SCIP. Table 3 lists all 53 measures by financial, customer, or process BSC perspective.

5.2. Multi-Level Balanced Scorecards (BSCs)

The 53 core and operational measures by BSC perspective provide an initial foundation for a BSC strategic approach to managing and controlling University Hospital's perioperative process. However, the strategic measures are at a high managerial level. Many other financial, customer, and process measures are available at lower tactical and even lower day-to-day operations levels. Perioperative stakeholders use the lower level measures to monitor and control perioperative process performance. For example, surgical location (e.g. GENOR, CVOR, HHOR, or CEFH) and/or surgical specialty (i.e. orthopedics) reflect tactical level performance measures. The following lists all 17 surgical specialty services (SSS) performed across the four surgical locations.

BURN: trauma burns
CV: cardio-vascular
ENT: ear, nose, and throat
GI: gastro-intestinal
GYN: obstetrics, oncology, incontinence
NEURO: neurological
OPH: Ophthalmology
ORAL: oral maxil facial
ORTHO: orthopedic, joint/device replacement
PLAS: plastic surgery
SURG ONC: surgical oncology
THOR: thoracic
TX: transplants (liver, renal)
TRAUMA: trauma, MASH
URO: urology
VASCA: vascular-arteries
VASULAR: blood vessels

University Hospital currently has 32 perioperative measures identified and defined at the tactical level to measure monthly perioperative

Table 2. Strategic outcomes

Strategic Outcome	Measures
Patient Safety	4
Patient Satisfaction	4
HCAHPS	3
Employee Satisfaction	2
Patient Throughput	4
Mortality/Readmissions	4
Financial	3
IGR Quality Measures	29 AMI-5 HF-8 PN-6 SCIP-10

Table 3. 53 strategic perioperative process measures

Time Outs Documented	Average Length of Stay (Days)	AMI- ACEI/ARB for LVSD	PN-Pneumonia Vaccinations
Hospital Nosocomial Infection Marker Rate (NIM Rate)	Length of Stay Index (Actual / Expected)	AMI- PCI within 90 min	PN-Antibiotic Selection
NIM Benchmarking Rating	Percent occupancy (Inpatients Units)	AMI- Readmission Rate	PN-Blood Cultures before ABX in UED
NIM Benchmarking Rating Change	Discharges by Noon	HF- Discharge Instructions-Activity	PN-Readmission Rate
Nurses kept you informed	Mortality (Number)	HF- Discharge Instructions-Diet	SCIP-Prophylactic ABX given within 1hr of incision
Staff sensitivity to inconveinence	Mortality Rate (deaths / total admits)	HF- Discharge Instructions-Weight Monitoring	SCIP-Prophylactic ABX d/c within 24/48hrs (Overall)
Staff addressed emotional needs	Mortality Index (Actual / Expected)	HF- Discharge Instructions-Symptoms Worsening	SCIP-Prophylactic ABX d/c within 48hrs (CV)
Response to concerns/complaints	Re-admissions	HF- Discharge Instructions-Follow-Up	SCIP-Prophylactic ABX d/c within 24hrs (Hips & Knees)
% definitely yes would recommend UH	Net Revenue / Adjusted Patient Day	HF- Discharge Instructions-Medications	SCIP-Prophylactic ABX d/c within 24hrs (Colon)
Pain Well Controlled (% Always)	CMI Medicare ONLY	HF-ACEI/ARB for LVSD	SCIP-Prophylactic ABX d/c within 24hrs (Vascular)
Nurse listened carefully to you (% Always)	Operating Margin	HF-Readmission Rate	SCIP-Prophylactic ABX d/c within 24hrs (GYNX)
RN Turnover Rate (%) (YTD)	AMI- Aspirin at Arrival	PN-ABX within 6hrs of arrival (overall)	SCIP-Post-Op Glucose
RN Recruitment Vacancy (%)	AMI- Beta Blocker at Discharge	PN-Flu Vaccinations	SCIP-Prophylactic VTE Assessment/Order
SCIP-Prophylactic VTE received			
Financial	Customer		Process

performance by surgical location and/or specialty. The CSIS captures, stores, or derives a majority of these measures. Similarly as with the strategic measures, each tactical measure maps to a process, definition, outcome, data source, data type, personnel responsible, reporting frequency, and control target. Table 4 lists specific tactical outcome categories and the number of associated measures. The corresponding 32 tactical measures reflect outcome categories that cover quality, satisfaction, financial, and IQR SCIP quality. Table 5 lists all 32 measures by financial, customer, or process BSC perspective.

At the day-to-day operations level, performance measures reflect more tallies, totals, and worksheets that are required by individual sub-process (i.e. PREP, PACU, CSS, etc.), surgical specialty, and/or by specific OR suite (i.e. Main OR 508). The granularity of performance measures at the day-to-day operations level allows aggregation at higher tactical and strategic levels. The multi-level BSC approach allows different perspectives (e.g. strategic, tactical, and/or day-to-day operations) of perioperative process performance as well as addressing end-to-end process performance.

The BSC for the day-to-day operations measures are more reflective of process components than end-to-end process segments as at the tactical level. The list of all day-to-day operations measures is too large to include in this paper, as most data elements within the CSIS are or are potential day-to-day operations measures. Table 6 lists examples of major day-to-day operations measures by BSC perspectives of financial, customer, and process.

Table 4. Tactical outcomes measured

Tactical Outcome	Measures
Quality	13
Satisfaction	2
Financial	7
IQR quality measures	SCIP-10

Table 5. Tactical measures

Financial	Customer		Process
Unit of Service (UOS)	Time Outs Documented	On Time Starts	SCIP-Prophylactic ABX given within 1hr of incision
Actual Supply $ / UOS	Brief Post Op Notes	#1 Delay Reason	SCIP-Prophylactic ABX d/c within 24/48hrs (Overall)
AS / UOS Variance	H&P 24hr update	% Case = Turn Time	SCIP-Prophylactic ABX d/c within 48hrs (CV)
CVOR+Perf Supply/UOS	Point of Use Sterilization	Turn Times under 45min	SCIP-Prophylactic ABX d/c within 24hrs (Hips & Knees)
CS / UOS Variance	Blood Admin	Preop-Nurse Ready Time	SCIP-Prophylactic ABX d/c within 24hrs (Colon)
7AM-7PM Case HRS / 8HR UTIL	Hair Removal	SCIP-Post-Op Glucose	SCIP-Prophylactic ABX d/c within 24hrs (Vascular)
Case Volume	PACU-LOS	SCIP-Prophylactic VTE Assess/Order	SCIP-Prophylactic ABX d/c within 24hrs (GYNX)
% Cases done by 5PM	Canceled Cases	PACU-Pain on DC	SCIP-Prophylactic VTE received

5.3. Perioperative Process Dashboards

Perioperative stakeholders pull BSC measures as needed. The strategic and tactical BSC measures reside on a secured, virtual drive accessible by any perioperative stakeholder who has sufficient rights and privileges within the CSIS. As previously mentioned, the majority of the day-to-day operations BSC measures reside within the CSIS with similar stakeholder access.

At the close of each monthly reporting period, Perioperative Services compiles the strategic, tactical, and day-to-day operations BSC measures into electronic dashboards that measure perioperative performance across each managerial level. These dashboards are then pushed out to update the BSC virtual drive as well as University Hospital administration, directors, and managers. Each University Hospital surgeon receives dashboards for their respective SSS and surgical locations. Team leaders also post the strategic and relevant tactical BSC dashboards in their specific areas. Therefore, BSC dashboards are pushed out monthly for stakeholder dissemination upward and downward.

Figure 4 illustrates an example of a strategic dashboard reflecting perioperative core measures aligned to University Hospital's strategic objectives. Each monthly measure is color coated to depict:

- **Green:** Measure is at or above target
- **Yellow:** An area of concern, as measure is within 10 points below target
- **Red:** Failing, as measure is below 10 points from target

Table 6. Day-to-day operations measures

Financial	Customer	Process
After Hour Cases	Time Outs	Cases done 7AM - 3PM
OR Time Used	Instrument Counts	Cases done 3PM - 5PM
%OR Use Time	OR Pauses	Cases done 5PM - 7PM
%Completed 7PM - 9PM	Average Case Time (Minutes)	% Completed 7AM - 3PM
Cases done 7PM - 9PM	Volume Shifts	% Completed 3PM - 5PM
Case Volume	Minute Shifts	% Completed 5PM - 7PM
Available Block Time (12 Hrs.)	Cases Turned	Remaining Cases
Block Time Utilization	% Turn Time Met	% Remaining Cases
Available Block Time (Minutes)	First Case Ontime Starts	Block Time
Minutes Blocked	On Time Starts	Total Cases
SSS Utilization	OR Suite Utilization	OR Suite Cases

The color-coding on each measure reflects opportunity for the BSC learning/growth perspective and improvement.

Figure 5 illustrates two examples of the 22 current tactical dashboards (i.e. 1 combined for all surgical locations, 4 individual surgical locations, and 17 SSS). The first tactical dashboard is a composite of the GENOR and CVOR surgical locations. The second tactical example is for the orthopedics SSS (e.g. ORTHO). ORTHO cases are performed in the surgical OR suites of GENOR and HHOR. All tactical dashboards use the same color code sequence of green, yellow, and red as noted with the strategic dashboards.

As of May 2013, there are 18 day-to-day operations dashboards used to generate the 22 tactical dashboards. Figure 6 contains examples of day-to-day operations dashboards. The first example in Figure 6 is a summary of late and OTS cases by OR suite by OR location for May 2012. The second example is a partial listing of SSS block time utilization by OR suite by day-of-week for May 2012. The third example shows surgical case completions by OR time slots (i.e. 7AM-3PM, 3PM-5PM, 5PM-7PM, 7PM-9PM, and remaining cases after 9PM) by OR location and in total.

Lastly, all dashboards are views of the original BSC data measures, stored in the CSIS or on the secured virtual drive. Perioperative stakeholders may manipulate data within each dashboard for task group analysis or graphing (e.g. data visualization), but the archived measures have read only access capabilities to ensure data integrity.

Figure 4. Strategic Dashboard Examples

	Core Measure Dashboard- FY2012								
Measures	**FYTD 12 Actual**	**FY 12 Target**	**Oct - 11**	**Nov - 11**	**Dec - 11**	**Jan - 12**	**Feb - 12**	**Mar - 12**	**Apr - 12**	**Status**
HEART FAILURE									
D/C Instructions-Activity	98%	100%	100% n=31	98% n=42	95% n=40	97.8% n=46	95.2% n=42	97.1% n=34	96.2% n=26	↑
D/C Instructions-Diet	98%	100%	100% n=31	98% n=42	95% n=40	97.8% n=46	95.2% n=42	97.1% n=34	96.2% n=26	↑
D/C Instructions-Weight Monitoring	98%	100%	100% n=31	98% n=42	95% n=40	97.8% n=46	95.2% n=42	97.1% n=34	96.2% n=26	↑
D/C Instructions-Symptoms Worseni	98%	100%	100% n=31	98% n=42	95% n=40	97.8% n=46	95.2% n=42	97.1% n=34	96.2% n=26	↑
D/C Instructions-Follow Up	100%	100%	100% n=31	100% n=42	100% n=40	100% n=46	100% n=42	100% n=34	100% n=26	↔
D/C Instructions-Medications	73%	100%	50% n=24	75% n=36	84.2% n=38	84.1% n=44	82.9% n=35	75% n=32	82.6% n=23	↑
ACEI/ARB for LVSD	98%	100%	100% n=16	97% n=28	100% n=26	95.5% n=22	100% n=19	100% n=14	100% n=13	↑
SCIP									
Proph ABX given within 1hr of surgery (All	99%	100%	98% n=177	98% n= 193	100% n=185	99.6% n= 225	98% n= 239	99% n=217	98.5% n=344	↔
Proph ABX d/c within 24/48hrs (All)	99%	100%	99% n=166	99% n=177	98% n=160	99.5% n= 203	99.5% n= 219	100% n=191	99% n=311	↓
Proph ABX d/c within 48hrs (CV)	99%	100%	100% n=39	98% n=42	97% n=56	100% n=50	100% n=37	100% n=37	98.3% n=58	↓
Proph ABX d/c within 24hrs(Hips & Knees)	99%	100%	100% n=44	97% n=34	100% n=22	98% n=47	100% n=55	100% n=23	100% n=54	↔
Proph ABX d/c within 24hrs (Colon)	100%	100%	100% n=17	100% n=27	100% n=15	100% n=22	100% n=35	100% n=42	96.7% n=61	↓
Proph ABX d/c within 24hrs (Vascular)	100%	100%	100% n=18	100% n=23	100% n=16	100% n= 26	97% n=36	100% n=23	100% n=18	↓
Proph ABX d/c within 24hrs (GYNX)	100%	100%	98% n=47	100% n=51	100% n=52	100% n=57	100% n=56	100% n=66	100% n=58	↑
Post Op Glucose (CV) <200	95%	99%	97% n=32	94% n=46	94% n=59	90% n=52	87% n= 35	92% n=37	91.4% n= 58	↑
Proph VTE Assessment/Order	99%	100%	100% n=124	100% n=124	100% n=104	100% n=139	100% n=160	100% n=145	99.6% n=248	↔
Proph VTE received	99%	100%	99% n=122	95% n=125	99% n=99	100% n=136	98% n= 152	99% n=142	98.8% n= 241	↓
BB Received Perioperative	97%	100%	95% n=78	96% n=80	92% n=75	99% n= 83	95% n= 78	97% n=59	98.6% n= 74	↑
Post Op Urinary Catheter Romoval	97%	100%	95% n= 81	98% n=103	97% n=98	96% n= 108	99% n=113	98% n=88	99.5% n= 187	↑

At or above target	Area of Concern	Failing Measure

For use in Univeristy Hospital's Quality Improvement Process. Privileged and confidential pursuant to the State Code, Section §6-533, §22-21

5.4. Data Visualization

Figure 7 illustrates examples of line charts representing perioperative KPI measures versus time. Charts are useful to identify trends in the financial, customer, and process BSC perspectives. The first four data visualization examples show OTS, UOS-total expenses, OR utilization, and completed cases 7AM-5PM from October 2008 to June 2011. The fifth example is one chart that shows OTS from October 2008 to December 2012. The sixth example shows Press-Ganey HCAPHS results for overall hospital and visitor/family ratings from Q3 2008 to Q1 2013.

All of the BSC measures at each managerial level can be pulled into a data visualization chart to report perioperative process performance. All six of the data visualization examples in Figure 7 show positive trends for financials, customer, and process perspectives of the BSC measures.

5.5. Goal Setting and Process Improvement Aligned to the Hospital Strategic Plan

The 2008 perioperative BPM initiative established BSC (e.g. financial, customer, and process) measures and a means to disseminate process feedback to perioperative stakeholders at the strategic, tactical, and operational levels.

However, the perioperative process is not the exclusive core process included in University Hospital Health System's strategic vision. Updated in 2010 and labeled AMC21, UHHS' strategic plan reaffirms the core healthcare industry standards coordinated and adopted by CMS and TJC, while

Figure 5. Tactical dashboard examples

GENOR & CVOR	FYTD 12 Actual	FY12 Target	Jan-12	Feb-12	Mar-12	Apr-12	Status
Quality							
Time Outs	100.0%	100.0%	[illegible]	[illegible]	[illegible]	[illegible]	↔
Brief Post Op Notes	91.9%	100.0%		93.8%	98.0%		↔
H&P 24hr update	96.8%	100.0%		[illegible]	98.4%	[illegible]	↔
On Time Starts	62.4%	70.0%	55.6%	66.1%	65.5%	62.7%	↓
% Case = Turn Time	20.6%	15.0%	[illegible]	[illegible]	[illegible]	[illegible]	↑
Turn Times under 45min	58.9%	50.0%	[illegible]	[illegible]	[illegible]	[illegible]	↑
Point of Use Sterilization %	15.8%	15.0%	13.0%	17.0%	[illegible]	[illegible]	↓
Blood Administration	6.3%		7.5%	5.7%	6.0%	6.1%	↑
Nursing							
Hair Removal	99.9%	100% non-Razor	99.9%	99.9%	99.9%	99.8%	↓
Preop Nurse Ready Time	45	<45 Min	43	43	45	47	↑
PACU-LOS	68.8%	<2 Hours	71.0%	55.5%	67.4%	61.8%	↓
PACU-Pain on DC	85.1%	<=5	83.5%	[illegible]	[illegible]	[illegible]	↑
SCIP							
Proph ABX d/c within 24h/48h (Overall)	96.3%	100.0%	99.5% n=203	99.5% n=219	[illegible]	99% n=311	↓
Proph ABX d/c within 48h (CV)	91.0%	100.0%	[illegible]	[illegible] n=37	[illegible] n=37	98.3% n=58	↓
Proph ABX d/c within 24h (Hips & Knees)	95.2%	100.0%	98% n=47	[illegible]	[illegible]	[illegible]	↔
Proph ABX d/c within 24h (Colon)	97.6%	100.0%	[illegible] n=22	[illegible]	[illegible]	96.7% n=61	↓
Proph ABX d/c within 24h (Vascular)	97.0%	100.0%	[illegible]	97% n=36	[illegible]	[illegible]	↔
Proph ABX d/c within 24h (GYNX)	99.1%	100.0%	[illegible]	[illegible]	[illegible]	[illegible]	↔
Satisfaction							
% Cases done by 5PM	88.5%	75.0%	[illegible]	[illegible]	[illegible]	[illegible]	↑
Canceled Cases	4.21%	5.0%	4.02%	4.00%	5.75%	6.60%	↑
Financial							
Actual Supply $ / UOS	$1,549.39		$1,691.48	$1,549.47	$1,656.51	$1,966.67	↑
Utilization	95.0%	100.0%	96.1%	[illegible]	87.7%	94.4%	↑
UOS	56613.8	69,628	6,969	6,895	7,146	7,212	↑
HS Case Volume	20,483		2,560	2,568	2,573	2,621	↑

Legend: At or above target · Area of Concern · Falling Measure

ORTHO	FYTD 12 Actual	FY12 Target	Jan-12	Feb-12	Mar-12	Apr-12	Status
Quality							
HHOR - On Time Starts	63.0%	70.0%	61.9%	54.6%	56.5%	72.7%	↑
GENOR - On Time Starts	59.5%	70.0%	56.6%	62.7%	61.0%	55.6%	↕
HHOR - #1 Delay Reason			Surgeon cases in multiple rooms	Surgeon cases in multiple rooms	Surgeon not available	Anesthesia - Block placed in Pre-op holding	
GENOR - #1 Delay Reason			Anesthesia Transport from ICU	Anesthesia - Block placed in	Added Case	Anesthesia - Block placed in	
HHOR - % Case = Turn Time		<10%	21.1%	17.9%	19.8%	28.5%	↑
GENOR - % Case = Turn Time	22.6%	<10%	24.6%	24.0%	28.0%	24.7%	↑
HHOR - Turn Times under 45min	70.1%	50.0%	[illegible]	[illegible]	[illegible]	[illegible]	↑
GENOR - Turn Times under 45min	71.0%	50.0%	19.0%	26.1%	24.1%	18.2%	↓
Satisfaction							
HHOR - % Cases done by 5PM	89.8%	75.0%	[illegible]	[illegible]	[illegible]	[illegible]	↑
GENOR - % Cases done by 5PM	65.0%	75.0%	70.8%	72.0%	64.1%	67.0%	↕
HHOR Canceled Cases	1.7%	5.0%	[illegible]	[illegible]	[illegible]	[illegible]	↑
GENOR Canceled Cases	10.9%	5.0%	9.70%	9.72%	[illegible]	[illegible]	↑
Financial							
GENOR							
7A-7P Case HRS / 8HR Utilization	134.8%	100.0%	[illegible]	[illegible]	[illegible]	[illegible]	↑
UOS (Hours)	1,253		166	161	183	126	↓
Case Volume	1,792		195	193	229	237	↑
HHOR							
7A-7P Case HRS / 8HR Utilization	86.1%	100.0%	94.0%	[illegible]	94.8%	[illegible]	↓
UOS (Hours)			303	724	359	709	
Case Volume			341	338	367	349	

** HHOR is transitioning to become the preferred location for scheduling and performing ORTHO SSS cases.

Legend: At or above target · Area of Concern · Falling Measure

complimenting core hospital process measures. Table 7 lists the foundation or strategic pillars that support AMC21 strategic goals. Furthermore, the vision within AMC21 is for UHHS to be the preferred academic medical center of the 21st century with characteristics where: a) patients want to come for care; b) employees want to work; c) faculty want to practice and conduct research; d) students, residents, and fellows want to learn; e) and donors want to give to a better future. These five characteristics in the UHHS vision exemplify the desired strategic outcomes of AMC21 goals and the four AMC21 strategic pillars reflect core BSC measures. Likewise, the perioperative BPM initiative nests within the overall execution of the AMC21 goals and vision. However, the UHHS strategic vision needed a more holistic BPM tool.

To align process improvements and stakeholder efforts with the AMC21 vision, UHHS administration also implemented an intranet-based goal setting and reporting tool to leverage existing process data via integrated IS and provide an extended business intelligence application layer across UHHS, similar to the perioperative

Table 7. UHHS' AMC21 strategic goals and pillars

AMC21 Strategic Pillars	AMC21 Strategic Goals
1. Quality 2. Satisfaction 3. Financial Performance 4. Knowledge Advancement	1. Delivering outstanding patient care 2. Developing advancements in scientific discovery and biomedical research 3. Providing a strong foundation of education and training for professionals

Figure 6. Day-to-day operations dashboards

General OR

Suite	Late	On Time	Total Cases
GENOR508	5	13	18
GENOR509	7	12	19
GENOR510	6	15	21
GENOR511	8	11	19
GENOR512	8	12	20
GENOR515	6	11	17
GENOR516	8	13	21
GENOR517	2	20	22
GENOR518	5	14	19
GENOR701	5	16	21
GENOR702	5	17	22
GENOR703	5	17	22
GENOR704	4	18	22
GENOR705	6	15	21
GENOR706	5	17	22
GENOR707	12	8	20
GENOR708	9	12	21
GENOR709	9	9	18
GENOR710	6	15	21
GENOR711	4	16	20
GENOR712	2	20	22
GENOR713	3	19	22
GENOR714	3	19	22
GENOR715	8	14	22
GENOR716	5	15	20
GENOR717	8	13	21
GENOR718	7	15	22
GENOR719	10	11	21
GENOR720	4	16	20
GENOR721	7	13	20
GENOR722	7	13	20
CYSTO	5	9	14
ENDO	4	5	9
GEN Total	198	463	661

GENOROn Time Starts: [redacted]

CVOR

Suite	Late	On Time	Total Cases
CVOR 501	4	9	13
CVOR 502	7	12	19
CVOR 503	6	10	16
CVOR 504	7	9	16
CVOR 505	11	7	18
CVOR 506	9	6	15
CVOR 507	4	11	15
CVOR 508	1	0	1
ENDO	4	2	6
CV Total	53	66	119

CVOR On Time Starts: 55.46%

CEFH

Suite	Late	On Time	Total Cases
CEFOR1	12	9	21
CEFOR2	12	9	21
CEFOR3	11	11	22
CEFOR4	5	15	20
CEFOR5	13	9	22
CEFOR6	13	10	23
CEFOR7	8	15	23
CEFOR8	7	13	20
CEFOR9	8	14	22
CEF Total	89	105	194

CEFH On Time Starts: 84.12%

HHOR

Suite	Late	On Time	Total Cases
HHGI01			0
HHGI02			0
HHOR	4	13	17
HHOR	2	16	18
HHOR	3	13	16
HHOR	6	14	20
HHOR	7	9	16
HHOR	8	11	19
HHOR	6	15	21
HHOR	6	15	21
HHOR09			0
HHOR1	2	7	9
HHOR11			0
HHOR1	4	8	12
HHOR1	3	13	16
HHOR1	2	17	19
HHOR1	3	11	14
HHOR1	2	6	8
HH Tot	58	168	226

HHOR On Time Starts: [redacted]

May 2012
Health System On Time Starts
66.83%

Block Time Utilization

May - 2012

Reflects Block changes made 10/1/2011
Indicated if blocked for a specific surgeon by name, otherwise by SSS
* Time adjusted with 2nd procedure record and reduced Holiday time
All time 7A-7P with 8HR denominator to equalize across services - Except CEFHOR

Overall Block Utilization 98.5%

Available Days	3.0 Monday	5.0 Tuesday	5.0 Wednesday	5.0 Thursday	4.0 Friday	22.0 Weekly Block Total	Weekly Room Total
Main OR 701	Trauma - 8	Surg Onc - 8	Surg Onc - 8	Trauma - 8	Trauma - 8	BLOCK TOTAL	ROOM TOTAL
Total Cases	9	4	11	8	13	45	57
Avg Case Time	170	305	193	103	173	189	169
Total Time	1531	1221	2124	825	2255	7956	9654
% of Utilization	106.32%	50.88%	88.50%	34.38%	117.45%	76.34%	91.42%
Main OR 702	SURG ONC - 8	GI - 8	SURG ONC - 8	Surg Onc - 8	SURG ONC - 8	BLOCK TOTAL	ROOM TOTAL
Total Cases	6	5	9	6	7	33	41
Avg Case Time	213	264	259	309	335	276	261
Total Time	1276	1321	2332	1853	2346	9128	10707
% of Utilization	88.61%	55.04%	97.17%	77.21%	122.19%	86.44%	101.39%
Main OR 703	GI - 12	GI - 12	GI - 12	GI - 12	GI - 12	BLOCK TOTAL	ROOM TOTAL
Total Cases	5	8	12	8	8	41	45
Avg Case Time	245	242	197	258	168	222	218
Total Time	1223	1935	2368	2064	1345	8935	9806
% of Utilization	84.93%	80.63%	98.67%	86.00%	78.05%	84.61%	92.86%

Data Element	Oct-11	Nov-11	Dec-11	Jan-12	Feb-12	Mar-12	Apr-12	May-12	FY12
GenOR Cases done 7AM - 3PM	1187	1169	1119	1222	1249	1226	1212	1238	9622
GenOR Cases done 3PM - 5PM	234	236	201	230	214	186	222	238	1761
GenOR Cases done 5PM - 7PM	123	146	121	129	121	124	148	134	1046
GenOR Cases done 7PM - 9PM	71	77	80	81	66	70	63	76	683
GenOR Remaining Cases	85	80	92	61	78	92	91	97	676
GenOR % Completed 7AM - 3PM	69.8%	68.4%	69.4%	70.9%	72.3%	72.2%	69.8%	69.5%	70.3%
GenOR % Completed 3PM - 5PM	13.8%	13.8%	12.5%	13.3%	12.4%	11.0%	12.8%	13.4%	12.9%
GenOR % Completed 5PM - 7PM	7.2%	8.5%	7.5%	7.5%	7.0%	7.3%	8.5%	7.5%	7.6%
GenOR % Completed 7PM - 9PM	4.2%	4.5%	5.0%	4.7%	3.8%	4.1%	3.6%	4.2%	4.3%
GenOR Remaining Case %	5.0%	4.7%	5.7%	3.5%	4.5%	5.4%	5.2%	5.4%	4.9%
All Cases done 7AM - 3PM	2754	2720	2599	2792	2800	2652	2670	2688	21675
All Cases done 3PM - 5PM	394	392	334	376	348	308	373	373	2898
All Cases done 5PM - 7PM	172	233	184	187	180	183	205	196	1540
All Cases done 7PM - 9PM	98	103	102	110	98	99	91	109	810
All Remaining Cases	103	105	113	79	102	119	111	123	855
All % Completed 7AM - 3PM	78.2%	76.6%	78.0%	78.8%	79.4%	78.9%	77.4%	77.0%	78.0%
All % Completed 3PM - 5PM	11.2%	11.0%	10.0%	10.6%	9.9%	9.2%	10.8%	10.7%	10.4%
All % Completed 5PM - 7PM	4.9%	6.6%	5.5%	5.3%	5.1%	5.4%	5.9%	5.6%	5.5%
All % Completed 7PM - 9PM	2.8%	2.9%	3.1%	3.1%	2.8%	2.9%	2.6%	3.1%	2.9%
All Remaining Case %	2.9%	3.0%	3.4%	2.2%	2.9%	3.5%	3.2%	3.5%	3.1%

Figure 7. KPI data visualization

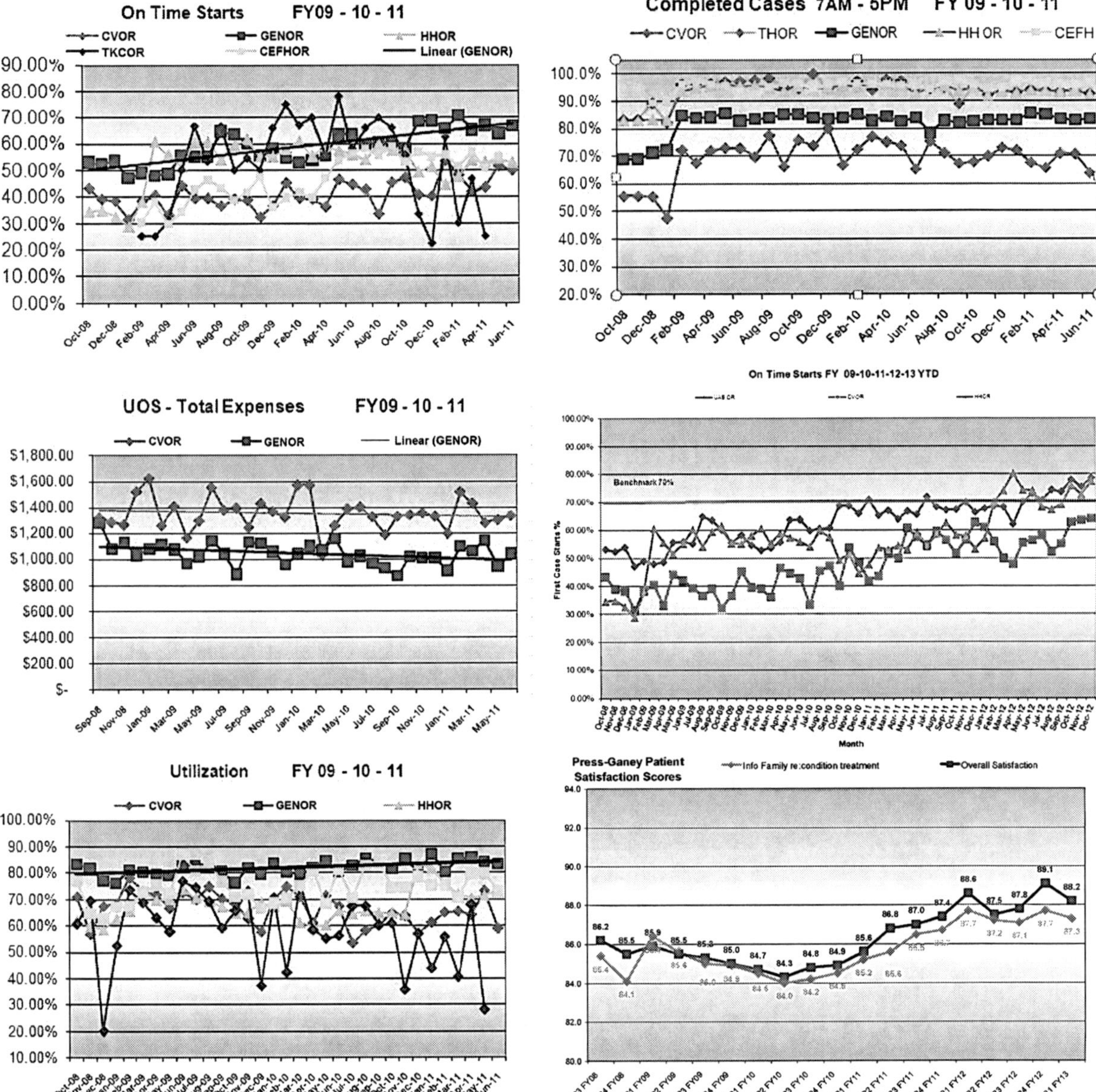

CSIS/BPM tool, but with an entire UHHS system focus. The "Reach for Excellence" (RFE) layer provides process management capabilities for qualitative and quantitative measures, across UHHS, measurable and aligned to AMC21 pillars and goals. The purpose for the RFE layer is to provide an objective tool to measure process and stakeholder performance toward strategic, tactical, and operational goals that support the AMC21 vision. Individual employee goal setting towards achieving AMC21 is a formalized RFE activity integrated into the UHHS employee evaluation and performance review process. As a result, all hospital stakeholders (e.g. physicians, surgeons, nurses, staff, and administrators) at strategic, tactical, and operational levels have action plans, RFE goals, and resulting merit increases that align with the AMC21 pillars, goals, and ultimately vision.

Rather than identify tactics, projects, or activities, RFE goals are quantitative, objective, aggressive, and realistic outcomes, where fewer rather than more is better. RFE goals will change focus as AMC21 progress advances. Consequently, each year UHHS administration reviews opportunities for improvement and identifies the most important outcomes needed. Many RFE goals do not change annually, as they are important outcomes for success. However, the iterative nature of the goal setting process yields aggressive targets for more familiar goals. As a result, administrators set goals so stakeholders focus on specific areas and the goal setting process aligns RFE process outcomes and stakeholder action to AMC21 strategy–a very powerful process management tool.

Figure 8 illustrates the 2012 AMC21 dashboard reflecting UHHS process measures aligned to AMC21 strategic pillars via RFE goals. The School of Medicine goals (9) are distinguishable from UHHS (15) and each goal carries a colorcoated rating and indicator on performance. RFE goals use the four strategic pillars as modified BSC categories to reflect and categorize where targeted opportunities align to the AMC21 vision and goals. The color-coded performance and rating hierarchy is as follows:

- **5:** Dark Green = Stretch (achieved about 20% of the time)
- **4:** Green = Partial Stretch (achieved about 50% of the time)
- **3:** Light Green = Target (achieved about 80% of the time)
- **2:** Yellow = Partial Accomplishment
- **1:** Red = No Accomplishment

The RFE strategic goals reflect multiple core UHHS processes that are necessary to achieve the AMC21 vision. Six 2012 goals had no or partial accomplishment while 18 had 80% or more accomplishment. Perioperative processes depicted previously in Figure 7 influenced portions of RFE goals across satisfaction, quality, and finance pillars that were achieved 80% of the time or better during 2012.

6. CONCLUSION

Empowered individuals, integrated IS, and a holistic framework for perioperative process management allows University Hospital to take control and improve its perioperative process. The BSC approach to identify process measures gives stakeholders an end-to-end (e.g. holistic) view for financial, customer, and process perspectives. Patients are clearly customers, as well as PACU is a customer to an OR suite, or an OR suite is a customer to PREP. Also, revenue or margins are clearly financial, as well as surgical cases performed between 7PM to 9PM or cases remaining after 9PM. Moreover, the RFE goal layer affords University Hospital opportunities for process improvement aligned to AMC21 vision. The modified BSC approach to BPM gives stakeholders an end-to-end (e.g. holistic) view for AMC21 pillars, RFE goals, and hospital strategy execution.

Adopting the holistic framework for BSC measures at strategic, tactical, and day-to-day operations levels further educates hospital stakeholders on the benefits of integrated IS for process measurement, control, and improvement. The cycle of analysis, evaluation, and synthesis reinforces communication and stimulates individual as well as collective organizational learning.

Our case study contributes to the healthcare IT literature by examining how CPI, BSC, performance dashboards, business analytics, and process management are applicable to the hospital environment. This study prescribes an a priori framework to foster their occurrence. This paper also fills a gap in the literature by describing how hospital process data is both a performance measure and a management tool.

Figure 8. AMC21 2012 pillars and RFE goals

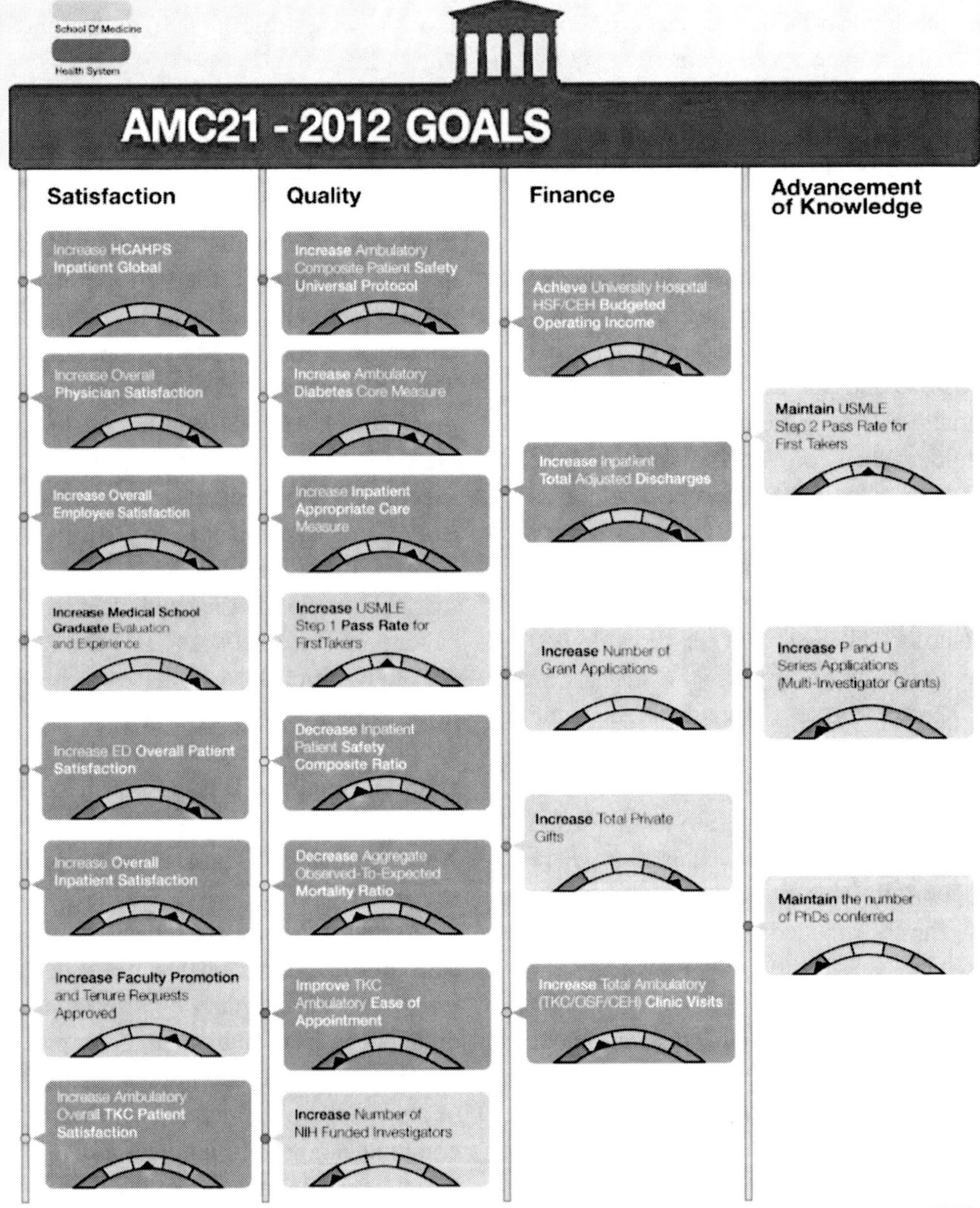

This study was limited to a single case, where future research should broaden the focus to address this issue along with others that the authors may have inadvertently overlooked. The case examples presented in this study can serve as momentum for healthcare BPM and strategy alignment methodology, comprehension, and extension. The study's results should be viewed as exploratory and in need of further confirmation. Researchers may choose to further or expand the investigation; while practitioners may apply the findings to create their own version of process management, control, and improvement aligned to strategy within the hospital environment.

REFERENCES

Ackoff, R. L. (1967). Management misinformation systems. *Management Science, 14*(4), 147–156. doi:10.1287/mnsc.14.4.B147

Albanese, M. P., Evans, D. A., Schantz, C. A., Bowen, M., Disbot, M., & Moffa, J. S. et al.. (2010). Engaging clinical nurses in quality and performance improvement activities. [PubMed]. *Nursing Administration Quarterly, 34*(3), 226–245. doi:10.1097/NAQ.0b013e3181e702ca

Barnes, M. (2010). 'Operating Room On-Time Starts and First Case of the Day. Thomson Group, 2. Retrieved February 15, 2013 from http://www.thomasgroup.com/eLibrary/Industry-Insights/Healthcare-and-Life-Sciences/Perioperative-Services.aspx

Bush, M., Lederer, A. L., Li, X., Palmisano, J., & Rao, S. (2009). The alignment of information systems with organizational objectives and strategies in health care. [PubMed]. *International Journal of Medical Informatics, 78*(7), 446–456. doi:10.1016/j.ijmedinf.2009.02.004

Catalano, K., & Fickenscher, K. (2007). Emerging technologies in the OR and their effect on perioperativeprofessionals. [PubMed]. *AORN Journal, 86*(6), 958–969. doi:10.1016/j.aorn.2007.07.007

CMS. (2005). Pay-for-Performance / Quality Incentives. 10. Retrieved May 15, 2013 from http://www.cms.gov/Regulations-and-Guidance/Guidance/FACA/downloads/tab_H.pdf

CMS. (2010). Medicare Hospital Quality Chartbook: 2010 Performance Report on Outcomes Measures. 44. Retrieved May 15, 2013 from http://www.cms.gov/Medicare/Quality-Initiatives-Patient-Assessment-Instruments/HospitalQualityInits/OutcomeMeasures.html

Eisenhardt, K. (1989). Building theories from case study research. *Academy of Management Review, 14*(4), 532–550.

Fairbanks, C. (2007). Using Six Sigma and Lean Methodologies to Improve OR Throughput. [PubMed]. *AORN Journal, 86*(1), 73–82. doi:10.1016/j.aorn.2007.06.011

Herzer, K. R., Mark, L. J., Michelson, J. D., Saletnik, L. A., & Lundquist, C. A. (2008). Designing and implementing a comprehensive quality and patient safety management model: A paradigm for perioperative improvement. *Journal of Patient Safety, 4*(2), 84–92. doi:10.1097/PTS.0b013e3181730863

Hospital Consumer Assessment of Healthcare Providers and Systems. (2012). HCAHPS Fact Sheet", 4. Retrieved May 15, 2013 from http://www.hcahpsonline.org/files/HCAHPS%20Fact%20Sheet%20May%202012.pdf

Jeston, J., & Nelis, J. (2008). *Business Process Management: Practical Guidelines to Successful Implementations* (2nd ed.). Burlington, MA: Elsevier, Ltd.

Kaplan, R., & Norton, D. (1996). *The Balanced Scorecard*. Boston: Harvard Business School Press.

Kruskal, J. B., Reedy, A., Pascal, L., Rosen, M. P., & Boiselle, P. M. (2012). Quality Initiatives: Lean Approach to Improving Performance and Efficiency in a Radiology Department. [PubMed]. *Radiographics, 32*(2), 573–587. doi:10.1148/rg.322115128

Kujala, J., Lillrank, P., Kronstrom, V., & Peltokorpi, A. (2006). Time-based management of patient processes. [PubMed]. *Journal of Health Organization and Management, 20*(6), 512–524. doi:10.1108/14777260610702262

Lindenauer, P. K., Remus, D., Roman, S., Rothberg, M. B., Benjamin, E. M., Ma, A., & Bratzler, D. W. (2007). Public Reporting and Pay for Performance in Hospital Quality Improvement. [PubMed]. *The New England Journal of Medicine, 356*(5), 486–496. doi:10.1056/NEJMsa064964

Luftman, J., & Ben-Zvi, T. (2010). Key issues for IT executives 2009: Difficult economy's impact on IT. *MIS Quarterly Executive, 9*(1), 49–59.

Macario, A., Vitez, T., Dunn, B., & McDonald, T. (1995). Analysis of hospital costs and charges for inpatient surgical care. [PubMed]. *Anesthesiology, 6*(83), 1138–1144. doi:10.1097/00000542-199512000-00002

Marjamaa, R., Vakkuri, A., & Kirvela, O. (2008). Operating room management: Why, how and by whom? [PubMed]. *Acta Anaesthesiologica Scandinavica, 52*(5), 596–600. doi:10.1111/j.1399-6576.2008.01618.x

Mazzella-Ebstein, A. M., & Saddul, R. (2004). Web-based Nurse Executive Dashboard. [PubMed]. *Journal of Nursing Care Quality, 19*(4), 307–315. doi:10.1097/00001786-200410000-00004

McClusker, J., Dendukuri, N., Cardinal, L., Katofsky, L., & Riccardi, M. (2005). Assessment of the work environment of multidisciplinary hospital staff. [PubMed]. *International Journal of Health Care Quality Assurance, 7*(18), 543–551. doi:10.1108/09526860510627229

Munroe, M. C., & Wheeler, B. R. (1980). Planning, critical success factors, and management's information requirements. *Management Information Systems Quarterly, 4*(4), 27–37. doi:10.2307/248958

National Quality Forum. (2008). Serious Reportable Events (SREs) Transparency, accountability critical to reducing medical errors and harm. 4. Retrieved May 15, 2013 from http://www.quality-forum.org/Publications/2008/10/Serious_Reportable_Events.aspx

Peters, J., & Blasco, T. (2004). Enhancing hospital performance through perioperative services. [PubMed]. *Physician Executive, 30*(6), 26–31.

PwC Health Research Institute. (2012). The future of the academic medical center: Strategies to avoid a meltdown. PricewaterhouseCoopers LLP, 44. Retrieved February 15, 2013 from http://www.pwc.com/us/en/health-industries/publications/the-future-of-academic-medical-centers.jhtml#

Rockart, J. F. (1979). Chief executives define their own data needs. [PubMed]. *Harvard Business Review, 57*(2), 81–93.

Tenner, A. R., & DeToro, I. J. (1997). *Process redesign: the implementation guide for managers.* Upper Saddle River, NJ: Prentice-Hall, Inc.

Thomson Group. (2010). Industry Insights: Perioperative Services, 2. Retrieved February 15, 2013 from via http://www.thomasgroup.com/eLibrary/Industry-Insights/Healthcare-and-Life-Sciences/Perioperative-Services.aspx

Turban, E., Sharda, R., Aronson, J., & King, D. (2008). *Business Intelligence: A managerial approach.* Upper Saddle River, New Jersey: Prentice Hall.

Walton, M. (1986). *The Deming Management Method.* New York: Dodd, Mead.

Wears, R., & Berg, M. (2005). Computer technology and clinical work: Still waiting for Godot. [PubMed]. *Journal of the American Medical Association, 293*(10), 1261–1263. doi:10.1001/jama.293.10.1261

Weber, R. (2004). The rhetoric of positivism versus interpretivism: A personal view. *Management Information Systems Quarterly, 28*(1), iii–xii.

Yin, R. K. (2003). *Case study research: Design and methods* (3rd ed.). Thousand Oaks, California: Sage Publications.

Zani, W. M. (1970). Blueprint for MIS. *Harvard Business Review, 48*(6), 85–90.

Zbinden, A. (2002). Introducing a Balanced Scorecard Management System in a University Anesthesiology Department. [PubMed]. *Medical Intelligence, 95*, 1731–1738.

Chapter 57
Using Mobile Technology to Address the 'Three Delays' to Reduce Maternal Mortality in Zanzibar

Rachel Hoy Deussom
IntraHealth International, USA

Marc Mitchell
Harvard School of Public Health, USA

Julia Dae Ruben
D-Tree International, USA

ABSTRACT

The hallmark article by Thaddeus and Maine (1994) presented a framework to reducing maternal mortality by addressing the delays: (1) deciding to seek care; (2) reaching care; and (3) receiving adequate care. This project developed a phone-based system used by traditional birth attendants to address the three delays in two districts in rural Zanzibar. Mobile phones provided: clinical algorithms to screen pregnant mothers for danger signs; phone numbers and mobile banking to arrange and pay for transportation; and contacts for health facility staff to alert them of referrals. 938 mothers participated in the "mHealth for Safer Deliveries" project. The intervention achieved a 71.0% facility delivery rate in the project zone, compared to the regional average of 32.0% (NBS and ICF Macro, 2011). This project demonstrated the effectiveness of mobile technology in addressing childbirth's three delays and its potential to impact maternal mortality in low-income countries.

BACKGROUND

Losing a mother to childbirth is a tragic loss to a family, community, and society. Worldwide, there were an estimated 287,000 maternal deaths in 2010 (UNFPA, UNICEF, WHO, and World Bank, 2012). The United Nations Millennium Development Goal 5, to reduce maternal mortality by 75%, will not be achieved in many countries (United Nations, 2012). This is in part due to the persistent

DOI: 10.4018/978-1-4666-8756-1.ch057

challenges of addressing the complex and diverse underlying determinants and causes that contribute to maternal mortality (Stokoe, 1991).

Reducing maternal mortality requires a co-ordinated, multi-pronged approach, including interventions at the family and community levels that involve efforts to improve female education, nutrition, and socioeconomic status (WHO, 1999; Jokhio et al, 2005; Kidney et al., 2009). In addition, high quality antenatal, obstetric, and postnatal services must be delivered by a functional health system that links the community and facility (Campbell and Graham, 2006). Only when demand for qualified care can be met by an adequate supply of qualified care do maternal health outcomes improve (Kidney et al., 2005).

The hallmark article by Thaddeus and Maine (1994; Maine et al., 1997) presented a compelling framework for reducing maternal mortality in low-income countries. The article suggested the following three delays to be critical barriers to reducing maternal mortality: (1) the delay in seeking care for the woman in labor; (2) the delay to arrange transportation and reach the health facility; and (3) the delay in receiving care at the health facility. Further, the theory states that reducing only one or two of the delays will not impact health outcomes; rather all three must be addressed in order to significantly reduce the high numbers of women and newborns who die in delivery and/or the postpartum period in low-income countries.

Many interventions aimed at reducing maternal mortality have been unsuccessful because they fell short of addressing the three delays in a comprehensive manner, thus failing to meet the complex needs of mother and child along the continuum of care, especially in resource-constrained contexts (Campbell & Graham, 2006; Prata et al., 2011; Hasan et al., 2013). Supply-side interventions in particular may not always reach the most vulnerable mothers. A joint statement from the World Health Organization, the United Nations Population Fund, the United Nations Children's

Fund, and the World Bank acknowledged, "[T]he settings where the problem of maternal mortality is most acute are precisely those where it is least likely to be accurately measured" (WHO, 1999, p. 10). Health systems may not always have an adequate monitoring and information system to track maternal deaths (Hill et al., 2007; Prata et al., 2011). The high-level Commission on Information and Accountability for Women's and Children's Health recommended that by 2015, all countries "have well-functioning health information systems that combine data from facilities, administrative sources, and surveys" (2011, p.2) in order to effectively improve maternal and child health and reduce mortality.

In Zanzibar, additional efforts are needed to improve maternal health indicators and address the three delays faced by women in childbirth. Zanzibar is a semi-autonomous part of the United Republic of Tanzania. It is composed of two islands, Unguja and Pemba, and a population of 1.3 million, of whom over two-thirds live in rural zones and half live on less than $2 per day (RGOZ MOHSW, 2010a). Zanzibar's population health is governed by an autonomous Ministry of Health and Social Welfare. Nearly 99% of the Zanzibari population is Muslim. In 2010, the maternal mortality ratio was estimated to be 454 per 100,000 live births (NBS and ICF Macro, 2011) The main causes of maternal death are hemorrhage, pregnancy-induced hypertension, obstructed labor, infection, and unsafe abortion (RGOZ MOHSW, 2010a).

In Zanzibar, the Ministry of Health is committed to improving maternal and neonatal health through its Reproductive and Child Health program. Zanzibar's 2006-2011 Health Sector Strategic Plan set reproductive and child health as a top priority. The ministry defined among its targets to increase the percentage of births delivered in health facilities to 60%. They proposed achieving this target through several core interventions, such as the early referral of obstetric emergencies, and improving the quality of delivery services at the district level–which includes enhancing delivery capacity at the primary health facility, secondary cottage hospitals, and tertiary hospital levels (RGOZ MOSHW, 2006). Further, in May 2012, Zanzibar's President Dr. Ali Mohamad Shein publicly declared that there would no longer be any child delivery fees in public hospitals (Yussef, 2012).

With regards to the first delay, the decision to seek care, the majority of Zanzibari women are not well informed of risk factors or danger signs in pregnancy, nor are they always adequately assessed for pre-existing health conditions or pregnancy-related risks prior to delivery. Over 95% of mothers in Zanzibar received antenatal care from a skilled provider over the course of their last pregnancy. However, only 17% of mothers were seen during their first trimester, and fewer than half all mothers (43%) completed four or more antenatal visits. Only 46% of rural Zanzibari women giving birth in the last five years reported being informed of signs of pregnancy complications during antenatal care (NBS and ICF Macro, 2011). The decision-makers in these women's families are often even less well informed about the possible risks that their wives or daughters-in-law face in pregnancy, childbirth, and the postpartum period.

Delays to seeking care after home birth are similar to those that families face during labor. Despite existing government guidelines for postnatal care (RGOZ MOH 2010b), families delivering at home do not generally decide seek care from a health professional in the first week after birth, when 60% of maternal deaths and 75% of neonatal deaths occur (Rogo et al., 2006; WHO 2012). In Zanzibar only 6% of women attend postnatal care within two days and only 7% within the first week after delivery (RGOZ MOHSW, 2010a). Primary reasons for not attending are: not receiving advice to go for a check-up; and not recognizing its importance (Mdungi, 2000; RGOZ MOH 2010b).

Particularly in rural Zanzibar, delays in arranging transport and arriving at health facilities are common for cultural, financial and logistical reasons. In a conservative Muslim context, it is the woman's husband, mother-in-law, or the head of household who usually grants permission for a laboring mother to travel to the health facility. These decision-makers are less likely to be informed about the health risks or pre-existing conditions that a mother may learn about during her antenatal consultations, and they are therefore less prepared for an adverse situation in birth should it arise. Discussions about transport to the health facility in a non-emergency event may not take place as frequently. As most mothers-in-law gave birth at home, in some households it may be assumed that this would also be the case for the pregnant mother.

In addition, procuring private transport to a health facility can be timely and costly, and often families will only consider it in the event of a serious medical emergency. However, by the time the event becomes an emergency, it is usually too late for the woman and/or her baby. Most rural families do not own a car and would prefer to save money for other aspects of the birth, such as food, clothing, or supplies. A family's ability to quickly mobilize the funds needed to procure emergency transport is generally limited. The cost of private transport may range between 10,000 and 60,000 Tanzanian shillings (USD$6-$37) to arrive at a health facility, depending on if it is a local primary health care unit or tertiary hospital. While mobile banking is common in urban areas, most rural areas have limited access to pay-points. In the event of an emergency, if families both decide to transport the pregnant mother to the health facility and are able to mobilize the funds for private transport, then they face the further logistical challenge of locating a driver and an available car with fuel. Often drivers are distrustful of providing emergency transport because they are not assured that they will be compensated for their services.

In Zanzibar, the third delay of receiving adequate care at a health facility is due to the limited preparedness and information that facility staffs have about incoming births, especially if the mother has had very limited contact with the facility during pregnancy. Too often a pregnant mother arrives without any advance notice. Facility staffs do not have information about her pregnancy history, medical conditions, or labor progression. If on-call staffs need to mobilize equipment or additional staff members to support the mother, critical time is spent doing so *after* the mother has arrived to the facility. In some facilities where few births took place, the facility was less likely to be well-staffed, which discouraged the surrounding community from seeking to deliver there. In the regions where this project was implemented–Unguja North and Pemba North–the most recent Demographic and Health Survey indicated that an average of 40.4% and 23.6% of women give birth in a health facility in these regions respectively (NBS and ICF Macro, 2011).

The Zanzibari public health system's ability to intervene and prevent the three delays is severely limited by its capacity to influence the factors described above, as much action and decision-making occurs at the family or community level. Efforts made by district health management teams to target services to high-risk mothers are limited due to the absence of reliable patient data, poor communication, limited funding, and limited ability to evaluate which interventions deliver the most effective results.

Many rural Zanzibari families engage traditional birth attendants to attend their home births; in project regions Unguja North and Pemba North, 42.8% and 73.2% of women give birth with the assistance of a traditional birth attendant (NBS and ICF Macro, 2011). With the exception of a few younger women with basic community health training who may also work as traditional birth attendants, the majority are older with no formal health training. Traditional birth attendants are well respected within their communities. Families generally reimburse them with a cash or in-kind gift of between 5,000-10,000 Tanzanian shillings ($3-6) for their services, which generally involve arriving at the family's home at the onset of active labor, providing massage and comfort measures

for the mother during delivery, administering delivery, and helping the family to clean up after the birth. They may also make daily visits to the mother in the days after birth. However, the linkages that these traditional birth attendants have with local health facilities, if any, are often informal and contextual, especially at secondary cottage hospitals, which cover a larger catchment area and have higher staff turnover.

In recent years, mobile health technology, or mHealth, has emerged as a means for improving service delivery and strengthening health information systems (DeRenzi et al., 2008; Mitchell et al., 2009). In addition, there is evidence that mobile phones have the potential increase access to communication to improve maternal and neonatal health services in developing country contexts (Noordam et al., 2011; Tamrat and Kachnowski, 2012; Mitchell et al., 2012). To this end, D-tree International worked with the Ministry of Health and local actors in rural Zanzibar to implement a mobile technology intervention to address the three delays that contribute to poor maternal health outcomes. Evidence has shown that traditional birth attendants can be effectively engaged to screen pregnant mothers and coordinate maternal referrals to health facilities (Sibley et al., 2004). Given the strong influence and role in home births that Zanzibar's traditional birth attendants have in their rural communities, we determined that it would be essential to involve them in this intervention.

Financed by the Bill and Melinda Gates Foundation, the "Cell-based protocols for safer deliveries" ("mHealth for Safer Deliveries") project used mobile technology to increase facility delivery and improve maternal health in two districts in rural Zanzibar, where the average facility delivery rate in these regions was 32.0% (NBS and ICF Macro, 2011). D-tree International implemented the project from November 2011 to December 2012 using an open source mobile health application, with the aim to reduce the three delays by decreasing the informational, logistical, and financial barriers to in-facility births and postnatal care.

METHODOLOGY

The mHealth for Safer Deliveries project aimed to address the three delays through the use of mobile technology in two health districts in Zanzibar. This was to be achieved through the development of several phone-based clinical algorithms that guided traditional birth attendants (the "users") to screen pregnant mothers for risk factors and counsel them to give birth at the appropriate facility; and recognize and refer women and their babies to the appropriate facility for complications during labor/delivery and the postnatal period. In addition to registering critical information about the mother, the mHealth application also allowed users to record family permissions ahead of time for transfer to the health facility, as well as store the mobile phone numbers of drivers and health staff to ensure timely arrangement of transportation and preparedness of health staff for the woman's arrival to the health facility. In addition, mobile banking accounts and a small communication top-up were put in place for users in order to pay for transport without handling cash and communicate freely with families, drivers, and health staff. Finally, the project engaged local leaders, reliable car owners, and other stakeholders to raise awareness for the intervention and pre-determine rates for transport, establishing community-based referral systems within which the mobile phone application could be used. The mHealth for Safer

Deliveries project intervention was subsequently implemented and monitored throughout the project intervention zone. *(See Table 1)*

DEVELOPING AND TESTING OF CLINICAL ALGORITHMS AND MOBILE DATA COLLECTION

Working with the Zanzibar Ministry of Health, we developed clinical algorithms that guided traditional birth attendants through a systematic screening process to identify women's risks and danger signs during pregnancy. Running on java-enabled Nokia phones, these algorithms registered pregnant mothers, screened them for risks, prompted the user to develop birth plans with the mothers for the appropriate level facility and–regardless of their risks–encouraged them to deliver at a facility. Mothers were also required to provide their antenatal care registration number as part of the screening, thus promoting earlier and more frequent antenatal care at their primary health facility.

Other algorithms assisted the same users to assess the mother's status during labor to ensure her timely transport to the appropriate facility; to assess mother and newborn for risks and refer as needed in the accidental event of a home delivery; and to screen and refer mother and newborn for any postpartum health issues within

Table 1. mHealth for Safer Deliveries project intervention zone in Zanzibar

Health District	Health Facilities (primary referral)	Cottage Hospitals (secondary referral)	Shehias (Villages) covered by intervention
North A	Nungwi	Kivunge	Nungwi
	Kidoti	Kivunge	Kidoti Fukuchani
Micheweni	Makangale	Micheweni	Makangale Mkia Ngombe
	Shumba vyamboni	Micheweni	Mihogoni Shumba vyamboni
	Tumbe	Micheweni	Tumbe Mashariki Tumbe Magharibi

one week after delivery. Software also included stored phone numbers of selected drivers with vehicles willing to transport pregnant women on an emergency basis, recorded permissions from husband and other relatives for emergency transfer, phone numbers of referral facilities to call when transfer was required and mobile banking to pay for transportation. *(See Figure 1)*

In order to assure high levels of quality and appropriateness, the central level Ministry of Health, as well as district health management teams and labor/delivery nurses in the referral health facilities reviewed the algorithms. This exercise also served to inform the health staffs of the kinds of information were being collected and thus available to them through the mobile health intervention. In addition, the project aimed to build a stronger and more formal relationship between the traditional birth attendants using the phone and the professional staffs at the health facilities, so as to enable dialogue, build trust, and develop more welcoming environment for mothers entering the facility. Built into the clinical algorithms were specific, pre-tested messages indicating to users as to when they should reach out to health facility staffs. The algorithms were field-tested and continuously refined at the start of the project.

TRAINING MOBILE PHONE USERS

The project trained 24 traditional birth attendants in the North A District, Unguja, and the Micheweni District, Pemba to use the mHealth application. These users were all female, ranging in age from 22 to 48 years of age. Most traditionally assisted

Figure 1. mHealth for Safer Deliveries Project: Clinical algorithms and data collected

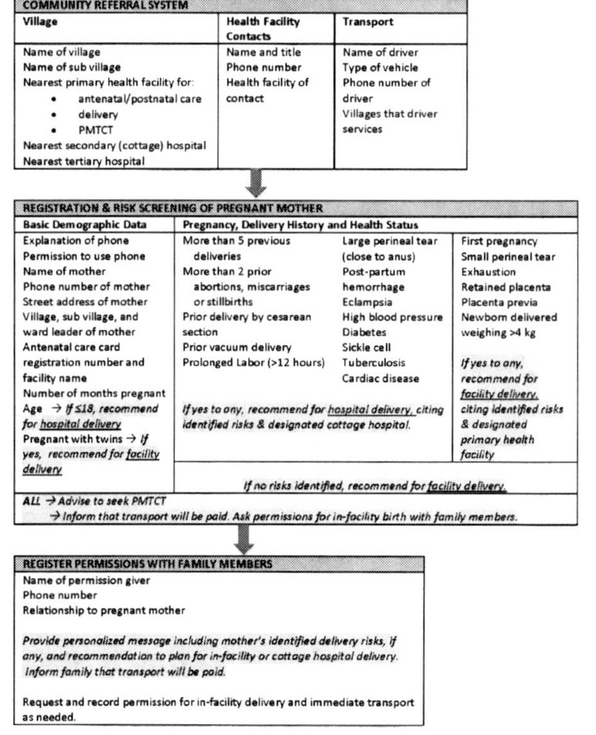

COMMUNITY REFERRAL SYSTEM

Village	Health Facility Contacts	Transport
Name of village Name of sub village Nearest primary health facility for: • antenatal/postnatal care • delivery • PMTCT Nearest secondary (cottage) hospital Nearest tertiary hospital	Name and title Phone number Health facility of contact	Name of driver Type of vehicle Phone number of driver Villages that driver services

REGISTRATION & RISK SCREENING OF PREGNANT MOTHER

Basic Demographic Data	Pregnancy, Delivery History and Health Status		
Explanation of phone Permission to use phone Name of mother Phone number of mother Street address of mother Village, sub village, and ward leader of mother Antenatal care card registration number and facility name Number of months pregnant Age → *If ≤18, recommend for hospital delivery* Pregnant with twins → *if yes, recommend for facility delivery*	More than 5 previous deliveries More than 2 prior abortions, miscarriages or stillbirths Prior delivery by cesarean section Prior vacuum delivery Prolonged Labor (>12 hours) *If yes to any, recommend for hospital delivery, citing identified risks & designated cottage hospital.*	Large perineal tear (close to anus) Post-partum hemorrhage Eclampsia High blood pressure Diabetes Sickle cell Tuberculosis Cardiac disease	First pregnancy Small perineal tear Exhaustion Retained placenta Placenta previa Newborn delivered weighing >4 kg *If yes to any, recommend for facility delivery, citing identified risks & designated primary health facility*
	If no risks identified, recommend for facility delivery.		
ALL → *Advise to seek PMTCT* → *Inform that transport will be paid. Ask permissions for in-facility birth with family members.*			

REGISTER PERMISSIONS WITH FAMILY MEMBERS

Name of permission giver
Phone number
Relationship to pregnant mother

Provide personalized message including mother's identified delivery risks, if any, and recommendation to plan for in-facility or cottage hospital delivery. Inform family that transport will be paid.

Request and record permission for in-facility delivery and immediate transport as needed.

DURING LABOR

Gestation age of baby <8 months Baby in breech position Labor lasting more than 12 hours Swollen face or hands	Severe headache or blurred vision Convulsion in the last 24 hours Bleeding
If any observed on arrival, transport immediately to health facility. Inform facility contact. *If none observed, transport to health facility when mother is ready.*	

IN EVENT OF ACCIDENTAL HOME DELIVERY

Advise to keep baby warm and dry. Massage mother's stomach below the navel to stop uterine bleeding every 15 minutes for next 4 hours.

If baby is: not crying blue	If baby is: pale yellow very small has congenital abnormality	If mother: bleeds through >1 kanga per hour is pale has abnormal breathing has fits has fever
Elevate baby's feet. Clean baby's mouth and nose. Transport immediately to health facility. Inform facility contact.	*Transport immediately to health facility. Inform facility contact.*	*Transport immediately to health facility. Inform facility contact.*

If neither baby nor mother referrals are needed, congratulate family for good health. Advise mother and family to:
Contact traditional birth attendant if anything changes
Repeat the stomach massage every hour for 24 hours
Breastfeed the baby now and as often as the baby wants
Keep the baby warm, directly against mother's or family member's skin
Plan to go to the health facility within 7 days

POSTPARTUM FOLLOW-UP

Confirm date, place, and person assisting delivery.

Assess mother for:		With mother, assess baby for:	
Fever Crying Excessive bleeding Exhaustion Severe abdominal Pain	Blurred vision Foul-smelling vaginal discharge Breast mastitis Breast cracking Sadness/hopelessness	Fever Infection Stiffness Convulsions Arching of back Excessive crying Inability to suckle Difficult or fast breathing Excessive vomiting Blue lips Pale pallor	Swollen eyes Yellow color Congenital abnormalities Skin rashes Bulging anterior fontanel Discharge from eyes Cord bleeding Red umbilical cord Abdominal distention If no urine passed If no bowel movement Severe diarrhea
If yes to any, transport to health facility, citing identified risks. Inform facility contact.		*If yes to any, transport to health facility, citing identified risks. Inform facility contact.*	
If no referral needed for mother or infant: Advise mother and family on: PMTCT Exclusive breastfeeding Visiting health facility within 4 days Good nutrition Rest Family planning			

deliveries, but in a few areas where it was difficult to find literate experienced traditional birth attendants, a younger, active community member with no experience assisting deliveries was chosen. Some were well versed at using cell phones while others had no experience at all. The 24 users received 2700c Nokia mobile phones that were loaded with the mHealth application, which ran offline and then transmitted data to a central server when the user initiated synchronization. They were trained in general use of the phone, such as calling, sending messages, and saving contacts, as well as use of the mHealth application for registering mothers, referring mothers to a health facility or hospital, and providing postnatal care. Finally, they were trained to submit data and pay for transport using mobile banking. After training, field visits continued on a regular basis to provide technical support to the users and continuously monitor the progress of the project, including its successes and challenges.

ENABLING MOBILE BANKING

The two islands of Zanzibar benefit from a widespread mobile network. We worked with a local mobile service provider, Zantel to establish mobile money accounts for all users through their Z-pesa mobile services, and to ensure that there were functional Z-pesa pay points near all health facilities. A monthly budget for each user was calculated based on the number of pregnant mothers that were expected to deliver that month, to include transport costs, a communication stipend for the user, and user compensation. This amount was then transferred to the users' mobile banking accounts. As referrals and postpartum visits were made, the users withdrew funds from the Z-pesa pay points. These timely transfers of the money led to smooth transactions and fast turnaround of payments. Funds were used to pay the drivers a predetermined fee for emergency transport. We also paid the users a fixed fee per birth (10,000

Tanzanian shillings, or $6). This was because transferring a mother to a facility meant the family for a home delivery would no longer reimburse the traditional birth attendant.

ENGAGING STAKEHOLDERS AND ESTABLISHING COMMUNITY-BASED REFERRAL SYSTEMS

We continuously informed the Zanzibar Ministry of Health, district health management teams and health facility staff about project progress through phone calls, visitations and monthly reports. Further, through a participatory approach, meetings were held in each district with village authorities, traditional birth attendants, drivers, and health facility staff. We introduced the project, invited participation, discussed expectations for each actor within the referral system, and provided estimated driving times and distances from each village to primary and secondary health facilities. The costs for each route were proposed by community members and negotiated by all stakeholders to ensure that rates were reasonable given market rates, fuel costs, distances to facilities, and road conditions. Health facility staff within the project intervention zone promoted the project during antenatal care consultations, obtaining permission from the mother for the traditional birth attendant to contact the mother directly or suggesting that the mother reach out to the traditional birth attendant within her community. The intervention developed and implemented by D-tree International was designed to strengthen and work within the existing health system to promote its economic viability for scale-up.

IMPLEMENTING AND MONITORING THE INTERVENTION

Registration of pregnant mothers began in the North A district of Unguja in November 2011 and in the Micheweni District of Pemba in February 2012. Registration continued through April 2012, while provision of support and transport for registered women continued through December 2012. Starting on a weekly, then biweekly, and finally monthly basis, project managers convened with users to troubleshoot any issues within the mobile application and learn about users' experiences with community members and in the field.

User data were transmitted from the phones via General Packet Radio Service to a cloud-based server. These data were then cleaned, and stored in an Access database. The database was used to evaluate data on maternal and newborn health outcomes, delivery locations, and the costs of referrals and deliveries.

RESULTS

The mHealth for Safer Deliveries project provided enhanced community-level outreach to pregnant mothers, reinforced knowledge of identified pregnancy risks and the importance of in-facility delivery within families, provided transport, and established more reliable access and communication to professional health care givers via the traditional birth attendants. Using mobile technology to address the three delays in rural Zanzibar resulted in in-facility birth rates of 71.0% among the pregnant mothers participating in the project. Nine villages in these two health districts developed community-based referral systems. Registered mothers benefitted from a coordinated system that improved their families' level of preparation and understanding of risks approaching delivery, helped them to plan for and coordinate transport to a health facility, and improved the preparedness of their service providers to deliver better care.

During project implementation 963 mothers were registered, of which 938 gave birth in the project area, leaving a 2.6% loss to follow-up. Of the 963 mothers, 433 were from the North A district of Unguja and 505 were from the Micheweni district

of Pemba. In North A, 328 (75.8%) births occurred in a health facility, and in Micheweni, 338 (66.9%) occurred in a health facility. During the project, we observed a substantial increase in the numbers of women delivering in a health facility compared to the Tanzania Demographic and Health Survey in-facility birth rate of 33.6% (NBS and ICF Macro 2011). Of the 938 mothers, 666 (71.0%) gave birth in health facilities, while 264 (28.1%) gave birth at home and 8 (0.9%) gave birth en route to the facility. There was one maternal death of a woman who gave birth at home, due a retained placenta and post-partum hemorrhage.

INCREASED FAMILY-LEVEL DEMAND FOR IN-FACILITY BIRTHS

The identification of risks via the mobile phone algorithm contributed to pregnant mothers' and their families' decision to seek care earlier on in pregnancy. Within the project intervention zone, there was high demand among rural Zanzibari families' to plan for an in-facility birth and seek professional health care during labor and delivery. The users successfully registered 963 pregnant mothers in the 5-month registration period. Almost immediately after the project began implementation, families approached our users to ask that their pregnant mothers be registered, some before they were even eligible to begin antenatal care. When registration ended, the requests continued. The high demand for in-facility births and postpartum care within the project intervention zone can be indicated by the following:

1. All but one pregnant mother consented to be included in the intervention and be screened for risks through use of the mobile phone application

2. 93% of household decision makers granted permission to the pregnant mother to plan for an in-facility delivery (67% under any condition; 26% only in an emergency)

3. 674 referrals were made for labor and delivery
4. 216 referrals were made for postpartum care (mother at risk)
5. 98 referrals were made for postnatal care (infant at risk)

The average age of the registered mothers was 25, ranging from 13 to 46 years of age. During the registration process, pregnant mothers were asked about their previous pregnancies and deliveries as well as a few basic questions about their medical history and general health. Of the mothers registered, *67% identified some health condition or risk that would especially require a facility delivery* (i.e., at least one low-level risk factor). Due to their medical or obstetrical history, almost half of women in the project (47%) had at least one higher risk that warranted a birth plan to deliver at a higher-level facility (i.e. a hospital). Of these women, 34 (3.6%) had high blood pressure. Approximately 36% of women had one or more problems during previous deliveries, including prolonged labor, eclampsia, perineal tear, exhaustion, delivery by cesarean section, or postpartum hemorrhage. Approximately 7% of women reported prior stillbirths, 5% reported prior abortions, and 12% reported prior miscarriages. *(See Table 2)*

In the Micheweni District, the two referral health facilities in the project intervention zone observed significant increases in their in-facility delivery rates. In the three months prior to the project, the Micheweni Cottage Hospital had an average of 44 births per month. By the end of the registration period, it averaged 67 births per

Table 2. Registered mothers' demographics and identified risks (N = 938)

	Minimum	Maximum	Mean	Median
Age	13	46	27	25
Pregnancies	1	15	4.25	4
Previous deliveries	0	14	3.9	3
Miscarriages	0	6	.19	0
Abortions	0	8	.08	0
Stillbirths	0	11	.23	0

Condition	Number	Percent	Condition	Number	Percent
More than 5 previous deliveries *	201	21.43	Sickle cell*	26	2.77
Prolonged labor*	184	19.62	Eclampsia*	22	2.35
First pregnancy	173	18.44	Prior vacuum delivery*	16	1.71
Small perineal tear	126	13.43	More than 2 prior miscarriages*	15	1.6
Exhaustion	81	8.64	Retained placenta	14	1.49
Prior delivery by cesarean section*	46	4.9	Placenta previa	12	1.28
Post-partum hemorrhage*	36	3.84	More than 2 prior stillbirths*	9	0.96
High blood pressure*	34	3.62	Newborn delivered weighing more than 4 kilos	7	0.75
Large perineal tear*	27	2.88	Cardiac disease*	6	0.64
Under age 18*	27	2.88	More than two prior abortions*	3	0.32
** Per Ministry of Health guidelines, this risk necessitates a hospital delivery*					

month, with 91 births recorded in March 2012 alone. Equally, the Makangale primary health care facility had an average of five births per month before the project began and 13 births during project implementation.

REDUCED DELAY IN ARRANGING AND RECEIVING TRANSPORT TO FACILITY

All project beneficiaries and health facility staff reported that the traditional birth attendants' presence, as well as their use of mobile banking to pay driver, significantly improved transport coordination, thus reducing laboring mothers' arrival time at health facilities and cottage hospitals. Moreover, many claimed that without the project they would not have been able to afford transport, and thus would have given birth at home.

For example, in April 2012, a mother named Mwanaidi was referred by user to Micheweni cottage hospital where she was supported through a prolonged labor and successfully delivered a healthy baby boy. On returning for a postpartum visit, Mwanaidi expressed thanks to the mHealth for Safer Deliveries project and attributed it to her family's health, stating that all of her past deliveries were unsuccessful home deliveries because she could not pay for transport. She indicated that she would no longer consider delivering at home for future pregnancies, no matter what the circumstance.

Of the mothers who did give birth at home during the project, most stated that the primary reason for their home delivery was due to their tardiness in notifying the traditional birth attendant that they were in labor. Many families were accustomed to calling the traditional birth attendant only after mothers demonstrated signs that she was progressing into active labor, as they had done prior to the intervention. Because these families had notified the traditional birth attendants so late in labor, health facility staff communicating with

the users via the mobile phone then determined that it would be unsafe for these mothers to be transported. These mothers still benefitted from the intervention due to users' communication with qualified health facility staff during delivery. In addition, the phone application included a clinical algorithm to assess the health of mother and newborn immediately after an accidental home birth, with the possibility to refer them to the facility afterwards as needed.

The average recurrent cost per delivery was approximately $22, of which $16 was for transportation and $6 was to reimburse the traditional birth attendant for her screening and referral role. The average recurrent cost per delivery was $21 in the North A District and $24 in the Micheweni District. Transport in Micheweni was slightly more expensive due to having remote villages with longer distances to facilities.

IMPROVED INFORMATION TO PROVIDE HIGHER QUALITY OF ANTENATAL, DELIVERY, AND POSTNATAL CARE

The mHealth for Safer Deliveries project provided key information to support timely, appropriate, high quality maternal, neonatal, and postnatal care. Because pregnant mothers' health and delivery risks and labor status were known by the health facility staff in advance of their arrival, staffs were better prepared to receive them. Communication by the mobile technology users to facilities also allowed them to ensure that qualified staffs were available and if not, they could easily arrange continued transport to another facility.

In terms of outcomes of the current pregnancy, 23% of women experienced some complications, most of which were not major. The most common conditions were exhaustion (6.6%), severe abdominal pain (4.9%), fever (4.5%), and depression (2.3%). As noted previously, one woman died from complications related to childbirth during a

Table 3. Postpartum and postnatal outcomes (N=938)

Postpartum Outcomes			Postnatal Outcomes					
Condition	N	%	Condition	N	%	Condition	N	%
Exhaustion	62	6.61	Fever	44	4.69	Pale pallor	4	0.43
Severe abdominal pain	46	4.9	Abdominal distention	24	2.56	Difficulty swallowing	4	0.43
Fever	42	4.48	Discharge in eyes	8	0.85	Infection	3	0.32
Feeling sad/ hopeless	22	2.35	Cord bleeding	8	0.85	Bulging fontanel	3	0.32
Excessive bleeding	21	2.24	Red umbilical cord	5	0.53	Convulsions	2	0.21
Breast mastitis	13	1.39	Fast breathing	4	0.43	Blue lips	2	0.21
Foul smelling discharge	9	0.96	Congenital abnormality	4	0.43	Yellow color	1	0.11
Breast cracking	7	0.75	Swollen eyes	4	0.43	Excessive vomiting	1	0.11
Blurred vision	5	0.53						

home delivery. Twenty-one mothers experienced excessive bleeding while 13 experienced breast mastitis. *(See Table 3)*

Regarding neonatal health outcomes, 10% of newborns experienced some sort of complication during or after birth. The most common issues were fever (4.7%) and abdominal distention (2.6%). Four infants had a congenital abnormality, three had infections, two experienced convulsions, and one had jaundice. There were 49 adverse outcomes, including 18 abortions, 24 stillbirths, and 7 neonatal deaths. *(See Table 4)* The causes of the neonatal deaths were asphyxiation (n=2), congenital abnormality (n=1), pre-term birth (n=1), and unknown (n=3).

Table 4. Birth outcomes at postpartum visit (N=938)

	Number	Percent
Healthy baby	889	94.8%
Abortion	18	1.9%
Stillbirth	24	2.6%
Death	7	0.7%
Total adverse outcomes	49	5.2%

61% of mothers received follow-up visits by a traditional birth attendant at home within one week after delivery to promote the family's continued access to care at a health facility, including post-partum and post-natal care, as well as family planning. In one documented case, a mother developed a high fever 24 hours after birth. Her linkages to the health facility were strong and the traditional birth attendant arranged transport and accompanied her to access care. Promoting clinical postnatal visits within seven days after delivery corresponds with the Zanzibar Ministry of Health guidelines.

The district health management teams benefitted from enhanced decision support systems through the mHealth application. During the project intervention period, their staff participated in regular meetings with mHealth users to learn more about the expectant mothers in their catchment areas. They had a better sense of which and how many mothers were due to give birth each month, the mothers' medical and pregnancy history, and they were systematically alerted by the users once the mothers were in labor. In interviewing six health facility nurses, all reported that they appreciated the call from the traditional birth attendant so that they could ensure that there was someone at the health facility to receive the woman and that they could be prepared for her condition. The staff reported that mothers who came in as a result of the project came in much earlier in the labor, at a time when they could more easily be helped if they were experiencing problems.

We interviewed 22 of the 24 traditional birth attendants to assess their mHealth user experience. All reported an increase in clients and reported the following results from the use of the phone-based tools: improved general knowledge (31%), improved knowledge about danger signs (27%), better understanding of the importance of obstetric history (14%), and chronic disease (5%). All reported satisfaction in using the phone; seven of the users reported that it was difficult to use the phone on the first day, but that they became comfortable using it shortly thereafter. It should be noted that not all of the traditional birth attendants had familiarity sending text messages before joining the project, so it is a significant achievement that they were able to become adept with the application during training for the project intervention.

We interviewed twenty participating mothers who delivered at health facilities to rank the factors that most influenced their decision to deliver there. They cited that the two most important factors were: the advice from traditional birth attendants on the importance of facility delivery and the availability of free transport. In addition, they reported being positively influenced by: the traditional birth attendants' frequent visits; identification of danger signs during labor; assistance in getting consent from family members to deliver at a facility; and the identification of health other risks in pregnancy.

DISCUSSION

The mHealth for Safer Deliveries project was effective in bringing 71% of participating women to give birth in the health facility by providing a comprehensive approach to address the underlying causes of the three delays that prevent women from having facility-based deliveries, compared to 33.6%, the regional average from the Demographic and Health Surveys (NBS and ICF Macro, 2011).

The following are factors that we believe contributed to its success:

1. *Greater engagement of family-based decision-makers.* Women and families received ongoing education and encouragement to seek care at the facility during the pre- and postnatal periods, as well as for delivery. Family decision-makers were involved earlier on in pregnancy so as to avoid transfer delays in an emergency situation. The mHealth application's personalized messages citing the mothers' risks that were actually identified through screening, and the actual name of the facility recommended for delivery helped support concrete decision-making.

2. *Enhanced role of the traditional birth attendants.* As the mobile technology users, they were given a legitimate role in the project as communicators and data collectors in lieu of their traditional role of delivering babies. The mHealth application provided the users with consistent messaging that supported the Ministry of Health's protocols. The traditional birth attendants were motivated to adapt the mHealth for Safer Deliveries project's approach because they felt they were providing a valued service to their communities. Their clients, the pregnant mothers and families, also appreciated their new role. Performance-based financial incentives to compensate for the traditional birth attendants' lost income from home deliveries reinforced their motivation to reach out to mothers and include them in the project.

3. *Improved communication, data collection, and information sharing linked with the formal health system.* The mobile technology

generated useful information, and encouraged communication, and used appropriate technology given the skill levels of stakeholders, infrastructure, and resources available. The one maternal death and seven infant deaths observed during the project intervention period highlight the importance for future perinatal interventions in Zanzibar. With the data collected by the mHealth for Safer Deliveries project, the Ministry of Health and its district health management team are now better equipped with population-level and case-specific data to support the development of evidence-based interventions. The potential for the traditional birth attendant to improve infant death rates is considered promising (Sibley et al., 2007; Falle et al., 2009).

4. *Provision of needed transport that the health system could not otherwise provide.* Difficulties accessing affordable and timely transport for routine or emergency deliveries emerged as a predominant barrier to many rural Zanzibari families. The first delay in consenting to the facility appeared to be less of an obstacle. In other contexts, this may not be the case, so the project's approach and use of the mobile technology must be adapted to each new context carefully, including for a planned application in India.

Future project monitoring is recommended to develop a better understanding of which elements or combinations of elements of the mobile technology (i.e. the screening protocols, provision of transportation, personal advice and contact with the traditional birth attendant, or family permissions) are most critical to the intervention's success. Further, investigation regarding the 25 pregnant mothers who were registered by the project but did not opt to deliver at a health facility at the onset of labor is also recommended.

Finally, the authors note that maternal mortality cannot be measured on a small scale. Given the time period and geographical scope of the project, the project opted to measure maternal health improvements via the proxy indicator of in-facility birth rates. Because no district-level data on in-facility birth rates in Zanzibar existed, project results were compared with reputable population-level data elicited by the Demographic and Health Surveys (NBS and ICF Macro, 2011). However, we recognize that the lack of a comparison group is a limitation, as we cannot prove an increase in facility delivery in real terms without using an appropriate comparison including a comparable denominator.

In conclusion, reducing maternal mortality has taken on new urgency with the publication of the Millennium Development Goals Report 2012 (UN, 2012) that showed that progress on MDG 5 (to improve maternal health) has been slow especially with regard to reducing maternal mortality in Africa and South Asia. A more comprehensive approach is needed to ensure that pregnant women receive proper counseling and care, deliver in a health facility that provides quality service, and have appropriate follow up care after the delivery. The mHealth intervention described in this paper presents the potential to reduce maternal mortality by increasing facility-based deliveries and providing protocol-based post-partum follow-up to infant and mother. While the numbers are small, the project's high facility-based delivery rate is highly suggestive of the potential benefit of mHealth on maternal and neonatal mortality.

REFERENCES

Campbell, O. M. R., & Graham, W. J. (2006). Strategies for reducing maternal mortality: getting on with what works. *Lancet, 368*, 1284–1299. doi:10.1016/S0140-6736(06)69381-1 PMID:17027735

Commission on Information and Accountability for Women's and Children's Health. (2011). *Keeping promises, measuring results*. Geneva, Switzerland: World Health Organization.

DeRenzi, B., Parikh, T., Mitchell, M., Chemba, M., Schellenberg, D., & Lesh, N. … Borriello, G. (2008). e-IMCI: Improving pediatric care in low-income countries. In *Proceedings of the SIGCHI Conference on Human Factors in Computing Systems* (pp. 753-762).

Falle, T. Y., Mullany, L. C., Thatte, N., Khatry, S. K., LeClerg, S. C., & Darmstadt, G. L. et al. (2009). Potential role of traditional birth attendants in neonatal healthcare in rural Southern Nepal. *Journal of Health, Population, and Nutrition, 27*(1), 53–61. PMID:19248648

Hasan, R., Hill, K., Reich, M., & Fink, G. (2013). Determinants of maternal healthcare utilization in Bangladesh, 1993-2007. In *Proceedings of the meeting of the Population Association of America*, Princeton, NJ.

Hill, K., Thomas, K., AbouZahr, C., Walker, N., Say, L., Inoue, M., & Suzuki, E. (2007). Estimates of maternal mortality worldwide between 1990 and 2005: as assessment of available data. *Lancet, 370*(9595), 1311–1319. doi:10.1016/S0140-6736(07)61572-4 PMID:17933645

Jokhio, A. H., Winter, H. R., & Cheng, K. K. (2005). An intervention involving traditional birth attendants and perinatal and maternal mortality in Pakistan. *The New England Journal of Medicine, 352*, 2091–2099. doi:10.1056/NEJMsa042830 PMID:15901862

Kidney, E., Winter, H. R., Khan, K. S., Gulmezoglu, A. M., Meads, C. A., Deeks, J. J., & MacArthur, C. (2009). Systematic review of effect of community-level interventions to reduce maternal mortality. *BMC Pregnancy and Childbirth, 9*(2). PMID:19154588

Maine, D., Murat, A., Ward, V., & Kamara, A. (1997). The three delays model. In *The design and evaluation of maternal mortality programs*. New York, NY: Center for Population and Family Health, Columbia University.

Mdungi, Z. N. (2000). *Reproductive and child health needs Assessment study – Analysis of focus group discussion*. Unpublished report submitted to the Zanzibar Safe Motherhood Program.

Mitchell, M., Getchell, M., Nkaka, M., van Esch, J., & Hedt, B. (2012). Perceived improvement in integrated management of childhood illness implementation through use of mobile technology: Qualitative evidence from a pilot study in Tanzania. *Journal of Health Communication, 17*, 118–127. doi:10.1080/10810730.2011.6491 05 PMID:22548605

Mitchell, M., Lesh, N., Cranmer, H., Fraser, H., Haivas, I., & Wolf, K. (2009). Improving care – improving access: The use of electronic decision support with AIDS patients in South Africa. *International Journal of Healthcare Technology and Management, 10*(3), 156–168. doi:10.1504/IJHTM.2009.025819

National Bureau of Statistics (NBS) [Tanzania] and ICF Macro. (2011.) *Tanzania demographic and health survey 2010*. Dar es Salaam, Tanzania: NBS and ICF Macro.

Noordam, A. C., Kuepper, B. M., Stekelenburg, J., & Milen, A. (2011). Improvement of maternal health services through the use of mobile phones. *Tropical Medicine & International Health, 16*, 622–626. doi:10.1111/j.1365-3156.2011.02747.x PMID:21342374

Prata, N., Passano, P., Sreenivas, A., & Gerdts, C. E. (2011). Maternal mortality in developing countries: Challenges in scaling-up priority interventions. *Women's Health (London, England), 6*(2), 311–327. doi:10.2217/whe.10.8 PMID:20187734

Rogo, K. O., Oucho, J., & Mwalali, P. (2006). Maternal mortality. In D. T. Jamison, R. G. Feachem, & M. W. Makgoba, et al. (Eds.), *Disease and mortality in Sub-Saharan Africa* (2nd ed.). Washington, DC: World Bank.

Sibley, L., Sipe, T. A., & Koblinsky, M. (2004). Does TBA training improve referral of obstetric complications: A review of the evidence. *Social Science & Medicine*, *59*(8), 1757–1768. doi:10.1016/j.socscimed.2004.02.009 PMID:15279931

Sibley, L. M., Sipe, T. A., Brown, C. M., Diallo, M. M., McNatt, K., & Habarta, N. (2007). Traditional birth attendant training for improving health behaviours and pregnancy outcomes. *Cochrane Database of Systematic Reviews*, *3*, CD005460. PMID:17636799

Stokoe, U. (1991). Determinants of maternal mortality in the developing world. *Aust N Z Obstet Gynaecol.*, *31*(1), 8–16. doi:10.1111/j.1479-828X.1991.tb02754.x PMID:1872781

Tamrat, T., & Kachnowski, S. (2012). Special delivery: An analysis of mhealth in maternal and newborn health programs and their outcomes around the world. *Maternal and Child Health Journal*, *16*(5), 1092–1101. doi:10.1007/s10995-011-0836-3 PMID:21688111

Thaddeus, S., & Maine, D. (1994). Too far to walk: Maternal mortality in context. *Sm. Sci. Med.*, *38*(8), 1091–1110. doi:10.1016/0277-9536(94)90226-7 PMID:8042057

The Revolutionary Government of Zanzibar, Ministry of Health. (2010a). *The Zanzibar strategy for growth and reduction of poverty: 2010-2015 (ZSGRP), Mkuza II. Zanzibar City.* Zanzibar, Tanzania: The Revolutionary Government of Zanzibar.

The Revolutionary Government of Zanzibar, Ministry of Health. (2010b). *Comprehensive postnatal maternal and newborn care guideline. Zanzibar City.* Zanzibar, Tanzania: The Revolutionary Government of Zanzibar.

The Revolutionary Government of Zanzibar, Ministry of Health and Social Welfare. (RGOZ MOHSW). (2006). Zanzibar health sector reform strategic plan II: 2006/07 – 2010/11. Zanzibar City, Zanzibar, Tanzania.

The United Nations. (2012). *The millennium development goals report 2012.* New York, NY: The United Nations.

UNFPA, UNICEF, WHO, World Bank. (2012). *Trends in maternal mortality: 1990-2010.* Geneva, Switzerland: the World Health Organization.

World Health Organization (WHO). (1999). *Reduction of maternal mortality: A Joint WHO/UNFPA/UNICEF/World bank statement.* Geneva, Switzerland: The World Health Organization.

World Health Organization (WHO). (2012). *Newborns: Reducing mortality. May 2012: Fact sheet N° 333.* Geneva, Switzerland. Retrieved February 25, 2013, from http://www.who.int/mediacentre/factsheets/fs333/en/index.html

Yussef, I. (2012). *Tanzania: Zanzibar intensified efforts to reduce maternal mortality.* May 23, 2012. Retrieved February 25, 2013, from http://allafrica.com/stories/201205230430.html

This work was previously published in the International Journal of User-Driven Healthcare (IJUDH), 4(1); edited by Rakesh Biswas, pages 33-47 copyright year 2014 by IGI Publishing (an imprint of IGI Global).

Chapter 58
Collaborative Participation in Personalized Health through Mobile Diaries

Pelin Arslan
Politecnico di Milano, INDACO Department, Italy & Massachusetts Institute of Technology, USA

ABSTRACT

Mobile and social media tools offer new opportunities for a more user centered, socially connected, and economically sustainable healthcare systems. A major focus of this chapter is to understand how to bring users to involve in their own everyday health management through mobile narratives, and new media as social platforms to incite social interaction in promoting healthier lifestyles. More in detail, the study discusses the utility of geo-located video diaries and social network, where the social interaction on the web and user-recorded video diaries create awareness and help subjects to self-reflect on their activities and aim to think for a health behavior change. The chapter experiences a focus project Locast Health Diary aims to provide a helpful set of tools for teen's risk at obesity to record their socio- psychological environment and everyday health routines through participatory workshops and evaluate the use of health diary tools for confronting obesity problems.

INTRODUCTION

Towards a Healthier Lifestyle through Mobile Interventions

Healthcare is in transition towards wellbeing in daily life of an individual. The concept of wellbeing derives from a healthier lifestyle requires a long-term relation with your everyday health, and co-producer with a good health status. With the improvement of mobile and social media technologies, health is moving forward for more participative, socially connected and economically sustainable solutions. Mobile technologies can help to manage everyday health, enable systems that can monitor, track, and respond to changing health status; and promote social health connections.

DOI: 10.4018/978-1-4666-8756-1.ch058

In todays health system three main issues have been considered: long-lasting chronic diseases and its burden to healthcare system, lack of consideration in patients' the socio-environmental factor in disease prevention, and the illness oriented approach of healthcare system where the patient is not regarded as a part of their solution.

Chronic Disease and Health Prevention

Chronic diseases are long duration illnesses and generally slowing progression such as heart disease, stroke, cancer, diabetes, and obesity. They require utilization of hospital services, medical sources and high necessity of healthcare providers, which results in high cost healthcare expenditure for both patients and/or government. Health damaging behaviors - particularly tobacco use, lack of physical activity, and poor eating habits – together with environmental problems are major contributors to chronic diseases.

However, these diseases are preventable and controllable by daily activities and changing 'unhealthy lifestyle choices.' Prevention requires a long-term management of everyday behaviors towards healthier habits such as eating nutritious foods, becoming more physically active and avoiding tobacco consumption. These self-manageable activities could prevent chronic diseases and therefore also prevent some of the important problems of the healthcare system. Self-managing an activity requires awareness of what you are doing and the mindset of whether what you are doing is right. As prior findings of the research (Arslan, 2012) shows that awareness of people's own behavior is the most underutilized health issue and being conscious of the situation anticipates an active participation in the prevention.

Patient Involvement in Health Management

Healthcare is a complex system where patients are not sufficiently considered as a relevant factor within the system. Rolyston (2004) states, "The biggest untapped resources in the health system are not doctors but users." The future of Healthcare in era of chronic disease shall turn on the full engagement of people in their own healthcare: the promotion of good health and prevention of illness. (Wanles, 2002) Active participation in long-term management with our own health would prevent chronic diseases; decrease health cost, enable more accessibility to services and decrease aging.

In order to answer social needs of today, information and communication technologies are becoming increasingly important in our life and are used in many areas of everyday healthcare-wellbeing context. Mobile phones are now a tool to access various applications and services from self-managing our health data by tracking and measuring our everyday activities to socializing in web platforms to generate collective action within a community. People who are a part of community have access to care and support from friends and neighbors. (Leadbitter & Cottam, 2004). Many scientists have done studies on understanding relations network and as Wing and Jeffery (1999) state that this network phenomenon might be exploited to spread positive health behaviors in part because people's perceptions of their own risk of illness may depend on the people around them. (Montgomery et al., 2003) As in Christakis (2008) work sharing information and experiences with other people socially allows them being motivated for a modification of their behavior. Participation and co-creation results in collaborative and distributed mobile interventions tapping into people's perceptions, expectations, desires, and motivations. It is also crucial as Zuboff & Maxmin (2002) argue that co-creation should provide people with the support they need to follow through on decisions. Being able to influence and guide people in their decision-making process we could possibly find opportunities for behavior change for healthier lifestyles.

Patients' Socio-Psychological Environment

There are so many influencing factors and clues about patients' lifestyle outside the hospital, which are not regarded by the medical experts due to their limited time availability with each patient and that, can also contribute to manage patients' life towards healthy behaviors. This patient's socio-psychological information gives additional information to medical experts for more complete chronic disease prevention.

This type of data is easier to be understood by the patient since he is more familiar to this language respecting to biophysical information where he might need a certain expertise or help by an expert to decode information to 'everyday language'. Helman (1995) claims that the patient is a network of physical and psychological functions and interacts with physical, biological, social, and symbolic. Traditionally, clinicians focus on the physical and biological aspects. Social and symbolic environments in which patients live and the meanings that patients derive from illness experiences often are not taken into account by contemporary biomedicine. As the World Health Organization (WHO) (1948) defines health as 'a state of a complete physical, mental and social well-being', we should not consider only the medical situation of the patient but also their everyday environment. This determinates an active engagement of patients in their health management and a more complete scene of individual's health pattern.

The objective of this chapter is to bring users to involve in their own health prevention through mobile narratives, and new media as social networks to incite social interaction in promoting healthier lifestyles. With the aim emphasizing the importance of socio-environmental factor, the following parts more in detail explores different ways of capturing information through guided video production as mobile diaries to incite for collaborative participation in a social platform. Social interaction on a web platform explores the collaborative participation in personalized health.

The chapter in particular proposes the methodology of participatory approach and the qualitative method as video diaries to collect and understand everyday human behavior with a focus project called Locast Health Diary. The focus project discusses and evaluates the use of geo-located video diaries and social network for developing awareness on teens with obesity at risk and self reflect upon their actions, which will consequently affect for their decision-making process for thinking towards a healthier behavior change.

BACKGROUND

Mobile Devices as a Support Tool for Personalized Healthcare Prevention

People's behaviors around mobile communication devices have certainly changed over the past decades.

The premise of around-device interaction where it takes beyond the physical constraints of a mobile device utilizes the space surrounding the device to provide richer input possibilities. Technological advancement in mobile technologies provides affordability, accessibility and usability that enable mobile phones to be used in various contexts. Today mobile devices are not just 'personal communication tools' but also own an additional role as measurement instruments, tracking health data, positioning location devices, monitoring conditions, posting and sharing multimedia content in health management and prevention areas.

The possibility to be continuously connected through mobile devices provides opportunities for reaching and engaging 'digital natives' in individuals' everyday health. In most of mobile applications in the market, the phone collects information automatically through its sensors as GPS, camera, microphone, accelerometer or wearable sensors can send their data directly to the phone, where captured physiological metrics can be sent off into the cloud and then to the physician, the user or the platform. Some other interventions involve educational and behavioral component where environmental data with images, audio and video content can be shared in a platform for health prevention or management. As an example, an application developed by Liu et al. (2011) helps adolescent migraine patients and their counselors manage migraine. This application provides on-demand access to audio, video and animated instructions to guide the learning and application of behavioral migraine management skills as well as a headache diary that allows adolescents and their counselors to monitor key migraine and medication use variables.

Connectivity through devices is everywhere at anytime allows for limitless interaction through people, information and places. Connectivity among people occurs through relationships and as a consequence roots of communities. Puikkonen et al. (2009) discusses that mobile phones are being used in many ways at the boundary of different levels of privacy. It is often the content that makes the phone feel personal (Venta et al., 2008), and handling other's device may be perceived as a violation of privacy. (Hakkila & Chatfield, 2005). However, mobile phones serve as objects play and artifacts for discussion, and in this role they can function as facilitators of social face-to-face interaction. Kindberg et al. (2005) and Taylor and Harper (2003) state that showing personal phone content to someone can facilitate ongoing conversation, provoke new topics, and increase the group cohesion through enjoyment of shared moments. It has been also shown that mobile phones with multimedia capabilities are used as platforms for expression and creativity. A field study experiment done by Puikkonen et al. (2008) with collaborative mobile video creation demonstrated that mobile phone video could function as a great tool for creativity, as groups of teenagers were inspired to produce and perform in their own mobile mini-movies. Therefore mobile devises are a common and accessible tool for participatory interventions.

Diaries as Self-Documentation Tools for a Healthier Lifestyle

There are many ways to collect data from patients' physical and environmental parameters. The diary study is a method to gather user experiences by having participants' record events as they happen.

Diary studies have been explored in literature reviews with many different media forms as photos, audio, video and text. Several studies have been published on the topic of capturing life experiences, such as wearable camera Sensecam (Gemmell et al., 2004); online media weblog (Kelliher, 2004); group story sharing (Appan et al., 2004); lifelogging (Sellen et al., 2007); capture and access (Abowd & Mynatt, 2000). All applications have their own limitations in terms of collecting, processing, and building, retrieving and expressing experiences by a specific target group. Carter and Mankoff (2005) have done a study about improvements of diary study contributing a tool to support media-based diary studies. They have found that images lead to more specific recall than any other medium, but that audio, in addition to making it easier for participants to capture information that does not have a visual representation, can be used secretly in situations in which participants do not feel comfortable using a photo to capture an event.

Diaries like self-documentation, including digital technologies, enrich participatory methods and account for users capacities, skills, and motivation. Self-reporting has been explored by Larson and Csikszentmihalyi (1983) as electronic sampling methods, Carter and Mankoff (2005), Gaver et al. (1999) as cultural probes, where participants are responsible for the data collection, gathering contextual data over-time and in situ, without the physical presence of researchers. Self-reporting can provide access into the private, personal and environmental aspects of people's lives that are often difficult, or impossible, to access through traditional methods such as observations or interviews. The personal reflection inherent in self-reporting makes aspects available that would otherwise remain tacit. Since so much of individuals' lives are routinized and automatic, it is not until we are asked to document or consider certain activities that we are able to identify key junctures in our own understanding of a behavior. This type of data collection usually occurs in one of two ways: participants answer predefined questions about events (feedback studies) or participants capture media that are then used as prompts for discussion in interviews (elicitation studies).

The use of video diaries in health interventions is mainly used for health decision consultation or to monitor patients' socio-environmental health patterns in a daily life. Diary like self-documentation as video consultation could be used for early diagnosis and follow-up care of diseases, for advice and instructions regarding assistive technology or as remote support for handling technical failures with artificial respiration equipment, thus contributing to both quality and efficiency of care. Video diaries in healthcare provide a more 'direct' understanding of participants' experiences than is afforded by data that are 'controlled' by the researcher. Some studies in similar areas explore the diary tool as a self-documentation and self-reflection of individuals' behavior. As Gibson (2005) has articulated how participants construct their video accounts provides a valuable source of analyzable data. As in the study of asthma by Rich (2000) Video Intervention Assessment was developed to determine whether medical information gathering might be augmented by video diaries created by patients to show clini-

cians the realities of managing chronic disease in the context of their lives. The unstructured user generated data is being analyzed by software by structuring in the postproduction. However, in this study huge amount of unstructured data collected by the patients 8 hours of their everyday life was difficult to analyze.

In another study by Klammer et al. (2010), a social media based user self-documentation with a collaborative online platform has been developed. This consisted of creating photos; short videos or texts about daily work situations where users thought video consultation would be used. The tool itself serves to collect data but also create collaborative awareness. As preliminary results of their research, participants told that they wanted more additional structure and guidance in documenting (i.e., more specific focus on what to look at work.). They did not know what exactly to show on video. It was not a lack of time or motivation, but this situation make participants to felt that the task put too much pressure on them, which relates to the documentation technique itself.

Both these two conditions are taken into account in Locast Health Video Diary tool, where the user through templates creates the video enables structure video creation and its content. The structures and guided content creation address obesity problems to create awareness while participants create their narratives through guided prompts or questions.

Another example of storytelling from this field is Mahmud et al. (2008) work on developing a home-based storytelling support system for Aphasics primarily intended to be used in their post rehabilitation period. The premise of their project is enabling Aphasics to share their daily stories will help them to become more active socially and to reengage in their preferred life style. The work includes passive capturing with a webcam application with a motion detection utility, which usually generates a huge collection of images of ongoing activities at the place. The camera uses a preprogrammed algorithm, which filters low-quality images. However, still there were images with no person in the photo, therefore filtering the photos to feed the story creation was a main challenge. Therefore the partner had provided subjects only content rich images for a story creation. This work also gives us insights to think opportunities how to utilize video as a story creation tool.

Over the last ten years digital, online and mobile technologies have been incorporated into self-reporting methods in a range of ways. These everyday tools can be easily integrated into people's daily lives and support the generation of a range of different media forms such as video, images, text and audio. Over the period of the study participants create collages, mind maps, videos and blog messages and send reports, which appear on the blog. They also receive prompts, questions and reminders via the mobile phone and the blog. In the literature (Hagen & Rowland, 2010)'s work is a particularly provocative, experiential and sensorial insight into participant's lives with people's own words in their day-to-day lives. Using their phone, participants capture images, text and audio and send to the blog throughout the day. Through these reports researcher can track events, locations, and participant's emotions across the days and weeks.

Over time, daily rhythms and habits emerge. As Masten and Plowman (2003) state the real-time reporting increases the sense of immersion in people's lives as we experience the activities 'as they happen'. This is complemented by more reflective accounts viewing the diaries via the blog or on the video camera. The use of video encourages in-depth descriptive accounts of events and surroundings from the participant's perspective.

Psychologists Csikszentmihalyi and Larson (1987) in their study state that they have recognized the need to monitor patients in situ versus asking a participant to recall an event a week or more after the fact. Previous studies show that many factors affect the memory of participants recalling past experiences. Recall can be caused by (i) the current emotional state of the participant,

(ii) the length of time the participant is asked to recall, (iii) the participant sitting in a foreign environment. The results of studies rely solely on participant's long-term memory. Instead of trying to account all of these, researchers can alleviate the issue by having participants' record events as they happen or immediately after. When the observer is the participant itself, awareness of time, physical environment, contracting experiences and social openings and barriers as outlined by Bruyn (1966) are elements that help participants to develop awareness.

Self-reporting studies can take many different forms and the degree of formal structure is one of the things that differentiates approaches and determines the type of material collected. For example in the Electronic Sampling Method approach known as ESM (Larson & Csikszent-mihalyi, 1983), the participant is directed to systematically log specific things at specific times. In more open-ended approaches such as the ones reported, data collection is only semi-structured around a particular topic. (Gaver, Dunne, & Pacenti, 1999; Hulkko, Mattelmäki, Virtanen, & Keinonen, 2004; Masten & Plowman, 2003; Palen & Salzman, 2002; Sanders, 2008) In this case participants are treated as active contributors and interpreters in the design process and select what, how and when to report. This encourages more playful and creative representations, important to an explorative and collaborative approach.

In addition to descriptions of events and activities, mobile diary reports also capture emotions, feelings and inner thoughts. The examples above show emotional reactions and descriptions of personal feelings at particular moments through words or metaphors or symbols. The process of self-reporting is an intervention designed to allow people to self-reflect and share aspects of their daily life; this process can also trigger participants to question their choices and everyday behaviors as discussed by Grinter and Eldridge (2001). These activities help to reveal emotional and infrastructural barriers to behavioral changes. As Hagen and Rowland (2010) found out in their study the results of the reports introduce the participants through their own words and images; illuminate the themes that have emerged and identify some future possibilities to be considered.

There is also a significant value in creating opportunities for co-interpretation of the material by practitioners and other actors of the project.

To combine self-diary studies with a group participation proposes a social component of self-documentation and inclusion of others in the process of self-reporting reflects a sense of control and ownership by participants over the process.

Social Platforms as an Infrastructure for Collaborative Health

The use of technology promotes collaboration between patients, their caregivers, medical professionals, and other stakeholders across healthcare in general, and in particular in public health promotion. Health 2.0 is defined by Hughes et al. (2008) as the use of a specific set of web tools (blogs, podcasts, tagging, search, wikis, etc.) by actors in healthcare including caregivers, patients, and scientists, using principles of open source, user-generated content and the power of networks in order to personalize healthcare, collaborate, and promote health education. These types of health platforms are being utilized for giving emotional support and information sharing, staying informed about medical education, managing a particular disease, providing quantified self tracking and clinical trial access. Health social networks such as DailyStrength, MedHelp, HealthChapter, MD-Junction, Experience Project, Peoplejam, and OrganizedWisdom, have become a powerful tool for bringing people with similar interests together to interact and share information. Other health social networks such as PatientsLikeMe, CureTogether focus on self-tracking and collaborative filtering to identify potentially related conditions patients that are in similar situations.

Social platforms could be an alternative support tools as traditional therapy sessions in support groups. Although, Cacioppo (2009), a neuroscientist at the University of Chicago, claims that social networking can foster feelings of sensitivity to disconnection, which can lead to loneliness, some other researchers discusses that this results in social connection. Burke et al. (2010) investigated a study about the directed communication between pairs-such as wall posts, comments and 'likes' and consumption of friends' content, including status updates, photos, and friends' conversation with other friends in Facebook. They have found that directed communication in social networking sites is associated with greater feelings of bonding social capital and lower loneliness, but has only modest relationship with bridging social capital, which is primarily related to overall friend network size. According to another author Field (2003, pp. 1-2) interaction in the social network enables people to build communities, to commit themselves to each other, and to knit the social fabric. A sense of belonging and the concrete experience of social networks, the relationships of trust and tolerance can be involved.

Social networks in healthcare as an important phenomena that not only provides platforms to share data but help users to connect with their parents, family and friends to get an emotional support during and after treatment. Social networks influence health behaviors as Christakis (2008) states, "Social support and a sense of belonging, being part of a social network, are a vital part of good health. People who are part of social networks are generally healthier than people who feel isolated. People who are part of a community have access to care and support from friends and neighbors. They also tend to have higher self-esteem and confidence from a sense of social belonging. Collaboration is vital for people to share and spread ideas and know-how." Centola (2010) in his experimental study shows that people with dense social networks are more likely to acquire new health practices.

Online social networking services are increasingly accessed through mobile devices equipped with location sensing technology. As Langheinrich (2009) state sharing real time location information raises important privacy concerns as discussed in Wagner et al. (2010) paper, there is an increasing amount of work understanding uses location privacy needs in ubiquitous systems including diary studies (Barkhuus, 2004); interviews (Hong & Landay, 2004); lab and field observation (Consolvo et al., 2005); survey (Khalil & Connelly, 2006).

Although there are privacy concerns about location awareness, it is an important issue to be considered in innovative interventions where the user could develop awareness and provide instant feedback mechanisms and real time-interventions while on the go.

Peltonen et al. (2007) state platforms that encourage active participation in media production create user experience in which a participant becomes increasingly aware and focused within the situation. As Rheingold (2007) state these characteristics give rise to the opportunity to use locative media as a supplementary tool for education around complex social topics in areas such as sustainability, community, and civic engagement. This encourages rethinking location-aware participatory media platforms for making the user the most highly involved actors within the participatory culture.

MAIN FOCUS OF THE CHAPTER

An Empirical Study on Obesity Prevention with Adolescents through Mobile Diaries: Locast Health Diary

The chapter focuses on an empirical study on obesity prevention with adolescents and discusses Locast Health Diary tools (the utility of mobile diaries, social networks and location-based technologies) and participatory methods to confront obesity problem.

Childhood Obesity as an Epidemic Phenomenon

The fast increasing incidence of overweight and obesity among adolescents demonstrates a global 'epidemic' in many countries of the World Health Organization. Nowadays its impact is estimated for the cause of 2-8% of health costs and 10-13% of deaths in adult age because obesity, in addition to causing various physical disabilities and psychological problems, can augment individuals' risk of developing future complications for their health. These teen-agers are developing "adult" diseases such as type 2 diabetes and hypertension, and are at increased risk for heart disease, stroke, certain types of cancer and other serious chronic conditions as obstructive sleep apnea, depression, hypoxemia (Eagle et al., 2009; Rochelle et al., 2011; Wang et al., 2011).

Obesity has been shown to have a substantial negative effect on longevity, reducing the length of life of people who are severely obese by an estimated 5 to 20 years. According to Koplan et al. (2005) state that the rising prevalence of obesity that has already occurred in the past 30 years is expected to lead to an elevated risk of a range of fatal and nonfatal conditions for these cohorts as they age. The study of Fontaine et al. (2003) shows that if the prevalence of obesity continues to rise, especially at younger ages, the negative effect on health and longevity in the coming decades could be much worse.

The medical expenses and indirect costs associated with obesity place a significant burden on a health care system. According to Robert Wood Johnson Foundation Center Report (2010) obese children cost the health care system roughly three times more than the average child. These trends suggest that the relative influence of obesity on the life expectancy of future generations could be markedly worse than it is for current generations. In other words, the life-shortening effect of obesity could rise from its current level of about one third to three fourths of a year to two to five years, or more, in the coming decades, as the obese who are now at younger ages carry their elevated risk of death into middle and older ages.

Causes, Incidences, and Risk Factors of Childhood Obesity

Obesity 'epidemic' is a complex issue with many interrelated factors involved in energy regulation and body weight. As Ogden et al. (2006) state that obesity is a significant public health problem and being obese is depending on variety of, genetic, environmental and behavioral factors, and leads to chronic diseases. It is not only a physical and physiological condition, but also relates to person's social and psychological environment, which triggers certain decisions and habits in their everyday life.

In this frame, among the most important aspects that can improve the risk of obesity in young adolescents, a great relevance is due to the food education (dietary) and the physical activity (active lifestyle). In particular, the underestimation of food portions, cheap unhealthy available food options, lifestyle habits as automotive and emotional eating, lack of recreational areas and low-self esteem that prevents to involve in social activities are considered as the main problems of obesity. Other additional factors that can contribute to this epidemic are related to the environment where these adolescents live (family habits, family income, ethical and cultural background, media influence, lifestyle choices but also outside factors as social and commercial opportunities, social media and relations, living/neighborhood conditions), their self-awareness and their personal involvement in their healing process.

From physiological factors it is important to consider emotional eating is one of the biggest problems of childhood obesity. People create emotional attachment to certain types of food due to its taste, color, and packaging. As Karremans et al. (2006) stated that thirst is a psychological goal. Being hungry and eating is not only depending on physical hunger but also psychological and emotional situation of the person.

Mindfulness eating is another fact that cause automotive eating without feeling that individual is feels full. This happens mostly while a person is doing a co-related activity such as watching TV, playing video games, browsing on Internet with full concentration that does not pay attention what and how much they eat. Social Isolation labeled with fat stigmatization is another problem factor that leads to psychological problems and sedentary lifestyle. As Crandall et al. (1994; 2001) state that fat stigmatization stems from a variety of factors, including negative attitudes and cultural beliefs that equate body fat with gluttony and laziness, and the belief that weight can be controlled with self-regulation. This negatively stereotyped image which results in social isolation.

Therefore having a complex multifactorial problem definition needs to have a more complimentary ways of collecting information. To manage and prevent a chronic disease as obesity, there are various levels of intervention as individual, family, medical, schools, community, environment and policy circles of influence. Mobile interventions will have the role of creating co-relations, transitions, and participative factors through these levels to increase efficiency and participation in prevention. By co-relating various actors in the system will promote a systematic solution, which confronts the complexity of obesity problem from a multifactorial aspects and bring mobile technology to revive with social aspects of a human being. In terms of improving health, from individual to policy level it is important to provide the right environment and incentives people to be able to make healthier choices and provide the skills and knowledge to manage their healthy life.

At individual level, it is important that individual makes healthier changes in habits, which are learning about appropriate portion sizes, consuming healthy snacks; learn new ways to manage stress or depression. Keeping a diary is a method tracking these activities consistently. A study from Kaiser Permanente's Center for Health Research (KPCHR) (2010) funded by the National Heart, Lung and Blood Institute at the National Institute of Health, where the study is the one of the largest and longest weight-loss maintenance trials ever conducted, finds that one of the most important things you can do is write down what you eat. According to KPCHR research lab studies show that those who kept daily food records lost twice as much weight as those who kept no records. The simple act of writing down what you eat encourages people to consume fewer calories.

In order to achieve progress in obesity prevention, the health system require changes in communities, homes, schools for food availability and distribution, marketing and advertising practices and the information environment.

Fighting with obesity is not an easy issue. To prevent and solve obesity problem, there are strategies in action at policy, environmental and community levels as well as strategies for individuals, schools, community and organizations: support groups; weight losing programs, dietician support, community health programs, fat camps and medical solutions such as laparoscopic gastric banding, gastric bypass surgery, all aims to prevent the epidemic obesity problem.

Mostly in scientific literature, obesity problem is considered from medical scientific groups, explored in studies regarding to physiological and genetically problem of obesity, where public health scientists explored obesity prevention in community programs with an educational approach. Recently, within the advancement and accessibility of mobile technology, technologists also aims to discover more solving the problem of obesity prevention through sensors and personalized health applications to track, measure health patterns, or create social health platforms. Health initiatives demonstrated successful scenarios with balance in energy expenditure and food intake as making healthy, nutritious foods and beverages more affordable and accessible; discouraging the consumption of unhealthy foods and beverages;

and achieving an appropriate caloric intake are all important strategies for preventing childhood obesity. However, it is becoming more crucial to create new synergies utilizing mobile tools to increase collaborative participation to develop personalized health interventions.

SOLUTIONS AND RECOMMENDATIONS

Locast Health Diary

Locast Health Diary uses participatory narrative technique as mobile diaries and location based platform to record users' socio-psychological environment and their everyday health routines. The project aims to provide a helpful set of tools tool for obese teens or teen's risk at obesity taking advantage of the Locast platform developed at MIT Mobile Experience Lab. This platform has been utilized in different application areas where the user participates in the content generation in civic engagement, street reporting, and sustainable education projects. In Locast Health Diary project, the platform has been redesigned and used for the obesity prevention study.

The primary aim is to help teens developing awareness of their daily habits and as a consequence, encourage them to change their behaviors towards a healthier life since the process of self-reporting allows people to self-reflect and share aspects of their daily life. As discussed by Grinter and Eldridge (2001) this process can also trigger participants to question their choices and everyday behaviors. More in detail, the purpose is to evaluate if Locast tools as the video diaries, the location based utility and the social interaction tools can be useful to self-reflection on everyday habits, behaviors and decisions. The secondary aim is to provide an effective instrument to nutritionists and educational experts to help teens to improve their actions in healthier behaviors. Psychologists Csikszentmihalyi and Larson (1987) state in their study that they have recognized the need to monitor patients in situ versus asking a participant to recall an event a week or more after the fact. Also the study of asthma conducted by Rich (2000) shows that medical information gathering might be augmented by video diaries created by patients to show clinicians the realities of managing individuals' own health.

Locast Health Diary is a personal diary for group participation through a location-based platform. This civic media tool enhances individuals' awareness of their everyday experiences while they are performing these activities and social dynamics- taking place around them. The system aims to understand obese teens' perception versus reality providing them tools to reflect on their problems and creating a network community that they could develop awareness by social interactions.

Video diaries, created by a mobile application, are used as a personal data collection system allows them to record their eating habits, physical exercises and social activities during the day. The diaries are visualized & shared in real-time on a location-based platform using mobile GPS receiver and location sensing technologies all recorded videos. The exchange of diary information affects health decision-making and creates a long-term behavioral change towards a healthier lifestyle. This web based platform supports social networks where teens can share experiences within the community.

Diaries are structured in templates where each template refers to a question. Each question is a specific area of intervention for obesity prevention outlined by medical experts during the exploration phase. The system allows teens control over 'what and how' data is collected. Templates offer flexibility to frame camera vision, the style of shooting video narratives, and content creation as how to tell their content and what to show in their environment. Through this supportive environment composed of social network and geo-located video diaries it is possible to monitor

teens' everyday habits, physical and emotional activities throughout the day.

Locast as a platform could address obesity problem through using three components: Video diaries, Social network and Location based map.

Video diaries are important for recording and reflecting teens' habits, choices and behaviors at the exact time of the activity performed. As mentioned in the diary studies part of this chapter, the memory of participants recalling past experiences at its most accurate state depends on their current emotional state, the exact time frame and in their current environment. (Csikszentmihalyi & Larson, 1987)

The video diary, which is a visual storytelling tool, could be useful to provide more "direct" understanding of participants' experiences. This visual narrative tool would not only help them to reflect on what they do in actual day but also give further information about their everyday life, for future collaborative decisions with a medical expert, a youth counselor or a health coach. The primary purpose is to use multimedia diaries to push teens' to develop awareness of their everyday eating and activity habits, as a consequence encourage them to change their behaviors towards a healthier lifestyle. In addition, the second purpose is to provide an effective instrument to nutritionists and educational experts to collect additional data to be aggregated to their medical parameters.

Location based technology allows understanding the co-relation between place, which is "individual's environment," and activity type. Individual's environment is correlated with the activity location is an important issue that needs to be considered in patients chronic disease prevention. Activity location visualized on a location based map help to map out the type of activity and services located in the neighborhood. Individuals' change of location depending on the activity during a time frame allows giving assumptions about individuals being active or passive during the day. All these properties of location based diaries; aim to give additional information both for the type of the activity and the individual choices.

Social Network is a place where social interaction and support occurs. One of the hypotheses in healthcare is to keep mental health positive, not something from negative to positive but making something positive to a more positive state to keep the psychological state of individual positive. There is a correlative relation between social support and physical health of an individual. According to Clark (2011) social support is one of most important factors in predicting the physical health and well-being of everyone, ranging from childhood through older adults. The absence of social support shows some disadvantage among the impacted individuals. In most cases, it can predict the deterioration of physical and mental health among the victims. The initial social support given is also a determining factor in successfully overcoming life stress.

Social network motivates individuals socially being active and a part of a community. Being a part of a community make them feel stronger and socially motivated to cope with their problems and also learn from others. However in chronic diseases, individuals take very personal their healthcare, therefore privacy and trust is an important issue to be considered due to sharing on a social platform. It depends on the personality,

psychological factors and ethical- cultural background of the individual where they might not want to show their personal life or some particular context of their life to other people even if they are their friends or families.

APPROACH TO COLLABORATIVE PARTICIPATION TO PERSONALIZED HEALTH – LOCAST HEALTH DIARY TOOLS

Health Diary Mobile Application

Mobile application allows teens to create their diaries from guided video creation technique. On the mobile Interface, 'Activity Log' and 'Casts' are two main elements, which allow teens to create their own diaries and share it on Locast Health Diary web platform (see Figure 1). 'Activity Log' includes categories of activities to capture in participants' environment mainly focused on eating, exercise and free time activities. 'Casts' are parts of recorded video created by teens while performing any categories from Activity Log.

From the secondary research results and medical expert discussions, it has been identified that the environment, the type of activity and the mood of the participant is important to confront obesity

Figure 1. Locast health diary mobile application

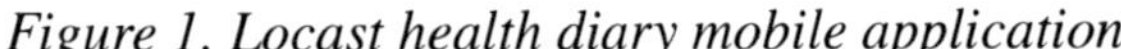

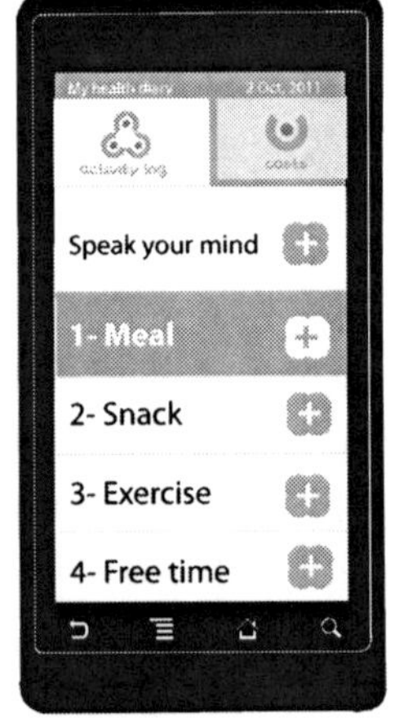

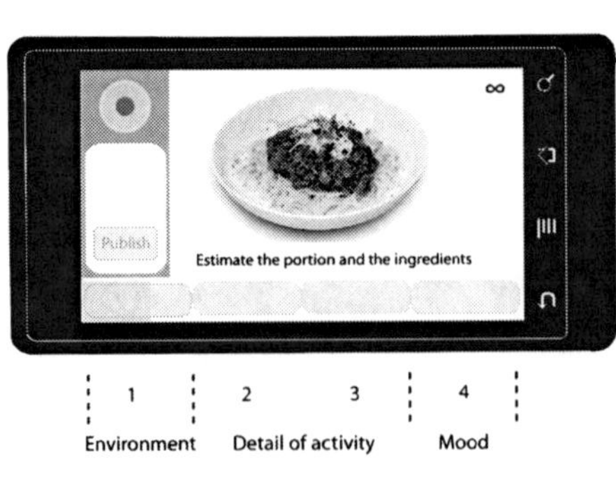

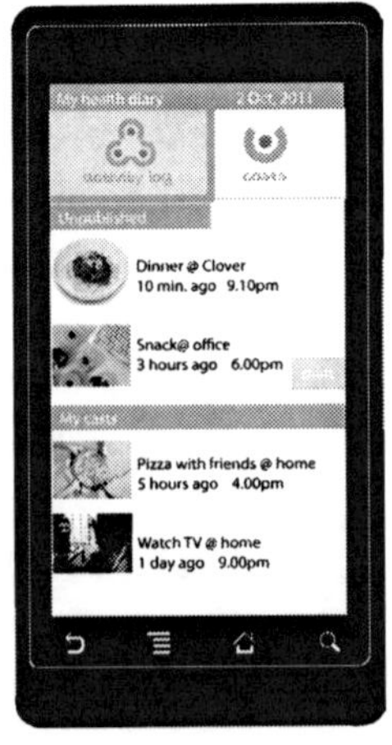

problem. During the design of data collection tool, it has been considered one of the obstacles in the Rich's Video Intervention Assessment (VIA) method (2000) is that unstructured user generated collected data was too much material to analyze. Therefore, the video creation tool has been structured and guided into Casts. Each cast has its own content, prompts and guidance within unlimited timeframe. All casts recording combines and produce the video itself that can be published in real-time on a social platform or can be viewed privately on the mobile interface.

The video content has been structured to capture three main issues to prevent obesity. Each video segment designed with an unlimited recording timeframe considering the results of the pilot study, where participants did not able to complete their narrative due to time restrictions on the cast creation.

1. **Environment:** Participants create a narrative about their physical and social atmosphere, describing the environmental factors, which contain information about the place and people in which participant is interacting or being surrounded with during the activity. In this segment participants are asked to describe their environment. The aim is to obtain data about where and with whom do participants' perform their activity (whether in a group or individual, and if participants are alone or in a social environment while performing their activity) gives us additional data about their environment and their engagement with social activities.

2. **Detail of activity:** These two parts of the video creation allow participants tell more detailed information about the type of activity they record. Providing indications and prompts, the aim is to gather data about the estimation of food portion and ingredients. As a sample, one indication to create this cast is asking them 'Show the proportion of the meal using your hand' or a question as 'if it

is a free time relaxing activity or a physical activity which requires energy consuming'.

3. Same as 2.

4. **Mood:** The last part but the most important is to understand their emotions on particular activities. This has been put as the last part as it would be friendlier to ask to the participant to express more about their feelings. The simple question 'Explain your mood' could help to collect important datasets about their emotional state of participants while performing the activity at that moment whether they are happy, sad, stressed, bored, energetic, tired, anxious, frustrated, lonely. The question aims to answer how does the participant feel and if the participant's voice confirm this mood or not.

Locast Health Diary Web Platform

The purpose of this web platform is to create a collaborative participation through social interactions towards healthier discussion forums. Locast Health Diary website is an important part of the system to develop awareness on teens where the platform allows viewing teens' own video or other participants' video and able to comment, like others' everyday diaries and video contents (see Figure 2). Through these geo-located videos, on the platform it is also possible to map out distribution of activities by different users or all the activities of the same user on the location based map.

The video content on the website has been organized according to data structure, tag management, and filtering prioritize. Diaries can be sorted out by most popular diaries, most recent diaries, and diaries in alphabetic order. There are 5 Web page layouts that are redesigned and modified of front hand according to the project. *Home Web page:* The webpage that includes all casts and activities; Community Web page: This webpage includes all profile of participants of the community; *My Diary Web page:* This webpage includes all "my casts" of a participant. There is

Figure 2. Locast health diary web platform and videos

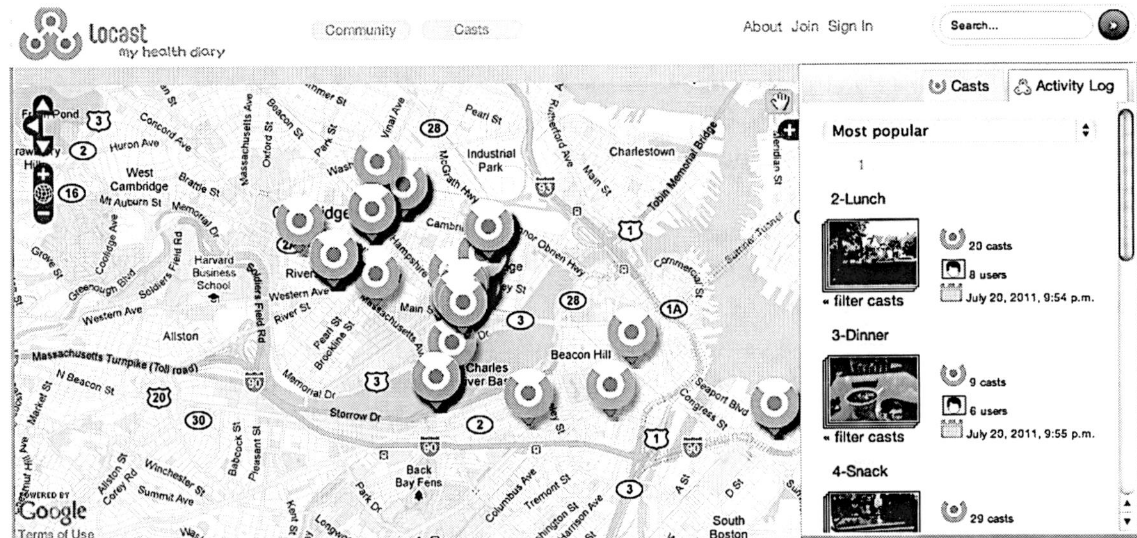

also a "profile info" and "diary timeline" to stream all casts of a 3-day diary of the participant; *Single Cast Web page:* This webpage includes single cast details and allow your interaction to the cast for editing, commenting, liking and viewing. If you click any cast on the webpage it will browse you to this webpage; *Activity Log Web page:* This webpage includes the activity description and all the casts related to this activity. It also allows you to see the "activity playlist", a sequence of playlist of casts.

In order to increase active engagement on the website, the web platform has been redesigned according to the social persuasion guidelines proposed by Kukkonen and Oinas (2011) and simplified for a more user friendly website. In order to support socially, a person will be more motivated to perform a target behavior if, he can use a system to observe others performing the behavior or in social comparison system users will have a greater motivation to perform the target behavior if they can compare their performance with the performance of others. On the platform, being able to viewing others' diaries and posting constructive comments to others' diaries, participants are more likely to perform target

behavior if they discern via the system that others are performing the behavior along with them where activity timeline and given assignments on the Locast website helped to create this type of social support.

Locast Health Diary Project Development

Locast Health Diary project has lasted 9 months through a five-step process of research, concept development, prototyping, deployment and evaluation. To develop the initial phase a secondary and primary research has been applied through semi-structured interviews with medical expert group of nutritionist, pediatrician and health coach who has expertise on childhood obesity interventions. Discussions and remarks have been made on Locast tools with medical experts to evaluate usefulness of video diaries, social network, and location based platform in order to confront obesity problem.

The results from the preliminary research with health experts show that underestimation of food portions, time-consuming traditional methods used by medical experts, no real-time data collection about mood while individuals performing activities inadequate information about social family history such as how their parents behave them, and how they force them to eat. Some of the discussions from the in-depth interviews:

Health coach discusses that "Awareness of their own behavior is the most underutilized health issue. Most of the people eat without paying attention what they eat. They are addictive, autopilot and automotive. We are eating in front of a computer while working, talking on the phone, and we are not focusing on the feeling of satisfaction the fullness of our stomach." Being aware of "am I hungry, why am I at this spot?" creates a mindful eating awareness of what they eat which leads to a behavioral change.

Nutritionist states that video diaries should be less threatening and more fun in comparison with a traditional written diary where they ask 3-day food logging of the type of food and how much they eat. The problem she state is "The traditional process is very time consuming. They fill out a paper, they think, and most of the time they do not give the right information but underestimate the fact. Portion is important. They don't get used to take a photo of their plate mostly; they forgot what and how much they eat. Most of the time patients underestimate the reality."

Pediatrician adds to this statement "When a doctor asks a question to the patient, patient most likely underestimate the answer, but through videos, they cannot lie and underestimate the fact. It is interesting to know what teens are thinking when their mom is making a meal or what is their mindset. I would like to see their script."

The expert group agreed that location based platform could be an opportunity to map out after school teen centers or any high school teen programs in the community, although there still might be privacy issues regarding to location based recordings. Furthermore it might be also useful to map out individual´s calorie consumption path, where are the best places they consume calorie or possibly be used to cluster the subjects as patient profile group, whether they live in the same neighborhood or different laces.

Another argument discussed was that the kids between 16-17 years old almost want to show their own TV show; they want them to be watched by other people. They could be aware of their behavior looking at their or others video. Another point is to understand their mindset in each health decision throughout the day. If they are being teased because they are overweight, or they choose that particular food because they are frustrated, or they stop by a fast food chain on the way from school to home, because they are aroused by the smell. The answer changes intervention target and approach to confront their problem.

The results from the secondary research shows that some of obese teens find a necessity to share their feelings and support each other in anonymous network environments such as blogs, social network sites, vblogs. Social motivation and self-esteem awareness, fat acceptance, family constraints are common trails to find in these blogs. The reason why they use mostly is to look for a motivational support, advise on certain medical topics, and to express their emotions and thought about the problem they confront in their life. As seen in the personal statements taken from the blogs shows that there is a high peer influence since they can encourage and provide solutions to each other. (i.e., for example, one obese seen another obese teen on the blog that is attending a yoga class and encouraged by this action and gave a decision to attend the same class as well.) Therefore, it has been a critical issue how to motivate teens to use Locast system where the ideas of creating a fun diary of their everyday activities are a way to enable participation and collaboration between each other.

Deployment with YES (Boston Youth Essential Center)

The Locast Health Diary has been experimented with participatory workshops and follow-up evaluation phase. The Locast Health Diary tools has been tested with teens participated at the obesity prevention program of YES.

This phase involved the participation of Boston Asian: Youth Essential Center (YES), which is a non- profit, community-based organization that aims to work collaboratively to provide services for youth as Prevention and Intervention programs. The aims of these programs address specific issues faced by youths and their families, and provide support and outreach for obesity prevention, diabetes, substance and tobacco abuse, which are funded from Federal Government Department of Health. Participants are selected among teens which are a part of 'Teens going Healthy' an obesity prevention program which helps teens to confront with obesity problems and teach participants to make healthier food choices, be better food shoppers, and incorporate sports and other physical activities into their schedules.

Participant observation recordings, pre and post project questionnaire surveys, visual and cognitive maps, structured and unstructured interviews with experts are being used as tools in the research process to investigate the usefulness of video diaries, the value of social network and the utility of location-based platform. Six teens, 2 female and 4 male aged between 14 and 18 years, involved in an obesity prevention program in Boston participated in the project together with a nutritionists, a youth counselors and an intermediate person as healthcare consultant. Subjects are involved in the study under the circumstances of the program voluntarily to try the application for wellbeing and active life rather than advertised as an obesity prevention tool.

To understand the utility of mobile diaries, social network, and location-based platform and to develop awareness on teens' perception, the workshop designed in three stages: perception, reality and future goals (see Figure 3). The aim is to compare the results of perception versus reality stage and which allows teens to design their future goals for a healthier lifestyle or a think for a behavior change.

Figure 3. Locast health diary project workshop

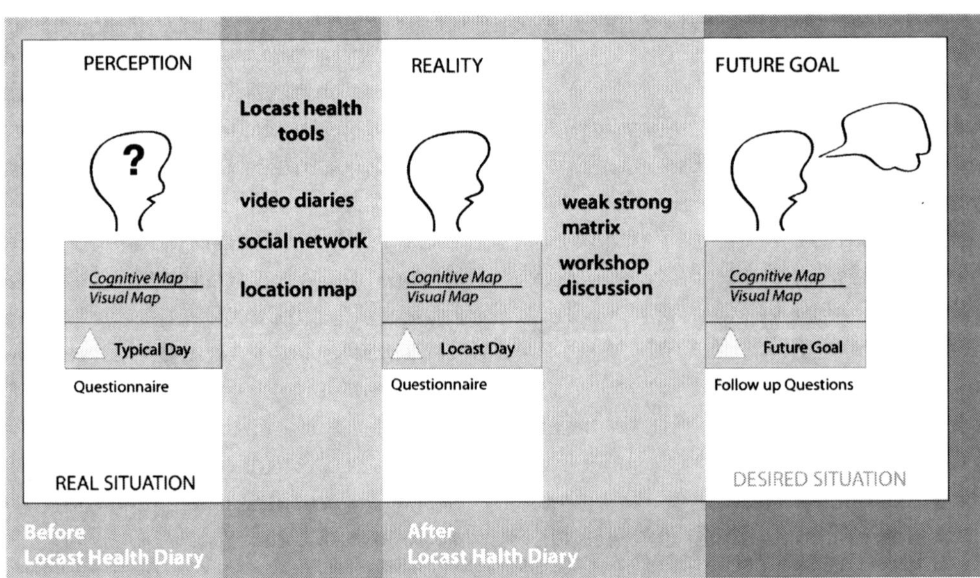

The experiment evolved in three stages: *Perception* stage allows understanding their current situation. Through questionnaires, and visual-cognitive maps the aim is to understand their perception of how teens think and they think to do. This will help to compare the past and present of their understanding and their doing. *Reality* stage aims to use Locast Health Dairy tools and try to gather their current behaviors. Locast health diary mobile application has been provided to teens through an explanatory workshop where they have logged their everyday activity through geo located- mobile video diaries for a week and interacted on the social network. *Future Goal* stage provides a discussion for group evaluation and self- reflection on their and others' diaries comparing their perception versus reality, which aims to define their future goal towards a healthier lifestyle and behaviors.

Locast tools helped to monitor the real environment and allowed teens to compare their perceived activities in their mindset and activities that they performed in their everyday life. Additional tools have been designed as cognitive and visual maps, weak and strong matrix, and questionnaires helped teens to analyze and compare *their typical day* and *Locast day* and create their *future goal* for a healthier lifestyle. In addition to these new tools, *video analysis card* is initially designed for the researcher aims to compare the results of participants' direct phrases with direct-subjective observation of their environment, and researchers interpretation of the collected data through video. As future steps, this tool could be utilized also for experts for review and evaluation.

Results from the Locast Health Diary Deployment

The six teens uploaded 66 videos on the Locast website *locast.mit.edu/healthdiary*, 26 casts are in the Meal category, 9 cast are in the Snack category, 19 casts are in the free-time category, 5 casts are in the Speak your mind category, and only 2 casts are in the Community category. 20 casts were the highest number recorded by one participant, 4 casts the lowest. It depends from a variety of issues as the age group and personality of the participant. For example two participants are 18 years old and they are 12th grade senior high school students; other three are 14-15 years old, 9th grade high school students. The oldest, mostly have a tight schoolwork and exams. They record their casts more complete and create a more constructive narrative; three participants mostly did not speak much or in an incomplete way, and record less casts than others.

The comparison between typical day and future goal day in visual and cognitive maps compiled by each participant shows that all participants developed awareness on unhealthy habits but two of them didn't want to change his behaviors in practice, although all of them state in the after project questionnaire they would want. According to questionnaires, they have all developed awareness on eating than exercise and free-time activities. Analyzing the interaction on the web using Locast tools, it is possible to see that teens developed more awareness viewing others video diaries than viewing their own. For example, one teen commented on other teens' video cast named 'Burger King for Lunch':

Don't eat tooo much. Fats are gona stack up in your blood vessels.

She has also commented in the discussion group, that viewing his videos where he was always eating fast food, discouraged her to eat fast food.

The utility of location-based map was more useful for researcher and experts to estimate teens' daily choices in community rather than the students. For example, one teen was eating his lunch in a fast food chain outside school, due to availability and proximity to his school, where he thinks that school lunch is not healthy and tasty. At this point, to move forward as next steps for a behavioral change, it is important to analyze whether if this teen does not have enough information about what a healthy food is, or the school lunch is apparently not tasty enough for teens.

Another important result from post questionnaire and discussion group is that the privacy concerns and motivation for recording diaries and sharing their content on the website. Some teens disagree that they felt comfortable recording their both eating and physical activity, however they somewhat agree that they felt comfortable seeing their own video on the website. Teens agree that technology was innovative and interesting to them and they did not encounter problems with the technology.

Consequently we are convinced that Locast Health Diary helps developing awareness however, without an expert participation it may not be sufficient to determinate behavioral change. As (Bhamra et al., 2008) states the elements of behavioral change, first user need to have intention where to develop awareness, which is derives from old habit to develop awareness and take into consideration for a behavior change. This project helps teens to clarify their behaviors and choices of their consideration for a positive change.

Focus group and expert interviews demonstrate that Locast Health can be an effective instrument for nutritionists, youth counselors and healthcare consultants in different ways. The teen's counselor proposed that Locast application could be applied as a longer-term program in Asian Youth Essential Center. The healthcare consultant at Tufts Community Wellness thinks that this could be applicable to other chronic disease conditions.

The clinical director and nutritionist works with obese teens at Center for Youth Wellness at Floating Hospital for Children indicated that they would like to be a part of a research proposal for grant, where they would like to test the Locast application on their obese patients. The Welcome project, Somerville, program director would like to apply Locast for other type of wellbeing projects as video voices of physical activities of community members. From the discussion with experts from different fields, it has been understand that the outcomes of this project envision many other application areas and research directions for different actors for the obesity prevention. For example, Locast Health Diary can be a discussion tool for educational expert, an additional food diary tool for nutritionist or used as an opportunity to implement in different health preventive-community related contexts for the community leaders.

Discussing with the expert team, the results show that medical expert see video diaries, as a complementary tool applicable to really get an idea of the portion sizes and the environmental factors to estimate teens' daily choices in community. For example, one teen was eating his lunch in a fast food chain outside school, due to availability and proximity to school, because he thinks that school lunch is not healthy and tasty. Educational expert see Locast Health Diary as a discussion tool able to monitor co-related activities and are interested in an extension of Locast Health Diary Project as a part of obesity prevention programs and its application also to other wellbeing projects. This is a relevant result of the project since further refinement of action research according to Jacobs et al. (1992, p. 431) is that the results obtained from the research should be relevant to the practice.

From user experience point of view, teens felt very comfortable using the Locast technology. They were able to do tasks on the website easily and very quick in learning technical functions of the mobile and website application. This is the advantageous way of deploying the study with teens since are eager to be familiar with the new technologies. However, it was relatively not comfortable for some teens to record in a social environment when they are with friends. One of the teen's feedbacks was "I didn't feel bored while recording but I did feel uncomfortable recording when other people are around me at first. It was awkward in school."

During the deployment there were system communication problems due to Internet connection, which results in saving casts as drafts rather than uploading them in real time. Although the quality of videos and sound properties were quite good, both from teens and also experts state that the quality of sound and videos could be better on the website to be able to analyze and understand the details in the recorded environment. The background noise is sometimes disturbing especially, recordings in social environment. The sound and video quality could be still improved on the website. Mobile phones record 5 MP, 2592 x 1944 pixels video recordings. When you record video on the mobile side it configures to the website by converting the right file size. The amount of lightweight file size needed to be configured from mobile to web transmission. It was a part of conversion process that converts videos from mobile to a web-friendly format. Therefore, there were video processing and synchronization problems from mobile to server and from server to website due to system communication error between Locast Web and Locast Mobile application. Although some of the casts could be seen on the mobile side, however they could not be seen on the website. The web developer had to re-process the videos to fix the problem. In addition to that creating four template-guided video was useful to structure the content and develop awareness on particular subjects, however sometimes ruins the fluency of narrative. One participant says, "the guided templates allows me to answer the questions asked more than telling a narrative of the description/mood and environment of the activity."

Participants' everyday communication tools and their social media preferences need to be taken into consideration. To get used to using a new platform in a frequent way requires time, effort and network. It was challenging in that sense for utilization of Locast website, which was a new platform for teens different from any other means of social sites. Therefore, this could possibly be integrated in one of their everyday social platform choice, which increases participation.

Another issue was teens' communication tools that they use every day. Teens did not get used to checking their emails on a daily routine but they were using more social networking sites such as Facebook (FB) and YouTube every day. It was not an easy to communicate with them directly without a second intermediate person as teens' counselor where he calls or meets them in his meeting sessions in the program. Therefore workshop sessions and posting an informative cast on the Locast website was more effective. For further studies, it is crucial to understand the best way to communicate with teens and design the deployment according to this fact.

FUTURE RESEARCH DIRECTIONS

Innovative care for chronic conditions is influenced and supported by integrated health organization, the broader community, and the policy environment. When the integration of the components is optimal, the patient, family becomes active participants in their care, supported by the community and healthcare team. New application areas could be included through mixing the different synergies of circles of influence in self-management of a chronic disease as defined by Clark and Patridge (2001) the influence on individual through these layers: self-management, family involvement, clinical expertise and systems, work and school support, community awareness, environmental health, and policy actions. The flexibility and adaptability of Health Diary tools could be used in in different areas of health prevention from environmental level to personalized level varying from wellbeing of communities to increase active life and healthy eating, quit smoking and drug addiction to prevent other type of chronic diseases as asthma, diabetes Type2, and migraine.

It is important to rethink the design process in different level of interventions and for targeted groups. For personalized health, diary tools could be utilized as an individual tool, which aims to develop awareness on individuals' health patterns in a more engaging and fun way. For community health programs, they could be used as a discussion and participative tool for prevention with longer-term objectives and help them to shape community members' future goal. For experts, the tools could be used as an alternative method to gather additional information about patients' social-psychological state throughout the day in their environment to be later aggregated with their medical parameters.

The age group of Locast Health Diary deployment 14-18 years old is very much interested in technology and quick to learn and adapt to their lifestyle. If this study was deployed for old people, than the application and the process should be considered according to the specific chronic disease prevention requirements and the targeted subject groups' needs and behaviors. As future steps, it is important to think about different target groups with different ages and other chronic disease applications. Another application area is targeting people with co-related chronic diseases such as aging people who have problem with obesity and diabetes Type 2. Utilizing video diaries aggregated with sensor systems to receive medical parameters could be a tool for experts for chronic disease prevention and management.

The guided template video production and a social engagement platform can be applied to many health problems where it is important to develop new impactful technologies to aim for healthy lifestyle in all levels of communities. The future step in this research field is to design new narrative and social media tools to allow user collect their own socio-psychological environmental data and help them to act upon to change their behavior in a long-term intervention.

The data collection tool through self-reporting and self-reflecting approach could be explored with the aim of collecting more meaningful data and more effective analysis tool. To improve the social interaction in the platform it is important to explore new models to increase engagement through the social connections in the web platform as well as using the video diaries to monitor and record their everyday health.

From methodological point of view, videos as a source of creating diaries are time-consuming but valuable source of information. We should look more optimized way of collecting and extracting knowledge out of that in healthcare prevention in order to gather different datasets of an individual. The question we could ask could be how we can use narrative approach and storytelling with using video as a means of capturing material to confront chronic disease problem. Qualitative information is valuable and we should integrate this datasets and increase feasibility and accuracy of the model of understanding individual behaviors from their point of view. The video analysis part could be take in one step further in order to analyze the tonality, frequency of the voice (i.e., Max Little's application helps to detect Parkinson's disease with 99 percent accuracy–in a 30 second phone call) or adding visual processing and video technologies to analyze the back-foreground areas. We can also try to quantify the qualitative information through scaling methods to allow user to rate their mood of their state or density of their pain at a scale. This will ease the data analysis to understand user behaviors.

Location based characteristics that influence health could be an additional datasets to be considered in the health prevention. Location based map could be extended and aggregated with other types of information such as environmental data as it has been done in the project of Bill DavenHall's TED talk on your health depends on where you live. Furthermore, location sensing technology could be aggregated within users' environment that integrates stakeholders, health providers, advertising, community service providers and having a real time feedback and healthy promotion mechanisms to change individuals' behavior towards a healthier decisions and habits.

As a conclusion, to advance in personalized services, which enable individuals, from the younger to the elder population, to become co-producers of their health and maintain good health status, further research directions could be explored such as (i) a "virtual individual" model, which comprises the personal characteristics of an individual (e.g., personal profile, preconditions, risk factors, unhealthy behaviors, preferences, physical activity, sleep, mental status etc.); (ii) advanced sensors to acquire data on lifestyle aspects, behavior and surrounding environment; (iii) intelligent systems for recognition of behavioral trends and prediction or early detection of health risks on the basis of heterogeneous data, including data acquired by sensors and individual self assessment; (iv) a supportive environment to engineer awareness about healthy behaviors, offer personalized guidance and provide support to behavioral change; (v) development of a new ecosystem of stakeholders, engaging also actors such as fitness, food and lighting industry, schools, health insurance companies, policy makers and media; (vi) innovation in organizational models and business models for ICT-enabled disease prevention.

CONCLUSION

The health system improvement is nowadays oriented towards new qualitative services that gain the same importance of the quantitative services, especially for young patients/individuals. The impact of these interventions is the potential reduction of the primary service because of the possibility of a continuous and real time connection between patients and caregivers through the creation of a real community. In such a community, patients are not only connected with physicians to plan the necessary visits, but at the same time they are connected to their responsive environment to be able to participate in their own health management.

In addition, social networks can create spontaneous confrontation between users, supported by the quantitative monitoring of their healing process. Patients can become sponsor of patients and build a friendly and scientific based community composed by all the involved stakeholders. This means an improvement of the quality of personalized services by the direct contact for patients, and the reduction of a more sustainable production for the industries (fitness, food and healthcare).

Changing a behavior of an individual requires many aspects of intervention and one of them is developing awareness and acting upon the problem through experts both from medical side as well as cognitive and psychological side. In order to understand such a complex phenomenon as behaviors of individuals with in its environment and its decision-making processes, it is important to correlate different type of information of individuals' lifestyle. The combination of this information could lead to a more complete solution set for behavior change, long term decisions and patterns both in individuals life but also in society's landscape towards long lasting life and healthier lifestyle.

With Locast Health Diary project, video diaries, created by a mobile application, visualized & shared in real-time on a location-based platform, provided the exchange of information among teens affected health decision-thinking with the aim to create a long-term behavioral change towards a healthier lifestyle. Geo-located mobile diaries and social network touch many points of the problems that has been stated at the beginning of the chapter which is the socio-psychological environment data collection, involvement of participants and the prevention of chronic disease through developing awareness on unhealthy habits to create future goals for healthier lifestyle. Results from this study show that it is not far to imagine the use of mobile technology and civic media creation as a tool to understand correlation of behaviors and encourage active participation in your own health. Locast Health Diary helps developing awareness however, without an expert participation it may not be sufficient to determinate behavioral change.

Despite the limited number of participants and the statement by Jacobs et al. (1992, p. 45) that action research "is characterized by the fact that problem solving, seen as renewed corrective actions, cannot be generalized, because it should comply with the criteria set for scientific character", however sharing process and qualitative outcomes of this project can be useful to other researchers as experiential knowledge base.

Privacy and trust is two critical points to be considered in health preventive interventions. There have been barriers of participation due to content and privacy in the social platform. In social networking sites to protect user privacy social networks usually provide different privacy levels that allow users to decide in their network who can view their profile, contact them, and add them to their list of contacts. In Locast Health Diary, all participants are already a part of the same prevention program; therefore they were a part of a large community, where the trust has been naturally created. Locast Health Diary social platform has created a specific community that has similar goals and interest within a larger community. The privacy on the mobile side allows user to decide whether to publish and share their diaries on the social platform or keep it as personal video on the mobile application. The privacy issue on the social platform has been more challenging where the web administrator controls and reviews all content published on the website. This protects the misuse of the shared content that might have negative effects among teens.

It is important as a designer to implement strategies and tools to produce a mutually agreeable outcome for all participants and nurture actors where they can take responsibility. As O'Brien (1998) states that to accomplish this, the researcher may necessitate adopting many different roles at various stages of the process as planner leader, catalyzer, teacher, listener, synthesizer, facilitator, designer, observer, and reporter. Due to the change in their role at different stages, the designer communicates with different actors as medical expert, educational expert, participants, and external intermediate person through using different research and design tools.

As a specific contribution of designer, it is important to create relations between actors through designers' creativity and intuitive competences. DiSalvo et al. (2007) argue that how communities and participants actually come to take up the systems of co-production is an obvious, yet under-addressed concern for designers. In discussing motivations for participation Botero and Saad-Sulonen (2008) highlight the value of working with existing communities around issues of community interest, but the role of designers may also extend to bringing the community 'into being' as part of the project. The capacity of translating and transforming ideas, desires, and the need of actors in visual representation forms is important to communicate through actors. The development of new tools to help both users and experts where for users to help them to modify behaviors, and gain awareness of their problems, on the other hand for expert to help them structure, synthesize and understand user behavior. As a designer, it is important to know how and in which phase to use visualization and communication methods to make participant understand things and which phase use research tools to collect data from the participants. For example in deployment phase, it is important that participant understand what to do, and in the evaluation phase designer need to know what to ask and how to gather information. Experts are integrated into the projects not as a team member but as an external collaborator. In concept development phase it is necessary to interact with different disciplines where the aim is to create innovative concept from different point of view, analyzing the collected ideas in realizable technology context, where most of the group discussions has occurred.

Standard tools as questionnaires (pre and post project) and interviews have been used to gain information from teens and experts. Locast video diary has been developed on the basis of the existing MIT platform to actively involve teens. Ad hoc Visual and cognitive maps organized in typical day, Locast day, future goal day making comparisons possible between perceived habits, real behaviors and future goals has been created to support communication between participants during focus group. Ad hoc Video Analysis Cards containing Reference Image, Observation of video content, Participant Answer, Researcher Interpretation has been generated to summarize information for nutritionists.

The system framework consists of three main functionalities which is to self report of the activity performed through mobile diaries, social-environmental monitoring of the subject in real time, and third as the sharing through a social platform to encourage for developing awareness and change for a healthier lifestyle through social connectivity and engagement. The aim is to develop awareness from a qualitative point of view, trying to make aware of individuals' perception, decisions and behaviors through self-reporting their activities in a narrative way (which is a way to collect information in a less visible way but more subjective and willingly way. Which might provide us more accurate information). There are lots of cases where people can track their collected quantitative data through mobile phones and monitor in visualized graphs to be aware of their activities and contribute to their decision-making. However, this type of applications might be less courage and motivating for people who has physical-psychological problem where involvement in their health management is becomes another important issue. Therefore, these types of tools should be encouraged and more integrated to individuals' lives (in this study obese teens at risk.)

As a partner for deployment or project development, it is not easy to involve health institutions as hospital due to bureaucratic agreements and time schedules. Firstly the medical experts do not have enough time for following and participating in research projects where it is difficult to schedule common working hours since the hospital settings primary goal is to cure patients. Secondly, in a hospital setting the interaction between medical experts and patients are more medical oriented, less concerned on socio-psychological level and less participative from patients' point of view. Thirdly, the patient privacy is highly protected and patient information is highly confidential. Due to protect the patient privacy, IRB- Intellectual Review Board- requires longer time to get approved from both collaborators.

Therefore, it is more likely and innovative to collaborate with community groups than in a hospital setting where participants would like to participate and privacy issues are depending on the participant itself. Community leaders are looking for new activities to innovate and educate their communities towards healthier lifestyle. This results in innovation, if we could focus on collaborative participation starting from personalized health to bring it towards community health interventions.

A Supportive Shared Environment to Self-Reflect Your Habits and Behaviors

It is crucial to rethink educational and proactive environments for individuals to create a new-generation of co-producers of health. Inviting participants to take the role of author and contributor prior to the development or specification of any particular mobile intervention and social platform creates the potential for a greater personal connection between innovative, participative and socially enriched mobile experiences towards a healthier lifestyle.

Creating a community helps to bring personalize health through collaborative participation into one step further to environmental level. The perfect community is thereby often portrayed as one in which individuals and groups naturally organize themselves to work to actively shape their shared environment, where people act together and '... participate in efforts to address their needs collectively' (Contractor and Peterson Bishop, 2000,

p. 152). This commonality and participation is what distinguishes a community from many other social groups. If we can start from the core and expand creating a community to aim to impact for environment, then we have a good direction to solve many health problems, mostly regarding to chronic disease from socio-environmental point of view.

Community is considered a positive symbiotic state invoking ideas of co-operation, lack of conflict and democratic decision-making (Robson, 2000, p. 71), As Wellman defines (1999) 'networked individualism', the building of social relationships, which are more fragmented, dispersed, and specialized than in previous social systems but over which their members can assert control and choice. Castells argues (1998) that the Internet is the most appropriate medium of communication in an emerging network society and that it will play an increasingly important role, not only in the way that people choose to communicate with each other but also in the way we form social relationships. Therefore, looking at the social rejection of people, who are obese, could be a way to approach to the problem. As Christakis and Fowler (2007) suggested social distance plays a stronger role than geographic distance in the spread of behaviors or norms associated with the obesity through use of, and exposure to, these new technologies, users will adopt new forms of behavior explicitly linked to the technology itself' (Rutter, 2001, p. 371).

There need to be more applications that concern group participation using mobile technologies. While new medical technologies will improve the practice of medicine to cure illnesses, it is critical to explore technologies that promote healthier lifestyle and social connections through supportive environments that proactively help people remain healthy, autonomous, and engaged in life.

The chapter tried to propose different tools and methods of narrative approach through using mobile video diaries to explore three main problems of healthcare. To understand and collect socio-environmental factors of individuals' lifestyle, to encourage patients participation and to design preventive interventions for chronic disease management could be confronted through social network, video diaries and location based technology. To reach this objective focus project Locast Health Diary proposed a collaborative participatory approach for personalized health through creating a health community to develop awareness and think individuals for a positive change.

ACKNOWLEDGMENT

I would like to express my gratitude to Federico Casalegno and MEL (Mobile Experience Lab) research team at Massachusetts Institute of Technology and Fiammetta Costa in TeDH (Technology and Design for Healthcare) research group at Politecnico di Milano. Special thanks to Boston Asian Youth Essential Center teens and workers, in particular YES youth counselor and Community Health Group health consultant at Tufts Medical Center for their contribution to Locast Health Diary Project.

REFERENCES

Abowd, G. (2000, Mar.). D., & Mynatt, E., D. (2000). *Charting past, present and future research in ubiquitous computing. ACM Transactions on Computer-Human Interaction*, 7(1), 29–58. doi:10.1145/344949.344988

Appan, P., Sundaram, H., & Birchfield, D. (2004). Communicating everyday experiences. In *Proceedings of the 1st ACM Workshop on Story Representation, Mechanism and Context*. New York: ACM.

Bhamra, T., Lilley, D., & Tang, T. (2008). Sustainable use: Changing Consumer Behavior through Product Design. In *Changing the Change: Design Visions*. Turin: Proposals and Tools.

Botero, A., & Saad-Sulonen, J. (2008). *Co-designing for new city-citizen interaction possibilities: Weaving prototypes and interventions in the design and development of Urban Mediator*. Proc. PDC 2008, 266-269.

Bruckner, H., & Bearman, P. S. (2005). After the promise: The STD consequences of adolescent virginity pledges. *The Journal of Adolescent Health*, *36*, 271–278. doi:10.1016/j.jadohealth.2005.01.005 PMID:15780782

Bruyn, S. (1966). *The human perspective in sociology: The methodology of participant observation*. Englewood Cliffs, NJ: Prentice-Hall.

Burke, M., Marlow, C., & Lento, T. (2010). Social network activity and social well-being. *ACM CHI 2010: Conference on Human Factors in Computing Systems* (pp. 1909-1912).

Carter, S., & Mankoff, J. (2005). When participants do the capturing: the role of media in diary studies. *Proc. CHI 2005* (pp. 899–908).

Christakis, N. A., & Fowler, J. H. (2007). The spread of obesity in a large social network over 32 years. *The New England Journal of Medicine*, *357*, 370–379. doi:10.1056/NEJMsa066082 PMID:17652652

Clark, C. M. (2011). *Relations Between Social Support and Physical Health Middle-Aged Adults*. Corey M Clark in Health San Francisco.

Consolvo, S., Everitt, K., Smith, I., & Landay, J. A. (2006). Design Requirements for Technologies that Encourage Physical Activity. *Proceedings of CHI 2006* (pp. 457-66). Montreal, Canada.

Contractor, N., & Bishop, A. P. (2000). Reconfiguring Community Networks. The Case of Prairie-Know. In T. Ishida & K. Isbister (Eds.), *Digital Cities, Technologies, Experiences and Future Perspectives*. Berlin, Heidelberg, New York: Springer-Verlag. doi:10.1007/3-540-46422-0_13

Cottam, H., & Leadbetter, C. (2004). *Red Paper 01: Health: Co-Creating Services*. London: Design Council.

Crandall, C. S. (1994). Prejudice against fat people: Ideology and self interest. *Journal of Personality and Social Psychology*, *66*, 882–894. doi:10.1037/0022-3514.66.5.882 PMID:8014833

Csikszentmihalyi, M., & Larson, R. (1987). Validity and reliability of the experience-sampling method. *The Journal of Nervous and Mental Disease*, *175*(9). doi:10.1097/00005053-198709000-00004 PMID:3655778

Ebbeling, C. B., Pawlak, D. B., & Ludwig, D. S. (2002). Childhood obesity: public-health crisis, common sense cure. *Lancet*, *360*(9331), 473–482. doi:10.1016/S0140-6736(02)09678-2 PMID:12241736

Fontaine, K. R., Redden, D. T., Wang, C., Westfall, A. O., & Allison, D. B. (2003). Years of life lost due to obesity. *Journal of the American Medical Association*, *289*, 187–193. doi:10.1001/jama.289.2.187 PMID:12517229

Gaver, B., Dunne, T., & Pacenti, E. (1999). Design: Cultural Probes. *Interaction*, *1999*, 21–29. doi:10.1145/291224.291235

Gemmell, J., Williams, L., Wood, K., Lueder, R., & Bell, G. (2004). Passive Capture and Ensuing Issues for a Personal Lifetime Store. In *Proceedings of the 1st ACM Workshop on Continuous Archival and Retrieval of Personal Experiences*. New York: ACM.

Gibson, E. B. (2005). Co-producing Video-diaries: The presence of the "Absent" researcher. *International Journal of Qualitative Methods, 4*, 2005.

Grinter, R. E., & Eldridge, M. (2001). y do tngrs luv 2 txt msg? In *Proceedings of the 7th European Conference on Computer-Supported Cooperative Work (ECSCW)* (pp. 219-238). Bonn, Germany.

Grinter, R., & Eldridge, M. (2003). Wan2tlk?: Everyday text messaging. *Proc. CHI 2003* (pp. 441-448). Ft Lauderdale, FL: ACM.

Hagen, P., & Rowland, N. (2010). *Mobile Diaries: Discovering Daily Life*. Johnny Holland.

Helman, C. (1995). *Culture, Health and Illness* (3rd ed.). Oxford, UK: Butterworth Heinemann.

Hughes, B., Joshi, I., & Wareham, J. (2008). Health 2.0 and Medicine 2.0: Tensions and Controversies in the Field. *Journal of Medical Internet Research, 10*(3), e23. Adapted from Jane Sarasohn-Kahn's "Wisdom of Patients" report, by Matthew Holt, Last updated June 6, 2008.

Jeffreys, M., & Lashof, J. (1991). Preparation for public health practice: into the twenty first century. In E. Fee & R. Acheson (Eds.), *A History of Education in Public Health. Health that Mocks the Doctors Rules* (pp. 314–335). Oxford, UK: Oxford University Press.

Karremansa, J. C., Stroebeb, W., & Clausb, J. (2006). Beyond Vicary's fantasies: The impact of subliminal priming and brand choice. *Journal of Experimental Social Psychology, 42*(6), 792–798. doi:10.1016/j.jesp.2005.12.002

Kelliher, A. (2004). Everyday Cinema. In *Proceedings of the 1st ACM Workshop on Story Representation, Mechanism and Context, SRMC'04* (pp. 59-62). New York: ACM.

Kindberg, T., Spasojevic, M., Fleck, R., & Sellen, A. (2005). The Ubiquitous Camera: An In-depth Study of Camera Phone Use. In *IEEE Pervasive Computing*. Piscataway, NJ: IEEE Educational Activities Department. doi:10.1109/MPRV.2005.42

Koplan, J. P., Liverman, C. T., & Kraak, V. I. (2005). *Preventing childhood obesity: health in the balance*. Washington, D.C.: National Academies Press. doi:10.1016/j.jada.2004.11.023

Kung, H. C., Hoyert, D. L., Xu, J. Q., & Murphy, S. L. (2008). Deaths: final data for 2005. *National Vital Statistics Reports 2008, 56*(10). Retrieved from http://www.cdc.gov/nchs/data/nvsr/nvsr56/nvsr56_10.pdf

Lehto, T. (2011). Oinas, & Kukkonen, H. (2011). Persuasive Features in Web-Based Alcohol and Smoking Interventions: A Systematic Review of the Literature. *Journal of Medical Internet Research, 13*(3), e46. Retrieved from http://www.jmir.org/2011/3/e46/ doi:10.2196/jmir.1559 PMID:21795238

Leivrouw, L. A. (2006). *Oppositional and activist new media: remediation, reconfiguration, participation.*

Mahmud, A. A., Aliakseyeu, D., & Martens, J. B. (2008). Enabling storytelling by Aphasics in an augmented home environment. *BCS-HCI '08 Proceedings of the 22nd British HCI Group Annual Conference on People and Computers: Culture, Creativity. Interaction, 2*, 3–6.

Manzini, E. (2002). Context-based wellbeing and the concept of regenerative solution: A conceptual framework for scenario building and sustainable solutions development. *The Journal of Sustainable Product Design, 2*, 141–148. doi:10.1023/B:JSPD.0000031026.11908.1d

Montgomery, G. H., Erblich, J., DiLorenzo, R., & Bovbjerg, D. H. (2003). Family and friends with disease: Their impact on perceived risk. *Preventive Medicine*, *37*, 242–249. doi:10.1016/S0091-7435(03)00120-8 PMID:12914830

O'Brien, R. (2001). Um exame da abordagem metodológica da pesquisa ação [An Overview of the Methodological Approach of Action Research]. In Roberto Richardson (Ed.), *Teoria e Prática da Pesquisa Ação [Theory and Practice of Action Research]*. João Pessoa, Brazil: Universidade Federal da Paraíba. (English version) Available: http://www.web.ca/~robrien/papers/arfinal.html

Ogden, C. L., Carroll, M. D., Curtin, L. R., Lamb, M. M., & Flegal, K. M. (2010). Prevalence of high body mass index in US children and adolescents, 2007-2008. *Journal of the American Medical Association*, *303*(3), 242–249. doi:10.1001/jama.2009.2012 PMID:20071470

Peltonen, P., Salovaara, A., Jacucci, G., Ilmonen, T., Ardito, C., Saarikko, P., & Batra, V. (2007). Extending Large Scale Event Participation with User Created Mobile Media on a Public Display. In *Proc. MUM 2007*. Oulu, Finland: IEEE.

Puikkonen, A., Venta, L., Beekhuyzen, J., & Hakkila, J. (2008). Playing, Performing, Reporting- A Case Study of Mobile Minimovies composed by Teenage Girls. *OZCHI 2008*.

Rheingold, H. (2007). Using Participatory Media and Public Voice to Encourage Civic Engagement. The John D. and Catherine T. MacArthur Foundation Series on Digital Media and learning (pp. 97-118).

Rich, M., Lamola, S., Amory, C., & Schneider, L. (2000, March). *Asthma in life context: Video Intervention/Prevention Assessment*. Pediatrics, Division of Adolescent/Young Adult Medicine [Boston, MA.]. *Childrens Hospital*, *105*(3Pt 1), 469–477.

Rich, M., Patashnick, J., & Chalfen, R. (2002). Visual illness narratives of asthma: explanatory models and health-related behavior. *American Journal of Health Behavior*, *26*(6), 442–453. doi:10.5993/AJHB.26.6.5 PMID:12437019

Robson, T. (2000). *The State and Community Action*. London: Pluto Press.

Rochelle, E., Garner, Feeny, D.H., Thompson, A., Bernier, J., McFarland, B.H. … Blanchard, C. (2011). Bodyweight, gender, and quality of life: A population-based longitudinal study. *Quality of Life Research*.

Rose, G., & Manderson, L. (n.d.). More than a breath of difference: Competing paradigms of asthma. *Anthropology & Medicine*, *7*(3), 335–350.

Rosson, M. B., & Carroll, J. M. (2002). *Usability Engineering: Scenario-based Development of Human-Computer Interaction*. London: Academic Press.

Royston, G., Dost, A., & Dick, P. (2004). *Healthcare Networks and Self-Care Support*. Unpublished paper, Department of Health Operational Research Branch.

Sanders, E. (2008). CoDesign. *International Journal of CoCreation in Design and the Arts*, *4*(1), 5–18.

Sanders, E., Brandt, E., & Binder, T. (2010). A framework for organizing the tools and techniques of participatory design. In *Proceedings of the 11th Biennial Participatory Design Conference (PDC '10)*. New York: ACM.

Sch[UNKNOWN ENTITY &odie;]n, D. A. (1983). *The Reflective Practitioner: How professionals think in action*. London: Temple Smith.

Sellen, A., Fogg, A., Aitken, M., Hodges, S., Rother, C., & Wood, K. (2007). Do Life-Logging Technologies Support Memory for the Past? An Experimental Study Using SenseCam. In *Proceedings of the ACM SIGCHI Conference on Human Factors in Computing Systems, CHI'07*. San Jose, CA: ACM.

Singh, G. K. et al. (2009). Neighborhood socio-economic conditions, built environments, and childhood obesity. *Health Affairs*, *29*(3), 503–512. doi:10.1377/hlthaff.2009.0730 PMID:20194993

Taylor, A. S., & Harper, R. (2003). The gift of the Gab?: A Design Oriented Sociology of Young People's Use of Mobiles. *Computer Supported Cooperative Work*, *12*(3), 267–296. doi:10.1023/A:1025091532662

Trasande, L., Liu, Y., Fryer, G., & Weitzman, M. (2009). *Effects of childhood obesity on hospital care and costs*, 1999-2005. *Health Affairs*, W751–W760. doi:10.1377/hlthaff.28.4.w751 PMID:19589800

Venta, L., Ahtinen, A., Ramiah, S., & Isomursu, M. (2008). 'My phone is a part of my soul' – How people bond with their Mobile phones. In Proc. Of UBICOMM 2008, Sep 2008.

Wagner, D., Lopez, M., Doria, A., Pavlyshak, I., Kostakos, V., Oakley, I., & Spiliotopolous, T. (2010). Hide and Seek: Location sharing practices with social media. Mobile HCI2010. Lisboa, Portugal.

Wanless, D. (2002). *Securing our Future Health: Taking a Long Term View*. London: HM Treasury.

Wellman, B. (2000). Physical Place and Cyber-Place: The rise of Networked Individualism. *Paper presented to Community Informatics: Connecting communities through the web*. University of Teesside, UK.

Wing, R. R., & Jeffery, R. W. (1999). Benefits of recruiting participants with friends and increasing social support for weight loss and maintenance. *Journal of Consulting and Clinical Psychology*, 67, 132–138. doi:10.1037/0022-006X.67.1.132 PMID:10028217

World Health Organization. (1948). Constitution of the World Health Organization. WHO: basic documents. Geneva.

Zuboff, S., & Maxmin, J. (2002). The Support Economy: Why corporations are failing individuals and the next episode of capitalism. Allen Lane, The Penguin Press, 2003, ISBN 0713993200

ADDITIONAL READING

Arnst, C. (2008). Health 2.0: *Patients as Partners*. Business Week 2008, http://www.businessweek.com/magazine/content/08_50/b4112058194219_page_2.htm (accessed December 4, 2008)

Arslan, P. (2013). *Service Design for Social Interaction. Applying Mobile Technologies for a Healthier Lifestyle*. PhD Dissertation. Presented in March 2013, Politecnico di Milano, Italy.

Carr, V., Sangiorgi, D., Buscher, M., Cooper, R., & Junginger, S. (2009). Clinicians as service designers? Reflections on current transformation in the UK health services. *First Nordic Conference on Service Design and Service Innovation*. Oslo, Norway.

Castells, M. (2002). The Rise of Network Society. *The Information Age: Economy and Society*, *1*, 2002.

Castells, M. et al. (2006). *Mobile Communication and Society: A Global Perspective*. Cambridge, MA: MIT Press.

Chiu, C., Chang, S., Chang, Y., Chu, H., Chen, C. C., Hsiao, F., & Ko, J. (2009). *Playful Bottle: A Mobile Social Persuasion System to Motivate Healthy Water Intake*. Orlando, FL: ACM. doi:10.1145/1620545.1620574

Chomitz, V. R. et al. (2010). Healthy Living Cambridge Kids: A Community-based Participatory Effort to Promote Healthy Weight and Fitness. *Obesity Journal*, *18*(1), 45–53. doi:10.1038/oby.2009.431

Clark, N. M., & Patridge, M. R. (2002). Strengthening Asthma Education to Enhance Disease Control. *Chest*, *121*(5), 1661–1669. doi:10.1378/chest.121.5.1661 PMID:12006458

Costa, F. G., Muschiato, S., Romero, M., Arslan, P., & Nam, G. (2010). *MOHE Mobile Health for pregnant, kids, adults and elderly. ICDC 2010, The First International Conference on Design Creativity*. Kyoto, Japan.

Delva, J., Johnston, L. D., & O'Malley, P. M. (2007). The Epidemiology of Overweight and Related Lifestyle Behaviors: Racial/Ethnic and Socioeconomic Status Differences Among American Youth. *American Journal of Preventive Medicine*, *33*(4S), S178–S186. doi:10.1016/j.amepre.2007.07.008 PMID:17884566

Dietz, W. H. (1998). Health Consequences of Obesity in Youth: Childhood Predictors of Adult Disease. *Pediatrics*, *101*(3 Pt 2), 518–525. PMID:12224658

Duncan, A. K., & Breslin, M. A. (2009). Innovating Health Care Delivery: The Design of Health Services. *The Journal of Business Strategy*, *30*(2/3), 13–20. doi:10.1108/02756660910942427

Economos, C. D., Hyatt, R. R., Goldberg, P. J., Must, A., Naumova, E. N., Collins, J. J., & Nelson, E. M. (2007). A community intervention reduces BMI z-score in children: Shape-up Somerville first year results. *Obesity (Silver Spring, Md.)*, *15*(5). doi:10.1038/oby.2007.155 PMID:17495210

Elizabeth, B., & Sanders, N. (2006). Scaffolds for Building Everyday Creativity. In J. Frascara (Ed.), *Design for Effective Communications: Creating Contexts for Clarity and Meaning*. New York: Allworth Press.

Fogg, B. J. (2003). *Persuasive Technology: Using Computers to Change What We Think and Do*. San Francisco, CA: Morgan Kaufmann Publishers.

Fogg, B.J. (2009). *A Behavior Model for Persuasive Design. Proceedings of the 4th International Conference on Persuasive Technology Persuasive 09*.

Fox, S. (2009). *The Social Life of Health Information*. June 11, 2009. Retrieved from: http://www.pewinternet.org/Reports/2009/8-The-Social-Life-of-Health-Information.aspx

Fox, S. (2010). *Mobile Health 2010*. Retrieved October 19, 2010, from http://pewinternet.org/Reports/2010/Mobile-Health-2010/Overview.aspx

Frost, J. H., Massagli, M. P., Wicks, P., & Heywood, J. (2008). How the social web supports patient experimentation with a new therapy: The demand for patient-controlled and patient-centered informatics. *AMIA... Annual Symposium Proceedings / AMIA Symposium. AMIA Symposium*, *6*, 217–221. PMID:18999176

Gortmaker, S. L., Must, A., Perrin, J. M., Sobol, A., & Dietz, W. H. (1993). Social and economic consequences of overweight in adolescence and young adulthood. *The New England Journal of Medicine*, *329*, 1008–1012. doi:10.1056/NEJM199309303291406 PMID:8366901

Grameen Foundation. (2009). *Mobile Technology for Community Health* (MoTeCH).

Hagen, P., & Robertson, T. (2010). Social Technologies: Challenges and Opportunities for Participation. In *Proceedings of PDC* (pp. 31-40).

Hawkes, N. (2005). *More people consult Google over Health. Times Online.*Retrieved from http://www.timesonline.co.uk/tol/news/uk/article530336.ece

Hicks, J., Ramanathan, N., Kim, D. H., Monibi, M., Selsky, J., Hansen, M. H., & Estrin, D. (2010). AndWellness: An open mobile system for activity and experience sampling. *Proceedings of Wireless Health, 2010*, 34–43.

Hofferth, S., & Jankuniene, Z. (2000, March–April). *Children's after-school activities.* Paper presented at the biennial meeting of the Society for Research on Adolescence. Chicago, IL.

Istepanian, R. S. (2006). MHEALTH: Emerging Mobile Health Systems. New York.

Kimm, S.Y., & Obarzanek, E. (2002). *Childhood obesity: A new pandemic of the new millennium.*

Kopelman, P. G. (2005). Clinical obesity in adults and children. In *Adults and Children.* Blackwell Publishing. doi:10.1002/9780470987087

Lenhart, A., Ling, R., Campbell, S., & Purcell, K. (2010). *Teens and Mobile Phones, Text messaging Explodes as Teens Embrace It as The Centerpiece of Their Communication Strategies with Friends.* Pew Research Center's Internet & American Life Project, April 20, 2010. Retrieved from: http://pewinternet.org/Reports/2010/Teens-and-Mobile-Phones.aspx.

Mamykina, L., & Mynatt, E. D., Davidson, P., R., Greenblatt, D., (2008). MAHI: Investigation of Social Scaffolding for Reflective Thinking in Diabetes Management, The proceedings of CHI 2008, Health and Wellness, April 5-10, Florence, Italy.

Mattelmäki, T. (2008). *Probing for co-exploring.* CoDesign. *International Journal of CoCreation in Design and the Arts, 4*(1), 65–78.

Miller, J., Rosenbloom, A., & Silverstein, J. (2004). Childhood obesity. *The Journal of Clinical Endocrinology and Metabolism, 89*(9), 4211–4218. doi:10.1210/jc.2004-0284 PMID:15356008

Moore, L. V., & Diez Roux, A. V. (2006, February). Association of Neighborhood Characteristics with the Location and Type of Food Stores. *American Journal of Public Health, 96*(2), 325–331. doi:10.2105/AJPH.2004.058040 PMID:16380567

Neumark-Sztainer, D., & Haines, J. (2004). Psychosocial and Behavioral Consequences of Obesity. In J. K. Thompson (Ed.), *Handbook of Eating Disorders and Obesity* (pp. 349–371). Hoboken, NJ: John Wiley & Sons.

Ogden, C. L., Flegal, K. M., & Carroll, M. D. et al. (2002, October). *Prevalence and Trends in Overweight Among US Children and* Adolescents, 1999-2000. *Journal of the American Medical Association, 288*(14), 1728–1732. doi:10.1001/jama.288.14.1728 PMID:12365956

Pediatrics, *110*(5), 1003–7. doi:. PMID 12415042.10.1542/peds.110.5.1003

Reason, P., & Bradbury, H. (Eds.). (2001). *Handbook of action research: Participative inquiry and practice.* London: Sage Publications.

Rich, M., Lamola, S., Amory, C., & Schneider, L. (2000, March). *Asthma in Life Context: Video Intervention/Prevention Assessment,* Pediatrics, Division of Adolescent/Young Adult Medicine [Boston, MA.]. *Childrens Hospital, 105*(3Pt 1), 469–477.

Sanders, E. B., & William, C. T. (2001). Harnessing People's Creativity: Ideation and Expression through Visual Communication. In J. Langford & D. McDonagh-Philp (Eds.), *Focus Groups: Supporting Effective Product Development.* Taylor and Francis.

Sangiorgi, D., Gillen, J., Junginger, S. & Whitham, R. (2010) *Personal development, participation and design. In ed. A. Yagou: special issue: Innovative Service Design for. All - part two.* Re-public -reimagining democracy: an online journal.

Smith, A. (2010). *Mobile Access Report 2010, Pew Internet and American Life Project*, Oct.19, 2010.http://www.pewinternet.org/Reports/2010/Mobile-Access-2010.aspx.

Smith, K. P., & Christakis, N. A. (2008, March 24). Social Networks and Health. *Annual Review of Sociology, 2008*(34), 405–429. doi:10.1146/annurev.soc.34.040507.134601

Trasande, L., Liu, Y., Fryer, G., & Weitzman, M. (2009). *Effects of childhood obesity on hospital care and costs,* 1999-2005. *Health Affairs,* W751–W760. doi:10.1377/hlthaff.28.4.w751 PMID:19589800

Troiano, R. P., Berrigan, D., & Dodd, K. W. et al. (2008, January). Physical Activity in the United States Measured by Accelerometer. *Medicine and Science in Sports and Exercise, 40*(1), 181–188. PMID:18091006

Wang, Y. C., McPherson, K., Marsh, T., Gortmaker, S. L., & Brown, M. (2011). Health and economic burden of the projected obesity trends in the USA and the UK. *Lancet, 378*(9793), 815–825. doi:10.1016/S0140-6736(11)60814-3 PMID:21872750

WHO. (2000). Obesity, Preventing and Managing the Global Epidemic. Report of a WHO Consultation. World Health Organization: Geneva, June 3-5-1997, 2000. 894.

World Health Organization. (2002). *The World Health Report 2002 - Reducing Risks, Promoting Healthy Life.* Geneva, 2002. Retrieved from: http://www.who.int/whr/2002/en/, accessed 21 March 2011.

KEY TERMS AND DEFINITIONS

Activity Log: Activity types performed by teen during their everyday life. Activity Log is Meal, Snack, Exercise, Chill Out, and Speak your mind.

Cast: A cast is a mobile narrative with 4-guided template recording. It is a single video with 4 shots in which each shot is titled with given tasks. They are location-based narratives.

Health Prevention: The preventive form of healthcare before it turns into chronic diseases.

Location-Based Platform: A platform that has a feature of location based map, using the GPS coordinates of the mobile phone.

Mobile Diary: Videos that are recorded through mobile phones features and compile as a diary. Refers visual narratives, all casts called 'a diary'.

Participative Health: An integrating approach where the aim is to involve all actors involved in creating and solving the specific health problem.

Socio-Environmental Factors of Health: The social and environmental factors of individuals' lifestyle.

Social Network: A community of people with the same interest interacts on a social platform for sharing experiences and health diaries.

Index

D

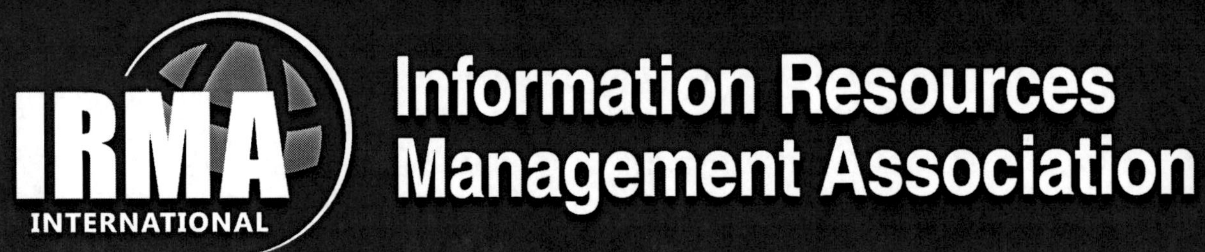

Become an IRMA Member

Members of the **Information Resources Management Association (IRMA)** understand the importance of community within their field of study. The Information Resources Management Association is an ideal venue through which professionals, students, and academicians can convene and share the latest industry innovations and scholarly research that is changing the field of information science and technology. Become a member today and enjoy the benefits of membership as well as the opportunity to collaborate and network with fellow experts in the field.

IRMA Membership Benefits:

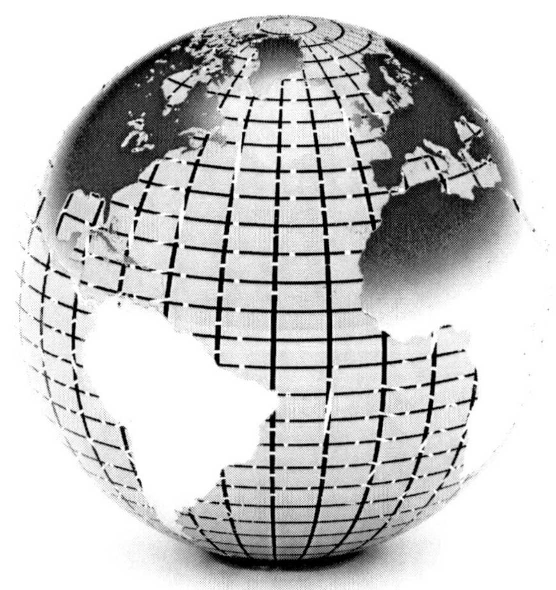

- **One FREE Journal Subscription**

- **30% Off Additional Journal Subscriptions**

- **20% Off Book Purchases**

- Updates on the latest events and research on Information Resources Management through the IRMA-L listserv.

- Updates on new open access and downloadable content added to Research IRM.

- A copy of the Information Technology Management Newsletter twice a year.

- A certificate of membership.

IRMA Membership $195

Scan code to visit irma-international.org and begin by selecting your free journal subscription.

Membership is good for one full year.

CPSIA information can be obtained at www.ICGtesting.com
Printed in the USA
LVOW09*0921160915

454396LV00013B/69/P